W0112582

Social Sciences for Healthcare Professionals

Social Sciences for Healthcare Professionals

Edited by

CHRIS ALLEN

University of Southampton, UK

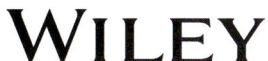

This edition first published 2026
© 2026 John Wiley & Sons Ltd

All rights reserved, including rights for text and data mining and training of artificial intelligence technologies or similar technologies. No part of this publication may be reproduced, stored in a retrieval system, or transmitted, in any form or by any means, electronic, mechanical, photocopying, recording or otherwise, except as permitted by law. Advice on how to obtain permission to reuse material from this title is available at http://www.wiley.com/go/permissions.

The right of Chris Allen to be identified as the author of the editorial material in this work has been asserted in accordance with law.

Registered Offices
John Wiley & Sons, Inc., 111 River Street, Hoboken, NJ 07030, USA
John Wiley & Sons Ltd, New Era House, 8 Oldlands Way, Bognor Regis, West Sussex, PO22 9NQ, UK

For details of our global editorial offices, customer services, and more information about Wiley products visit us at www.wiley.com.

The manufacturer's authorized representative according to the EU General Product Safety Regulation is Wiley-VCH GmbH, Boschstr. 12, 69469 Weinheim, Germany, e-mail: Product_Safety@wiley.com.

Wiley also publishes its books in a variety of electronic formats and by print-on-demand. Some content that appears in standard print versions of this book may not be available in other formats.

Trademarks: Wiley and the Wiley logo are trademarks or registered trademarks of John Wiley & Sons, Inc. and/or its affiliates in the United States and other countries and may not be used without written permission. All other trademarks are the property of their respective owners. John Wiley & Sons, Inc. is not associated with any product or vendor mentioned in this book.

Limit of Liability/Disclaimer of Warranty
The contents of this work are intended to further general scientific research, understanding, and discussion only and are not intended and should not be relied upon as recommending or promoting scientific method, diagnosis, or treatment by physicians for any particular patient. In view of ongoing research, equipment modifications, changes in governmental regulations, and the constant flow of information relating to the use of medicines, equipment, and devices, the reader is urged to review and evaluate the information provided in the package insert or instructions for each medicine, equipment, or device for, among other things, any changes in the instructions or indication of usage and for added warnings and precautions. While the publisher and authors have used their best efforts in preparing this work, they make no representations or warranties with respect to the accuracy or completeness of the contents of this work and specifically disclaim all warranties, including without limitation any implied warranties of merchantability or fitness for a particular purpose. No warranty may be created or extended by sales representatives, written sales materials or promotional statements for this work. This work is sold with the understanding that the publisher is not engaged in rendering professional services. The advice and strategies contained herein may not be suitable for your situation. You should consult with a specialist where appropriate. The fact that an organization, website, or product is referred to in this work as a citation and/or potential source of further information does not mean that the publisher and authors endorse the information or services the organization, website, or product may provide or recommendations it may make. Further, readers should be aware that websites listed in this work may have changed or disappeared between when this work was written and when it is read. Neither the publisher nor authors shall be liable for any loss of profit or any other commercial damages, including but not limited to special, incidental, consequential, or other damages.

Library of Congress Cataloging-in-Publication Data Applied for

Paperback ISBN: 9781394186341

Cover Design: Wiley
Cover Image: © Angelina Bambina/stock.adobe.com

Set in 9.5/12.5pt SourceSansPro by Straive, Pondicherry, India

Printed and bound by CPI Group (UK) Ltd, Croydon, CR0 4YY

C9781394186341_260825

Contents

List of Contributors

Chris Allen
School of Health Sciences
University of Southampton
Southampton
UK

Louise Baxter
Faculty of Arts and Humanities
University College London
London
UK

Lynn Calman
School of Health Sciences
University of Southampton
Southampton
UK

Matt Flynn
School of Health Sciences
University of Southampton
Southampton
UK

Assaf Givati
Department of Population Health Sciences
King's College London
London
UK

Erica Goddard
School of Health, Wellbeing & Social Care
The Open University
Milton Keynes
UK

Janine Hall
School of Health and Social Wellbeing
University of the West of England
Bristol
UK

Simon Hall
School of Health Sciences
University of Southampton
Southampton
UK

Gilly Mancz
School of Health Sciences
University of Southampton
Southampton
UK

Cheryl Metcalf
School of Healthcare Enterprise and Innovation
University of Southampton
Southampton
UK

Eloise Monger
School of Health Sciences
University of Southampton
Southampton
UK

Ellen Kitson-Reynolds
School of Health Sciences
University of Southampton
Southampton
UK

Robert Slinn
Department of Social Sciences
A maintained Secondary School and Sixth Form College
Southampton
UK

Jasmine Snowden
School of Health Sciences
University of Southampton
Southampton
UK

Neil Summers

School of Health, Wellbeing & Social Care

The Open University

Milton Keynes

UK

Lindsay Welch

Faculty of Health and Social Sciences

Bournemouth University

Bournemouth

UK

Sam Woodnutt

School of Health Sciences

University of Southampton

Southampton

UK

I completed my nursing training in 2010, before going on to work as a Staff Nurse at a local general hospital, specifically working in an acute care for older person's medical ward. My training, which was clinically excellent, as with many other healthcare professional programmes at the time, largely followed the biomedical model. People were 'well' until they became 'unwell', at which point, it was the role of healthcare, and healthcare professionals specifically, to make them 'well'. Health promotion and public health were already well established by this time. Aspects of these were taught, of course, but these were generally the side dish to biomedicine's main course, and very much took a back seat to more reactionary care. The social sciences were visible, but barely, and rarely related back to the social context of health and healthcare, and how people found themselves in the position of needing healthcare in the first place.

As such, the healthcare professional role I was socialized into was largely directed by biomedicine. I was very familiar and comfortable with a range of acute care presentations and what was needed including a range of pharmacological interventions, alongside the fundamentals of care, that have rightfully become an essential feature of hospital and community healthcare: fluid balance, nutrition, skin integrity, etc. As Florence Nightingale famously emphasised, the importance of hospitals not harming the sick, has and will continue to remain at the core of what healthcare professionals do. However, healthcare has become significantly more complex since then. Florence Nightingale, alongside other key thinkers of her time, was able to identify the social causes of ill health. The recognition of relationships between poor living and working conditions are by no means new, but increasingly, the social context of care is necessitating new ways of thinking about health and how healthcare is delivered, and in my view, how healthcare professionals are trained and supported.

As a healthcare professional, I have been very fortunate to have been socialised into the social sciences over years of further study. First, in Gerontology, where I was first able to see and really grasp the importance of health across the life course and determining later-life health and wellbeing. Then, later, through a PhD in Health Sciences, which had a specific focus on technology and social networks in the context of chronic condition management. Many of the theories and concepts I was able to engage with arose from the social sciences and have been incredibly powerful in shaping my thinking about health, and what is important in terms of supporting individuals and populations. Overtime, and through these academic and clinical experiences, I have seen that health is about more than being in a hospital stuck to an IV drip. Working in the community, including supporting those who were vulnerable, and who had significant multimorbidity, showed me firsthand how people's social contexts shaped their health, making it more likely they would become unwell, but also then making it more challenging for them to engage with healthcare and manage their health conditions with the material and social resources they were able to access.

All these experiences have supported my social understanding of health and illness, and through this socialization, I have been able to see where my healthcare professional education (as clinically brilliant as it was at the time), was lacking. Important social science contributions such as how health and disease are understood, how physical and mental health is classified and how this relates to the care people are able to access, how healthcare systems are set up and who is advantaged and disadvantaged by their design, how health inequalities manifest and how they can be addressed, and the impact this has on people's care. Other vital contributions have changed and continue to change how society responds to people and groups, such as the social model of disability, which has influenced how impairment and disability are seen in society, drawing attention to the unjust barriers people face to full social and economic participation, alongside inclusion health, which is directing focus towards those experiencing social exclusion and extremely poor health outcomes in our communities.

Finally, healthcare professionals are taking on an increased role in health behavior change, and social science has contributed very significantly to our understanding of people's health behaviors and how they can be best supported to make positive changes. Health behavior in particular provides an important example of why this book has included the main social sciences, as opposed to simply focusing on one discipline. Because health behavior is determined by so many things, it can only really be understood through engagement with work across the social sciences, such as that offered by Psychology, Sociology and Economics. Only by understanding these, can we make sense of people's behaviors and how they can be best supported to change them. The many and varied contributions across the social sciences are hugely important in informing how support is provided to people wanting to make a change, and healthcare professionals need to be able to engage with this work, in order to support people's behavior change using evidence-based approaches.

However, many important contributions from the social sciences are published in their own disciplinary specific journals and are often written using a language and vocabulary that can make it difficult for those outside of that specific discipline to interpret and subsequently engage with important core concepts and in turn, use these to support and underpin their practice. Busy healthcare professionals at the front end of care are unlikely to hunt out papers published in social science specific journals, no matter how relevant these papers might be to their care. This is where my motivations for this writing this book emerged, to offer healthcare professionals a broader and wider understanding of health and its many and varied influences. The issues most healthcare systems around the world currently face cannot be solved with one discipline working in isolation, and instead, it is vital that healthcare professionals are able to access some of the most important contributions of the social sciences in one place, and in a format that allows these sometimes quite abstract concepts, to be translated into everyday clinical practice, where they can be used to improve care, reduce inequalities and improve the health of individuals and populations.

Acknowledgements

First, I would like to thank all of those who have dedicated their time, effort, energy and expertise to contributing to this book. Your many and varied contributions have helped shape this book and particularly its clinical relevance. I would also like to thank all those healthcare professionals I have had the privilege of teaching the Social Sciences to over many years. Your contributions to lectures, feedback on content, lively debate and discussion have helped shape this book more than you would believe, ensuring its current and fits the needs of healthcare students. You continue to teach me everyday, and for that I am grateful.

Thanks also to my employer and brilliant colleagues, many of whom have supported this book, either directly or indirectly through our many and varied debates over the years. Preparation of this book was supported by the University of Southampton Faculty of Medicine/Faculty of Environmental and Life Sciences Writing Retreat (July 2025). Special thanks for making this time available. There are a few colleagues who have been particularly influential in shaping my interest in the Social Sciences and who deserve special recognition. Professor Athina Vlachantoni, you provided me with the foundations and showed me the importance of the life course in shaping later-life health. Thanks to my brilliant PhD supervisors: Professor Anne Rogers, Professor Anne Kennedy and Dr Ivaylo Vassilev. Our many supervisions have continued to shape my thinking. You have all taught me that health is about more than simply making people better when they fall ill, alongside the importance of people's social support and community networks to maintaining health and wellbeing. Professor Anne Kennedy, I miss you, and your loss is still felt. Your legacy continues in your significant contributions to health and wellbeing that you have made, including in the social sciences.

Wiley, as a publisher, you have been incredibly supportive of this project from its inception. As a first-time book editor finding my feet in the world of book publishing, you took a chance on me; you have been incredibly patient, supportive and motivating (often at just the right time). You have supported my personal development and, through that, the development of this book. Special thanks to Tom Marriott, who took this project on, and to Bhavya Boopathi and Christabel Daniel Raj for your unwavering support throughout the editing process, for being approachable, responsive and supportive.

Thank you to my mum, for proofreading and providing valuable feedback on the chapters. Finally, the biggest thanks goes to my wonderful family. Taking on a project this size, with two young girls under six, has been a significant undertaking (more than I had appreciated when I enthusiastically took this project on two years ago). Thank you to my amazing wife, Helen, who has been supportive of the many weekends and late evenings worked to bring this project to its conclusion. I could not have done this without you taking on a disproportionate share of child-rearing. I owe you a huge debt of gratitude. Florence and Niamh, I am so proud of you and the girls you are becoming.

CHAPTER 1

An Introduction to Social Sciences for Healthcare Professionals

Chris Allen

School of Health Sciences, University of Southampton, Southampton, UK

How to Use This Book

This book provides an overview across its 20 chapters of the aspects of the social sciences most relevant to informing your practice as healthcare professionals now, and in the future. As a summary of some of the social sciences' largest bodies of work to date, crossing disciplines as diverse as Sociology, Psychology and Economics, this book provides readers with an overview of these disciplines work that has the most relevance to healthcare professionals in an accessible and easy to digest format. It is worth emphasising that all of these are large disciplines (and their sub-disciplines) and comfortably fill entire textbooks. As such, this book's chapters are intended as an introduction to some of the social sciences' most important contributions to health and healthcare. You can read this book's chapters in any order you like or you can start from **chapter 2**. A few of the chapters are particularly interrelated and we have highlighted these, both in this introduction and within the chapters themselves. In most of the chapters, we have provided opportunities to 'stop and think', and there are a number of case studies within this book that are intended to help you reflect on your own learning and relate the discussion and contents to your own practice and observations.

What Are the Social Sciences?

Sociology and Medical Sociology

Sociology is a scientific discipline that is concerned with the study of human societies, the institutions that as a society we build and the social relationships and processes that emerge from these (Giddens and Sutton, 2017, Scambler, 2018). A particular focus of sociology is understanding the unequal distribution of status, power and resources within a society that sees some having significant advantages and some having significant disadvantages, as well as the various social processes that influence and lead to such differences occurring (Giddens and Sutton, 2017).

Much of this applies to health too, and medical sociology (sometimes referred to as the sociology of health and illness) is simply the sociological study of health and illness (Allan, 2016, Barry and Yuill, 2022, Scambler, 2018). How health is constructed and seen in a society, as well as the health inequalities that exist between different individuals and groups, and the sometimes significant differences that exist relating to access to safe and effective healthcare (Scambler, 2018, Barry and Yuill, 2022). Medical sociology has also had a long interest in the healthcare professions, including the relative differences in terms of power and status afforded to different professional groups (Crinson, 2018), as well as how healthcare systems are seen and understood within a broader social system (Mays, 2018). Sociologies contributions to all of this, and more are considered throughout this book.

Psychology and Health Psychology

Psychology, and in particular its sub-discipline Health Psychology, is another scientific discipline. As a broad discipline, it is generally most concerned with our minds, our thoughts, our behaviours, as well as how we make decisions (Gross, 2015, Marks et al., 2020, Ogden, 2023). Essentially, how we think, and how we behave (Gross, 2015, Marks et al., 2020,

Social Sciences for Healthcare Professionals, First Edition. Edited by Chris Allen.
© 2026 John Wiley & Sons Ltd. Published 2026 by John Wiley & Sons Ltd.

Ogden, 2023). This relates to and influences our health in several ways, many of which are explored throughout this book. For example, how we think can influence our behaviours and our behaviours can be influenced by those we are in contact with (Marks et al., 2020, Ogden, 2023).

This can affect the health-enhancing or health-harming behaviours we follow (such as drinking too much and smoking), and how we think about these behaviours, including whether we have the belief or motivation to change them (Marks et al., 2020, Michie et al., 2011, Michie et al., 2024, Ogden, 2023). It can also influence how we feel about our social relationships and the social contact that we have (Cacioppo and Cacioppo, 2018). From a health systems and organisational perspective, it can also shape how well we work with, or indeed how well we are able to lead others (Northouse, 2022, Salas et al., 2018a, Salas et al., 2018b), both of which are increasingly recognised as being important to healthcare delivery. Psychology's contributions to all of this, and more are considered throughout this book.

Economics and Health Economics

Economics is the study of human behaviour, especially relating to the production, distribution and consumption of scarce resources – notably goods and services (Sloman et al., 2022). Health economics is also concerned with these, but in the context of health and healthcare provision for individuals and populations (Glied and Smith, 2011, Wiseman, 2011). Generally, we want people to consume healthcare when they need it, but as healthcare is generally seen as being finite (i.e. there are only so many hospital beds, healthcare professionals, drugs, etc. to go around), we do not want people to overconsume it when it is not needed (Glied and Smith, 2011, Koohi Rostamkalaee et al., 2022). With scarce goods, economic decision-making can be hugely important in determining what is and what is not funded, and economists are often concerned with how to maximise utility, by considering the tangible health benefits that arise through the consumption of healthcare, often when several alternative options exist (Feng et al., 2020, Glied and Smith, 2011, Rand and Kesselheim, 2021, Wiseman, 2011). The positive impacts of health consumption can of course relate to health outcomes, but can also relate to wider impacts on society, such as increased labour market productivity and reduced time off work, and these outcomes can have a reciprocal impact on health, as wider determinants (Dahlgren and Whitehead, 2021). Of course, all this consumption can impact on our planet, its resources and its ability to sustain life in a fair, just and equitable way (Raworth, 2017, Raworth, 2018).

As with psychology, economics is often also concerned with how people make decisions (especially decisions around consumption), particularly within behavioural economics (Glied and Smith, 2011, Sloman et al., 2022, Thaler and Sunstein, 2009). For example, much attention is often paid to how changing the price of products based on their harmful or helpful impacts on health may change patterns of consumption (known as elasticity), such as increasing the price of alcohol to deter consumption, or subsidising gym memberships to encourage uptake (Clements et al., 2022, Glied and Smith, 2011, Sloman et al., 2022). Economics' contributions to all of this, and more are considered throughout this book.

So Why the Social Sciences?

Even outside of healthcare, your everyday experiences, and the experiences of those that you meet, are influenced by social, anthropological, psychological, economic and political influences. This book will introduce you to many of these and provide you with the underpinning social science knowledge to be able to make socially sensitive decisions in the care that you give, whatever healthcare role you do. As a healthcare professional, much of the care that you deliver will be shaped by these, and often in unexpected ways. Essentially, in your role as a healthcare professional, you must work within a set of complex and interconnected social conditions and structures that shape and influence how care is set up, organised and delivered.

So why is this all relevant to you, as a healthcare professional, or aspirant healthcare professional? Don't you just want to make people better? Isn't this largely a matter of biology and medicine? The short answer – no. This book provides a longer answer and will hopefully show that sickness and health are cultural and social experiences that are influenced by many complex and interrelated social processes. The delivery of healthcare is essentially a social activity that is determined by many of these processes across societies many layers.

A Patient's Journey: The Social Sciences in Action

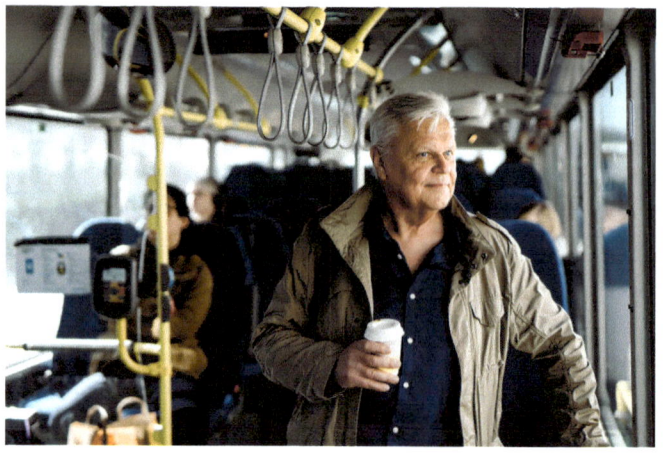

Source: Maskot/Adobe Stock Photos.

Barry is 58 and works in an office as a supervisor. He has recently divorced and lives on his own in a dank flat in the middle of town. Since his divorce six months ago, he has largely neglected himself and mostly just works. He has occasional contact with his sister, who is supportive, but apart from that he only really speaks to people at work (mostly his direct reports and his manager), as well as the local shopkeeper. It is a Friday, and Barry heads off to work, as he does every Friday.

Barry catches the 8:21 bus, which normally gets him to his office in about 20 minutes. Swiping his season ticket, he stands near the front of the bus next to another office worker who he occasionally speaks to; transactional, nothing too much. A 'hi' there, a nod here. Suddenly Barry begins to feel very funny and collapses into the aisle. A helpful bystander alerts the driver, the bus stops and Barry is tended too by bystanders. Someone calls an ambulance, and paramedics arrive at the scene and believe Barry to have had a stroke. They let the local Emergency Department know that they will be bringing Barry to hospital, under a blue light, and that they should expect to receive Barry in around 10 minutes. During the transit, the paramedics monitor his vital signs, pulse, blood pressure, levels of consciousness, etc. His levels of consciousness are poor, and he is slurring his speech, and tending to lean to one side. On arrival at the hospital, the paramedics transfer Barry's care to the Emergency Department team, who run through their various protocols and processes, and get him an urgent CT brain scan to determine if he has had a stroke, and what type of stroke he has had. This is an important information as it determines how Barry should be treated. Following this, Barry is diagnosed with an ischemic cerebrovascular accident (CVA), caused by a blockage to oxygenated blood flow to his brain. The decision is made to administer a drug delivered into his veins in the hope it will break down any clot that has caused a blockage, restoring blood oxygen flow to the affected areas of his brain. The treatment is partially successful, and in the weeks that follow, with the support of nurses, doctors, physiotherapists and occupational therapists, amongst others within the multi-disciplinary teams across the hospital, and with input from various community healthcare teams, Barry is ready to be discharged home to his flat. Whilst Barry is well enough to go home, the stroke has resulted in some damage to his brain, which has resulted in Barry having some physical, cognitive and sensory impairments that he will likely have to live with for the rest of his life. Three months later, Barry returns to work on a 'phased return'.

This is Barry's story. A story that many of you will be very familiar with.

So where are the social sciences and why are they relevant here? After all, wasn't Barry's recovery mostly through medicine? Wasn't it mostly healthcare professionals that put him back on his feet, got him home and back to work? All of these played a vital role, clearly, but this book will show you that Barry's story is actually incomplete; as too is the story of the healthcare professionals, healthcare system and wider society that provided his care. The social sciences can help us fill in the gaps in Barry's story, helping us understand, prevent and support Barry and his health, so that as a society, and in

particular as healthcare professionals we are better placed to provide equitable care for all, and may even be able to prevent people like Barry collapsing on the bus in the first place. In the next section, we will step you through the book and how it will help you complete Barry's story.

Completing Barry's Story

Part 1: Understanding Health, Healthcare Systems and the Healthcare Workforce

In **chapter 2**, an overview of social theory and social research methods is provided. What you will see in this chapter, and alongside the rest of the book, is that social theory and social research methods are important to understanding how society works (Clark et al., 2021, Kislov et al., 2019) – and within the rest of this book, you will see diverse theories that have helped make sense of society and people's situations, as well as a range of methods that have been used to test or create these theories in many contexts with relevance to health. These can ultimately help us as a society to improve people's care and situations.

In **chapter 3**, we introduce you to the concept of 'health'. Barry, in his story, is clearly unwell. But defining health and disease is tricky, but nonetheless important, as it guides societies in thinking about who needs care, as well as how health is understood and delivered (Larsen, 2021, Leonardi, 2018, Schramme, 2023). It also guides what societies should prioritise or focus on (Larsen, 2021, Leonardi, 2018, Schramme, 2023). In fact, as we show in this chapter, how we think about health might even be relevant in preventing Barry from becoming unwell in the first place, and what aspects of Barry's care are seen as most important. This chapter also discusses the various ways health has been classified, and why classifications of health and disease matter (Clark et al., 2017, Harrison et al., 2021).

In **chapter 4**, we move on to consider health in the context of mental ill health. This chapter tracks the social changes that relate to mental ill health, including its identification and management (Rogers and Pilgrim, 2021), alongside the concept of deviance (something that sets someone apart) (Henry, 2018). Barry is presenting with a physical health issue, but poor mental health makes it more likely for people like Barry to find themselves in this position (Fiorillo et al., 2023, Kivimäki et al., 2020). In addition, experiencing a stroke makes it more likely Barry will experience poor mental health and poor well-being (Damsbo et al., 2020, Towfighi et al., 2017). The impact society has had on the various ways mental ill health has been viewed are considered, and how this might impact on how people like Barry are seen (Rogers and Pilgrim, 2021), alongside some prominent models in mental health practice (Beck and Fleming, 2021, Burns, 2020, Davidson, 2016, Middleton and

Moncrieff, 2019), and how these relate to the care that those presenting with mental ill health receive from a diverse range of backgrounds and experiences.

In **chapter 5**, we turn our attention to health economics, and the political economy, and consider in more depth the health systems that provide care to people like Barry. This chapter looks at some different healthcare systems that exist around the world and considers how these differences relate to how care is financed, what care people can access and what people like Barry must pay for it (if anything) (Anandaciva, 2023, Braithwaite et al., 2020, Britnell, 2015, Papanicolas and Cylus, 2015). The importance of countries working towards universal health coverage to ensure periods of ill health such as that experienced by Barry do not result in catastrophic healthcare expenditure is also considered (Wagstaff and Neelsen, 2020). In **chapter 6**, we move on to consider the healthcare professionals that work within these healthcare systems to care for people like Barry, highlighting some of the current challenges that exist relating to global healthcare workforce shortages (Boniol et al., 2022), and the relevance of this to meeting current and future healthcare needs. This chapter also considers how people end up in positions of care and what it means to be a 'healthcare professional'; how this has changed over time, as well as the differences in how professionals are seen and the differences in terms of the power and status that have been afforded to the different healthcare professions overtime (Saks, 2016).

Part 2: Meeting Population Health Needs and Health Inequalities

Various demographic and epidemiological transitions have made Barry's situation more common in most societies. In **chapter 7**, these demographic and epidemiolocal transitions are discussed, alongside the challenges they present global healthcare systems with (Omran, 2005, Weisz and Olszynko-Gryn, 2010). These changes have meant that people are living longer, and more often with increased morbidity (Bury and Taylor, 2008, Taylor and Bury, 2007). The impact such changes are likely to have on health systems, and society more generally are considered, alongside the importance of people like Barry being supported to take on a greater role in the management of their own health once they have become unwell, alongside healthcare professionals (Bury and Taylor, 2008, Taylor and Bury, 2007).

Whilst anyone can find themselves in Barry's position, research consistently demonstrates increased early morbidity and mortality in those from lower socio-economic status groups (Bartley, 2017, Marmot et al., 2020). Differences in longevity and health outcomes are unequally experienced, and in **chapter 8**, readers are introduced to the social determinants of health (Dahlgren and Whitehead, 2021), and health inequalities (Marmot et al., 2020). Various explanations are considered that explain why those from lower socio-economic groups are more

likely to experience early mortality and morbidity than those in higher-status groups (Bartley, 2017, McCartney et al., 2019, Wami et al., 2020). In **chapter 9**, bias and stigma are introduced as concepts that explain why some within a society experience various forms of disadvantage, including poorer care, based on their real or perceived differences (Hatzenbuehler et al., 2013, Phelan et al., 2008, Scambler, 2009, Tyler and Slater, 2018). These differences can result in people like Barry being more or less likely to receive emergency care, as well as influencing the quality of care they are able to access, and these differences can amount to discrimination, leading to poorer health outcomes, alongside reduced social and economic opportunities (Hatzenbuehler et al., 2013).

In **chapter 10**, some groups that are particularly vulnerable to being socially excluded are considered (Aldridge et al., 2018, Luchenski et al., 2018, Marmot, 2018, Tweed et al., 2022), alongside the consideration of how their needs can be better met by healthcare professionals, healthcare systems and society more generally. Those with a physical, mental, cognitive or sensory impairment are often excluded and disabled by society, and in **chapter 11**, the needs of those with impairments are considered, alongside the impact that society itself has on the lives of those living with such differences, often making it significantly (and unnecessarily) harder to participate fully in social and economic life, and access healthcare, through healthcare systems poorly accommodating the needs of those with impairments across their lives (Oliver, 2013).

Part 3: Understanding Health Behaviours, Health Behaviour Change and Public Health

Of course, people like Barry can just be unlucky, and many of those who engage in unhealthy behaviours do not go on to have a stroke. However, global burden of disease studies consistently highlights the impact of health behaviours on non-communicable diseases and mortality (Afshin et al., 2019, Degenhardt et al., 2018, Katzmarzyk et al., 2022, Khan Minhas et al., 2024, Shield et al., 2020). **Chapters 12 and 13** consider why people engage in behaviours (such as drinking too much alcohol, smoking, being physically inactive or having a poor diet) that they know are unhealthy and that may lead to poor health outcomes, as well as how we can support individuals through various behaviour change techniques and interventions that seek to elicit change at the level of individuals. In this chapter, approaches that are particularly common in clinical practice, such as motivational interviewing and making every contact count are considered alongside their respective evidence bases (Frost et al., 2018, Nichol et al., 2024, Parchment et al., 2023, Rodrigues et al., 2024). These techniques may be effective in supporting people like Barry to change behaviours that could be harming their health. Of course, behaviours, including Barry's occur within a social context (Christakis and Fowler, 2013, Kickbusch et al., 2016, McCartney et al., 2019

Wami et al., 2020, WHO, 2023). This social context can make behaviour change difficult, especially where people lack the resources they need to change their behaviour and where behaviours are so often influenced by society, its institutions, as well as those within it. In **chapter 14**, we move beyond behaviour change at the level of individuals and consider how whole populations can be supported to change their behaviours through various population-level interventions, that may work to incentivise, disincentivise, restrict and even ban certain unhealthy behaviours. As part of this chapter, a whole systems approach to public health is considered (Danielli et al., 2023, Davey et al., 2022), alongside consideration of the relationship between our health and well-being and the health of our planet (Raworth, 2017, Raworth, 2018).

Part 4: Social and Community Networks, Loneliness and Social Prescribing

Our social networks influence our health and lives in a number of ways across the life course (Christakis and Fowler, 2013, Granovetter, 1973, Rogers et al., 2014). They give us access to needed social, material and economic resources in good and bad health and also shape our health behaviours. In **chapter 15**, we introduce the life course approach and highlight the importance of earlier life stages on later life health and opportunities. Preceding Barry's stroke are a set of social network circumstances that are unique to him. How well supported he was in his early years relates to how well he is able to build and maintain relationships later in his life, as well as the economic resources that he is able to accumulate. His social network also has a significant impact on the health behaviours that he himself follows, with evidence consistently highlighting that unhealthy behaviours spread through social networks (Christakis and Fowler, 2008, Christakis and Fowler, 2013, Rosenquist et al., 2010). In **chapter 16**, the public health issue of social isolation and loneliness is introduced. Prior to the stroke, Barry's lack of social contact, especially if more contact was desired, may have actually increased his risk of becoming unwell (Cacioppo and Cacioppo, 2018, Holt-Lunstad, 2018). Of course, Barry's new situation also places him at an increased risk of experiencing social isolation and loneliness, with new impairments making it harder for him to reach out to maintain and connect with new social ties (Macdonald et al., 2018), and

can also lead to poorer health, social and economic outcomes. In **chapter 16**, we turn to social prescribing as one approach that is being increasingly used to support those who are lonely, alongside those presenting with other social needs, through connecting people to a range of activities within their local communities (Chatterjee et al., 2018, Husk et al., 2020).

Part 5: Leading Safe and Effective Care in Increasingly Changing Healthcare Systems

When Barry first accessed healthcare following his stroke, he was very vulnerable and was reliant on healthcare professionals like you being able to meet his needs safely and effectively. He was reliant on healthcare systems having safe work systems (Carayon et al., 2020, Holden et al., 2013) and strong leadership (Wu et al., 2024), and this is the focus of **chapter 18**. Barry's needs are complex and cannot be met by one healthcare professional working in isolation (Kerrissey et al., 2023, Sanford et al., 2024, Shuffler and Carter, 2018). Even just getting to a hospital involved the coordinated efforts of multiple healthcare professionals working within a multi-team system, where communication and other teamwork processes can have a significant impact on the quality and safety of care that Barry was able to receive (Salas et al., 2018b). It is the healthcare teams and teamwork processes that are the focus of **chapter 19**. Finally, Barry's care was reliant on healthcare professionals being able to use various health technologies effectively. In **chapter 20**, the place and importance of health technology and innovations are considered, alongside the importance of them being designed responsibly, and with the needs of intended users considered in their design to ensure that they can be used safely and effectively to enhance the care of people like Barry (Greenhalgh et al., 2017, Topol, 2019). Of course, Barry is just one person. The exact social influences and needs of those accessing care will vary from person to person, based on a range of complex and interrelated social processes and influences. This book is intended to help you give socially responsive care by considering social context, and across this book, you will have the opportunity to apply this learning to the diverse needs of a range of people across a wide range of settings and clinical contexts.

References

Afshin, A., Sur, P. J., Fay, K. A., Cornaby, L., Ferrara, G., Salama, J. S., Mullany, E. C., Abate, K. H., Abbafati, C., Abebe, Z., Afarideh, M., Aggarwal, A., Agrawal, S., Akinyemiju, T., Alahdab, F., Bacha, U., Bachman, V. F., Badali, H., Badawi, A., Bensenor, I. M., Bernabe, E., Biadgilign, S. K. K., Biryukov, S. H., Cahill, L. E., Carrero, J. J., Cercy,

K. M., Dandona, L., Dandona, R., Dang, A. K., Degefa, M. G., El Sayed Zaki, M., Esteghamati, A., Esteghamati, S., Fanzo, J., Farinha, C. S. E. S., Farvid, M. S., Farzadfar, F., Feigin, V. L., Fernandes, J. C., Flor, L. S., Foigt, N. A., Forouzanfar, M. H., Ganji, M., Geleijnse, J. M., Gillum, R. F., Goulart, A. C., Grosso, G.,

Guessous, I., Hamidi, S., Hankey, G. J., Harikrishnan, S., Hassen, H. Y., Hay, S. I., Hoang, C. L., Horino, M., Ikeda, N., Islami, F., Jackson, M. D., James, S. L., Johansson, L., Jonas, J. B., Kasaeian, A., Khader, Y. S., Khalil, I. A., Khang, Y.-H., Kimokoti, R. W., Kokubo, Y., Kumar, G. A., Lallukka, T., Lopez, A. D., Lorkowski, S., Lotufo, P. A., Lozano, R., Malekzadeh, R., März, W., Meier, T., Melaku, Y. A., Mendoza, W., Mensink, G. B. M., Micha, R., Miller, T. R., Mirarefin, M., Mohan, V., Mokdad, A. H., Mozaffarian, D., Nagel, G., Naghavi, M., Nguyen, C. T., Nixon, M. R., Ong, K. L., Pereira, D. M., Poustchi, H., Qorbani, M., Rai, R. K., Razo-García, C., Rehm, C. D., Rivera, J. A., Rodríguez-Ramírez, S., Roshandel, G., Roth, G. A., et al. 2019. Health effects of dietary risks in 195 countries, 1990–2017: a systematic analysis for the Global Burden of Disease Study 2017. *The Lancet*, 393, 1958–1972.

Aldridge, R. W., Story, A., Hwang, S. W., Nordentoft, M., Luchenski, S. A., Hartwell, G., Tweed, E. J., Lewer, D., Vittal Katikireddi, S. & Hayward, A. C. 2018. Morbidity and mortality in homeless individuals, prisoners, sex workers, and individuals with substance use disorders in high-income countries: a systematic review and meta-analysis. *Lancet*, 391, 241–250.

Allan, H. 2016. *Understanding Sociology in Nursing*, London: Sage Publications.

Anandaciva, S. 2023. How Does the NHS Compare to the Health Care Systems of Other Countries? The King's Fund.

Barry, A. & Yuill, C. 2022. *Understanding the Sociology of Health*, London: Sage.

Bartley, M. 2017. *Health Inequality: An Introduction to Concepts Theories and Methods*, Cambridge Polity.

Beck, J. S. & Fleming, S. 2021. A brief history of Aaron T. Beck, MD, and cognitive behavior therapy. *Clinical Psychology in Europe*, 3, e6701.

Boniol, M., Kunjumen, T., Nair, T. S., Siyam, A., Campbell, J. & Diallo, K. 2022. The global health workforce stock and distribution in 2020 and 2030: a threat to equity and 'universal' health coverage? *BMJ Global Health*, 7, e009316.

Braithwaite, J., Tran, Y., Ellis, L. A. & Westbrook, J. 2020. Inside the black box of comparative national healthcare performance in 35 OECD countries: issues of culture, systems performance and sustainability. *PLoS One*, 15, e0239776.

Britnell, M. 2015. *In Search of the Perfect Health System*, Palgrave Macmillan.

Burns, T. 2020. A history of antipsychiatry in four books. *Lancet Psychiatry*, 7, 312–314.

Bury, M. & Taylor, D. 2008. Towards a theory of care transition: from medical dominance to managed consumerism. *Social Theory & Health*, 6, 201–219.

Cacioppo, J. T. & Cacioppo, S. 2018. The growing problem of loneliness. *Lancet*, 391, 426.

Carayon, P., Wooldridge, A., Hoonakker, P., Hundt, A. S. & Kelly, M. M. 2020. SEIPS 3.0: human-centered design of the patient journey for patient safety. *Applied Ergonomics*, 84, 103033.

Chatterjee, H. J., Camic, P. M., Lockyer, B. & Thomson, L. J. M. 2018. Non-clinical community interventions: a systematised review of social prescribing schemes. *Arts & Health*, 10, 97–123.

Christakis, N. A. & Fowler, J. H. 2008. The collective dynamics of smoking in a large social network. *New England Journal of Medicine*, 358, 2249–2258.

Christakis, N. A. & Fowler, J. H. 2013. Social contagion theory: examining dynamic social networks and human behavior. *Statistics in Medicine*, 32, 556–577.

Clark, L. A., Cuthbert, B., Lewis-Fernández, R., Narrow, W. E. & Reed, G. M. 2017. Three approaches to understanding and classifying mental disorder: ICD-11, DSM-5, and the National Institute of Mental Health's research domain criteria (RDoC). *Psychological Science in the Public Interest*, 18, 72–145.

Clark, T., Foster, L., Sloan, L. & Bryman, A. 2021. *Social Research Methods*, Oxford University Press.

Clements, K. W., Mariano, M. J. M., Verikios, G. & Wong, B. 2022. How elastic is alcohol consumption? *Economic Analysis and Policy*, 76, 568–581.

Crinson, I. 2018. The health professions and professional practice. *In:* Scambler, G. (ed.) *Sociology as Applied to Health and Medicine*, Bloomsbury.

Dahlgren, G. & Whitehead, M. 2021. The Dahlgren-Whitehead model of health determinants: 30 years on and still chasing rainbows. *Public Health*, 199, 20–24.

Damsbo, A. G., Kraglund, K. L., Buttenschøn, H. N., Johnsen, S. P., Andersen, G. & Mortensen, J. K. 2020. Predictors for wellbeing and characteristics of mental health after stroke. *Journal of Affective Disorders*, 264, 358–364.

Danielli, S., Ashrafian, H. & Darzi, A. 2023. Healthy city: global systematic scoping review of city initiatives to improve health with policy recommendations. *BMC Public Health*, 23, 1277.

Davey, F., Mcgowan, V., Birch, J., Kuhn, I., Lahiri, A., Gkiouleka, A., Arora, A., Sowden, S., Bambra, C. & Ford, J. 2022. Levelling up health: a practical, evidence-based framework for reducing health inequalities. *Public Health in Practice*, 4, 100322.

Davidson, L. 2016. The recovery movement: implications for mental health care and enabling people to participate fully in life. *Health Affairs*, 35, 1091–1097.

Degenhardt, L., Charlson, F., Ferrari, A., Santomauro, D., Erskine, H., Mantilla-Herrara, A., Whiteford, H., Leung, J., Naghavi, M. & Griswold, M. 2018. The global burden of disease attributable to alcohol and drug use in 195 countries and territories, 1990–2016: a systematic analysis for the Global Burden of Disease Study 2016. *The Lancet Psychiatry*, 5, 987–1012.

Feng, X., Kim, D. D., Cohen, J. T., Neumann, P. J. & Ollendorf, D. A. 2020. Using QALYs versus DALYs to measure cost-effectiveness: how much does it matter? *International Journal of Technology Assessment in Health Care*, 36, 96–103.

Fiorillo, A., De Girolamo, G., Simunovic, I. F., Gureje, O., Isaac, M., Lloyd, C., Mari, J., Patel, V., Reif, A., Starostina, E., Summergrad, P. & Sartorius, N. 2023. The relationship between physical and mental health: an update from the WPA Working Group on Managing Comorbidity of Mental and Physical Health. *World Psychiatry*, 22, 169–170.

Frost, H., Campbell, P., Maxwell, M., O'carroll, R. E., Dombrowski, S. U., Williams, B., Cheyne, H., Coles, E. & Pollock, A. 2018. Effectiveness of motivational interviewing on adult behaviour change in health and social care settings: a systematic review of reviews. *PLoS One*, 13, e0204890.

Giddens, A. & Sutton, P. 2017. *Sociology*, Cambridge: Polity Press.

Glied, S. & Smith, P. 2011. *The Oxford Handbook of Health Economics*, Oxford University Press.

Granovetter, M. S. 1973. The strength of weak ties. *American Journal of Sociology*, 78, 1360–1380.

Greenhalgh, T., Wherton, J., Papoutsi, C., Lynch, J., Hughes, G., A'court, C., Hinder, S., Fahy, N., Procter, R. & Shaw, S. 2017. Beyond adoption: a new framework for theorizing and evaluating nonadoption, abandonment, and challenges to the scale-up, spread, and sustainability of health and care technologies. *Journal of Medical Internet Research*, 19, e367.

Gross, R. 2015. *Psychology: The Science of Mind and Behaviour*, London: Hodder Education.

Harrison, J. E., Weber, S., Jakob, R. & Chute, C. G. 2021. ICD-11: an international classification of diseases for the twenty-first century. *BMC Medical Informatics and Decision Making*, 21, 206.

Hatzenbuehler, M. L., Phelan, J. C. & Link, B. G. 2013. Stigma as a fundamental cause of population health inequalities. *American Journal of Public Health*, 103, 813–821.

Henry, S. 2018. *Social Deviance*, John Wiley & Sons.

Holden, R. J., Carayon, P., Gurses, A. P., Hoonakker, P., Hundt, A. S., Ozok, A. A. & Rivera-Rodriguez, A. J. 2013. SEIPS 2.0: a human factors framework for studying and improving the work of healthcare professionals and patients. *Ergonomics*, 56, 1669–1686.

Holt-Lunstad, J. 2018. The potential public health relevance of social isolation and loneliness: prevalence, epidemiology, and risk factors. *Public Policy & Aging Report*, 27, 127–130.

Husk, K., Blockley, K., Lovell, R., Bethel, A., Lang, I., Byng, R. & Garside, R. 2020. What approaches to social prescribing work, for whom, and in what circumstances? A realist review. *Health & Social Care in the Community*, 28, 309–324.

Katzmarzyk, P. T., Friedenreich, C., Shiroma, E. J. & Lee, I.-M. 2022. Physical inactivity and non-communicable disease burden in low-income, middle-income and high-income countries. *British Journal of Sports Medicine*, 56, 101–106.

Kerrissey, M., Novikov, Z., Tietschert, M., Phillips, R. & Singer, S. J. 2023. The ambiguity of "we": perceptions of teaming in dynamic environments and their implications. *Social Science & Medicine*, 320, 115678.

Khan Minhas, A. M., Sedhom, R., Jean, E. D., Shapiro, M. D., Panza, J. A., Alam, M., Virani, S. S., Ballantyne, C. M. & Abramov, D. 2024. Global burden of cardiovascular disease attributable to smoking, 1990–2019: an analysis of the 2019 Global Burden of Disease Study. *European Journal of Preventive Cardiology*, 31, 1123–1131.

Kickbusch, I., Allen, L. & Franz, C. 2016. The commercial determinants of health. *The Lancet Global Health*, 4, e895–e896.

Kislov, R., Pope, C., Martin, G. P. & Wilson, P. M. 2019. Harnessing the power of theorising in implementation science. *Implementation Science*, 14, 103.

Kivimäki, M., Batty, G. D., Pentti, J., Shipley, M. J., Sipilä, P. N., Nyberg, S. T., Suominen, S. B., Oksanen, T., Stenholm, S., Virtanen, M., Marmot, M. G., Singh-Manoux, A., Brunner, E. J., Lindbohm, J. V., Ferrie, J. E. & Vahtera, J. 2020. Association between socioeconomic status and the development of mental and physical health conditions in adulthood: a multi-cohort study. *The Lancet Public Health*, 5, e140–e149.

Koohi Rostamkalaee, Z., Jafari, M. & Gorji, H. A. 2022. A systematic review of strategies used for controlling consumer moral hazard in health systems. *BMC Health Services Research*, 22, 1260.

Larsen, L. T. 2021. Not merely the absence of disease: a genealogy of the WHO's positive health definition. *History of the Human Sciences*, 35, 111–131.

Leonardi, F. 2018. The definition of health: towards new perspectives. *International Journal of Health Services*, 48, 735–748.

Luchenski, S., Maguire, N., Aldridge, R. W., Hayward, A., Story, A., Perri, P., Withers, J., Clint, S., Fitzpatrick, S. & Hewett, N. 2018. What works in inclusion health: overview of effective interventions for marginalised and excluded populations. *The Lancet*, 391, 266–280.

Macdonald, S. J., Deacon, L., Nixon, J., Akintola, A., Gillingham, A., Kent, J., Ellis, G., Mathews, D., Ismail, A., Sullivan, S., Dore, S. & Highmore, L. 2018. 'The invisible enemy': disability, loneliness and isolation. *Disability & Society*, 33, 1138–1159.

Marks, D., Murray, M. & Estacio, E. V. 2020. *Health Psychology: Theory, Research and Practice*, Sage.

Marmot, M. 2018. Inclusion health: addressing the causes of the causes. *The Lancet*, 391, 186–188.

Marmot, M., Allen, J., Boyce, T., Goldblatt, P. & Morrison, J. 2020. Health Equity in England: The Marmot Review 10 Years On. The Health Foundation Available: **www.health.org.uk/reports-and-analysis/ reports/health-equity-in-england-the-marmot-review-10-years-on-0** [Accessed].

Mays, N. 2018. Health care systems. *In:* Scambler, G. (ed.) *Sociology as Applied to Health and Medicine*, Bloomsbury.

Mccartney, G., Bartley, M., Dundas, R., Katikireddi, S. V., Mitchell, R., Popham, F., Walsh, D. & Wami, W. 2019. Theorising social class and its application to the study of health inequalities. *SSM - Population Health*, 7, 100315.

Michie, S., Atkins, L. & West, R. 2024. *The Behaviour Change Wheel*, Silverback publishing.

Michie, S., Van Stralen, M. M. & West, R. 2011. The behaviour change wheel: a new method for characterising and designing behaviour change interventions. *Implementation Science*, 6, 42.

Middleton, H. & Moncrieff, J. 2019. Critical psychiatry: a brief overview. *BJPsych Advances*, 25, 47–54.

Nichol, B., Haighton, C., Wilson, R. & Rodrigues, A. M. 2024. Enhancing making every contact count (MECC) training and delivery for the third and social economy (TSE) sector: a strategic behavioural analysis. *Psychology & Health*, 1–32.

Northouse, P. 2022. *Leadership: Theory and Practice*, Sage.

Ogden, J. 2023. *Health Psychology*, Maidenhead: Open University Press.

Oliver, M. 2013. The social model of disability: thirty years on. *Disability & Society*, 28, 1024–1026.

Omran, A. R. 2005. The epidemiologic transition: a theory of the epidemiology of population change. 1971. *The Milbank Quarterly*, 83, 731–757.

Papanicolas, I. & Cylus, J. 2015. Comparison of health systems performance. *In:* Kuhlmann, E., Blank, R., Bourgeault, I. & Wendt, C. (eds.) *The Palgrave International Handbook of Healthcare Policy and Governance*, Basingstoke: Palgrave Macmillan.

Parchment, A., Lawrence, W., Perry, R., Rahman, E., Townsend, N., Wainwright, E. & Wainwright, D. 2023. Making every contact count and healthy conversation skills as very brief or brief behaviour change interventions: a scoping review. *Journal of Public Health*, 31, 1017–1034.

Phelan, J. C., Link, B. G. & Dovidio, J. F. 2008. Stigma and prejudice: one animal or two? *Social Science & Medicine*, 67, 358–367.

Rand, L. Z. & Kesselheim, A. S. 2021. Controversy over using quality-adjusted life-years in cost-effectiveness analyses: a systematic literature review. *Health Affairs*, 40, 1402–1410.

Raworth, K. 2017. A doughnut for the Anthropocene: humanity's compass in the 21st century. *The Lancet Planetary Health*, 1, e48–e49.

Raworth, K. 2018. *Doughnut Economics: Seven Ways to Think like a 21st-Century Economist*, Penguin.

Rodrigues, A. M., Nichol, B., Wilson, R., Charlton, C., Gibson, B., Finch, T., Haighton, C., Maniatopoulos, G., Giles, E., Harrison, D., Orange, D., Robson, C. & Harland, J. 2024. Mapping regional implementation of 'making every contact count': mixed-methods evaluation of implementation stage, strategies, barriers and facilitators of implementation. *BMJ Open*, 14, e084208.

Rogers, A., Brooks, H., Vassilev, I., Kennedy, A., Blickem, C. & Reeves, D. 2014. Why less may be more: a mixed methods study of the work and relatedness of 'weak ties' in supporting long-term condition self-management. *Implementation Science*, 9, 19.

Rogers, A. & Pilgrim, D. 2021. *A Sociology of Mental Health and Illness*, 6th Edition, McGraw-Hill Education (UK).

Rosenquist, J. N., Murabito, J., Fowler, J. H. & Christakis, N. A. 2010. The spread of alcohol consumption behavior in a large social network. *Annals of Internal Medicine*, 152, 426–433.

Saks, M. 2016. A review of theories of professions, organizations and society: the case for neo-Weberianism, neo-institutionalism and eclecticism. *Journal of Professions and Organization*, 3, 170–187.

Salas, E., Reyes, D. L. & Mcdaniel, S. H. 2018a. The science of teamwork: progress, reflections, and the road ahead. *The American Psychologist*, 73, 593–600.

Salas, E., Zajac, S. & Marlow, S. L. 2018b. Transforming health care one team at a time: ten observations and the trail ahead. *Group & Organization Management*, 43, 357–381.

Sanford, N., Lavelle, M., Markiewicz, O., Reedy, G., Rafferty, D. A. M., Darzi, L. A. & Anderson, J. E. 2024. Decoding healthcare teamwork: a typology of hospital teams. *Journal of Interprofessional Care*, 38, 602–611.

Scambler, G. 2009. Health-related stigma. *Sociology of Health & Illness*, 31, 441–455.

Scambler, G. 2018. *Sociology as Applied to Health and Medicine*, London: Palgrave.

Schramme, T. 2023. Health as complete well-being: the WHO definition and beyond. *Public Health Ethics*, 16, 210–218.

Shield, K., Manthey, J., Rylett, M., Probst, C., Wettlaufer, A., Parry, C. D. & Rehm, J. 2020. National, regional, and global burdens of disease from 2000 to 2016 attributable to alcohol use: a comparative risk assessment study. *The Lancet Public Health*, 5, e51–e61.

Shuffler, M. L. & Carter, D. R. 2018. Teamwork situated in multiteam systems: key lessons learned and future opportunities. *The American Psychologist*, 73, 390–406.

Sloman, J., Garratt, D. & Guest, J. 2022. *Economics*, Harlow: Pearson.

Taylor, D. & Bury, M. 2007. Chronic illness, expert patients and care transition. *Sociology of Health & Illness*, 29, 27–45.

Thaler, R. & Sunstein, C. 2009. *Nudge: Improving Decisions about Health, Wealth and Happiness*, Penguin.

Topol, E. 2019. Preparing the healthcare workforce to deliver the digital future. NHS Health Education England Available: **https://topol.hee.nhs.uk** [Accessed].

Towfighi, A., Ovbiagele, B., El Husseini, N., Hackett, M. L., Jorge, R. E., Kissela, B. M., Mitchell, P. H., Skolarus, L. E., Whooley, M. A. & Williams, L. S. 2017. Poststroke depression: a scientific statement for healthcare professionals from the American Heart Association/ American Stroke Association. *Stroke*, 48, e30–e43.

Tweed, E. J., Popham, F., Thomson, H. & Katikireddi, S. V. 2022. Including 'inclusion health'? A discourse analysis of health inequalities policy reviews. *Critical Public Health*, 32, 700–712.

Tyler, I. & Slater, T. 2018. Rethinking the sociology of stigma. *The Sociological Review*, 66, 721–743.

Wagstaff, A. & Neelsen, S. 2020. A comprehensive assessment of universal health coverage in 111 countries: a retrospective observational study. *The Lancet Global Health*, 8, e39–e49.

Wami, W., Mccartney, G., Bartley, M., Buchanan, D., Dundas, R., Katikireddi, S. V., Mitchell, R. & Walsh, D. 2020. Theory driven analysis of social class and health outcomes using UK nationally representative longitudinal data. *International Journal for Equity in Health*, 19, 193.

Weisz, G. & Olszynko-Gryn, J. 2010. The theory of epidemiologic transition: the origins of a citation classic. *Journal of the History of Medicine and Allied Sciences*, 65, 287–326.

WHO. 2023. Commercial determinants of health. World Health Organization. Available: **https://www.who.int/news-room/fact-sheets/detail/commercial-determinants-of-health** [Accessed].

Wiseman, V. 2011. Key concepts in health economics. *In:* Guinness, L. & Wiseman, V. (eds.) *Introduction to Health Economics*, McGraw-Hill Education.

Wu, Y., Awang, S. R., Ahmad, T. & You, C. 2024. A systematic review of leadership styles in healthcare sector: insights and future directions. *Geriatric Nursing*, 59, 48–59.

PART 1

Understanding Health, Healthcare Systems, and the Healthcare Workforce

Social Theory, Social Research Methods and Health in the Context of Society and Care

Chris Allen[1] and Assaf Givati[2]

[1] *School of Health Sciences, University of Southampton, Southampton, UK*
[2] *Department of Population Health Sciences, King's College London, London, UK*

Introduction

This chapter will help you to contextualise some of the social research observations that will be discussed throughout this book and begin to consider their relevance to health and well-being. During this chapter, you will be introduced to some of the social sciences' key concepts, thinkers, debates and methods, and how these have been used in answering small (micro) and big (macro) questions about society and social life; as well as concerns in between (meso). This chapter will equip you with the basic tools that you need in order to understand and engage with research and academic literature across the social sciences and consider how we know what we know about the social world and how we might learn more about it in the future.

To understand the complex social world that we inhabit, and its intersections with health and well-being, social scientists use systematic observations to develop concepts and theories that explain the social world around us and how it works. After reading this chapter, you will understand the meaning of the terms *concept*, *theory* and *paradigm* and the way these are used and generated through social science research. You will also have the opportunity to consider some of the main seminal social theories and consider their relevance to health and well-being. Finally, you will gain an overview of some of the overarching methods commonly used to study the social world.

LEARNING OUTCOMES

By the end of this chapter, you will be able to:

- Understand the importance of social science and social theory in understanding the social world from different levels and different perspectives.
- Recognise the relevance of theory to improving understandings of the social world and how it works.
- Understand the different levels of theory that exist.
- Recognise some of the main grand theories that are used in the social sciences, their relevance to health and their relevance to the development and testing of mid-range and programme theories.
- Understand the two broad research approaches that are used to better understand the social world.

Social Sciences for Healthcare Professionals, First Edition. Edited by Chris Allen.
© 2026 John Wiley & Sons Ltd. Published 2026 by John Wiley & Sons Ltd.

What Is a Theory?

> ### Key Terms and Definitions
>
> **Concept:**   Is an abstract general idea or understanding of something. In social science, concepts capture realities in society, for example, 'social class' or 'stigma'. These provide the building blocks for theories.
>
> **Theories:**   Relate to a set of concepts and their relationships and seek to explain how the social world works.
>
> **Paradigms:**   Are broad philosophical assumptions about the way that we see and approach the world.

To understand why concepts and theories are so important to the development of well-thought-through, robust and well-established strategies and interventions in health, it is important to consider the way social sciences' explanations are developed. The social sciences include several disciplines and their sub-disciplines (e.g. medical sociology) that are quite different from one another in the way they observe and examine social life; but they also have some significant commonalities, otherwise they would not be all grouped together as *social sciences*. The social sciences are used to understand our complex and evolving social world, how it is created, what structures it has and how individuals within it interact with one another, how they think, how they make decisions and how they behave. These understandings about how the social world works have relevance to how we think about, understand and seek to improve health and well-being in our society.

The starting point in social sciences is that whilst we all have certain ideas and beliefs about the way our lives and the way our behaviour are shaped by our social environment, there is a difference between our common-sense understandings of it and the way social science explanations are developed (Green and Thorogood, 2014, Schutt, 2018). As our common-sense understandings are often based solely on our own experiences and interpretations, rather than what actually happens, they tend to be a product of our own interactions and personal accounts with the world around us over the course of our lives. This judgement whereby we rely on past experiences and social cues to develop logical reasoning, is often informed by stereotypes, various biases and incomplete information. Immersing ourselves in theory, helps us to move away from our common-sense interpretation of the world to an analytical observation that goes beyond our own personal experiences and impressions (Dillon, 2020). To fully understand our social world, we must ask critical questions, collect empirical findings about it and generate theories based on those findings (Chijioke et al., 2020, Green and Thorogood, 2014).

Theories in the social sciences seek to explain a social phenomenon and how or why it arises. They seek to explain the way something *is* in a society (Chijioke et al., 2020, Pettigrew, 1997). Theories can highlight where meaningful interaction exists between variables and can help us create processes, models or ways of thinking that allow us to make sense of, or explain how and why these variables interact with one another in the way that they do (Chijioke et al., 2020, Pettigrew, 1997). Essentially this helps us create testable propositions or hypotheses about how different aspects of society work (Allan, 2006). We can use this knowledge to help us make sense of or explain things that have happened in the past, or to make some predictions about what might happen in the future (Chijioke et al., 2020, Kislov et al., 2019). *Good* theories provide researchers with well-defined, organised and empirically supported perspectives, or 'lenses', through which we can examine complicated societal problems and issues (Reeves et al., 2008). The starting point to theorising more generally is asking *critical* questions and familiarising ourselves with a body of academic literature so that we become aware of the knowledge, the research base, and the various discourses (how things are discussed) that exist, to develop an in-depth understanding of it. By developing such critical awareness, we are able to position ourselves in relation to these areas of concern and therefore understand where common sense accounts of it come from, and where they may be limited. All of this helps us to advance our practice, whether in clinical or academic settings, by casting a light on what social interactions and processes we understand through empirical observation, as well as the ones we still do not know enough about.

Concepts typically refer to the general ideas that serve as the building blocks of the broader theory that characterises aspects of society (Monaghan and Gabe, 2022). For example, the concepts 'autonomy' and 'dominance' are important in understanding the roles of professions in society; especially in relation to healthcare professions (explored in chapter 6). By conducting empirical research and drawing on connections between such concepts, social scientists generate *theories* and conceptual frameworks. Through this, we can then put our ideas and explanations to the test – rather than simply drawing on our own personal experiences or common-sense understandings. Through this, fairer, more accurate understandings can be identified and examined (Clark et al., 2021, Green and Thorogood, 2014). As we explore in this chapter, we can use qualitative and quantitative research methods to examine our social world, and the body of empirical evidence that emerges through these can lead to the further development of theories. This evidence can lead to existing theories being rejected, amended or refined in a continuous process as shown in Figure 2.1.

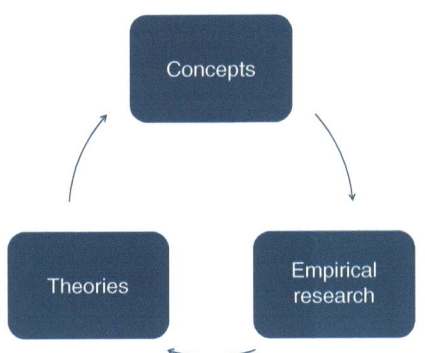

FIGURE 2.1 The relationships between concepts, empirical research, and theory.

Understanding Theories Through Levels of Abstraction

Society and our social lives are incredibly layered and complex – with many parts and interrelated processes. Because there are so many aspects of society we could look at, well-defined theory helps us to understand what to look at, how we should study it and how we should understand it.

Why Is This Needed?

Because describing the social reality around us through facts and figures in isolation does not explain the social reality that it amounts to. How do we know, for example, whether the fact that most health professionals are female is a good thing? Is it right that some signs and symptoms are classified as a disease, whereas others are not? Or how do we decide if it is fair who must pay for care? To answer such questions, we need to make some assumptions about the social world. Moreover, as we shall see, these assumptions depend on the perspective that we take.

Grand Theories

Some of the most significant theories in the social sciences are relatively simply stated, allowing knowledge to emerge that provides a schema to explain what might otherwise remain a confusing, messy bundle of events and activities (Damschroder, 2020). There is often considerable value in theories being simply stated, as it allows them to be used to unpick a broad range of observed social phenomena. Theories at the highest level of abstraction are often called 'Grand Theories' or paradigms; their breadth provides a framework through which

we can think about some of society's largest issues – providing a worldview and language that can be applied to a range and diversity of social contexts (Davidoff et al., 2015). These are in the form of our basic assumptions of the social world. They typically aim to provide an overarching schema for how things work.

Mid-Range Theories

Since society is composed of so many different people, groups, institutions and social processes, a grand theory (paradigm) cannot possibly explain it through a handful of variables that seek to explain how all aspects of that society works. To bridge this gap, what is often needed are 'mid-range' theories. Boudon, who wrote extensively on the use of mid-range theories argued that:

> it is hopeless and quixotic to try to determine the overarching independent variable that would operate in all social processes, or to determine the essential feature of social structure, or to find out the two, three, or four concepts…that would be sufficient to analyse all of social phenomena. (Boudon, 1991, p. 519)

The aim of mid-range theories is typically to integrate theory and empirical research. Theories can be developed from an empirical phenomenon, which allows the general observations about the social world that we create to be tested and verified by data. So grand theories provide an overarching perspective to understand and to study society, mid-range theories help to bridge this wider perspective with more concrete empirical data in relation to more concrete circumstances whilst still being useful in a range of different contexts (Brodie et al., 2011, Davidoff et al., 2015).

Programme Theories

We can then use 'small' or programme theories to consider how a specific policy, regulation or intervention may work in a specific social context (Kislov et al., 2019). These are sometimes also referred to as logic models, or theories of change (Funnell and Rogers, 2011, Mills et al., 2019). Programme theories were largely pioneered by evaluation scientists, largely through realist evaluation and synthesis, and have become important in implementation science, service improvement and public health with whole books being dedicated to it (Funnell and Rogers, 2011, Pawson et al., 2005, Pawson and Tilly, 1997). Programme theories can help us think about specific features of a programme or intervention and how they might work to address the issue they are seeking to, by making it clear what features of an intervention are potentially important – through which we can then test these assumptions through research (Funnell and Rogers, 2011, Skivington et al., 2021). Programme theories – once we have 'surfaced them' – for example, through searching the literature to determine exactly how something might work – can help us understand what to look at and how to evaluate its impact (Mark, 2023). Middle-range theories can be visible in some of these explanations for why aspects of a programme or intervention work in the way that they do (Shearn et al., 2017). We can use programme theories to explore the connections between context, mechanisms and outcomes (Greenhalgh and Manzano, 2022, Pawson, 2013). One programme theory we particularly like, not least because it adds some light humour to a chapter about social theory, is the 'Dishy David Beckham Theory' (Pawson and Sridharan, 2009). This programme theory considered whether replacing the media exposure of unhealthy but attractive role models such as rockstars, with healthy but equally as attractive sports stars, might improve the health behaviours of teenagers. Spoiler alert – it didn't. Essentially programme theories help us to consider the theoretical basis for an intervention – what exactly

is involved in the intervention and how does this relate to the outcomes that are observed? This helps us consider how the intervention works, for who and in what context – and perhaps most importantly to what extent (Funnell and Rogers, 2011, Pawson et al., 2005, Pawson and Tilly, 1997).

How Grand, Mid-Range and Programme Theories Work Together

Here we can think about levels of abstraction as how close we are getting to what we are observing. A good way to think about the levels of abstraction is landscape or aerial photography. Let's assume that the picture includes some of societies' institutions such as shops, schools, universities and hospitals, rather than the scenery of say a deserted hilly valley.

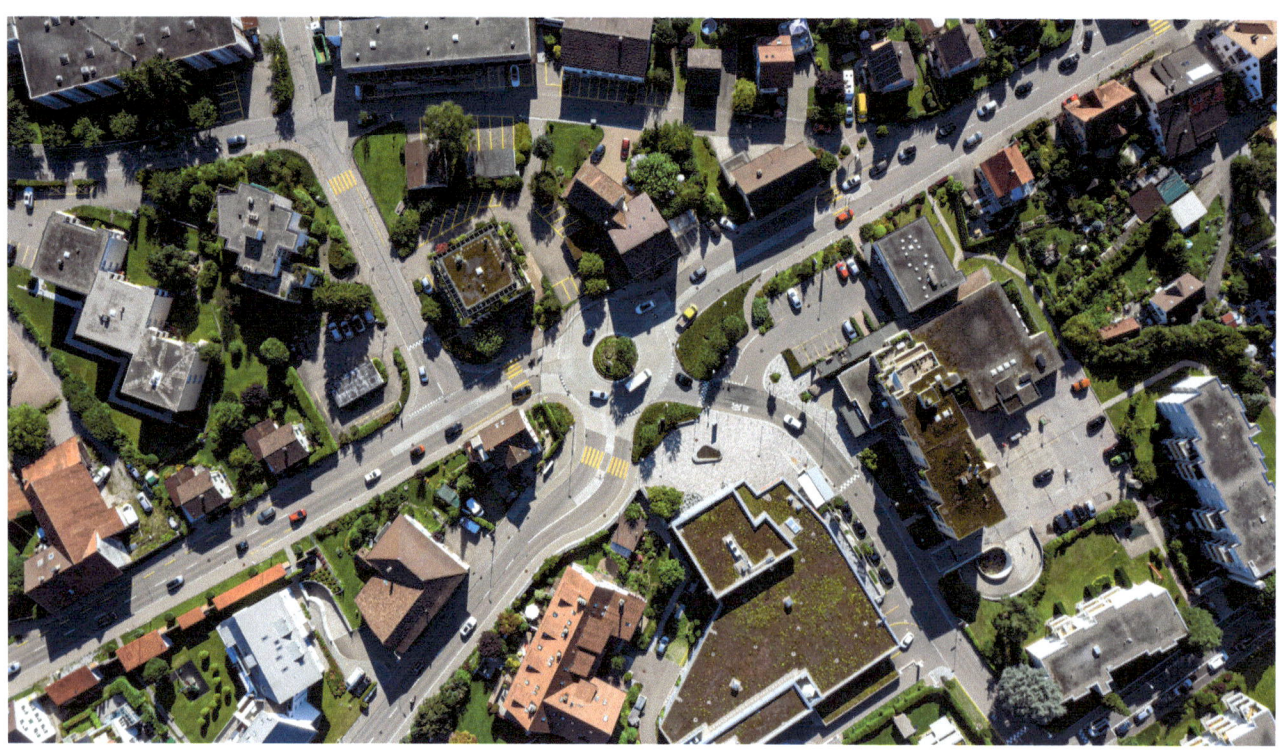

Source: Florian/Adobe Stock Photos.

With a good landscape or aerial photograph, you might be able to capture a fair bit about that society and how it generally operates. For example, some overarching rules, a schema; but what you capture and infer from your observations might not be that concrete, detailed or even particularly focussed. You might be able to make some general inferences about how people interact with one another, and how they interact with that society's institutions. From this wide or high perspective, any assertions are also hard to dispute, as at this level, it is tricky to create any type of real testable hypothesis. However, by zooming in on some of the photograph's details, you can potentially see the ebbs and flows of society in a particular place, space and context. You can explore the specific details and the intricacies of society, the people within it, and its institutions, its processes and causal relationships.

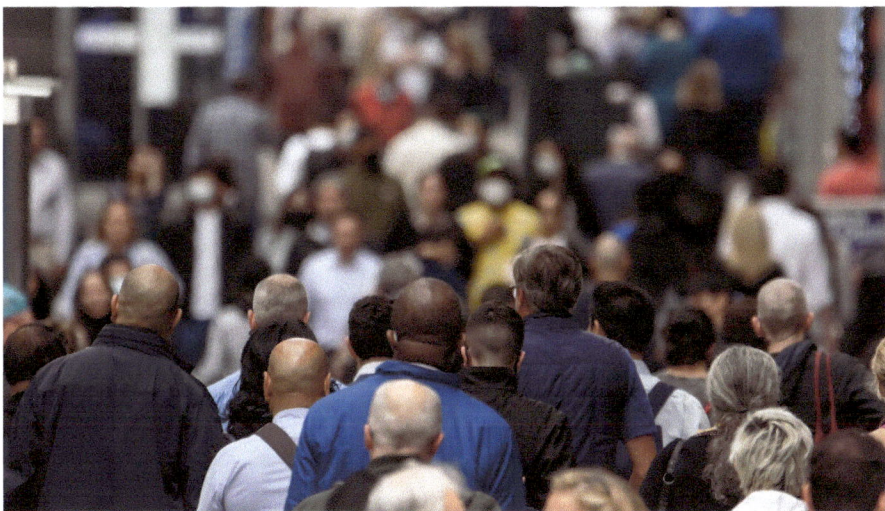

Source: blvdone/Adobe Stock Photos.

As you zoom in and look at different aspects, the tools you will need to understand what is going on will likely need to change, for example, in the social sciences, these tools can be the methods that you use which will be theoretically informed, which may include different types of data collection and analysis techniques. Sometimes the tools you need will be obvious, but often you will need to look at the tools that other people have used, and this will help you compare what you have observed, with what they have. By changing your tools to look at some of the picture's most fascinating parts, things will likely come into greater focus, and the knowledge that you gain, might in turn deepen your understanding of how things work in the picture as a whole; helping you to revise, or tinker with some of the theory at the higher levels, where it no longer fits with your new understanding about how that society works. Of course, where something about a society is undesirable and where we want to intervene to change it – we need to think about what specific features of a society we want to change, what we should do to change them and how we will know if the intervention has led to the intended outcomes. This is where programme theories are useful.

In summary, grand theories provide different perspectives on the way we observe and research society, from which mid-range and programme theories are developed. Mid-range theories are designed to engage more closely with the study of more concrete aspects and circumstances of social processes and interactions and are arguably more practical to you in your roles as healthcare professionals, whether that be in relation to clinical practice, research or service improvement due to their portability and applicability to a range of different contexts. Programme theories allow you to consider the specific components of a programme or intervention and understand how they work to bring about a specific change or outcome.

Most of the theories covered throughout this book can be considered mid-range theories, with the exemption of the grand theories discussed in this chapter. It is worth highlighting that the boundaries to different levels of theories are generally not clear-cut – some programme theories might be considered mid-range theories, for example, and in some literature these terms are used interchangeably (Shearn et al., 2017), and mid-range theories, may be composed of several related programme theories (Kislov et al., 2019). Programme theories can also use mid-range theories to explain aspects of an intervention and how they work (Shearn et al., 2017).

To help you make the distinction between the different theories that you may encounter, Davidoff (2015), offers a 'rule of thumb' typology of theories. Table 2.1 offers a summary of these different levels of theory, alongside some of their defining features and key characteristics.

The relationships and roles of 'small' or 'programme theories', 'mid-range' or 'large' theories and 'grand theories' within the 'scientific circle or enquiry' are shown in Figure 2.2, which we have adapted from the work of Brodie et al. (2011).

As the figure illustrates well – the knowledge gained through empirical observation at the lower levels of abstraction (i.e. programme theories) can be used to revise and refine higher-level theories to make them better fit with any new understandings that have emerged through empirical testing and observations.

Macro, Meso and Micro Levels

Alongside the level of abstraction, social science theories can also be characterised by their micro, meso or macro perspective. These levels frequently reflect the study of differing priorities within society (Sawatzky et al., 2021). For example, when considering quality of life and overall well-being (an important thread throughout this book) at a macro level we can consider the way the political system in a country influences healthcare policy intending to promote quality of life across the whole sector. This might also include broader considerations about how society sees illness, and where priorities should lie (Sawatzky et al., 2021). This will influence the meso level where we can consider how organisations as a whole work to better enhance the quality of care that they provide, with a view to promoting quality of life and well-being, as well as the micro level such as how healthcare professionals interact with those in their care, how they consider

TABLE 2.1 Levels of theory.

	Definition	Characteristics	Types and examples	Level of abstraction
Grand theories	Aim to explain a complete understanding of the social world and all its constituent parts.	High level of abstraction. Provides overarching perspectives or 'maps' for observing and analysing society. Not very specific – difficult to operationalise. Difficult to study – society is complex, and multiple aspects hang together within a society, that are challenging to isolate and test using scientific methods.	Overarching theoretical perspectives through which the social world is seen and understood through. For example, classics such functionalism and conflict theory, discussed below, as well as system complexity and rational choice. Many of these are 'theoretical oeuvres of sociological classics' (Kislov et al., 2019, p. 2) like Marx and Durkheim.	
Mid-range (sometimes referred to as 'Big') theories	Theories that sit between our general everyday observations, questions and hypothesis that we might generate about how something is, and the overarching assertions offered by grand theories to understand the overarching social word and everything in it.	Better aligned to be tested empirically than grand theories. Consider mechanisms and social processes that can be tested. Often influenced by one or more grand theory.	Diffusion of innovations (Rogers et al., 2014) Normalisation process theory (Murray et al., 2010). Social capital theory (Lin, 2002) Social cognitive theory (Bandura, 2001)	
'Small' or programme theories	Theories that consider how a specific intervention might function in a given social context. For example, a behaviour change intervention, aimed at reducing a harmful health behaviour in a target population. These are specific to a particular programme or intervention – though may have similarities with similar programmes and interventions.	Practical and accessible. Provides concrete working models that can be tested empirically. Can test assumptions about how interventions work, which can allow us to look at the merits of different aspects of an intervention. Can easily be modified in response to empirical data.	Programme theories of individual health interventions	

Source: Adapted from Kislov et al. (2019).

an individual's goals of their treatment and how these are negotiated between healthcare professionals, individual patients and their families (Bracher et al., 2020, Sawatzky et al., 2021).

Macro Approaches: How Does Society Work?

Many overarching paradigms seek to explain how society works. Within the constraints of this chapter, we cannot explain all of these, so instead, we will focus on some of the most influential ones whilst highlighting their relevance to understanding health.

Functionalism

Structural functionalism principally focusses on social systems, stability, social roles, and order (Barry and Yuill, 2022, Dillon, 2020). The basic principles of Structural Functionalism are the maintenance of social stability, through the collective functioning of social structures (Barry and Yuill, 2022, Dillon, 2020). By social structure of society, we refer to its components including social institutions, norms and values, which

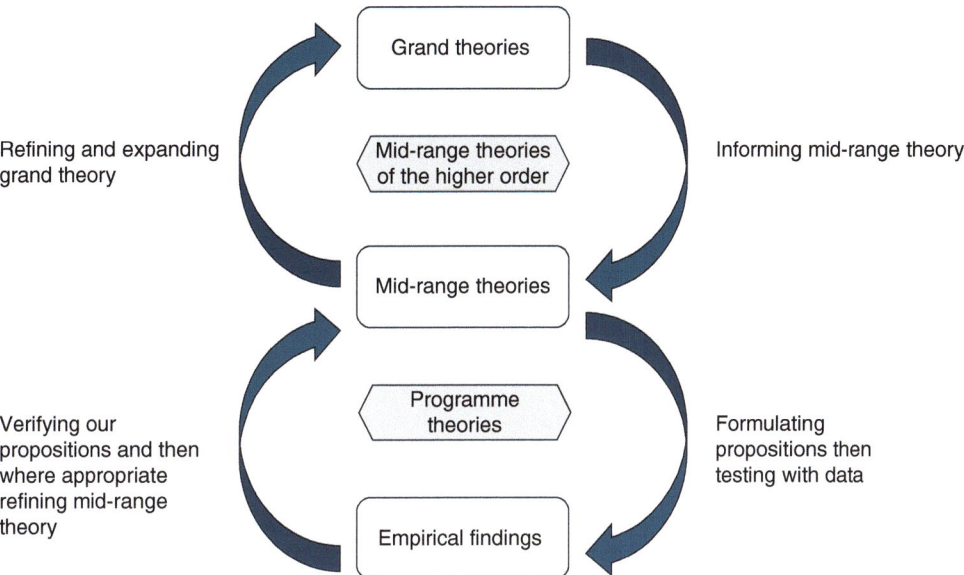

FIGURE 2.2   The relationship and roles of 'small' or 'programme theories', 'mid-range' or 'large' theories and 'grand theories' within the 'scientific circle of enquiry'. **Source:** Adapted from Kislov et al. (2019).

are interconnected and interdependent. Through their roles in society, these components together contribute to the emergence of social patterns that maintain the balanced and stable functioning of society (Barry and Yuill, 2022).

Early sociologists such as Émile Durkheim (1858–1915) and before him, Auguste Comte (1798–1857) and Harriet Martineau (1802–1876) believed that the study of society should be a scientific discipline (Dillon, 2020). Functionalists believed that society's normal and abnormal functionings in particular, could be understood using scientific methods (Dillon, 2020). Durkheim likened Sociology to other scientific disciplines, referring to *society* as an *organism*; formed of different *component parts* that need to work together for the organism to function effectively (Baert and Da Silva, 2010, Dillon, 2020, Levine, 1995). The functionalist perspective suggests that every structure has a function that meets the needs of a society, and each has a role in maintaining the smooth functioning of that society. All these structures are suggested to work together to maintain an equilibrium through functional unity (Willis et al., 2007). An example of a structure within this framework is institutions, which are any system that meets the needs of society, such as healthcare and education systems. Merton (1968), in his seminal book highlighted that institutions have both manifest (intended) as well as latent functions (i.e. functions that are not the main focus, but that are still relevant to how a society works) (Merton, 1968). A manifest function of the healthcare system is to prevent, detect and treat disease. A latent function of the healthcare system is to ensure that members of society are well enough to perform their family and occupational roles.

Alongside the importance of society's institutions are its 'social facts'. This term was defined by the Sociologist Émile Durkheim who conceptualised social facts as the values, cultural norms and social structures that exist beyond any one individual and exert social control over how people act and behave (Dillon, 2020). These are constructs, ways of thinking and acting as part of social interactions, informal rules that direct behaviour in groups and societies, and that exist as social expectations (Baert and Da Silva, 2010, Dillon, 2020). Norms of a society are hard to act against and when people do act against them, there is usually some kind of disapproval or sanction be it formally, such as if a crime has been committed, or informally, such as when you have acted in a way others might disprove of such as failing to attend a medical or dentist appointment, or attending a job interview late, in shorts, flip flops and a t-shirt (Dillon, 2020).

Structural functionalism has been a dominant approach in sociology; however, over time, its applicability to contemporary social theory and its popularity has waned (Belgrave and Charmaz, 2015). One of the most important contributors to structural functionalism was Talcott Parsons (1902–1979), who contributed to the development and conceptualisation of this paradigm, including in the field of health and healthcare. Very notable, was Parson's famous conceptualisation of 'the sick role' which we discuss next.

Talcott Parsons: The Sick Role

Whilst recognising that all societies have people who become unwell, Parsons viewed 'good health' as being one of many prerequisites for a well-functioning society. If too many people are unwell at the same time, then the 'Social System' becomes destabilised, or 'dysfunctional', since when people become unwell their capacity to perform other expected roles such as within the family and society more generally reduces (Willis, 2015). Parsonian thinking suggests that a stable functioning society requires those who are temporally incapacitated through poor health, must return to good health as soon as possible. In his book *The Social System*, Parsons (1951) described illness as a form of sanctioned 'deviance'. He proposed that whilst it is not 'normal' to be sick, society allows it, provided certain conditions are met. Under the 'Sick Role', people have certain rights. Whilst these are influenced by social and political contexts, these rights afford people support and make them temporarily exempt from having to carry out their normal social roles and responsibilities. For example, the sick role assumes that people do not have to work or care for their families when they are temporarily incapacitated (Willis, 2015).

In return for the affordances society offers you when you are unwell, when you are sick, you also have certain obligations through what Parsons described as 'a social contract'. You should behave in ways that support your return to health; you are allowed to be sick, but not for too long; and the time spent being unwell should be appropriate to the severity of your condition. Moreover, when you are sick, you are expected to seek medical care and be compliant with recommended treatments (Varul, 2010). In this model, the providers of care are dominant over those who are unwell, who are expected to be passive and willing recipients of the care they receive. This perspective assumes that doing so allows the sick to quickly become better and to recommence their previous important societal roles and responsibilities.

As you may have noticed, some of the assumptions inherent in the sick role do not align with contemporary healthcare needs or provision, and therefore it has been subject to critique and expansion (Cheshire et al., 2021, Rier, 2000, Varul, 2010). This is particularly the case in the context of chronic illness, whereby individual responsibility is emphasised, a return to fitness is not always possible, the condition will need to be managed across a life course, and therefore people are often not able to (and may not want to) remove themselves from their other roles and responsibilities to exclusively tend to their health and the demands of society and healthcare (Allen et al., 2020, Cheshire et al., 2021, Hallowell et al., 2015, Vassilev et al., 2017). Parsons also felt that 'true sickness', was largely unavoidable, which does not align well with our current understanding of the social determinants of health or our current focus on preventing ill health through health promotion and protection; both of which are explored in later chapters. The main contribution of Parsons' Sick Role to our understanding of health and illness are: first, the notion that sickness is a social role rather than merely changes in the biological body as we will unpack in the next chapter, and second, that the sick role has cultural and historical contexts; the experience of being ill isn't necessarily the same everywhere. Therefore, despite its shortcomings, it is still seen as a useful perspective.

Conflict Theory

A chief concern of sociology, and indeed its subdiscipline medical sociology, is the distribution of power within a society. This is the centre of concern in the second macro theory, Conflict Theory. The foundation for conflict theory was laid by two of the founders of sociological thinking, Karl Marx (1818–1883) and Max Weber (1864–1920), and it was developed further by a host of important sociologists thereafter. Conflict Theory sees society as characterized by inequalities and conflicts between parts of society which derive from differences in power, resources and social status (Barry and Yuill, 2022). This involves continuous competition between social groups and the relationships of dominance and subordination between them.

Marx saw class, an important sociological concept, as a social group whose members share the same relationships to the means of production (Barry and Yuill, 2022, Collyer, 2015, Giddens, 1973). In societies with social stratification, he argued that there are two major social classes: the ruling capitalist class, or bourgeoisie, and the subject class, or proletariat, which are definable in terms of ownership and non-ownership of resources (Barry and Yuill, 2022, Collyer, 2015). This relationship, and specifically the power of the ruling class over the subject class leads to exploitation, inequality and conflict (Collyer, 2015).

Despite the foundations for this grand theory being laid more than 150 years ago, its advances especially that relating to power and inequalities remain highly relevant to how we understand health and wellbeing now. Marx was principally concerned about how historical and social factors shape, and influence people's everyday lives and the opportunities people have (Collyer, 2015). Marx and his long-time collaborator Friedrich Engels (1820–1895) lived at a time before the social determinants of health were fully understood, yet they were able to connect poor living and working conditions with health; arguing that the situations society put its poorest members in, contributed to them becoming unwell (Das, 2022).

Conflict theory, as a grand theory can act as a broad lens through which disadvantages can be explored, and as such, has become popular in sociology, and its medical sociology subdiscipline. It informs contemporary theories that have helped consider the different power and opportunities afforded by sex and gender, race and ethnicity, and social class, across and within societies. The notions of social stratification and class are essential concepts to the understanding of social health inequalities which are explored later in this book.

Micro Approaches: How Does Society Work?

Symbolic Interactionism

Symbolic Interactionism, a micro theory, is considered one of the three main sociological paradigms. Associated with the social psychologist George Mead (1863–1931), the focus of the theory is on the meanings attached to human interaction, both verbal and nonverbal, and to symbols (Dillon, 2020). Communication is the central point of the theory's interest; conceptualised as the exchange of meaning through language and symbols, it is seen as the means through which people make sense of the social world around them (Dillon, 2020). The theory was developed largely in response to the predominant 'passivity' of the macro level grand theories of the time, that suggested that society was something that 'happens' to us, with little opportunity to determine or shape it (Carter and Fuller, 2016). The term Symbolic Interactionism was coined by Blumer, a student of Mead's, to reflect the premise that humans interact with things in the social world around them based on the meanings ascribed to those things (Dillon, 2020).

A society's 'symbols' are products of our interactions with one another, and therefore represent a shared meaning for whatever that particular symbol relates to (Carter and Fuller, 2016). Symbols can take many forms; for example, a patient information sheet can be seen by patients as helpful or encouraging, and to their healthcare professionals as an object that might help someone better manage their health and their condition. As such, human behaviour is a product of both internal processes such as how we think, how we make decisions and how we act or react, as well as our external environment, such as the impact of other individuals, and social structures on these internal processes. How a person acts, reacts or behaves in a given context, relates to the meaning that situation has for them, and these are often developed through interactions with others, with their environment and with themselves (Burbank and Martins, 2010). For example, an individual might observe how other people react towards them or to other people who are similar to them, in relation to some perceived difference they may have such as, for example, a physical, mental, cognitive or sensory impairment; and taken with other cues from these interactions, and from their environment, may perceive that society values those who are living with such differences as less than those who are not (Link et al., 2015). In the context of healthcare professionals, these interactions may create and reinforce status and hierarchy, leading to professional groups being seen in very different ways, and often creating paternalistic and imbalanced relationships between and amongst healthcare professionals, and those seeking care. Symbolic interactionism can also help us to understand how people come to understand what behaviours are expected of them in different social contexts including in care, through their perceptions of the situation, and their interactions with other people (often called the reference group) in that culture and environment (Dillon, 2020, Goffman, 1959). And finally, symbolic interactionism might explain why certain behaviours cluster in some groups and in some places – for example, taking part in unhealthy behaviours because it has shared value and meaning with other members of that group, or with particular places (Hefler and Carter, 2019, Skjælaaen, 2016).

As with all grand theories, symbolic interactionism has its limitations. Notably, it deals far less with some of the macro elements that shape a society, and that shape many of the behaviours that people engage with. However, its specific focus on everyday interactions and behaviours, makes it useful for the study of health (Cersosimo, 2024).

Table 2.2 summarises broadly the focus of the three main grand theories discussed and their broad healthcare perspectives.

Social Research Methods

Of course, as we have alluded to, theory should inform how we do research, by guiding us to what we should examine, and how we should examine it. In guiding our thinking, theory may

TABLE 2.2   **Summary of grand theories and their relevance to health.**

Grand theory	Level	Focus	Relevance to health
Structural functionalism	Macro	How each part of a society works together to maintain an ordered and well-functioning society overtime.	Good health and effective medical care are essential for the smooth functioning of society.
			When we become unwell, we have certain rights, but also certain obligations. We have to follow the medical instruction and therefore hierarchical relationships can exist between healthcare professionals and patients. Illness is a social concept, as well as a biological one.
Conflict theory	Macro	Considers the different relations to capital and power and how these result in differences in the resources people have, how they are treated, as well as what their living and working conditions are like.	Highlights the power differences that exist between different groups and individuals within a society and their impact on different living and working conditions, different access to resources and the impact of these on social and health inequalities.
Symbolic interactionism	Micro	Considers the symbolic meanings attributed to interactions with people, objects and the environment.	Health and illness are social constructions. Society defines what constitutes health, illness and disease.
			Having a difference such as an impairment, or a health condition can change how you anticipate people responding to you, as well as how they do respond.

also help us identify things within the data that we might have otherwise overlooked, or not seen as being significant. In turn, the findings of research should be used to help us to modify our theories, and thus advance our respective fields of study. To do this, we need robust research methods – so that we know the findings reflect as much as possible, what is going on, allowing us to make valid statements about the way things are and the way things are not.

If we look at claims that health is distributed unevenly across a population, we need empirical evidence to prove that this is the case. We might observe that people from lower socio-economic status groups tend to have poorer health outcomes than those who are wealthier, or that people with a learning disability, face barriers to accessing physical healthcare. However, without a method to look at this in a robust and systematic way, these remain merely common-sense observations. We cannot say for sure that these observations happen more generally, or to what magnitude, and as a result, we cannot put measures in place to reduce inequality and improve access to care for those who are disadvantaged. In fact, we do know that these social issues exist through well-conducted research – and this has also helped us better understand some of the underlying causes of these issues and thus begin to address them (Bambra et al., 2010, Davey et al., 2022, Whittle et al., 2018).

Most discoveries about the social world are relatively small and incremental – there are very few 'eureka' moments. But over time, even these small and incremental contributions build a more coherent and meaningful picture of our social world and how it all works and fits together. The social sciences use two broad approaches, or research paradigms, to understanding our social world, these are quantitative and qualitative approaches, as well as mixed methods approaches, which use aspects of both (Clark et al., 2021). Within these broad approaches, various methods are used to help us get a better view and understanding of society, which can be employed at macro, micro and meso levels. The relative merits and limitations of each *paradigm* have been the subject of often fierce debate for some time (Gage, 1989). What we hope to show you in this chapter's closing section, is how both broad approaches are useful to helping us better understand our social world.

We will close this chapter, and in a way, open the rest of this book, by considering these two broad approaches to research: quantitative research methods which reflect a positivist paradigm, and qualitative research methods which are grounded in an interpretivist paradigm. A useful starting point to explore research approaches in social sciences is Andrew Bryman's Social Research Methods (Clark et al., 2021). Our summary of positivism and interpretivism below is necessarily limited in scope and therefore, only serves to ground our discussion of theorising within this chapter. We hope that it will enable you to recognise these diverse types of research, and the knowledge they bring, in the examples that we will provide throughout the rest of this book.

Positivism (Quantitative Methods)

In the social sciences, quantitative research is useful in helping us to understand things objectively. Quantitative data is typically in a numerical form that can be counted or tallied up, and can be analysed mathematically, and sometimes using statistics. It is useful in measuring differences – such as differences in cancer screening rates in different ethnicities, and understanding the relationship between variables statistically, for example, the relationships between family wealth and attending university.

The basic premise is that if something cannot be measured using valid instruments and tools, we cannot know for certain that it exists. Therefore, quantitative research tends to ask quite narrow questions that are observable either with our own senses, or drawing on specialist tools, or scales. In the social sciences, there are many 'validated' instruments which are measurement tools that have been tested and deemed to appropriately measure what they are meant to, through which what is being studied, examined or observed can be recorded in a systematic and transparent way.

However, quantitative research is often less able to provide us with context for the reason why observed events occur. Society, as we have seen in this chapter is complex, nuanced and multilayered. Much of it we cannot test in the same way as we would in the natural sciences through quantifiable measurable categories and we often cannot control and isolate variables in the same way as we can in the natural sciences. However, quantitative research is still incredibly useful in determining patterns and the effects of interventions – for example helping us identify the demographic differences of those attending cancer screening. Quantitative methods, however, cannot help us understand much about *why* certain groups are less likely to attend cancer screening and what the reasons and factors behind their reduced uptake might be. To understand the latter, we often must directly interview people within these groups to understand their experiences and perceptions from their own perspective, and to learn how these experiences guide the decisions they make about accessing care.

Interpretivism (Qualitative Methods)

In the social sciences, qualitative research methods help us to understand people's experiences, the meanings they ascribe to these experiences, and how they make sense of the social world – in other words, it reaches the places that quantitative research cannot (Pope and Mays, 1995). Qualitative data is often, but not always, in the form of words, which are often obtained from interviews that researchers must interpret. As a result, qualitative research is more subjective in the sense that it reflects peoples' own unique and unstandardised views and experiences of the world around them. One of the challenges of qualitative research is that it is naturally less standardised compared to quantitative research in the way that data is collected and analysed. One researcher's interpretation of someone else's articulation of their experience may vary from researcher to researcher and will likely be influenced by their own perspective of whatever is being looked at, and therefore may be more prone to bias.

Historically seen as less scientific, qualitative research is now recognised as being incredibly important in helping us better understand social phenomena – that is, what is actually going on from the perspectives of those experiencing it.

The key premises of this research paradigm are:

a. to represent the studied population's own perspective and experience of the social world around them and

b. to represent this perspective in the context of the social world in which they are a part of – where they live and work.

Where questions such as how smoking impacts on life expectancy are typically answered using quantitative methods, qualitative research can help us understand the experiences of smokers; why they smoke, and why they find it difficult to quit. If we then use our knowledge to design interventions that might help people give up smoking, we can then use quantitative methods to measure how effective the intervention is in reducing rates of smoking, whilst qualitative methods can be used to understand how the intervention was experienced and factors affecting participation and compliance with that intervention.

Clinical Considerations

- Theories help us understand our social worlds and how social life impacts health and health outcomes.

- Well-known grand theories, some of which were developed hundreds of years ago, still have relevance to understanding health and illness today.
- Theories are not static and untouchable. They are subject to constant revision, as new information and understandings emerge.
- Quantitative and qualitative research approaches can be used to help us gain new understandings about our social world and its impact on health.
- Quantitative research can help us identify associations, or areas of need, as well as the effectiveness of interventions in addressing these.
- Qualitative research can help us understand people's experiences and perspectives helping us better understand how health is experienced and how people can be better supported.

Conclusion

In this chapter, you have been introduced to concepts, theories, and paradigms. We have discussed how theory and research are used to generate a better understanding of our social world and how it relates to health and well-being. The chapter has provided an overview of the different levels of theory and how these relate to our understanding of the social world and how knowledge about it is gained. It has introduced you to three prominent grand theories and highlighted where these are useful to generating understanding about our social world and in particular health, and where they may be more limited. Finally, this chapter highlighted two broad research paradigms that we can use alongside theory, to help us consolidate and develop our understandings of how the social world works.

References

Allan, K. 2006. *Contemporary Social and Sociological Theory: Visualising Social Worlds*, Pine Forge Press.

Allen, C., Vassilev, I., Kennedy, A. & Rogers, A. 2020. The work and relatedness of ties mediated online in supporting long-term condition self-management. *Sociology of Health & Illness*, 42, 579–595.

Baert, P. & Da Silva, F. 2010. *Social Theory in the Twentieth Century and Beyond*, Polity.

Bambra, C., Gibson, M., Sowden, A., Wright, K., Whitehead, M. & Petticrew, M. 2010. Tackling the wider social determinants of health and health inequalities: evidence from systematic reviews. *Journal of Epidemiology and Community Health*, 64, 284.

Bandura, A. 2001. Social cognitive theory: An agentic perspective. *Annual Review of Psychology*, 52, 1–26.

Barry, A. & Yuill, C. 2022. *Understanding the Sociology of Health*, London: Sage.

Belgrave, L. L. & Charmaz, K. 2015. *The Palgrave Handbook of Social Theory in Health*, Illness and Medicine: Palgrave Handbooks.

Boudon, R. 1991. What middle-range theories are. *Contemporary Sociology*, 20, 519–522.

Bracher, M., Stewart, S., Reidy, C., Allen, C., Townsend, K. & Brindle, L. 2020. Partner involvement in treatment-related decision making in triadic clinical consultations – A systematic review of qualitative and quantitative studies. *Patient Education and Counseling*, 103, 245–253.

Brodie, R. J., Saren, M. & Pels, J. 2011. Theorizing about the service dominant logic: the bridging role of middle range theory. *Marketing Theory*, 11, 75–91.

Burbank, P. M. & Martins, D. C. 2010. Symbolic interactionism and critical perspective: divergent or synergistic? *Nursing Philosophy*, 11, 25–41.

Carter, M. J. & Fuller, C. 2016. Symbols, meaning, and action: the past, present, and future of symbolic interactionism. *Current Sociology*, 64, 931–961.

Cersosimo, G. 2024. Medicine, health, and illness. *In: The Oxford Handbook of Symbolic Interactionism*, Oxford University Press.

Cheshire, A., Ridge, D., Clark, L. V. & White, P. D. 2021. Sick of the sick role: narratives of what "Recovery" means to people With CFS/ME. *Qualitative Health Research*, 31, 298–308.

Chijioke, O. C., Ikechukwu, A. & Aloysius, A. 2020. Understanding theory in social science research: public administration in perspective. *Teaching Public Administration*, 39, 156–174.

Clark, T., Foster, L., Sloan, L. & Bryman, A. 2021. *Social Research Methods*, Oxford University Press.

Collyer, F. 2015. Karl Marx and Friedreich Engels: Capitalism, health and the healthcare industry. *In: The Palgrave Handbook of Social Theory in Health, Illness and Medicine*, Palgrave Macmillan.

Damschroder, L. J. 2020. Clarity out of chaos: use of theory in implementation research. *Psychiatry Research*, 283, 112461.

Das, R. J. 2022. Capital, capitalism and health. *Critical Sociology*, 49, 395–414.

Davey, F., Mcgowan, V., Birch, J., Kuhn, I., Lahiri, A., Gkiouleka, A., Arora, A., Sowden, S., Bambra, C. & Ford, J. 2022. Levelling up health: a practical, evidence-based framework for reducing health inequalities. *Public Health in Practice*, 4, 100322.

Davidoff, F., Dixon-Woods, M., Leviton, L. & Michie, S. 2015. Demystifying theory and its use in improvement. *BMJ Quality and Safety*, 24, 228–238.

Dillon, M. 2020. *Introduction to sociological theory: Theorists, concepts, and their applicability to the twenty-first century*, John Wiley & Sons.

Funnell, S. C. & Rogers, P. J. 2011. *Purposeful program theory: Effective use of theories of change and logic models*, John Wiley & Sons.

Gage, N. L. 1989. The paradigm wars and their aftermath: a "Historical" sketch of research on teaching since 1989. *Educational Researcher*, 18, 4–10.

Giddens, A. 1973. *Capitalism and Modern Social Theory*, Cambridge University Press.

Goffman, E. 1959. *The Presentation of Self in Everyday Life*, Bantam Doubleday Dell Publishing Group.

Green, J. & Thorogood, N. 2014. *Qualitative methods for health research*, Sage publications.

Greenhalgh, J. & Manzano, A. 2022. Understanding 'context' in realist evaluation and synthesis. *International Journal of Social Research Methodology*, 25, 583–595.

Hallowell, N., Heiniger, L., Baylock, B., Price, M., Butow, P. & KConFab Psychosocial Group on behalf of the KConFab Investigators 2015. Rehabilitating the sick role: the experiences of high-risk women who undergo risk reducing breast surgery. *Health Sociology Review*, 24, 186–198.

Hefler, M. & Carter, S. M. 2019. Smoking to fit a stigmatised identity? A qualitative study of marginalised young people in Australia. *Health*, 23, 306–324.

Kislov, R., Pope, C., Martin, G. P. & Wilson, P. M. 2019. Harnessing the power of theorising in implementation science. *Implementation Science*, 14, 103.

Levine, D. N. 1995. The Organism Metaphor in Sociology. *Social Research*, 62, 239–265.

Lin, N. 2002. *Social capital: A theory of social structure and action*, Cambridge University Press.

Link, B. G., Wells, J., Phelan, J. C. & Yang, L. 2015. Understanding the importance of "symbolic interaction stigma": how expectations about the reactions of others adds to the burden of mental illness stigma. *Psychiatric Rehabilitation Journal*, 38, 117–124.

Mark, M. M. 2023. Surfacing, as well as testing, "elliptical assumptions" in a theory of change: Principled discovery. *Evaluation and Program Planning*, 97, 102266.

Merton, R. 1968. *Social Theory and Social Structure*, Simon and Schuster.

Mills, T., Lawton, R. & Sheard, L. 2019. Advancing complexity science in healthcare research: the logic of logic models. *BMC Medical Research Methodology*, 19, 1–11.

Monaghan, L. & Gabe, J. 2022. *Key Concepts in Medical Sociology*, Sage.

Murray, E., Treweek, S., Pope, C., Macfarlane, A., Ballini, L., Dowrick, C., Finch, T., Kennedy, A., Mair, F. & O'donnell, C., Ong, B. N., Rapley, T., Rogers, A. & May, C. 2010. Normalisation process theory: a framework for developing, evaluating and implementing complex interventions. *BMC Medicine*, 8, 63.

Parsons, T. 1951. *The Social System England*, Routledge.

Pawson, R. 2013. The Science of Evaluation: A Realist Manifesto.

Pawson, R., Greenhalgh, T., Harvey, G. & Walshe, K. 2005. Realist review-a new method of systematic review designed for complex policy interventions. *Journal of Health Services Research & Policy*, 10, 21–34.

Pawson, R. & Sridharan, S. 2009. 43Theory-driven evaluation of public health programmes. *In:* Killoran, A. & Kelly, M. P. (eds.) *Evidence-Based Public Health: Effectiveness and Efficiency*, Oxford University Press.

Pawson, R. & Tilly, N. 1997. *Realist Evaluation*, London: Sage.

Pettigrew, P. 1997. *How to Think Like a Social Scientist*, Pearson.

Pope, C. & Mays, N. 1995. Qualitative Research: reaching the parts other methods cannot reach: an introduction to qualitative methods in health and health services research. *BMJ*, 311, 42–45.

Reeves, S., Albert, M., Kuper, A. & Hodges, B. D. 2008. Why use theories in qualitative research? *BMJ*, 337, a949.

Rier, D. 2000. The missing voice of the critically ill: a medical sociologist's first-person account. *Sociology of Health & Illness*, 22, 68–93.

Rogers, E. M., Singhal, A. & Quinlan, M. M. 2014. Diffusion of innovations. *In: An Integrated Approach to Communication Theory and Research*, Routledge.

Sawatzky, R., Kwon, J. Y., Barclay, R., Chauhan, C., Frank, L., Van Den Hout, W. B., Nielsen, L. K., Nolte, S. & Sprangers, M. A. G. 2021. Implications of response shift for micro-, meso-, and macro-level healthcare decision-making using results of patient-reported outcome measures. *Quality of Life Research*, 30, 3343–3357.

Schutt, R. K. 2018. *Investigating the Social World: The Process and Practice of Research*, Sage publications.

Shearn, K., Allmark, P., Piercy, H. & Hirst, J. 2017. Building realist program theory for large complex and messy interventions. *International Journal of Qualitative Methods*, 16, 1609406917741796.

Skivington, K., Matthews, L., Simpson, S. A., Craig, P., Baird, J., Blazeby, J. M., Boyd, K. A., Craig, N., French, D. P. & Mcintosh, E. 2021. A new framework for developing and evaluating complex interventions: update of Medical Research Council guidance. *BMJ*, 374.

Skjælaaen, Ø. 2016. How to be a good alcoholic. *Symbolic Interaction*, 39, 252–267.

Varul, M. Z. 2010. Talcott Parsons, the sick role and chronic illness. *Body & Society*, 16, 72–94.

Vassilev, I., Rogers, A., Todorova, E., Kennedy, A. & Roukova, P. 2017. The articulation of neoliberalism: narratives of experience of chronic illness management in Bulgaria and the UK. *Sociology of Health & Illness*, 39, 349–364.

Whittle, E. L., Fisher, K. R., Reppermund, S., Lenroot, R. & Trollor, J. 2018. Barriers and enablers to accessing mental health services for people with intellectual disability: a scoping review. *Journal of Mental Health Research in Intellectual Disabilities*, 11, 69–102.

Willis, E. 2015. *In:* Collyer, F. (ed.) *Talcott Parsons: His legacy and the sociology of health and illness*, Palgrave Macmillan.

Willis, K., Daly, J., Kealy, M., Small, R., Koutroulis, G., Green, J., Gibbs, L. & Thomas, S. 2007. The essential role of social theory in qualitative public health research. *Australian and New Zealand Journal of Public Health*, 31, 438–443.

CHAPTER 3

What Is Health and Disease Why Do Definitions and Classifications of It Matter?

Chris Allen

School of Health Sciences, University of Southampton, Southampton, UK

Introduction

How health is seen and understood matters. As a social construct, health has been defined in several ways, and its meaning changes over time in line with a society's values, norms and culture. In this chapter, we will explore why. As healthcare professionals, you are clearly interested in health. Whether that is promoting health, preventing disease or providing care to someone who has become acutely or chronically unwell. Health is the central feature of your role and your work; what is prioritised and what is not. Definitions of health have relevance to how your role interacts with individuals and with society; what is seen and treated as a disease, and what is not, and why this is relevant to the healthcare and support that people have available to them, as well as how appropriate (or not) this care is. Definitions of disease also influence how reactive or proactive healthcare is.

In this chapter, you will have the opportunity to consider the most prominent lenses through which health is considered, including the medical (deficit model), and the bio-psychosocial model. We will also introduce you to salutogensis, and more recent positive health concepts, such as capabilities-based approaches, that seek to promote health and support people to live well. You will also have the opportunity to consider the different ways physical and mental health, as well as impairments, have come to be classified, such as through the World Health Organization's International Classification of Disease (ICD), the International Classification of Functioning, Disability and Health (ICF) and the Diagnostic and Statistical Manual of Mental Disorders (DSM). Such classification systems highlight that what is, and what is not considered a disease is socially constructed and subject to change over time, in response to changes in societies concern with different issues, and increased medical knowledge. However, there can also be concern that aspects of everyday life can inappropriately be moved into the domain of medicine, through medicalisation; another concept explored in this chapter. Finally, we explore the case of medically contested conditions, where people struggle to have their experiences seen, alongside the challenges of proving poor health, and the impact this might have on someone's access to support.

LEARNING OUTCOMES

By the end of this chapter, you will be able to:

- Compare and understand the different definitions of health and how they shape our understanding of health and disease in populations.
- Recognise how these various definitions influence what is prioritised and which aspects of social life fall within the remit of health and care.
- Recognise the various disease classification systems that are commonly used and their relevance to the classification and treatment of disease.
- Understand the relevance of different disease thresholds and how changes in these impact who is and who is not seen as being unwell and needing care.
- Understand the various tensions that can emerge through such classification systems and debates.

Social Sciences for Healthcare Professionals, First Edition. Edited by Chris Allen.
© 2026 John Wiley & Sons Ltd. Published 2026 by John Wiley & Sons Ltd.

What Is Health and Well-Being?

> ## Key Terms and Definitions
>
> **Biomedical model:**   Health is purely the absence of a disease. If you do not have a disease, you are healthy. When you become unwell, it is the role of healthcare to identify the cause and address this to return you to health.
>
> **Biopsychosocial model:**   Sees health as the product of biological, psychological and social factors.
>
> **Illness:**   Something that may give someone unwelcome symptoms and makes people feel unwell.
>
> **Disease:**   Something that is abnormal in either the structure or the function of a part of the human body that may make someone feel unwell.
>
> **Well-being:**   Generally being satisfied with life, having more positive affect (such as happiness) than negative affect (such as sadness) and having a sense of purpose and meaning.
>
> **Sign:**   This is something that can be observed by others, either through a physical assessment or some other type of diagnostic test, for example, a blood test.
>
> **Symptom:**   A symptom is something that people themselves experience, for example, pain.
>
> **Medicalisation:**   This is a process that involves behaviours, feelings and other human experiences that were not previously within the scope of medicine, falling within that remit.
>
> **Overdiagnosis:**   The diagnosis of a disease based on an identified abnormality that is unlikely to cause someone any issues during their anticipated life course.

In approaching this chapter, we must first start with some important considerations about what health is. Over many years, there have been several efforts to neatly define health. Even now, physical and mental health are defined in several ways (Alejandro and Laura, 2008, Laurie et al., 2015, Leonardi, 2018, Schramme, 2023, van Druten et al., 2022). Definitions of health and classifications of disease are quite significant, as they fundamentally shape how health and disease are thought about across macro and micro levels of society, and this has implications for health policy, healthcare services and frontline clinical practice and care. As we explored in the previous chapter, health is a social construct. Our social world has a significant role in shaping what is, and what is not considered a 'disease', as well as shaping how we respond to issues that may fall on either side of the various definitions relating to health, illness and disease. Because of this, definitions can have implications for the boundaries that are set around who

gets care, and who does not, how much government support someone might be entitled to; as well as how people think about their own health and how well they are; and even who is responsible for it.

Considerations around what defines health and disease are not new. But to avoid a deep dive into the full history of our human understanding of health and illness, we start with how our understanding of health was constructed in the 19th and early 20th centuries. At this time, health was largely seen as relating to the absence of a specific disease. No disease, you were deemed healthy (Larson, 1999, Willis and Elmer, 2011). This way of thinking about health suggests that we should think about the body as though it were a machine. Aspects of our bodies can break, and when they do, we should attempt to fix these through, for example, medicine or other therapeutic interventions (Larson, 1999, Willis and Elmer, 2011). There is little mention of addressing the underlying causes in this definition, or about helping people achieve what they want to achieve. Under such a definition, health only becomes relevant where there is a clear identifiable cause for someone's suffering or issue that we can address. Such a definition is narrow, missing the social, cultural and psychological domains of health, that we now know to be most important (Bambra et al., 2010, Bambra, 2022, Davey et al., 2022, Holt-Lunstad et al., 2015, Marmot et al., 2008, Marmot et al., 2020). Because a clear identifiable cause for someone's state is required (i.e. a sign – something that can be seen or detected), this view of health also misses those suffering from illnesses such as Myalgic Encephalomyelitis (ME), Chronic Fatigue Syndrome (CFS) and Fibromyalgia, where there is currently no identifiable cause (Geraghty and Esmail, 2016, Wessely et al., 1999), but very real symptoms (something that is experienced), and may well have an underlying cause that is just not yet known. This approach to health is known as the medical model, which has largely dominated healthcare delivery in western developed nations, and currently includes mental health as well as physical health, through the field of psychiatry.

Shifting Perspectives on Health

In 1948, in the ashes and embers of the Second World War, there was a relatively significant shift in thinking about health, which occurred through the United Nations (UN) ratification of the World Health Organization[1] (WHO) (Alejandro and Laura, 2008). In this year, WHO defined health as: 'a state of complete physical, mental and social well-being and not merely the absence of disease or infirmity' (p. 100). The inclusion of mental and social health and well-being was at the time radical but has since gone someway to changing how people think about health and what

---

[1] The WHO is an agency of the United Nations and is governed by the World Health Assembly which has a specific responsibility toward global public health.

exactly it entails (Schramme, 2023). Health is not just about not having a disease, and this very broad definition makes most of what we experience relevant to health. However, it arguably makes health rather hard to achieve. After all, is it even possible for people to obtain 'complete' physical, mental and social well-being, especially now in the context of increasing life courses and increasing prevalence of chronic illnesses that require ongoing management for much of people's lives (Bury, 1982, Bury and Taylor, 2008, May et al., 2014, Salisbury, 2012, Taylor and Bury, 2007, Vassilev et al., 2011, Vassilev et al., 2014). In addition, the breadth of this definition, and its lack of precision, also makes it hard to measure health using it (Leonardi, 2018). Taken at face value, and particularly in the use of the term 'complete', this definition suggests most of us are unhealthy most of the time, especially where general well-being is concerned, as we all encounter negative events and experiences throughout the course of our lives that lead to negative affect (such as sadness) (Huber et al., 2011, Leonardi, 2018). With everything having the potential to fall under the domain of medicine as healthcare's dominant profession, as we will go on to explore, there have been concerns surrounding attempts to 'medicalise' what might otherwise be seen as normal human experiences and emotions such as grief, unhappiness, loneliness and ageing (Bandini, 2015, Busfield, 2017, Dowrick and Frances, 2013, Cacioppo and Cacioppo, 2015, Jovicic and McPherson, 2020, McLennan and Ulijaszek, 2018). When negative events and experiences happen, it would be unusual to not be upset by them, after all, this is a common and usual human response. What we generally need when these events and experiences happen is supportive personal networks (as we explore in Chapter 15), and ways to build our own personal resistance, rather than healthcare trying to make us *'better'*.

However, what academics such as Schramme (2023) argue was really implied by the definition, was that holistic health involves physical, mental and social health taken together (i.e. 'complete[2]'). As other academics such as Larsen (2021) have highlighted, the definition and its architects primarily sought to move understandings of health beyond medicine. In this context, medicine, which was reactive and generally addressed physical health issues alone, began to be concerned with other aspects of health, such as psychological and social, and importantly became more concerned with preventing ill health. In addition, the definition has been particularly impactful in highlighting health as a fundamental right, and one significant impact of seeing health in this way is that societies have a responsibility to address incomplete health (Schramme, 2023). Because the definition is broad, any number of issues where they have the potential to impact on an individuals' physical, psychological or social well-being should be addressed (Schramme, 2023). Essentially, this definition challenges societies to consider the broader determinants of health (covered in Chapter 8), and to achieve such an ambition, governments

alongside the other social institutions that shape people's living and working conditions, have to become involved in the health and well-being of populations (Alejandro and Laura, 2008, Larsen, 2021).

Health as a 'Resource'

Since the initial WHO definition, further definitions have followed, including in the Ottawa Charter, where health is highlighted as 'a resource for everyday life, not the objective of living' (WHO, 1986). Under this definition, health is a *capacity* or an *asset* that can help us live the lives that we value. The definition further included that: 'health is a positive concept, emphasizing social and personal resources, as well as physical capacities'; continuing to include both physical and mental health, whilst also emphasizing the importance of social and personal resources and individual capacities, which throughout this book, we will highlight the importance of.

This is where the definitions provided by the WHO are perhaps most useful.

Utopic and aspirational, yes, of course. But important in framing how societies should see and support health.

Such a view of health has reorientated societies away from seeing health solely through the lens of disease and pathology (as in the biomedical approach), towards a more holistic understanding of what makes (and keeps) us *well*, as well as emphasising the importance of this to all our daily lives.

Even now, there is no one accepted definition of health (Alejandro and Laura, 2008, Kontos, 2011, Laurie et al., 2015, Leonardi, 2018, Schramme, 2023). It is unlikely that any uniform definition will ever exist, after all, definitions need to be able to adequately capture a concept, and the concept of health is incredibly complex and difficult to capture precisely.

The Biopsychosocial Model

Whilst as we will show, there are different perspectives on health, definitions tend to fall into two categories. These are the biomedical model (outlined above) and the more holistic biopsychosocial model, which emerged largely in response to concerns, particularly from American Psychiatrist George Engel (1913–1999), around seeing health through the lens of biomedicine alone (Engel, 1977, Wade and Halligan, 2017). Whilst not intending to replace the biomedical model entirely, Engels argued that it did not encourage consideration of the other aspects of health highlighted as being important in more holistic definitions of illness, such as those provided by the WHO. In contrast to the medical model, this way of thinking about health encourages us to think about illness (e.g. where someone feels unwell) where there is no identifiable cause or something that can be detected – which is common, especially in the context of mental ill health (Rogers and Pilgrim, 2021). The

[2] For example, you can have a 'complete' house, without having the 'perfect' house, as long as all of the constituent parts are there – in the case of health, this is physical, mental, and social well-being.

biopsychosocial model is useful in considering the broader context of health and its many and varied influences.

Let's consider this in the context of Chronic Obstructive Pulmonary Disease (COPD). In the case of COPD, biomedical, psychological and social factors are interrelated. Our knowledge and understanding of COPD highlights that it is an obstructive lung disease (Chapman et al., 2021). It is a *'disease'* because it is characterised by detectable altered changes to a person's physiology. These bodily changes make it harder for those with the condition to breathe, especially on exertion, due to either chronic inflammation of the person's airways or damage to their alveoli (the tiny air sacs in a person's lungs) (Chapman et al., 2021). The impact – poorer gaseous exchange, leading to breathlessness, especially on exertion. All these biomedical changes are detectable[3] (but only because we have the science to do so) – but they cannot necessarily be reversed, as is the case with chronic illness more generally.

Psychosocial factors are also heavily involved in both the genesis and later the management of COPD, including the steps taken to prevent the condition from getting worse (such as smoking cessation) and following recommended interventions such as pulmonary rehabilitation and broader self-management (Gardiner and Singh, 2022, Kock et al., 2022, Rogers and Pilgrim, 2024). Those in lower socio-economic groups are at an increased risk of COPD, in part due to increased engagement in smoking tobacco, a trend that is likely to continue (Song et al., 2021), and continued smoking following a COPD diagnosis is associated with particularly poor health outcomes (Tashkin, 2021). Such a behaviour, as we will explore later in this book is related to an individual's own psychology (personality, emotions, coping strategies), their personal characteristics and existing health, their social networks and their broader living and working conditions (Christakis and Fowler, 2008, Joyner et al., 2018, Kock et al., 2022, Pearce et al., 2016). If we adopted a purely medical model, we would overlook much of what is making someone unwell – only ever acting reactively as a result. We can provide medicines to alleviate symptoms (e.g. inhalers that may help with breathlessness) and in part manage the condition, but without consideration of the broader system, medical intervention can only ever be minimally effective and will likely not meet people's holistic needs either.

Salutogenesis and Positive Health

As we have shown, the WHO definitions, particularly that set out in the Ottawa Charter (1986), clearly incorporate positive health states; and further definitions of 'positive health' have increased in prominence (Seligman, 2008), including salutogenesis, and the capabilities approach, as well as an increased focus on personal well-being. These generally differ from deficit approaches, as they mostly focus on whether people have the resources and opportunities to live in the way that they want to, and that people can live valued lives, even where deficit models might suggest that they are 'unwell'.

Salutogenesis

Salutogenesis can be considered as an 'umbrella term' that draws together many different aspects of 'positive health' such as quality of life and general well-being, and resistance to challenging life events and experiences (Idan et al., 2017). Where the biomedical model might be seen as a deficit model, salutogenesis involves considering the origins of *health*, rather than considering the origins of *disease* through its 'ease-dis-ease continuum' and its fundamental question: 'how can this person be helped to move toward greater health?' (Antonovsky, 1979, Antonovsky, 1996, Antonovsky and Sagy, 2022). Essentially, what do we want to create in terms of health and human potential? This is a fundamental shift away from seeing health through the lens of disease and something that must be 'fixed' (being reactive), towards creating health (being proactive) (Becker et al., 2010, Idan et al., 2017, Mittelmark et al., 2022).

It is generally recognised that some people cope better than others when confronted with the same challenging situations and even the same underlying pathology and disease (Idan et al., 2017, Mittelmark et al., 2022). As we will go onto unpack later in this book, this is because people likely have very different (inequitable) health 'reserves'. Salutogensis emphasises the importance of these reserves and considers how these can be improved in individuals and populations to move people towards greater health. A key feature of the salutogenic approach is the emphasised importance of a 'sense of coherence', which is typically gained through 'general resistance resources', essentially, what might also be seen as various forms of capital, that can be protective, such as increased knowledge and resources (Bauer et al., 2019, Idan et al., 2017, Mittelmark et al., 2017, Mittelmark et al., 2022). Having a high sense of coherence has been shown to be protective in a number of studies (Boeckxstaens et al., 2016, Drageset et al., 2008) and as we will explore in later chapters (specifically chapter 8), status and wealth in particular are highly related to health outcomes. In particular, salutogenesis has paved the way for asset-based models that look towards improving the health of individuals and populations through the identification of individual and community 'assets', and drawing on these to move individuals and populations towards greater health and well-being (Morgan, 2014, Tine Van et al., 2019).

Capability Approaches

The capabilities approach is another way of thinking about health and health priorities. It has become increasingly important in reorientating our focus on condition management towards supporting people to live well with a disease, which

---

[3] Of course, the thresholds for what detectable changes count as a specific disease are socially defined and as we will go on to explore, are themselves subject to revision in response to new understandings of diseases emerging.

has become increasingly important in the context of increasing chronic illness (Entwistle et al., 2018). Amartya Sens (1933–), who developed the approach, alongside other academics who have refined it, most notably Martha Nussbaum (1947–), are generally concerned with whether people have what they need to live a life that they value (Entwistle et al., 2018, Owens et al., 2022). People can have resources, for example money, but this is only useful if they can use these to do the things they want to be able to do and be the person who they want to be. Whilst there are slightly different flavours of the capabilities approach, all relate to the importance of valued 'doings' and 'beings' (Robeyns, 2016, Sen, 2014).

This has particular relevance to how we think about health and what the main priorities of health should be (Entwistle et al., 2018). People can have aids, such as assistance aids, but these are only seen as useful if they allow people to do the things they want to do and be the people they want to become (referred to as functionings) (Entwistle et al., 2018). Each of us has our own 'capability sets', these are the things that allow us to do the things we want to do or be the people we want to be (i.e. our functionings). This capability is influenced by several things, including our own personal characteristics, the resources (or commodities) that we have access to and our social environments (Entwistle et al., 2018). We can have lots of resources, but we might not be able to translate these resources into desired functionings. For example, a person may have access to a computer, but without having the necessary knowledge and skills, they might not be able to extract the kind of utility that they wish to from this resource (such as connecting with new people, getting an education or finding a job).

Functionings can relate to meeting basic needs (such as being safe, having access to secure housing and sanitation), but they can also relate to the fulfilment of more complex needs such as being happy (an increasingly studied phenomenon), and being free from embarrassment, shame or stigma. By adopting a capabilities approach, we can reorientate our focus away from simply correcting health issues when they emerge (which in the context of chronic illness, is generally not even possible), towards equipping people with the necessary tools that they need to live a life that they value, and helping them use these tools to be who they want to be, and do the things that they want to do, despite having a disease or impairment (Entwistle et al., 2018).

So How Should Health Be Seen and Understood?

Health is a complex concept and is itself a product of cultural and social norms. Because these are different and change over time, even within the same country (e.g. the biomedical model and bio-psychosocial models co-exist in western industrialised societies, have done so for some time and will likely continue too), there is a lack of consensus as to what health is, and no unifying definition currently exists. Health concepts may well need to be context-specific drawing on what is seen as important to clinicians, as well as patients and service users themselves in different health settings and contexts (Leonardi, 2018). Several definitions of health help us to understand its different aspects, from prevention, through to detection and treatment, and help us to consider what our priorities should be, both in relation to reactive care and more proactive care (what is sometimes referred to as upstream prevention), that might prevent people from becoming unwell in the first place. In the ongoing management of those with chronic disease, broader conceptualisations of health are perhaps more useful, and it is essential that definitions here allow for the prioritisation of living well with limitations imposed by the condition and recognition that the condition cannot be cured. One definition of health cannot effectively cover the full range of macro–micro-level health considerations – but as Leonardi (2018) suggests that we should perhaps consider health as our ability to manage 'malaise' states such as being upset, or feeling sorrow, and well-being in response to events and our environment – essentially the capability to cope and to manage, and this is something that societies can work towards achieving for everyone.

Whilst there are many overarching definitions of health and these are often quite broad, we still need disease classification systems that allow us to identify conditions, and provide appropriate treatments to help alleviate suffering, when this is appropriate and wanted. To understand diseases so that we can prevent, detect and treat them, there needs to be some kind of valid classification system that pulls together a collection of abnormalities into distinct disease classifications. In this next section, we outline some of the most common ways that disease and impairment have been classified – most notably the ICD, the DSM and the ICF.

Disease Classifications

Being diagnosed with a health condition usually involves the following steps. An individual enters a healthcare facility (such as a hospital) with symptoms (things they experience and feel) and sometimes signs (things that others can see or detect, sometimes using various technologies) and they leave with a diagnosis (a label that attempts to capture their 'ill'). But the diagnosis that they leave with, is not always as clear cut as you might think. Classification of disease is powerful and is shaped by biomedical science, alongside social processes (Green et al., 2022, Wadmann, 2023). The process of diagnosis can involve tension and sensitivity. Having a name given to something that is being experienced can influence how people feel about themselves and also how others feel and respond towards them. It can also influence who gets what care, and who provides it, as well as influencing living and working conditions, and how people are treated in the labour market. In short, decisions about what is, and what is not a disease, are incredibly important and therefore often contentious.

Labels are powerful and being given a diagnosis can have positive and negative psychosocial and treatment-related consequences. The nature and extent of these consequences can relate to how well a person feels, how the condition was detected, and of course the condition itself (Sims et al., 2021). After all, being diagnosed with the common cold, is significantly less impactful than say, being diagnosed with a life-limiting, life-shortening and stigmatised condition. Thresholds for conditions are often not clear cut and defining thresholds should therefore involve careful consideration as to the potential benefits (access to treatment, access to support) and the potential harms that any diagnostic label might bring, to the individual and their families and to healthcare systems and society more generally (Sims et al., 2021). Bringing something within the realm of medicine, invariably involves costs and social impacts (in terms of treatments, time of work, etc.), and these need to be carefully balanced with any potential benefits.

The International Classification of Diseases (ICD)

The ICD is now in its 11th version (WHO, 2019), highlighting that what constitutes a disease can change over time in response to biomedical understandings and social responses to people's differences. It has become the main mechanism through which global comparisons can be made in relation to morbidity and mortality, and much of what is known about patterns of disease worldwide is known through the ICD (Harrison et al., 2021). However, the ICD is not without its criticisms. For example, the ICD has generally defined diseases as mutually exclusive, despite often considerable overlap and increasing prevalence of multi-morbidity (having more than one condition). This may be appropriate for some diseases, for example, where a specific pathogen causes a specific disease, but less appropriate for most chronic conditions, which often share similar underlying social determinants and often exist co-morbidly (Levine et al., 2014). There have also been tensions about what is and what is not included as a 'disease' within the ICD, as we will explore later in this chapter.

Classifying Mental Health and the DSM

Whilst our understanding of some of the causes of mental ill health and its presentations has improved, much of our knowledge remains incomplete, making classification arguably more challenging. Whilst social determinants are relevant to most health conditions, conditions such as cancers, COPD and ischemic heart disease can generally still be related to clear pathological pathways in ways that many mental health conditions cannot (Rogers and Pilgrim, 2021). For example, in the case of COPD, we can see that smoking causes irreversible damage to a person's lungs, which results in them experiencing breathlessness, alongside the other signs and symptoms of the disease. Most mental health disorders (as we explore in the following chapter) on the other hand generally lack a clearly discernible central cause, often arising from a mixture of inter-related biological, psychosocial, behavioural and cultural causes, and this makes classification challenging and at times contentious (Rogers and Pilgrim, 2021).

Mental health disorders are included in the ICD but are also classified in the American Psychiatric Association Diagnostic and Statistical DSM, now in its fifth iteration (DSM-5) (Clark et al., 2017). Classification within these is largely based on signs (what we can see – e.g. observable behaviours) and symptoms (what the person experiences – typically their thoughts and feelings) which can relate to several classifications, because in the context of mental ill health, these are rarely exclusive, and there is often considerable overlap in different presentations (Clark et al., 2017). The recent introduction of ICD-11 involved efforts to harmonise the classification of disorders between the two bodies – but there remain differences in the classification of conditions between the two – and some disorders are absent from the ICD and the DSM-5 (First et al., 2021).

International Classification of Functioning, Disability and Health (ICF)

The ICF, produced by the WHO (2001), is the main international standard for the classification of functioning and disability, and it provides a framework for measuring functioning and disability of individuals and of populations, largely within the framework of the biopsychosocial model of health and the social model of disability (explored in more depth in Chapter 11) which highlights that it is not people's impairments or differences that disable them, but is instead the unfair treatment and inaccessibility of society that results in their disability (Oliver, 2013). The dominance of both the medical model and the more recent social model of disability makes the classification of functioning and disability tricky, and at times contentious (Bickenback, 2020). However, alongside the demographic and epidemiological transitions, that we explore in Chapter 7, it is widely recognised that an increasing number of people will have impairments in most societies, and therefore, it is relevant to have a standardised way whereby epidemiological data on the levels of disability within a society can be adequately captured, and then used to guide decision-making about best ways to support individuals and societies (Bickenback, 2020). The ICF provides this and has been informed by the work of those living with impairments, activists, healthcare professionals and academics from across the social sciences (Bickenback, 2020). As with the social model of disability, and the definition of disability within the United Nations Convention on the Rights of Persons with Disabilities, the ICF sees disability as the interaction between a person's impairments (physical, mental, intellectual, sensory, etc.) and their environment (UN, 2007).

Medicalisation, Over Medicalisation and Overdiagnosis

Advances in our knowledge and understanding of human health and behaviour have resulted in more patterns of signs and symptoms being pulled together into formal disease classifications; with such conditions frequently falling under the domain of medicine, which has also gained increased knowledge in how to manage these. This is essentially the main lens through which healthcare professionals and the lay public have come to understand health and illness (Barry and Yuill, 2022, Conrad and Barker, 2010). Countless times, such advancements have allowed people to be diagnosed, and therefore treated. So, such advances are often hugely positive. Whole conditions (e.g. smallpox) have been eradicated almost entirely through such advances.

Many conditions do clearly require medical intervention, and many interventions have been shown to alleviate great suffering and increase the quality of life for many people. However, as we have highlighted, the WHO's broad definition of health has the potential to pull many aspects of individual and community life into the realms of medicine (Kaczmarek, 2019, Parens, 2013, Vogt et al., 2016), and therefore alongside such positives, are concerns that medicine (through medicalisation), and pharmaceuticals (through pharmaceuticalisation), have crept into aspects of our daily lives, where most would feel they do not belong, where they serve little benefit and where they may actually cause harm (Parens, 2013).

As a concept medicalisation emerged in the 1970s when medicine was perhaps at its most dominant, largely through Ivan Illich's highly influential book *Limits to medicine: medical nemesis* (Dew et al., 2016, Illich, 1975). Illich argued that medicine posed a threat to society through 'iatrogenesis', whereby a medical intervention is offered for a social or personal presentation that is unlikely to help and might even bring about harm. Concerns were also raised about medicine being used as a form of social control (Zola, 1972). Illich, alongside others, believed that issues such as childbirth, ageing and dying were fundamental human experiences, that did not require medical oversight and that medicines involvement might actually render people and societies less capable of dealing with what might otherwise be seen as natural and inevitable processes; simply part of being a human (Ballard and Elston, 2005, Clark, 2002).

There are countless examples of human behaviours, presentations and experiences being medicalised, for example, male pattern baldness (for which, you can have surgery – a hair transplant, and for which, you can now take finasteride, a drug traditionally used to treat prostate issues in men) (Gupta et al., 2022, Vañó-Galván et al., 2023), and obesity (for which you can also have surgery – liposuction, gastric bands, etc., and can also take medications such as liraglutide and semaglutide to curb hunger) (Arterburn et al., 2020, Pi-Sunyer et al., 2015, Wilding John et al., 2021). Or similarly, whilst less common, they can be demedicalised, for example, homosexuality, which was once criminalised (and continues to be in some countries), and appeared in several versions of the DSM and ICD, even as recently as 1992, as a pathologised condition deemed to require quite horrific 'treatments', such as chemical castration and aversion therapy (Dew et al., 2016, Drescher, 2015, Smith et al., 2004). Homosexuality was both decriminalised (in most western industrialised countries) and demedicalised through widescale political action and changing societal views around sexuality (Drescher, 2015). Suicide provides another example of how societal attitudes change, at one stage criminalised in the United Kingdom, then medicalised, shifting societies focus from sanctions to support, which is generally believed may lead to less overall suicide (as people may seek less lethal means, and be more open to, and more likely to be able to access support from their communities) (Lew et al., 2022, Tait and Carpenter, 2016). Medicalisation can also change how people see themselves and how others respond to them, including the extent to which they feel and receive stigma (a concept we explore later in this book) (Kvaale et al., 2013). As one example, alcohol use disorder (AUD) is now a recognised condition, and therefore those with the condition are seen as unwell and needing support; removing some of the negative moral evaluations they might have otherwise received from themselves and from others, prior to this (Conrad, 2013).

Decisions about what falls under the domain of medicine, and what does not, have wide-reaching impacts. These decisions influence who in society should respond (i.e. police, social worker, healthcare professional), and what the response should be (i.e. punishment, support, etc.). As social constructs, the boundary between a legitimate medical condition requiring treatment and a non-medicalised condition is far from clear cut, especially where there is a lack of a clear underlying disease process, or a limited ability to see one where it might exist (such as through limitations in science). The constant revision of what is vs what is not a medical issue suggests that medicalisation should be seen as a continuum; and one that reflects societies changing attitudes and values towards differences, alongside changes in our ability to detect abnormalities and understand their impact on health (Conrad and Barker, 2010, van Dijk et al., 2016).

Social science has provided many comprehensive critiques of medicalisation and pharmaceutalisation over the years and these have largely focused on the concern that through medicines dominance, the profession had been able to extend its relevance and remit into experiences that might otherwise be seen as 'normal', or even deviant, but not in such a way as should be a concern of medicine (Abraham, 2010). There are various ways medicalisation has been conceptualised, but they generally point towards 'mission creep' and making something the responsibility of medicine or expanding medicines remit into everyday life (van Dijk et al., 2020). Medicine in this context is seen as a 'quick fix' for normal albeit sometimes unpleasant or undesired issues, which expands the role of both medicine (through medicalisation) and its primary intervention, pharmaceuticals (in a process often referred to as pharmaceutisiation) and comes with a cost to those becoming patients,[4] and to the healthcare system and society more generally, because more people end up 'needing' and receiving treatment (Bell and Figert, 2012, Conrad et al., 2010).

Medicine's role in much of everyday life and health in particular is clearly important in shaping the societies in which we live (Rose, 2007). However, much of Illich's original arguments that we should be 'liberated' from medicine have not stood the test of time. As healthcare professionals, you would likely have some concerns if medicine was sidelined altogether – and this would set most societies back. There is after all no doubt that medicine has now alleviated a great deal of human suffering and has been the driving force for lots of human progress in relation to our understanding of health and disease, how we look after ourselves and the generally better living and working conditions much of humanity now enjoys (Rose, 2007). In the context of death and dying, which was one of Illich's initial concerns, medicine and healthcare are often essential in ensuring people are supported to have a comfortable and dignified death. Whilst this book necessarily emphasises the importance of the social and positive health approaches, we are careful not to do this at the expense of the biomedical approach, which has been successful in helping to identify, diagnose and treat life-limiting and life-changing conditions, bringing about increased longevity and improvements to population health that society as a whole has benefited from.

However, a key challenge that is examined throughout this book is that when issues are seen as being responsive to medicine, healthcare and systems have tended to focus on its management through medicine (i.e. reactionary) rather than seeking to understand and take action in response to the complex social, psychological and economic problems that *really* lead to increased risks and exposures, negative health behaviours and poorer health-related outcomes (i.e. preventative) (Leonardi, 2018).

Does Medicine Want to Be Dominant Through Medicalisation?

Probably not. There are likely different actors involved in medicalisation. For example, diagnosis of ADHD has expanded, but this has not occurred because of medicines wish for this condition to fall under its remit, but has instead arguably occurred through the voices of parents and teachers actively seeking diagnosis through the perceived deviance, disruption and

challenge presented by children in their care (Francis, 2012, Frigerio et al., 2013, Gray Brunton et al., 2014). As others have highlighted, the profession of medicine is generally not now the main driver for medicalisation, and the basic drivers are now often general market forces, and those seeking medical care for themselves (such as patient movements), or for those they care about (Barker, 2011, Conrad, 2005).

Medicalisation and Overdiagnosis

Diagnostic criteria can be expanded and often is. This usually happens through a greater understanding of the disease or disorder, alongside societies level of concern relating to these conditions (Hofmann, 2016, Kaczmarek, 2019). Movement of diagnostic thresholds can though lead to overdiagnosis, which is a related concept to medicalisation. It relates to the detection and treatment of harmless abnormalities and presentations that result in otherwise healthy people being diagnosed with a medical condition (Hofmann, 2016). Diagnostic advances and precision medicine have the potential to make overdiagnosis more common – with more decisions about which abnormalities are clinically important needing to be made (Vogt et al., 2019). Disease thresholds, as diagnostic criteria, are socially constructed (Conrad and Barker, 2010), and exactly where disease thresholds are set can be contentious, as it can turn people who are otherwise well into patients requiring treatment with all the associated burdens (to the patient, to the healthcare system and to society as a whole). As we discuss later in this book (in Chapters 12–14 specifically), prevention programmes are a cornerstone of public health and in the context of screening programmes, these invariably involve decisions about what abnormalities are and are not concerning. The thresholds for detectable changes are not static and can change as our knowledge changes; for example, the diagnostic threshold for gestational diabetes has recently changed (Sexton et al., 2018) and significant concerns have been raised about using different thresholds for different people, for example, in the context of race, such as how the estimated glomerular filtration rate is used to determine kidney function (Vyas et al., 2020). It is widely understood that high blood pressure is related to morbidity and mortality, but the exact thresholds through which someone should be treated medically, rather than through, for example, addressing the underlying causes, are socially produced (albeit, guided by epidemiological data), for example, a blood pressure of 139/75 in someone who is otherwise deemed low risk, might not hit a threshold for medication, but a blood pressure of 140/75, might. Relatively small increases and decreases in exactly where the threshold sits can result in increases or decreases in how many people are 'sick' and take medication for a given abnormality.

Lastly, whilst the extremes of Illich's concerns do not fit with our current healthcare focus, he did argue that laypeople should have increased input into how the disease is classified and treated (Tomes, 2007). In this regard – society and many healthcare systems have addressed Illich's concerns. The patient voice and recognition of their expertise have rightly

---

[4] Medicalisation can lead to people's health status changing overnight, even where there have been no discernable changes to themselves, or how they are presenting, in response to how diseases are classified.

become far more significant than they once were, especially in a research context, and in priority setting and health technology assessment (Castro et al., 2016, Gagnon et al., 2021, Steffensen et al., 2022). As we explore in Chapter 7, patients are being expected to increasingly self-manage and patients themselves are often now the drivers for medicalisation, because there is a recognition that diagnosis can legitimise suffering and allow access to needed support and resources. Doctor–patient interactions are increasingly being performed on a more even footing, in which patients, and their families (where appropriate), are embraced as partners in their care, rather than subordinate and passive recipients of medicine and its overreach.

Invisible Illness: Felt but Not Seen

Whilst medicalisation focusses on bringing normal human experiences into the realm of medicine, many struggle to have their symptoms recognised, or to be diagnosed with anything despite their suffering. For these people, the process of medicalisation can be important in having their troubling symptoms seen, validated and therefore treated (Dumit, 2006).

Gaslighting has been adopted as a critique of medicine relatively recently, including in the context of female reproductive health, and long covid (Au et al., 2022, Fetters, 2018, Sebring, 2021). Gaslighting refers to a form of manipulation that makes someone question whether what they are experiencing is 'real'. Long covid provides an interesting example, as it is not dissimilar to conditions that have been dismissed or contested in the past, for example, ME or CFS, but has become hard to ignore due to the large numbers of people suffering from it. Symptoms for those suffering include fatigue, general weakness, muscle aches and pains, brain fog, alongside more serious symptoms causing long-term physical and cognitive disability (Lopez-Leon et al., 2021, ONS, 2023, Ziauddeen et al., 2022). The impact of long covid on the day-to-day lives of those experiencing it is significant, with people reporting difficulties working, taking part in leisure activities, keeping up with household tasks and caring for themselves and those people they normally provide care to (Ziauddeen et al., 2022).

In the early stages of the pandemic, those suffering with symptoms of long covid were themselves highly influential in having it recognised as a specific medical condition requiring care and support (Callard and Perego, 2021, Turner et al., 2023). As with other medically contested conditions (i.e. conditions with symptoms experienced by those with it, but with no signs that others can see and where no test exists that allows us to 'detect' whether someone has it), those suffering with long covid, turned to the support of others with similar experiences to make their shared experiences visible, make sense of it and have their symptoms validated (Callard and Perego, 2021, Miyake and Martin, 2021, Rushforth et al., 2021, Turner et al., 2023). Like other medically contested conditions, those with long covid

have experienced a lack of recognition from the healthcare system (Au et al., 2022), through ignorance, and because their conditions do not fit well within the medical model, which demands an underlying detectable and treatable pathology.

Health, Disability and Personal Independence Payments

One final area of contention relating to the definition, and classification of disease and impairment relates to who gets what types of support, including financial support. Whose claim to welfare support is 'legitimate,' and whose is not? Concern as to whether people are 'deserving' of state support, and the perceived ease through which people are suggested to be able to access financial support that they might not in fact need is very visible in TV portrayals of benefit claimants in the media (e.g. in TV shows such as Benefits Street).

Yet proving need is often far from straightforward for applicants. This is particularly evident in the United Kingdom, and through the implementation of Personal Independence Payments (PIP) in 2013, which replaced the previous Disability Living Allowance, with a narrower eligibility criteria, excluding some with previous entitlement, and with a requirement for regular medical assessments (carried out by healthcare professionals)[5]. Research has demonstrated that the process of 'proving' entitlement, and therefore, proving a health issue, is highly stressful and is associated with worsening mental health and suicide (Barr et al., 2016, Ploetner et al., 2020, Roberts et al., 2022). We do not have the space to unpick the full range and diversity of criticisms directed towards the benefits system and towards PIP and its implementation, of which there are many, including those captured by the impactful 'I, Daniel Blake' (in which Daniel is deemed not fit to work, having had a heart attack, but deemed fit enough to not be entitled to health-related benefits). However, many of these do have specific relevance to some of the tensions that arise through the definitions and classifications that we have discussed in this chapter. For example, that the process of claiming is largely underpinned by a deficit (or biomedical) model, that health can be difficult to adequately capture, that assessments tend to be overly medicalised, that assessments tend to focus primarily on physical health as opposed to mental health, that even with the suggestion that eligibility can be objectively measured, that those with higher social and cultural capital can steer the process in way that increases their odds of success and that the process generally fails to account for peoples own experiences of health, or the resources (or lack of) that they have available to them.

---

[5] These assessments were contracted out to private companies, to assess potential claimants for this benefit, on behalf of the state.

Clinical Considerations

- How we define health can influence what the focus of health and healthcare is. This can include whether the focus is upstream prevention or downstream reactive treatments and interventions for conditions that people already have.

- Holistic definitions of health are important because they orientate healthcare and healthcare systems towards addressing the social determinants of health and towards upstream prevention.

- Disease categorisation and thresholds are socially produced. Whilst advances in science allow us to recognise potentially significant abnormalities that might lead to increased risk of morbidity and mortality, what is and what is not classified as a disease is subject to change over time, influencing what care people are able to access and who is and is not seen as being unwell.

- It can be hard to have some conditions recognised as a specific disease and this can have implications on how much support people are able to access.

Conclusion

In this chapter, various definitions of health have been provided, alongside some of the recent history attached to changes in how health is seen. Dominant models of health have been introduced, such as the medical model and the biopsychosocial model, alongside positive health approaches, such as salutogenesis, and other approaches that have led to health and care priorities being reconsidered. The main ways physical and mental health, as well as impairment, are classified, have also been introduced, alongside medicalisation and overdiagnosis, and the challenges some face in terms of proving 'ill health'. In a way, this chapter serves as one final introduction to the rest of this book, as understanding health, including broader definitions of health that see health as an asset, and not just merely the absence of disease, has resulted in the increased involvement of the social sciences in supporting the health of individuals and of whole populations.

References

Abraham, J. 2010. Pharmaceuticalization of society in context: theoretical, empirical and health dimensions. *Sociology*, 44, 603–622.

Alejandro, R. J. & Laura, O. G. 2008. How should health be defined? *BMJ*, 337, a2900.

Antonovsky, A. 1979. Health, stress, and coping. *New perspectives on mental and physical well-being*, 12–37.

Antonovsky, A. 1996. The salutogenic model as a theory to guide health promotion. *Health Promotion International*, 11, 11–18.

Antonovsky, A. & Sagy, S. 2022. Aaron Antonovsky (1923–1994): The Personal, Ideological, and Intellectual Genesis of Salutogenesis. *In:* Mittelmark, M. B., Bauer, G. F., Vaandrager, L., Pelikan, J. M., Sagy, S., Eriksson, M., Lindström, B. & Meier Magistretti, C. (eds.) *The Handbook of Salutogenesis*, Cham: Springer International Publishing.

Arterburn, D. E., Telem, D. A., Kushner, R. F. & Courcoulas, A. P. 2020. Benefits and risks of bariatric surgery in adults: a review. *JAMA*, 324, 879–887.

Au, L., Capotescu, C., Eyal, G. & Finestone, G. 2022. Long covid and medical gaslighting: dismissal, delayed diagnosis, and deferred treatment. *SSM - Qualitative Research in Health*, 2, 100167.

Ballard, K. & Elston, M. A. 2005. Medicalisation: a multi-dimensional concept. *Social Theory & Health*, 3, 228–241.

Bambra, C. 2022. Placing intersectional inequalities in health. *Health & Place*, 75, 102761.

Bambra, C., Gibson, M., Sowden, A., Wright, K., Whitehead, M. & Petticrew, M. 2010. Tackling the wider social determinants of health and health inequalities: evidence from systematic reviews. *Journal of Epidemiology and Community Health*, 64, 284.

Bandini, J. 2015. The Medicalization of Bereavement: (Ab)normal Grief in the DSM-5. *Death Studies*, 39, 347–352.

Barker, K. K. 2011. Listening to Lyrica: contested illnesses and pharmaceutical determinism. *Social Science & Medicine*, 73, 833–842.

Barr, B., Taylor-Robinson, D., Stuckler, D., Loopstra, R., Reeves, A. & Whitehead, M. 2016. 'First, do no harm': are disability assessments associated with adverse trends in mental health? A longitudinal ecological study. *Journal of Epidemiology and Community Health*, 70, 339–345.

Barry, A. & Yuill, C. 2022. *Understanding the Sociology of Health*, London: Sage.

Bauer, G. F., Roy, M., Bakibinga, P., Contu, P., Downe, S., Eriksson, M., Espnes, G. A., Jensen, B. B., Juvinya Canal, D., Lindström, B., Mana, A., Mittelmark, M. B., Morgan, A. R., Pelikan, J. M., Saboga-Nunes, L., Sagy, S., Shorey, S., Vaandrager, L. & Vinje, H. F. 2019. Future directions for the concept of salutogenesis: a position article. *Health Promotion International*, 35, 187–195.

Becker, C. M., Glascoff, M. A. & Felts, W. M. 2010. Salutogenesis 30 years later: where do we go from here? *International Electronic Journal of Health Education*, 13, 25–32.

Bell, S. E. & Figert, A. E. 2012. Medicalization and pharmaceuticalization at the intersections: looking backward, sideways and forward. *Social Science & Medicine*, 75, 775–783.

Bickenback, J. 2020. The ICF and its relationship to disability studies. *In:* Watson, N. & Vehmas, S. (eds.) *Routledge Handbook of disability Studies*, Routledge.

Boeckxstaens, P., Vaes, B., De Sutter, A., Aujoulat, I., Van Pottelbergh, G., Matheï, C. & Degryse, J.-M. 2016. A high sense of coherence as protection against adverse health outcomes in patients aged 80 years and older. *The Annals of Family Medicine*, 14, 337–343.

Bury, M. 1982. Chronic illness as biographical disruption. *Sociology of Health & Illness*, 4, 167–182.

Bury, M. & Taylor, D. 2008. Towards a theory of care transition: from medical dominance to managed consumerism. *Social Theory & Health*, 6, 201–219.

Busfield, J. 2017. The concept of medicalisation reassessed. *Sociology of Health & Illness*, 39, 759–774.

Cacioppo, S. & Cacioppo, J. T. 2015. Why may allopregnanolone help alleviate loneliness? *Medical Hypotheses*, 85, 947–952.

Callard, F. & Perego, E. 2021. How and why patients made Long Covid. *Social Science & Medicine*, 268, 113426.

Castro, E. M., Van Regenmortel, T., Vanhaecht, K., Sermeus, W. & Van Hecke, A. 2016. Patient empowerment, patient participation and patient-centeredness in hospital care: a concept analysis based on a literature review. *Patient Education and Counseling*, 99, 1923–1939.

Chapman, S. J., Robinson, G. V., Shrimanker, R., Turnbull, C. D. & Wrightson, J. M. 2021. *Oxford Handbook of Respiratory Medicine*, 4th Edition, Oxford University Press.

Christakis, N. A. & Fowler, J. H. 2008. The collective dynamics of smoking in a large social network. *New England Journal of Medicine*, 358, 2249–2258.

Clark, D. 2002. Between hope and acceptance: the medicalisation of dying. *BMJ*, 324, 905–907.

Clark, L. A., Cuthbert, B., Lewis-Fernández, R., Narrow, W. E. & Reed, G. M. 2017. Three approaches to understanding and classifying mental disorder: ICD-11, DSM-5, and the national institute of mental health's research domain criteria (RDoC). *Psychological Science in the Public Interest*, 18, 72–145.

Conrad, P. 2005. The shifting engines of medicalization. *Journal of Health and Social Behavior*, 46, 3–14.

Conrad, P. 2013. Medicalization: Changing contours, characteristics, and contexts. *In: Medical Sociology on the Move: New Directions in Theory*, Springer.

Conrad, P. & Barker, K. K. 2010. The social construction of illness: Key insights and policy implications. *Journal of Health and Social Behavior*, 51, S67–S79.

Conrad, P., Mackie, T. & Mehrotra, A. 2010. Estimating the costs of medicalization. *Social Science & Medicine*, 70, 1943–1947.

Davey, F., Mcgowan, V., Birch, J., Kuhn, I., Lahiri, A., Gkiouleka, A., Arora, A., Sowden, S., Bambra, C. & Ford, J. 2022. Levelling up health: a practical, evidence-based framework for reducing health inequalities. *Public Health in Practice*, 4, 100322.

Dew, K., Scott, A. & Kirkman, A. 2016. Medicalization and Contested Illnesses. *In:* Dew, K., Scott, A. & Kirkman, A. (eds.) *Social, Political and Cultural Dimensions of Health*, Cham: Springer International Publishing.

Dowrick, C. & Frances, A. 2013. Medicalising unhappiness: new classification of depression risks more patients being put on drug treatment from which they will not benefit. *BMJ*, 347.

Drageset, J., Nygaard, H. A., Eide, G. E., Bondevik, M., Nortvedt, M. W. & Natvig, G. K. 2008. Sense of coherence as a resource in relation to health-related quality of life among mentally intact nursing home residents – a questionnaire study. *Health and Quality of Life Outcomes*, 6, 1–9.

Drescher, J. 2015. Out of DSM: depathologizing homosexuality. *Behavioral Sciences (Basel)*, 5, 565–575.

Dumit, J. 2006. Illnesses you have to fight to get: facts as forces in uncertain, emergent illnesses. *Social Science & Medicine*, 62, 577–590.

Engel, G. L. 1977. The need for a new medical model: a challenge for biomedicine. *Science*, 196, 129–136.

Entwistle, V. A., Cribb, A. & Owens, J. 2018. Why health and social care support for people with long-term conditions should be oriented towards enabling them to live well. *Health Care Analysis*, 26, 48–65.

Fetters, A. 2018. *The doctor doesn't listen to her. But the media is starting to*. [Online]. The Atlantic Available: https://www.theatlantic.com/family/archive/2018/08/womens-health-care-gaslighting/567149/ [Accessed].

First, M. B., Gaebel, W., Maj, M., Stein, D. J., Kogan, C. S., Saunders, J. B., Poznyak, V. B., Gureje, O., Lewis-Fernández, R., Maercker, A., Brewin, C. R., Cloitre, M., Claudino, A., Pike, K. M., Baird, G., Skuse, D., Krueger, R. B., Briken, P., Burke, J. D., Lochman, J. E., Evans, S. C., Woods, D. W. & Reed, G. M. 2021. An organization- and category-level comparison of diagnostic requirements for mental disorders in ICD-11 and DSM-5. *World Psychiatry*, 20, 34–51.

Francis, A. 2012. Stigma in an era of medicalisation and anxious parenting: how proximity and culpability shape middle-class parents' experiences of disgrace. *Sociology of Health & Illness*, 34, 927–942.

Frigerio, A., Montali, L. & Fine, M. 2013. Attention deficit/hyperactivity disorder blame game: a study on the positioning of professionals, teachers and parents. *Health*, 17, 584–604.

Gagnon, M.-P., Dipankui, M. T., Poder, T. G., Payne-Gagnon, J., Mbemba, G. & Beretta, V. 2021. Patient and public involvement in health technology assessment: update of a systematic review of international experiences. *International Journal of Technology Assessment in Health Care*, 37, e36.

Gardiner, L. & Singh, S. 2022. Inequality in Pulmonary Rehabilitation - The challenges magnified by the COVID-19 pandemic. *Chronic Respiratory Disease*, 19, 14799731221104098.

Geraghty, K. J. & Esmail, A. 2016. Chronic fatigue syndrome: is the biopsychosocial model responsible for patient dissatisfaction and harm? *British Journal of General Practice*, 66, 437–438.

Gray Brunton, C., Mcvittie, C., Ellison, M. & Willock, J. 2014. Negotiating parental accountability in the face of uncertainty for attention-deficit hyperactivity disorder. *Qualitative Health Research*, 24, 242–253.

Green, S., Carusi, A. & Hoeyer, K. 2022. Plastic diagnostics: the remaking of disease and evidence in personalized medicine. *Social Science & Medicine*, 304, 112318.

Gupta, A. K., Venkataraman, M., Talukder, M. & Bamimore, M. A. 2022. Finasteride for hair loss: a review. *Journal of Dermatological Treatment*, 33, 1938–1946.

Harrison, J. E., Weber, S., Jakob, R. & Chute, C. G. 2021. ICD-11: an international classification of diseases for the twenty-first century. *BMC Medical Informatics and Decision Making*, 21, 206.

Hofmann, B. 2016. Medicalization and overdiagnosis: different but alike. *Medicine, Health Care, and Philosophy*, 19, 253–264.

Holt-Lunstad, J., Smith, T. B., Baker, M., Harris, T. & Stephenson, D. 2015. Loneliness and social isolation as risk factors for mortality: a meta-analytic review. *Perspectives on Psychological Science*, 10, 227–237.

Huber, M., Knottnerus, J. A., Green, L., Van Der Horst, H., Jadad, A. R., Kromhout, D., Leonard, B., Lorig, K., Loureiro, M. I. & Van Der Meer, J. W. 2011. How should we define health? *BMJ*, 343.

Idan, O., Eriksson, M. & Al-Yagon, M. 2017. The salutogenic model: the role of generalized resistance resources. The handbook of salutogenesis, Cham (CH): Springer; 57–69.

Illich, I. 1975. *Medical Nemesis: The Expropriation Of Health*, Australian Broadcasting Commission, Science Programmes Unit Sydney.

Jovicic, A. & Mcpherson, S. 2020. To support and not to cure: general practitioner management of loneliness. *Health & Social Care in the Community*, 28, 376–384.

Joyner, C., Rhodes, R. E. & Loprinzi, P. D. 2018. The prospective association between the five factor personality model with health behaviors and health behavior clusters. *Europe's Journal of Psychology*, 14, 880–896.

Kaczmarek, E. 2019. How to distinguish medicalization from over-medicalization? *Medicine, Health Care, and Philosophy*, 22, 119–128.

Kock, L., Brown, J., Shahab, L., Tattan-Birch, H., Moore, G. & Cox, S. 2022. Inequalities in smoking and quitting-related outcomes among adults with and without children in the household 2013-2019: a population survey in England. *Nicotine & Tobacco Research*, 24, 690–698.

Kontos, N. 2011. Perspective: biomedicine--menace or straw man? Reexamining the biopsychosocial argument. *Academic Medicine*, 86, 509–515.

Kvaale, E. P., Haslam, N. & Gottdiener, W. H. 2013. The 'side effects' of medicalization: a meta-analytic review of how biogenetic explanations affect stigma. *Clinical Psychology Review*, 33, 782–794.

Larsen, L. T. 2021. Not merely the absence of disease: a genealogy of the WHO's positive health definition. *History of the Human Sciences*, 35, 111–131.

Larson, J. S. 1999. The conceptualization of health. *Medical Care Research and Review*, 56, 123–136.

Laurie, A. M., Skye, P. B., Karen, R., Zachary, D., Cheolsoon, L., Emma, W. & Kwame, M. 2015. What is mental health? Evidence towards a new definition from a mixed methods multidisciplinary international survey. *BMJ Open*, 5, e007079.

Leonardi, F. 2018. The definition of health: towards new perspectives. *International Journal of Health Services*, 48, 735–748.

Levine, R. S., Kilbourne, B. A., Rust, G. S., Langston, M. A., Husaini, B. A., Gittner, L. S., Sanderson, M. & Hennekens, C. H. 2014. Social determinants and the classification of disease: descriptive epidemiology of selected socially mediated disease constellations. *PLoS One*, 9, e110271.

Lew, B., Lester, D., Mustapha, F. I., Yip, P., Chen, Y.-Y., Panirselvam, R. R., Hassan, A. S., In, S., Chan, L. F., Ibrahim, N., Chan, C. M. H. & Siau, C. S. 2022. Decriminalizing suicide attempt in the 21st century: an examination of suicide rates in countries that penalize suicide, a critical review. *BMC Psychiatry*, 22, 424.

Lopez-Leon, S., Wegman-Ostrosky, T., Perelman, C., Sepulveda, R., Rebolledo, P. A., Cuapio, A. & Villapol, S. 2021. More than 50 long-term effects of COVID-19: a systematic review and meta-analysis. *Scientific Reports*, 11, 16144.

Marmot, M., Allen, J., Boyce, T., Goldblatt, P. & Morrison, J. 2020. *Health Equity in England: The Marmot Review 10 Years On*. The Health Foundation Available: https://www.health.org.uk/publications/reports/the-marmot-review-10-years-on [Accessed].

Marmot, M., Friel, S., Bell, R., Houweling, T. A. J. & Taylor, S. 2008. Closing the gap in a generation: health equity through action on the social determinants of health. *The Lancet*, 372, 1661–1669.

May, C. R., Eton, D. T., Boehmer, K., Gallacher, K., Hunt, K., Macdonald, S., Mair, F. S., May, C. M., Montori, V. M., Richardson, A., Rogers, A. E. & Shippee, N. 2014. Rethinking the patient: using Burden of Treatment Theory to understand the changing dynamics of illness. *BMC Health Services Research*, 14, 281.

Mclennan, A. K. & Ulijaszek, S. J. 2018. Beware the medicalisation of loneliness. *The Lancet*, 391, 1480.

Mittelmark, M. B., Bauer, G. F., Vaandrager, L., Pelikan, J. M., Sagy, S., Eriksson, M., Lindström, B. & Meier Magistretti, C. 2022. *The Handbook of Salutogenesis*, Cham (CH): Springer.

Mittelmark, M. B., Bull, T. & Bouwman, L. 2017. Emerging ideas relevant to the salutogenic model of health. The Handbook of Salutogenesis. Cham (CH): Springer, 45–56.

Miyake, E. & Martin, S. 2021. Long Covid: online patient narratives, public health communication and vaccine hesitancy. *Digital Health*, 7, 20552076211059649.

Morgan, A. 2014. *Revisiting the Asset Model: A Clarification of Ideas and Terms*, London, England: Sage Publications Sage UK.

Oliver, M. 2013. The social model of disability: thirty years on. *Disability & Society*, 28, 1024–1026.

ONS. 2023. *Prevalence of ongoing symptoms following coronavirus (COVID-19) infection in the UK*. Available: https://www.ons.gov.uk/peoplepopulationandcommunity/healthandsocialcare/conditionsanddiseases/bulletins/prevalenceofongoingsymptomsfollowingcoronaviruscovid19infectionintheuk/2february2023 [Accessed].

Owens, J., Entwistle, V. A., Craven, L. K. & Conradie, I. 2022. Understanding and investigating relationality in the capability approach. *Journal for the Theory of Social Behaviour*, 52, 86–104.

Parens, E. 2013. On good and bad forms of medicalization. *Bioethics*, 27, 28–35.

Pearce, J., Rind, E., Shortt, N., Tisch, C. & Mitchell, R. 2016. Tobacco retail environments and social inequalities in individual-level smoking and cessation among Scottish adults. *Nicotine & Tobacco Research*, 18, 138–146.

Pi-Sunyer, X., Astrup, A., Fujioka, K., Greenway, F., Halpern, A., Krempf, M., Lau David, C. W., Le Roux Carel, W., Violante Ortiz, R., Jensen Christine, B. & Wilding John, P. H. 2015. A randomized, controlled trial of 3.0 mg of Liraglutide in weight management. *New England Journal of Medicine*, 373, 11–22.

Ploetner, C., Telford, M., Brækkan, K., Mullen, K., Turnbull, S., Gumley, A. & Allan, S. 2020. Understanding and improving the experience of claiming social security for mental health problems in the west of Scotland: a participatory social welfare study. *Journal of Community Psychology*, 48, 675–692.

Roberts, H., Stuart, S. R., Allan, S. & Gumley, A. 2022. 'It's Like the Sword of Damocles' – A trauma-informed framework analysis of individuals' experiences of assessment for the personal independence payment benefit in the UK. *Journal of Social Policy*, 1–16.

Robeyns, I. 2016. Capabilitarianism. *Journal of Human Development and Capabilities*, 17, 397–414.

Rogers, A. & Pilgrim, D. 2021. *A Sociology of Mental Health and Illness*, 6th Edition, McGraw-Hill Education (UK).

Rogers, A. & Pilgrim, D. 2024. *Living with Health Inequalities*, Routledge.

Rose, N. 2007. Beyond medicalisation. *Lancet*, 369, 700–702.

Rushforth, A., Ladds, E., Wieringa, S., Taylor, S., Husain, L. & Greenhalgh, T. 2021. Long Covid – The illness narratives. *Social Science & Medicine*, 286, 114326.

Salisbury, C. 2012. Multimorbidity: redesigning health care for people who use it. *The Lancet*, 380, 7–9.

Schramme, T. 2023. Health as complete well-being: the WHO definition and beyond. *Public Health Ethics*, 16, 210–218.

Sebring, J. C. H. 2021. Towards a sociological understanding of medical gaslighting in western health care. *Sociology of Health & Illness*, 43, 1951–1964.

Seligman, M. E. 2008. Positive health. *Applied Psychology*, 57, 3–18.

Sen, A. 2014. Development as Freedom (1999). *In: The Globalization and development Reader: Perspectives on Development and Global Change*, 525.

Sexton, H., Heal, C., Banks, J. & Braniff, K. 2018. Impact of new diagnostic criteria for gestational diabetes. *Journal of Obstetrics and Gynaecology Research*, 44, 425–431.

Sims, R., Michaleff, Z. A., Glasziou, P. & Thomas, R. 2021. Consequences of a diagnostic label: a systematic scoping review and thematic framework. *Frontiers in Public Health*, 9, 725877.

Smith, G., Bartlett, A. & King, M. 2004. Treatments of homosexuality in Britain since the 1950s--an oral history: the experience of patients. *BMJ*, 328, 427.

Song, F., Elwell-Sutton, T., Naughton, F. & Gentry, S. 2021. Future smoking prevalence by socioeconomic status in England: a computational modelling study. *Tobacco Control*, 30, 380.

Steffensen, M. B., Matzen, C. L. & Wadmann, S. 2022. Patient participation in priority setting: co-existing participant roles. *Social Science & Medicine*, 294, 114713.

Tait, G. & Carpenter, B. 2016. The continuing implications of the 'crime' of suicide: a brief history of the present. *International Journal of Law in Context*, 12, 210–224.

Tashkin, D. P. 2021. Smoking cessation in COPD: confronting the challenge. *Internal and Emergency Medicine*, 16, 545–547.

Taylor, D. & Bury, M. 2007. Chronic illness, expert patients and care transition. *Sociology of Health & Illness*, 29, 27–45.

Tine Van, B., Nuwan Darshana, W., Antony, M. & Steven, M. 2019. Health assets in a global context: a systematic review of the literature. *BMJ Open*, 9, e023810.

Tomes, N. 2007. Patient empowerment and the dilemmas of late-modern medicalisation. *The Lancet*, 369, 698–700.

Turner, M., Beckwith, H., Spratt, T., Vallejos, E. P. & Coughlan, B. 2023. The #longcovid revolution: a reflexive thematic analysis. *Social Science & Medicine*, 333, 116130.

UN 2007. Convention on the Rights of Persons with Disabilities.

Van Dijk, W., Faber, M. J., Tanke, M. A., Jeurissen, P. P. & Westert, G. P. 2016. Medicalisation and overdiagnosis: what society does to medicine. *International Journal of Health Policy and Management*, 5, 619–622.

Van Dijk, W., Meinders, M. J., Tanke, M. A. C., Westert, G. P. & Jeurissen, P. P. T. 2020. Medicalization defined in empirical contexts - A scoping review. *International Journal of Health Policy and Management*, 9, 327–334.

Van Druten, V. P., Bartels, E. A., Van De Mheen, D., De Vries, E., Kerckhoffs, A. P. M. & Nahar-Van Venrooij, L. M. W. 2022. Concepts of health in different contexts: a scoping review. *BMC Health Services Research*, 22, 389.

Vañó-Galván, S., Bisanga, C. N., Bouhanna, P., Farjo, B., Gambino, V., Meyer-González, T. & Silyuk, T. 2023. An international expert consensus statement focusing on pre and post hair transplantation care. *Journal of Dermatological Treatment*, 34, 2232065.

Vassilev, I., Rogers, A., Kennedy, A. & Koetsenruijter, J. 2014. The influence of social networks on self-management support: a metasynthesis. *BMC Public Health*, 14, 719.

Vassilev, I., Rogers, A., Sanders, C., Kennedy, A., Blickem, C., Protheroe, J., Bower, P., Kirk, S., Chew-Graham, C. & Morris, R. 2011. Social networks, social capital and chronic illness self-management: a realist review. *Chronic Illness*, 7, 60–86.

Vogt, H., Green, S., Ekstrøm, C. T. & Brodersen, J. 2019. How precision medicine and screening with big data could increase overdiagnosis. *BMJ*, 366, l5270.

Vogt, H., Hofmann, B. & Getz, L. 2016. The new holism: P4 systems medicine and the medicalization of health and life itself. *Medicine, Health Care, and Philosophy*, 19, 307–323.

Vyas, D. A., Eisenstein, L. G. & Jones, D. S. 2020. *Hidden in plain sight—reconsidering the use of race correction in clinical algorithms*, Mass Medical Soc.

Wade, D. T. & Halligan, P. W. 2017. The biopsychosocial model of illness: a model whose time has come. *Clinical Rehabilitation*, 31, 995–1004.

Wadmann, S. 2023. Disease classification: a framework for analysis of contemporary developments in precision medicine. *SSM - Qualitative Research in Health*, 3, 100217.

Wessely, S., Nimnuan, C. & Sharpe, M. 1999. Functional somatic syndromes: one or many? *The Lancet*, 354, 936–939.

WHO. 1986. *Ottawa charter for health promotion* [Online]. World Health Organization Available: https://www.who.int/publications/i/item/WH-1987 [Accessed].

WHO. 2001. *International classification of functioning, disability and health* [Online]. World Health Organization. Available: https://iris.who.int/handle/10665/42407 [Accessed].

Wilding John, P. H., Batterham Rachel, L., Calanna, S., Davies, M., Van Gaal Luc, F., Lingvay, I., Mcgowan Barbara, M., Rosenstock, J., Tran Marie, T. D., Wadden Thomas, A., Wharton, S., Yokote, K., Zeuthen, N. & Kushner Robert, F. 2021. Once-weekly semaglutide in adults with overweight or obesity. *New England Journal of Medicine*, 384, 989–1002.

Willis, K. & Elmer, S. 2011. *Society, Culture and Health*, Oxford University Press.

Ziauddeen, N., Gurdasani, D., O'hara, M. E., Hastie, C., Roderick, P., Yao, G. & Alwan, N. A. 2022. Characteristics and impact of Long Covid: findings from an online survey. *PLoS One*, 17, e0264331.

Zola, I. K. 1972. Medicine as an institution of social control. *The Sociological Review*, 20, 487–504.

CHAPTER 4

The Social Science of Mental Health and Illness

Samuel Woodnutt, Simon Hall, and Chris Allen

School of Health Sciences, University of Southampton, Southampton, UK

Introduction

In this chapter, we move beyond our previous chapter's consideration of health more broadly and turn our attention specifically to mental health. Mental health is gaining increased focus and discussion in all domains of public life, especially in the context of health and well-being. Over the last few decades, public health messaging in wealthier societies in particular has increasingly incorporated mental health alongside physical health, and it is hoped that the increased awareness and focus on mental health, will in time, help mental ill health receive the same attention or 'parity of esteem' as physical health.

In this chapter, you will gain an understanding of current mental health concepts and clinical practice, as well as the social and historical contexts that have shaped it from the 1700s through to today. We will examine the lenses through which mental ill health is viewed and will consider some of the most prominent models in current mental health practice. Through this, we will highlight how these models and our thinking around mental health have evolved over time and have been shaped by our social worlds. The social factors that influence the identification, diagnosis, management and care of those presenting with a range of mental health issues from diverse backgrounds and experiences are also explored.

LEARNING OUTCOMES

By the end of this chapter, you will be able to:

- Recognise and understand some of the determinants of poor mental health, including the impact of stressful working and living conditions, alongside some of the protective factors such as access to material and social resources.

- Consider the role of society and social life in shaping what mental health is and how those with poor mental health are seen and cared for.

- Consider the different ways mental health has been seen and understood across time, including how it is currently understood and classified.

- Understand the importance of patient voice, advocacy and activism.

- Consider a range of clinical interventions that are underpinned by the social sciences, including cognitive behavioural therapy and sandplay therapy.

Stress, Vulnerability and Mental Health

> ### Key Terms and Definitions
>
> **Social deviance:** Simply means that someone is different in terms of their behaviours or in terms of their characteristics. They 'deviate' from the 'norm' (Henry, 2018).
>
> **Labelling:** Labels are socially constructed representations of deviance (Link et al., 1989).
>
> **Stigma:** Something that categorises someone apart from the society in which they live in a way that discredits or devalues them (Scambler, 2009).
>
> **Total institution:** Where people with similar characteristics and sometimes their caregivers are cut off from society in a way that allows the institution to fully dictate how people live (Goodman, 2013).

Social Sciences for Healthcare Professionals, First Edition. Edited by Chris Allen.
© 2026 John Wiley & Sons Ltd. Published 2026 by John Wiley & Sons Ltd.

At the start of this chapter, we would like you to take a moment to think about what mental health is to you. Your answer, to some extent, will be unique. We suggest seeing mental health as our emotional fuel; what we need to get through each day. Taking the metaphor of a vehicle, we have a fixed capacity for fuel, which is used during all our daily activities.

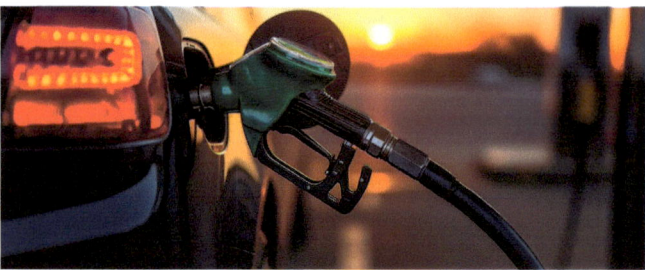

Source: Cheewynn/Adobe Stock Photos.

This means that we need to also monitor how full our fuel tank is and act when it is beginning to empty. As with vehicles, all our fuel tanks and engines are different; and we all travel different distances and cover different terrains. Tasks that barely have an impact on some can significantly drain the energy of others or may be impassable. Some may have supportive social networks and resources that help them keep their tanks full (i.e. resistance resources), whilst others may have less supportive relationships which may in fact deplete their fuel. Being unwell, both physically and mentally, can have an impact on how efficient we are. When we are more unwell, even basic tasks can drain our tanks far quicker. Some people may not be aware of their fuel level or the activities that would normally provide them with fuel may no longer be as effective. Some may run out of fuel altogether, leading them to become unwell. This metaphor is the basis of the *stress-vulnerability model* (Demke, 2022, Zubin and Spring, 1977).

> ### Stop and Think: What Factors Determine the Size of Your Tank?
>
> Some factors that you may have considered include:
>
> - Your relationships and their quality
> - Your broader social network
> - Your friends and family
> - Your hobbies and cherished activities
> - Your physical health
> - Your resources
> - Your job or occupation
>
> All these factors relate to our social world – the people we have who are supportive, the things that we do that we enjoy, our physical health (which alongside mental health is socially determined), the resources we have access to, whether or not we are employed and the quality of that employment.

> When preparing for a difficult journey, what can you do to help you retain your fuel?
>
> - *This could be planning an activity or time where you do something that is enriching – if you were travelling far, you would plan when to stop your vehicle for fuel.*
>
> What factors might drain your fuel more quickly?
>
> - *This could be how sensitive you are to the emotions that you are currently feeling (identifying what might make you vulnerable to stress).*

Mental health is all about our emotions and behaviours which may largely relate to our emotional capacity and how much fuel we have. This is a good way of thinking about our own support needs, as well as the mental health needs of others. However, as we will discuss throughout this chapter, mental health is incredibly entangled with many domains of social life. How it is seen in a society, how it is diagnosed, how it is treated and what support people can access. All of this happens within a social context that is subject to change and revision over time, including our perceptions of what 'normal' is.

Mental Health, Social Deviance and the Law

When our mental health is poor, we can act and behave in ways that society may see as unusual. Such behaviour may be seen as 'socially deviant'. Émile Durkheim (1858–1917) is largely credited with coining the concept of 'social deviance' (Durkheim, 2005). Now, it typically refers to individuals or groups whose behaviours or characteristics mark them out as being in some way different (or 'deviant') from the norms of a given society or culture (Henry, 2018). Certainly, most do not want to be labelled as 'deviant' and deviance is normally viewed as negative within a society – as something transgressive and therefore subject to stigma and/or punishment. For many behaviours and characteristics, this is true – people can be and are excluded from many aspects of a society (including healthcare) based on perceived differences (as we will expand upon in chapters 9–11 specifically). But really, as a concept, 'social deviance' just highlights that a person's behaviour or characteristics are different to what society sees as being 'normal' and in any given society there will always be people who fall outside of the 'norm'. This can include behaviours that are unwanted – such as criminality, or more simple acts such as wearing unusual or 'quirky' clothes. Not following healthy behaviours, especially if society's expectations are that you do, can also be seen as deviant (van der Horst et al., 2021). The recent COVID-19 pandemic demonstrated this phenomenon – as the baseline for our preoccupation with hygiene, cleanliness and what we touch changed because of the presence of infectious disease. Prior to the pandemic, it was unusual to see someone wearing a face covering in some cultures (but very usual in others) or for people to carry their own hand hygiene fluid. However, some behaviours that are commonly associated with mental ill health (such as becoming socially withdrawn, or having an excessive preoccupation with cleaning) become 'normal' during pandemics.

Being subject to constant revision, what is and what is not 'deviant' is usually dependent on time, the particular setting, the underlying culture, as well as the shared values and beliefs of a given society. Media play a large role in setting the tone for what is 'normal', and it is common for the media to poorly portray mental ill health, which in turn creates stereotypes (Klin and Lemish, 2008). This not only sets people with these conditions apart but also simplifies or exaggerates how they present, and their experiences. In the context of mental health, underlying culture and social values are central to the conceptualisation of illness. Whilst this can be difficult to see within the culture you are living in, it is clearly visible in historical contexts. Behaviour that is unexpected or unusual is typically associated with mental illness – largely because this deviates from the societal 'norm'.

Criminality is one poignant example of deviance, where there are shared cultural values that certain behaviours are 'wrong' or unfavourable and that these behaviours inhibit the functioning of a society. Criminal behaviour is commonly associated with stigma and punishment (Hirschfield and Piquero, 2010). For example, theft is considered a deviant behaviour – and the agreed view of theft is that it is something that should be punished. Laws themselves are updated and changed in accordance with changes in society and how behaviours and characteristics are seen and viewed. For example, as highlighted in the previous chapter, suicide was illegal in many countries in the first half of the 20th century, before being incorporated into broader health definitions (Kevin Chien-Chang et al., 2022). This also provides an example of how the language used in relation to mental health can be problematic, especially when it becomes entangled with the law as this language has the potential to endure, even when the law is later changed. Language can be suggestive of stigma, such as reference to acts of mental ill health as relating to an offence – as in 'commit suicide' – despite suicide no longer being an offence in most wealthy industrialised societies (Kevin Chien-Chang et al., 2022). In the context of physical health, it would be highly unusual to say that someone 'committed' diabetes, in the same way as people still commonly refer to suicide. The word 'commit' in English is associated with offending behaviour; hence the movement away from this to 'death by suicide' or 'died by suicide' in recognition that this is no longer a criminal act and should demand the same levels of care, support and empathy as all other needs (Canetto, 2021, Joiner, 2016).

Stop and Think: The Social Determinants of Suicide

Émile Durkheim's seminal study of suicide was one of the first social science studies to use systematic methods to examine our social world (Durkheim, 2005). Durkheim believed that there was a relationship between a societies structure – specifically its levels of social integration, and the risk of people in that society attempting or completing suicide. He found that societies where people felt more alone and less connected to their society had an increased suicide risk. The decision to attempt or complete suicide is personal and multifactorial – but identifying broader social determinants using a scientific method was revolutionary at the time and paved the way for social sciences more sophisticated methods for examining the social world as well as highlighting the influence of society to suicidal behaviours.

The social determinants of suicide are now widely studied. Thomas Joiner is notable in his dominant theory around suicidal thinking and behaviour (Joiner, 2016). The Interpersonal Theory of Suicide posits three main components, two of which are fundamentally social in nature. Joiner asserts that someone who perceives themselves as a burden on others (perceived burdensomeness) and who feels they do not belong (thwarted belongingness – not dissimilar to Durkheim's theory of social integration) is at high risk of developing suicidal ruminations. The final component suggests that through exposure over time, some people lose their instinctive fear of pain or death. Joiner's theory begins to explain why suicides may occur in greater volumes in certain demographic populations or industries – people who may be exposed at a greater rate to pain and/or death, and thus may lose their instinctive fear – such as soldiers exposed to war, refugees and people working in the police or emergency services, healthcare and agricultural workers (Arif et al., 2021, Awan et al., 2021, Cogo et al., 2022, Klingelschmidt et al., 2018, Moradi et al., 2021). However, recent evidence suggests such trends can be reversed through targeted support and intervention, for example, currently serving UK armed forces personnel may now have lower rates of suicide than the general population (Roberts et al., 2024).

There have also been suggestions that suicidal behaviours are socially contagious (known as the Werther effect).[1] Suicides can occur in clusters, and one suicide can lead to similar behaviours in others – whereby suicide is

---

[1] The term 'Werther effect' came from a 1774 Goethe novel, in which the titular character died by suicide, with others in the story subsequently imitating his death (Kim et al., 2023).

attempted or completed using similar methods (Haw et al., 2013). Awareness of the social contagion that can follow a death by suicide has resulted in strict reporting guidelines in the media around suicide (Duncan and Luce, 2020).

Besides guidelines for the reporting of suicides, there are other public health interventions that can be used to deter attempted suicide and prevent completed suicide.

Access to means is a common thread in suicide prevention and influences the regulation of certain substances, firearms or other means. Greater firearm regulation in countries, whilst not lowering the overall suicide rate, is correlated with less firearm-related suicides (Langmann, 2021). Medicines have also received regulatory changes to limit the risk of suicide. In the United Kingdom, paracetamol, which can be obtained without a prescription, has had changes in regulation since the 1990s. There are now restrictions on the quantity that can be purchased in one place and it must be sold in 'blister packs' (Hawton, 2002). Through making the process of obtaining and releasing the medication laborious, there is greater 'thinking time' that allows someone to change their mind or receive intervention, and research suggests that this might be effective because suicidal thoughts are often temporary (Joiner, 2016).

Systematic reviews have suggested that relatively simple acts such as the installation of barriers at known jumping sites may reduce attempts, though such interventions may bring about unintended negative effects, such as reducing opportunities for someone to be spotted and therefore receive help (Chamberlain and Woodnutt, 2024, Okolie et al., 2020).

There are many distinctions and technicalities involved in upholding the rights of those who may not be able to make decisions about their own care and, therefore, care that is directed through societies' law institutions can result in ethical and moral dilemmas (Sugiura et al., 2020). Such issues comfortably fill entire books and can only be summarised here to illustrate how society, and in particular the law influences the care of those with mental ill health. The legal system, a product of society and a social institution, continues to play a pivotal role in how mental ill health care is seen and treated. Mental and physical health issues often entail different rights and responsibilities. Unlike physical health, most countries that have mental health services have laws that are designed to protect people and provide treatment through legislation that mandates treatment when a person is incapacitated (Sheridan Rains et al., 2019). In western societies, a very different contract of care exists between mental and physical healthcare. In physical healthcare, most laws relate to people's rights to accessing care, whereas in mental health, these laws are joined with laws mandating engagement with services (Barkhuizen et al., 2020), for example, the Mental Capacity Act (2005). It is relevant to highlight that the threshold for enforced treatment in any context should be proportionate to the risk of not treating, and a person's right to have autonomy over their decisions (Code of Practice: Mental Health Act, 1983). However, a common factor in laws around the world is the inability to use the law to treat a physical condition for someone with mental ill health unless the two are intertwined (Code of Practice: Mental Health Act, 1983). If someone has schizophrenia and diabetes, the law may not allow enforced treatment for diabetes, unless the person is at risk of death, but might for schizophrenia depending on their capacity to make decisions (Code of Practice: Mental Health Act, 1983).

How Does Society Care for Those Who Are Mentally Unwell?

Mental Health, the Illness Framework and Psychiatry

As with health more generally, there continues to be debate around a variety of approaches as to what mental ill health is, how to conceptualise it and therefore how to treat it. To fully understand the differences and disagreement in modern management of mental ill health, it is important to understand social and historical contexts.

Psychiatry, as with other specialties within medicine tends to conceptualise mental illness through a biomedical or illness framework lens (as shown in chapter 3). As with physical health, medicine is a dominant profession in mental health through its sub-discipline of psychiatry. Through this lens, psychiatry seeks to identify what is different, likely harmful, and suggest or impose a course of treatment to 'fix' it (Rogers and Pilgrim, 2021). In some contexts, there is a biological basis for someone's behaviour or feelings changing, for example: detectable biological causes such as altered blood sugar, acute infections and intoxication can bring about changes in how we present, and how conscious we are, that might lead to our behaviour deviating from accepted norms or that may cause others concern (Brown et al., 2019, Kim et al., 2022). We can detect these abnormalities and can often 'treat' the underlying cause. Some changes to our mental state are associated with detectable physical changes to a person's brain, for example, Lewy body dementia (Sanghvi et al., 2020). In addition, negative emotions and patterns of stress are linked with physical illness and altered biochemical markers (Hsiao et al., 2023, Kivimäki and Steptoe, 2018, Miola et al., 2021). However, often there are no clear indicators that biological changes or imbalances account for someone's mood or emotions. For example, one dominant and widely believed theory of depression is that it is caused by lower serotonin concentrations or activity in the brain. A recent meta-analysis highlights that there is no clear evidence that such a relationship exists, despite such widespread beliefs existing in the population, including in professionals and laypeople (Moncrieff et al., 2023). That no known specific biological or, indeed, psychological markers exist to aid the diagnosis of mental illness is a now widely recognised issue within mental health – yet mental health is included in diagnostic classification systems like the DSM-5, and ICD, alongside physical health conditions that typically do have recognised underlying aetiological processes and known markers highlighting disease (Timimi, 2014).

The illness model has its foundation in the work of German physician Emil Kraepelin, who was the first known adopter of the approach which involved monitoring someone, recording notes and then inferring brain disease based on their behaviour (Bentall, 2004, Engstrom and Kendler, 2015). Whilst Kraepelin's formulation of mental illness as premature dementia (termed dementia praecox) has since been largely dismissed, his contribution to the process of psychiatry helped western societies in particular move away from the belief that mental illness was a moral failing, to a belief that mental illness had signs and symptoms that were distinct enough to allow for classification, and arose from a pathological issue that could be treated (Engstrom and Kendler, 2015).

Unfortunately, one significant consequence of this model was the development and use of very aggressive treatments such as electroconvulsive therapy (also known as ECT) and insulin shock therapy that were largely ineffective for those who were mentally unwell (Brannon and Graham, 1955, Faria, 2013). These primarily occurred in an attempt to move beyond the use of warehouse-style asylums, through approaches to 'fix' the underlying cause of people's behaviours and distress. Where such treatment was ineffective, more aggressive surgical procedures (psychosurgery) began to be used in an attempt to fix an underlying pathology – such as lobotomy, a procedure in which connections within the frontal lobe are severed in order to reduce unwanted behaviours (such as distress or aggression) (Faria, 2013). Essentially, this approach sought to surgically alter the disturbed mind without fully understanding what exactly it was that needed to be fixed, inadvertently causing significant harms including changes in personality and reduced functional ability to those receiving them. At the time, proponents of psychosurgery were celebrated, without clear empirical evidence that it improved people's mental ill health, although the expectation for evidence-based practice was significantly different from today (Caruso and Sheehan, 2017). The advent of antipsychotic

medication in the 1950s is associated with a reduction in psychosurgery (Caruso and Sheehan, 2017), although surgical routes to the management of mental ill health still exist in the form of deep-brain stimulation (Figee et al., 2022), although these are not widely available, and reserved for severe cases.

Despite a biomedical approach being common, most mental illnesses do not have a clear detectable cause or biological explanation (Rogers and Pilgrim, 2021). As we explored in the previous chapter, this makes diagnosis challenging despite recognised classification manuals such as the DSM and ICD existing. Conditions such as depression and anxiety may run in families (Dunn et al., 2015), but there is as yet, no concrete evidence that these conditions are exclusively, or even in part biologically caused (Moncrieff et al., 2023) and influences such as people's personal characteristics and traits, alongside the quality and quantity of social relationships are recognised as being increasingly relevant – all of which may result in increased mental health diagnoses within families (Wang et al., 2023).

Whilst diagnosis as with physical illness continues to largely be the domain of medicine, some of today's mental health services have no regular medical involvement (in the form of a psychiatrist) or are not led by one – suggesting an embrace of more a psycho-social approaches to management (Johns et al., 2019, Porter et al., 2024, Wakefield et al., 2021). As one example, the United Kingdom's Improving Access to Psychological Therapy (IAPT) programme,[2] aimed at those with common mental illnesses such as depression, anxiety and obsessive–compulsive disorder, is led by psychologists rather than psychiatrists (Howells et al., 2020). In Canada, 'BounceBack', a similar self-help, coach-assisted telephone programme has been deployed and has demonstrated positive recovery rates (Schumann et al., 2024). In such services, diagnosis is used, but its relevance is much less emphasised than in somatic care (Howells et al., 2020). What matters most is the person and their circumstances – two people can have the same diagnosis but hugely different presentations and needs. Social factors such as where someone lives, what they have access to and who they live with are better indicators of hospital admission or discharge than diagnosis or illness alone (Davoren et al., 2015, Tulloch et al., 2011).

A Brief History of Mental Healthcare as a Social Paradigm

Hippocrates (c.460–c.370 BC) is credited with providing the model of 'humourism' in health and medicine (Marcum, 2015). Humourism suggests that the body is composed of four bodily

[2] The Improving Access to Psychological Therapy (IAPT) service seeks to formulate and provide structured therapy on a one-to-one basis alongside group-work (Porter et al., 2024, Wakefield et al., 2021).

fluids that must balance – when these fluids are not balanced, ill health follows. This was arguably the first conceptual departure from deity or superstition-related ill-health (such as 'being cursed'), with a focus on underlying bodily causes for ill health that could be managed and controlled. However, in western societies, supernatural and pseudo-scientific beliefs continued in mental health well into the 20th century (Bentall, 2004). A significant move towards seeing mental ill health as body-related first occurred in 19th-century Europe with the founders of modern psychiatry (Bentall, 2004). The word 'melancholy' (which is no longer used, but was commonly used in the 18th and 19th centuries to describe the sadness and other symptoms of depression, psychosis or unexplained physical discomfort) is related to humourism: 'melanc' and melancholy were old words to describe 'black bile', one of the four bodily fluids in humourism (Ross and Margolis, 2018).

Until the 18th century, those with mental ill health were often chained to walls in locked asylums – considered afflicted through demonic possession or other supernatural means. Asylums were largely created to remove those afflicted with poor mental health, who were seen as beyond treatment, from society and were largely self-sufficient communes (Carpenter, 2010, Carpenter, 2013). It was not just those who were mentally unwell who were removed to such institutions, but also those whose behaviours deviated from societies' expectations about how people at the time should behave – such as bearing children out of wedlock, sexual promiscuity, displaying strong emotions and those using alcohol or other illicit substances (Rehling and Moncrieff, 2021). Whilst peoples institutionalisation was generally involuntary and often involved barbaric treatment,[3] asylums were generally seen as a place for those who were troubled to seek 'asylum' from their disturbances (Braslow, 2023, Tasca et al., 2012).

Alongside conceptualising causes of mental ill health as moral, efforts were later made to provide more compassionate care through decreased use of restriction and the provision of a role within a self-contained society. Early 19th-century treatment became less focused on containment, and more on meaningful community development, in which everyone had a stake (Jay, 2016). At the centre of these communities, the value in occupation was embraced, and this included the promotion of activities such as craft making, gardening and industrial therapies. Staff were employed if they had skill in a musical instrument – or another entertainment-based way of calming the disturbed mind (Carpenter, 2013). Essentially, this group of people,

who largely reflected individuals living outside of societal values, were given lives outside of wider society as a form of segregation. Alongside the patients living in the hospital, housing largely contained the care staff whose lives were intertwined with those of the asylum's patients, in what would become referred to as 'total institutions' (Goffman, 1961).

Consideration of the brain in isolation from other factors typified most care in the early to mid-20th-century asylums (Bentall, 2010); felt by many to be inhumane, cruel and epistemically unjust – in that patient views were informed by 'madness', and therefore not valid. Whilst diagnoses may have become more sophisticated (aided by disease classification systems such as DSM and ICD), and reasons for admission have changed in parallel with a significant reduction to inpatient bed availability and the recognition of the value of community care (Giménez-Díez et al., 2020, Lamb et al., 2020), recent literature has highlighted care that is epistemically unjust (Kidd et al., 2022), and that is totalitarian with healthcare facilities, particularly in meeting the needs of some vulnerable patient groups, not having fully moved away from being 'Total Institutions' (Hope et al., 2022).

Early Psychology Within Modern Society and Cognitive Behavioural Therapy

Psychoanalysis

At the turn of the 20th century, psychiatrists like Sigmund Freud (1856–1939) and Carl Jung (1875–1961) pioneered a form of mental healthcare that looked inwards at meaning. Jung believed that mental illness is related to a lack of balance and harmony within the individual's psyche. He proposed the concept of the 'collective unconscious', which is a shared reservoir of archetypal images and experiences that all humans inherit (Jung, 1936). According to Jung, mental disturbances could arise when the individual is not in touch with these deeper, symbolic aspects of their unconsciousness (Jung, 1936). This led to the belief that therapy should avoid trying to treat surface-level symptoms and behaviour, but should instead focus on the 'root cause' of the presentation. This root cause was felt to be held deep in the unconscious part of our minds, and trapped due to previous trauma(s). Its influence can be dependent on the relationship with the social interpretation of this root cause or the collective values, beliefs and stigma held by society – called the collective unconscious (Jung, 1936).

---

[3] For example, women whose behavior deviated from socially agreed norms, tended to be associated with hysteria or supernatural factors such as witchcraft Tasca, C., Rapetti, M., Carta, M. G. & Fadda, B. 2012. Women and hysteria in the history of mental health. *Clinical Practice and Epidemiology in Mental Health*, 8, 110–9.

Jung's Influence on Current Practice

Linked to Freud's psychoanalysis movement, Jung pioneered analytic psychology. His work has been influential across many fields including healthcare, medicine, literature, philosophy, anthropology and psychology (Wehr, 1987).

Freud and Jung both focused on psychodynamic forms of therapy – this means focusing on the unconscious processes that may motivate someone's behaviour and/or actions. In modern mental health practice, Jung's approach is particularly useful in a health context when people are unable to verbalise their experiences (Kegerreis and Midgley, 2014). This may be because the patients are children (who may not possess the language skills to communicate fully), due to a developmental need, or another reason that inhibits the person's ability to form, process and communicate thoughts and feelings to others.

Sandplay Therapy

Sandplay therapy is one psychotherapeutic method that can be applied to working with children, adolescents and adults (Roesler, 2019). As an approach, sandplay therapy was used largely from the 1920s, when British paediatrician Margaret Lowenfeld identified it as a developmentally appropriate way to allow children to express their emotional and psychological inner worlds (Lowenfeld, 1979). Significantly influenced by the work of Jung, the approach has since been further developed by others, for example, Dora Kalff (2004). The sandplay approach is based on Jung's approach on the symbolic meaning people ascribe to their feelings and their context (Jung and Hull, 1990). Jung believed that all things have a symbolic meaning behind them called 'archetypes' – and that these are often shared in a collective unconscious (Jung and Hull, 1990). If we consider a lion as an example, we can assume its archetype to be proud, strong and loyal. These positive qualities are often accompanied with its 'shadow' archetype connotations such as scary, fierce or being a killer. A form of therapy used in mental healthcare involves asking people to use a tray that has been filled with sand and choose items (normally from a large range of toys, figures, stones, gems or other items) to populate the tray and show either a given subject (such as 'school'), a significant moment in their life (such as 'when someone close passed away') or a broad topic like 'your world'.

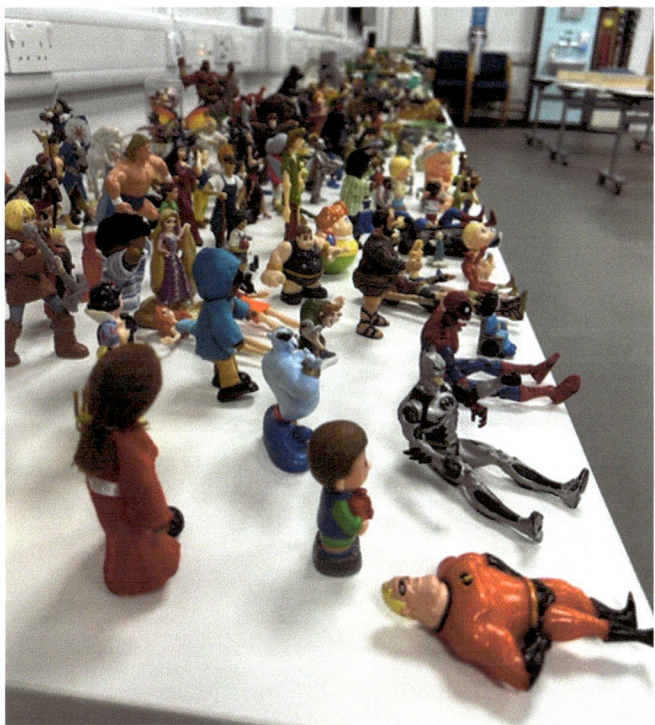

In sandtray therapy, a therapist supports the person to populate the tray and then uses this as a platform to understand that individual's 'world' and make sense of what this person is trying to communicate through enquiry-based conversation and questions to clarify the meaning ascribed to different objects (Homeyer and Sweeney, 2022).

For example, imagine a child is making a tray called 'my life at home' and they decide to pick up some animal figures to represent them and their family. The child chooses:

- A small monkey to represent themselves
- A large gorilla to represent their father
- A deer to represent their mother

We may start to think of archetypes about how this child has represented their family:

- That they perceive themselves as 'cheeky' or 'naughty' and in some ways like their father.
- That they see their father as 'strong' but also potentially 'scary'.
- That they see their mother as 'easily frightened' and/or 'elegant'.

Such an approach can therefore reveal a lot about a child's social support and their needs. A therapist would then work with the child by asking questions to arrive at a point where they feel they understand what the child is trying to communicate. This could also include how the figures are positioned in relation to each other (e.g. is mum 'hiding' behind dad or hiding the child from the father). Sand tray therapy has been found to be an effective approach in reducing emotional and behavioural problems in children with mental health and other chronic health conditions (Tan et al., 2021, Nickum and Lewis Purgason, 2017).

Behaviourism

Cognitive psychiatry also evolved during the 20th century, through prominent figures such as Burrhus Frederic Skinner (1904–1990) and Ivan Pavlov (1849–1936). Behaviourism started to link factors such as impulses, feelings, emotions, behaviours and choices (Watson, 2017). Skinner and Pavlov both experimented with animals – modifying (operating on) the animal or their environment and observing the behaviour. Pavlov's experiments with dogs are particularly well known (Adams, 2019, Kohler, 1962): They involved ringing a bell every time he fed a dog and monitoring the dog's salivation levels. Overtime the dog would begin to salivate upon hearing the bell without the presence of food, that is, it had formed an 'association' between the bell and food. This association was called 'classical conditioning'

(Blackman, 2022). This way of looking at the mind's interaction with the world forms part of our understanding of modern mental ill health – for example, a soldier with post-traumatic stress disorder who becomes alarmed upon hearing a loud noise as this is associated with explosives, guns or warfare (Shively and Perl, 2012). In this scenario of trauma, the soldier may *feel* as if they are actually at war – whereas in reality, the loud noise could be something that is harmless, such as someone dropping an item in the street, a car backfiring or a firework going off.

Behaviourism's notions of the mind interacting with stimulus and conditioning arguably helped form the basis of the most widely available form of talking therapy today: cognitive behavioural therapy (CBT); which is often credited to the American Psychologist Aaron Beck (1921–2021) (Beck and Fleming, 2021). CBT, a process highlighted in Figure 4.1,

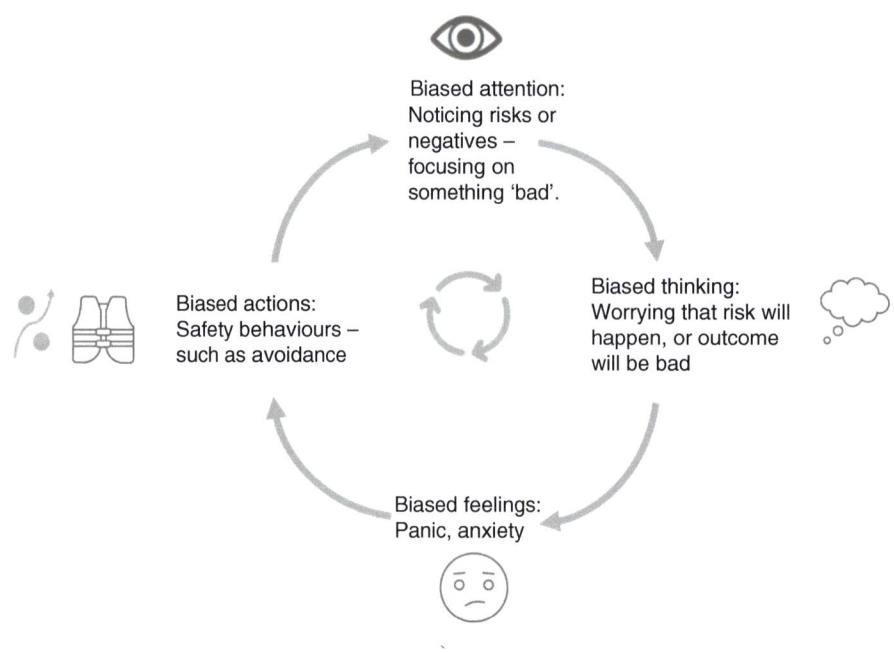

FIGURE 4.1 Cognitive behavioural therapy.

attempts to identify and map the processes underneath depressed or anxious moods. It considers less overt stimulus than food or explosions, through looking at thought-based stimulus, the perception of social interactions, and thought-based responses (López-López et al., 2019).

Critical Views on Psychiatry and Mental Health Treatment

Psychiatry now has a significant countermovement – often referred to as 'Antipsychiatry', that seeks to undermine its central principles (Burns, 2020). Psychiatrists from the 1960s and 1970s such as RD Laing (1927–1989) or Thomas Szasz (1920–2012) questioned the central ideas of psychiatry (Burns, 2020). Key areas of criticism were psychiatry's attempts to 'pathologize', and therefore socially control behaviour and morals in society through diagnosis and labelling – as opposed to seeing these emotions as normal and expected human emotions and responses (Davies, 2013, Davies, 2021). Those engaging with this view largely see human distress as a normal human response to wider societal issues such as oppression, alienation or general human suffering that can be alleviated not through treatment, but through addressing the underlying social determinants that are thought to have brought about the suffering in the first place. In essence, suffering can be alleviated not through the interventions of healthcare, but through addressing these broader social issues (Davies, 2013).

Power Threat Meaning Framework

Whilst society defines what is and what is not an illness or disease, disease classification in mental health is particularly challenging as most conditions do not have a clearly detectable underlying cause that can be fixed. For example, diabetes and cardiovascular disease have agreed biomedical markers that highlight risk, or that someone is unwell. In the context of mental health, such diagnostic certainty is often not possible.

Though the term antipsychiatry is less used, modern movements such as the 'Critical Psychiatry Network', continue to question the validity of diagnostic processes such as that proposed by the DSM-5 and ICD, and seek to instead understand human distress (Middleton and Moncrieff, 2019). Alternatives to diagnostic manuals (e.g. the DSM and the ICD), such as the Power Threat Meaning Framework (Johnstone and Boyle, 2018) emphasise a 'formulation' based approach – highlighting the person's context as the central focus, rather than seeking to elicit symptoms and fit these into a neatly defined objective classification system such as those in the DSM or ICD. However, as with many aspects of the critique of medicalisation more generally, there are wider ethical issues with this and times when it is important and necessary for someone to have a diagnosis – such as care pathways for personality disorder in the United Kingdom (Flynn et al., 2019).

Other examples exist, particularly in areas where people require health insurance to fund care, as some degree of uniform governance to the diagnostic and treatment process is likely needed to satisfy insurance requirements; though insurance-based health coverage is associated with mental health inequalities (Wang and Xie, 2019). Even in countries with free universal healthcare coverage diagnosis can help to determine who gets care, and what care they get – for example, in the UK NICE guidance is available for many diagnosed mental health conditions (NICE, 2014, NICE, 2022).

> ## Rosenhan's (1973) study 'on being sane in insane places'
>
> In Rosenhan's (1973) now seminal study 'On being sane in insane places' eight confederate patients posed as 'insane'. They did this by telling healthcare professionals that they heard voices uttering words like 'thud'. Apart from this symptom, the pseudo-patients gave true accounts of themselves and acted otherwise 'normally' (Rosenhan, 1973). They were admitted to a psychiatric hospital, where they claimed they no longer heard voices. However, the way people came to perceive them meant that their initially declared symptoms led healthcare professionals to label them as 'insane' at which point proving their 'sanity' became challenging (Rosenhan, 1973).
>
> There was an outcry from psychiatrists in particular following Rosenhan's study as it highlighted the highly subjective nature of their work and their ability to make accurate diagnoses of mental ill health and how those deemed mentally unwell were managed (Agarwal, 2023). In the 50 years since Rosenhan's work, the management of mental ill health has evolved alongside diagnostic manuals, guidance and process have been refined several times in response to our continuously improving knowledge of mental health. Whilst we cannot say Rosenhan's work is indicative of health services today, it does highlight some of the uncertainty around mental healthcare and conflicting views that exist within psychiatry and mental health; some of which have been discussed in this chapter.

The Birth of the Recovery Movement

The diagnostic framework has faced criticism, including from recipients of mental healthcare themselves, through its lack of focus on recovery and person-centeredness (Chamberlin, 1978, Deegan, 1992). The emerging concept of 'recovery', and rejection of diagnostic labelling predominantly originated from those with lived experience of diagnostic categorisation and mental ill health (Deegan, 1988, Leete, 1989, Unzicker, 1989). Alongside this, have been lay and professional concerns and scepticism that mental health diagnostic classification systems like the DSM-5 focus on deficits, rather than strengths, and classify people rather than conditions (Flanagan and Davidson, 2007). They have also been highlighted as unnecessarily pathologizing normal human experiences – arguably to the benefit of the profession of psychiatry and the pharmaceutical industry (Pavlo et al., 2019, Timimi, 2014).

Traditionally, mental ill health has largely been seen as a life-long remitting and relapsing illness – and not something someone was expected to make a full recovery from. Hence, diagnostic labels once they have been given, have the capability to endure. However, people's own narratives have highlighted that they can recover from mental ill health and live valued fulfilling lives, even without having much, or indeed any professional mental health involvement (Davidson, 2016). Recovery, as a movement, introduced the idea that recovery from illness was possible, and that the meaning of recovery is derived from the individual and not the clinician – and this notion is supported by evidence that many people with a mental health diagnosis do indeed recover, or at least learn to manage their condition in such way as ensuring it only minimally disrupts daily life (Davidson, 2016).

In 1988 Patricia Deegan wrote 'Recovery: The lived experience of rehabilitation' (Deegan, 1988). This was arguably the first articulation of today's recovery movement. But this movement was not necessarily created, or indeed anything 'new', but was instead a mobilisation of alternative philosophies that highlighted the rights of people with mental ill health to be able to participate in all aspects of society, and a shift in mental health service delivery towards supporting those with a serious mental illness to be supported away from institutions, and in their own homes in everyday life (Davidson, 2016, Hopper et al., 2007). This notion of recovery-orientated practice highlighted that the care of mental health should no longer be viewed as a prescription of mass institutionalisation and treatments. This requires a paradigm shift away from focussing on what people cannot do (i.e. their deficits – as seen in the illness model), and instead, we focus on what people can do (i.e. their capabilities and their strengths) (Perkins and Slade, 2012, Rapp and Goscha, 2006). Recovery today is about individualised approaches that help people to develop new purposes and meanings to their lives beyond their limitations. As such 'recovery' should not seek to fix underlying issues – as this may not be possible – but instead support people to live valued lives despite these (Cruwys et al., 2020).

Modern (Integrated) Approaches in Current Health Contexts (4Ps Formulation)

A common method of case formulation, which is a collaborative process between service users and healthcare professionals to arrive at a shared understanding of someone through many aspects of their life, is the 4Ps model (Predisposing, Precipitating, Perpetuating and Protective Factors) (Cox, 2020; Henderson & Martin, 2014). This is a method to organise and help clinicians focus on the aspects of someone's mental health that are relevant to their presentation. When combined with the biopsychosocial model (introduced in the previous chapter) (Adler, 2009, Engel, 1977), as highlighted through the example in the table below, this allows us to see a more nuanced and multifactorial approach to mental health – essentially a way of mapping the biological, psychological and social factors that may predispose (put someone at increased risk of developing mental ill health), precipitate (make an episode of ill health more likely to occur), perpetuate (make an episode of ill health more likely to continue) and protect (make an episode of ill health less likely, or more likely to resolve) someone's mental health. In this model, social factors are given equal focus with biological and psychological factors – in other words, this places the person within their whole context and does not seek to isolate a specific biological or psychological process as a cause for ill health (as with the illness framework) (Table 4.1).

Formulation helps clinicians because someone with mental ill health may not be able to identify and manage factors relevant to their episode of ill health (Rainforth and Laurenson, 2014). Most mental health assessments use a form of interview, where there are some planned questions but also space for the interviewer to expand on any issues that may arise, using a Socratic method (Clark and Egan, 2015). The formulation-based approach allows as many factors as possible to be explored, whereas a rating scale or tool may limit the focus of the interviewer (Chan et al., 2016). From an objective, litigious or insurer perspective provision of care would be more problematic without a diagnosis. However, this type of assessment provides a generally more comprehensive foundation to plan appropriate care.

TABLE 4.1   The 4Ps model combined with the biopsychosocial model – the table has been completed with some examples of factors that may contribute to someone's mental health.

	Biological	Psychological	Social
Predisposing	Genetics Physical status Co-occurring (or co-morbid) conditions Childhood development trauma (Ahmed-Leitao et al., 2016)	Identity Personality Patterns of behaviour and ways of thinking Ways of coping with stress Sense of self/self-esteem Trauma	Family and peer relationships (including how they are formed and maintained) Cultural influences (including ethnicity, religion, etc) Education

TABLE 4.1   *(continued)*

	Biological	Psychological	Social
Precipitating	Drug/alcohol use Physical health status Medication use (e.g. concordance)	Adopted or predicted responses to stressors Emotional intensity Triggers (such as from trauma)	Acute stressors (e.g. work, finances, study, peer/family relationships Rejection (Joiner, 2016)
Perpetuating	Drug/alcohol use Medication use (e.g. concordance)	Insight into self Patterns of coping Self-stigma Self-esteem	Social relationships Stigma
Protective	Medication use	Resilience Healthy ways of coping Hope for the future Sense of agency (feeling of control over actions and consequences)	Relationships with others

Stop and Think: Formulation in Mental Health

Below is an example of a 4Ps formulation of someone who would likely meet the DSM-5 diagnostic criteria for depression.

Read the vignette and try to identify the biopsychosocial factors that have predisposed and precipitated, are perpetuating and are protective of this episode of mental ill health. The below is written using a first-person narrative, an approach that is consistent with mental healthcare planning in some areas.

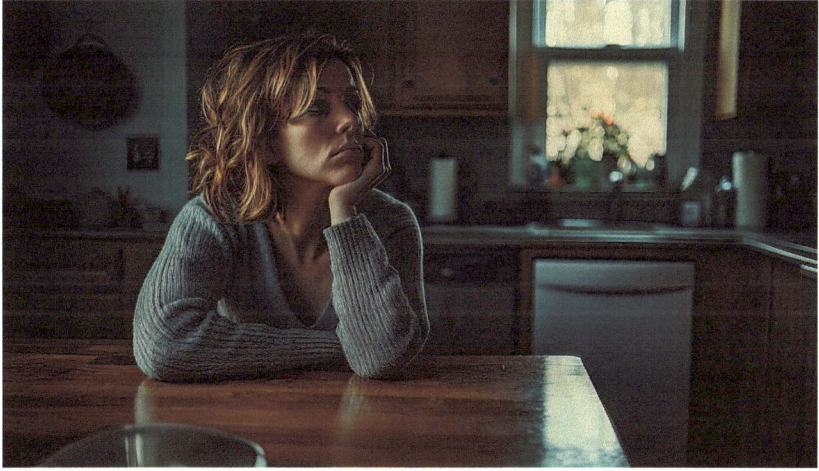

Source: Art Fusion/Adobe Stock Photos.

Predisposing Factors

Growing up, my father would drink alcohol frequently and often stay out late. He would argue with my mother and sometimes there would be physical fights in the house. My older sister left home at the age of 15 and I spent a long time in the house by myself. Due to my mother's long working hours, I needed to cook for myself. I avoided being in communal areas of the house when my parents were around. All these experiences and possible genetic factors have predisposed me to be someone who avoids others and conflicts. I felt worthless a lot, and malnutrition during my teenage years probably contributed to me not developing or thriving at the rate I should have done.

Precipitating Factors

Prior to this episode of low mood, I was in a relationship and working a job. I drink alcohol frequently as my parents never really gave me a good model of how to cope with emotions. Work stress started to get to me and I drank more and more to cope. My partner got frustrated with me spending more money on alcohol and we used to argue- so they left. In a way I rejected her as I wanted to avoid the conflict. It also feels more normal for me to be alone, and I don't feel like I deserve closeness with anyone because I don't really know what it feels like. If I start to feel close to someone, I feel scared and want to reject them.

Perpetuating Factors

I continue to drink alcohol heavily as there is no reason not to – it's just me at home. I am being performance-managed at work and some days I call in sick just to avoid it. I don't sleep very well, and I have racing thoughts throughout the night. Isolating myself makes me feel safe. I don't feel like I enjoy anything anymore, and I struggle to concentrate so I've stopped doing any hobbies in the house. A loss of sleep, alcohol consumption and low mood may have made it more likely for my brain to 'default' to depressed ways of thinking. As a result, I have probably developed a bias towards seeing things in a depressing way. If my phone rings I feel scared before I know who it is. I say no to anything social before I know any details about it.

Protective Factors

My relationship with my sister is distant but she cares for me and calls every Sunday. I've promised her I wouldn't do anything to harm myself. I have agreed with my care team that I will contact them in the event I feel suicidal or want to hurt myself. I always try and take my medication and rarely miss a dose.

ANSWERS

	Biological	Psychological	Social
Predisposing	Neglect – malnutrition in early years Genetics – father's alcohol use	Sense of self – worthlessness Avoidance as a way of coping as a child	Isolation Struggled to make secure attachments with family members
Precipitating	Alcohol use Physical health status Medication use (e.g. concordance)	Avoidance Using alcohol to cope	Work stress Relationship stress Financial stressors
Perpetuating	Alcohol use	Avoidance of emotional bonds and relationships Ways of looking at the world and self	Work-related performance and stress
Protective	Medicine concordance Possible family history of treatment response	Active engagement with safety planning Sense of agency	Relationship with sister Engaged with a care team

Clinical Considerations

- People's risk of mental ill health is determined by many factors, including the social determinants of health.

- How mental health is seen and understood has changed over time. Even now, there are several ways in which mental health is seen and understood.

- Antipsychiatry and recovery movements, which have involved significant activism, are contributing to recent changing perceptions around mental ill health.

- Mental health and physical health often entail different rights and responsibilities.

- People can have the same mental health diagnosis, but hugely different circumstances and needs.

- Social views around mental ill health can result in stereotypes that not only set people apart, but also simplify or exaggerate their experiences.

- The contributions of the social sciences underpin many well-known interventions in mental health, such as CBT and sand-play therapy.

- Mental health assessment should incorporate social, psychological and biological factors.

Conclusion

In this chapter, we have highlighted the historical and social contexts around mental health care. As we have highlighted, there continues to be significant tension and differences in perspectives in mental health conceptualisation, treatment and care. Psychiatry remains an arm of medicine where there remains some significant disagreement about how to approach diagnosis, care and treatment. The evolution of mental health –

from supernatural origins to a more integrated and pragmatic approach, can be traced throughout history. However, social values around normality and deviance of behaviour still influence the categorisation of mental ill health in the absence of definitive or objective tests that can prove an objective diagnosis. The social context for an individual is paramount to understanding their mental health needs and good assessment of mental health incorporates a range of lenses such as those outlined in this chapter – considering biological, psychological and social aspects as they relate to someone's presentation.

References

Adams, M. 2019. The kingdom of dogs: understanding Pavlov's experiments as human–animal relationships. *Theory & Psychology*, 30, 121–141.

Adler, R. H. 2009. Engel's biopsychosocial model is still relevant today. *Journal of Psychosomatic Research*, 67, 607–611.

Agarwal, A. 2023. "On being sane in insane places" . . . it is a work half done. *Indian Journal of Psychiatry*, 65, 601–603.

Ahmed-Leitao, F., Spies, G., Van Den Heuvel, L. & Seedat, S. 2016. Hippocampal and amygdala volumes in adults with posttraumatic stress disorder secondary to childhood abuse or maltreatment: a systematic review. *Psychiatry Research: Neuroimaging*, 256, 33–43.

Arif, A. A., Adeyemi, O., Laditka, S. B., Laditka, J. N. & Borders, T. 2021. Suicide mortality rates in farm-related occupations and the agriculture industry in the United States. *American Journal of Industrial Medicine*, 64, 960–968.

Awan, S., Diwan, M. N., Aamir, A., Allahuddin, Z., Irfan, M., Carano, A., Vellante, F., Ventriglio, A., Fornaro, M., Valchera, A., Pettorruso, M., Martinotti, G., Di Giannantonio, M., Ullah, I. & De Berardis, D. 2021. Suicide in healthcare workers: determinants, challenges, and the impact of Covid-19. *Frontiers in Psychiatry*, 12, 792925.

Barkhuizen, W., Cullen, A. E., Shetty, H., Pritchard, M., Stewart, R., Mcguire, P. & Patel, R. 2020. Community treatment orders and associations with readmission rates and duration of psychiatric hospital admission: a controlled electronic case register study. *BMJ Open*, 10, e035121.

Beck, J. S. & Fleming, S. 2021. A brief history of Aaron T. Beck, MD, and cognitive behavior therapy. *Clinical Psychology in Europe*, 3, e6701.

Bentall, R. 2004. *Madness Explained: Psychosis and Human Nature*, Penguin.

Bentall, R. 2010. *Doctoring the Mind: Why Psychiatric Treatment Fails*, London, UK: Penguin.

Blackman, D. 2022. Conditioned suppression and the effects of classical conditioning on operant behavior. *In*: Honig, W. K. & Staddon, J. E. R. (eds.) *Handbook of Operant Behavior*, New York: Routledge, 340–363.

Brannon, E. P. & Graham, W. L. 1955. Intensive insulin shock therapy—a five-year survey. *American Journal of Psychiatry*, 111, 659–663.

Braslow, J. 2023. *Mental Illness and Bodily Cures: Psychiatric Treatment in the First Half of the Twentieth Century*, University of California Press.

Brown, J. B., Reichert, S. M., Valliere, Y., Webster-Bogaert, S., Ratzki-Leewing, A., Ryan, B. L. & Harris, S. B. 2019. Living with hypoglyce-

mia: an exploration of patients' emotions: qualitative findings from the InHypo-DM study, Canada. *Diabetes Spectrum: A Publication of the American Diabetes Association*, 32, 270–276.

Burns, T. 2020. A history of antipsychiatry in four books. *Lancet Psychiatry*, 7, 312–314.

Canetto, S. S. 2021. Language, culture, gender, and intersectionalities in suicide theory, research, and prevention: challenges and changes. *Suicide & Life-Threatening Behavior*, 51, 1045–1054.

Carpenter, D. 2013. Rewriting the Asylum. *In*: Araoz, G., Alves, F. & Jaworski, K. (eds.) *Rethinking Madness: Interdisciplinary and Multicultural Reflections*, Brill.

Carpenter, D. T. 2010. Above all a patient should never be terrified: an examination of mental health care and treatment in Hampshire 1845–1914. University of Portsmouth, Portsmouth.

Caruso, J. P. & Sheehan, J. P. 2017. Psychosurgery, ethics, and media: a history of Walter Freeman and the lobotomy. *Neurosurgical Focus*, 43, E6.

Chamberlain, B. & Woodnutt, S. 2024. Systematic review of suicide prevention from jumping in public locations. *Mental Health Practice*, 28(1).

Chamberlin, J. 1978. *On Our Own: Patient-Controlled Alternatives to the Mental Health System*, New York: McGraw Hill.

Chan, M. K., Bhatti, H., Meader, N., Stockton, S., Evans, J., O'connor, R. C., Kapur, N. & Kendall, T. 2016. Predicting suicide following self-harm: systematic review of risk factors and risk scales. *The British Journal of Psychiatry*, 209, 277–283.

Clark, G. I. & Egan, S. J. 2015. The Socratic method in cognitive behavioural therapy: a narrative review. *Cognitive Therapy and Research*, 39, 863–879.

Code of Practice: Mental Health Act (1983). UK Government. https://www.gov.uk/government/publications/code-of-practice-mental-health-act-1983.

Cogo, E., Murray, M., Villanueva, G., Hamel, C., Garner, P., Senior, S. L. & Henschke, N. 2022. Suicide rates and suicidal behaviour in displaced people: a systematic review. *PLoS One*, 17, e0263797.

Cox, L. 2020. Use of individual formulation in mental health practice. *Mental Health Practice*, 24(1).

Cruwys, T., Stewart, B., Buckley, L., Gumley, J. & Scholz, B. 2020. The recovery model in chronic mental health: a community-based investigation of social identity processes. *Psychiatry Research*, 291, 113241.

Davidson, L. 2016. The recovery movement: implications for mental health care and enabling people to participate fully in life. *Health Affairs*, 35, 1091–1097.

Davies, J. 2013. *Cracked: Why Psychiatry is Doing More Harm than Good*, Icon books Ltd..

Davies, J. 2021. *Sedated: How Modern Capitalism Created Our Mental Health Crisis*, Atlantic Books.

Davoren, M., Byrne, O., O'connell, P., O'neill, H., O'reilly, K. & Kennedy, H. G. 2015. Factors affecting length of stay in forensic hospital setting: need for therapeutic security and course of admission. *BMC Psychiatry*, 15, 301.

Deegan, P. E. 1988. Recovery: the lived experience of rehabilitation. *Psychosocial Rehabilitation Journal*, 11, 11–19.

Deegan, P. E. 1992. The independent living movement and people with psychiatric disabilities: taking back control over our own lives. *Psychosocial Rehabilitation Journal*, 15, 3.

Demke, E. 2022. The vulnerability-stress-model-holding up the construct of the faulty individual in the light of challenges to the medical model of mental distress. *Frontiers in Sociology*, 7, 833987.

Duncan, S. & Luce, A. 2020. Using the responsible suicide reporting model to increase adherence to global media reporting guidelines. *Journalism*, 23, 1132–1148.

Dunn, E. C., Brown, R. C., Dai, Y., Rosand, J., Nugent, N. R., Amstadter, A. B. & Smoller, J. W. 2015. Genetic determinants of depression: recent findings and future directions. *Harvard Review of Psychiatry*, 23, 1–18.

Durkheim, E. 2005. *Suicide: A study in sociology*, Routledge.

Engel, G. L. 1977. The need for a new medical model: a challenge for biomedicine. *Science*, 196, 129–136.

Engstrom, E. J. & Kendler, K. S. 2015. Emil Kraepelin: icon and reality. *The American Journal of Psychiatry*, 172, 1190–1196.

Faria, M. A., Jr. 2013. Violence, mental illness, and the brain - a brief history of psychosurgery: part 1 - from trephination to lobotomy. *Surgical Neurology International*, 4, 49.

Figee, M., Riva-Posse, P., Choi, K. S., Bederson, L., Mayberg, H. S. & Kopell, B. H. 2022. Deep brain stimulation for depression. *Neurotherapeutics*, 19, 1229–1245.

Flanagan, E. H. & Davidson, L. 2007. "Schizophrenics," "borderlines," and the lingering legacy of misplaced concreteness: an examination of the persistent misconception that the DSM classifies people instead of disorders. *Psychiatry: Interpersonal and Biological Processes*, 70, 100–112.

Flynn, S., Raphael, J., Graney, J., Nyathi, T., Williams, A., Kapur, N., Appleby, L. & Shaw, J. 2019. The personality disorder patient pathway: service user and clinical perspectives. *Personality and Mental Health*, 13, 134–143.

Giménez-Díez, D., Maldonado Alía, R., Rodríguez Jiménez, S., Granel, N., Torrent Solà, L. & Bernabeu-Tamayo, M. D. 2020. Treating mental health crises at home: patient satisfaction with home nursing care. *Journal of Psychiatric and Mental Health Nursing*, 27, 246–257.

Goffman, E. 1961. *Asylums*, New York: Doubleday/Anchor.

Goodman, B. 2013. Erving Goffman and the total institution. *Nurse Education Today*, 33, 81–82.

Haw, C., Hawton, K., Niedzwiedz, C. & Platt, S. 2013. Suicide clusters: a review of risk factors and mechanisms. *Suicide and Life-threatening Behavior*, 43, 97–108.

Hawton, K. 2002. United Kingdom legislation on pack sizes of analgesics: background, rationale, and effects on suicide and deliberate self-harm. *Suicide & Life-Threatening Behavior*, 32, 223–229.

Henderson, S. A. & Martin, A. 2014. Case Formulation and Integration of Information in Child and Adolescent Mental Health. *In*: Rey, J. M. (ed.) *IACAPAP e-Textbook of Child and Adolescent Mental Health*, Geneva: International Association for Child and Adolescent Psychiatry and Allied Professions.

Henry, S. 2018. *Social deviance*, John Wiley & Sons.

Hirschfield, P. J. & Piquero, A. R. 2010. Normalization and legitimation: modeling stigmatizing attitudes toward ex-offenders. *Criminology*, 48, 27–55.

Homeyer, L. & Sweeney, D. 2022. *Sandtray Therapy: A Practical Manual*, Routledge.

Hope, J., Schoonhoven, L., Griffiths, P., Gould, L. & Bridges, J. 2022. 'I'll put up with things for a long time before I need to call anybody': face work, the Total Institution and the perpetuation of care inequalities. *Sociology of Health & Illness*, 44, 469–487.

Hopper, K., Harrison, G., Janca, A. & Sartorius, N. 2007. *Recovery from Schizophrenia: An International Perspective: A Report from the WHO Collaborative Project, the International Study of Schizophrenia*, New York, NY, US: Oxford University Press.

Howells, L., Rose, A., Gee, B., Clarke, T., Carroll, B., Harbrow, S., Oliver, C. & Wilson, J. 2020. Evaluation of a non-diagnostic 'psychology of emotions' group intervention within a UK youth IAPT service: a mixed-methods approach. *Behavioural and Cognitive Psychotherapy*, 48, 129–141.

Hsiao, F. Y., Peng, L. N., Lee, W. J. & Chen, L. K. 2023. Sex-specific impacts of social isolation on loneliness, depressive symptoms, cognitive impairment, and biomarkers: results from the social environment and biomarker of aging study. *Archives of Gerontology and Geriatrics*, 106, 104872.

Jay, M. 2016. *This Way Madness Lies: The Asylum and Beyond*, Thames and Hudson Ltd.

Johns, L., Jolley, S., Garety, P., Khondoker, M., Fornells-Ambrojo, M., Onwumere, J., Peters, E., Milosh, C., Brabban, A. & Byrne, M. 2019. Improving Access to psychological therapies for people with severe mental illness (IAPT-SMI): lessons from the South London and Maudsley psychosis demonstration site. *Behaviour Research and Therapy*, 116, 104–110.

Johnstone, L. & Boyle, M. 2018. The power threat meaning framework: an alternative nondiagnostic conceptual system. *Journal of Humanistic Psychology*, 0022167818793289.

Joiner, T. 2016. *Why People Die by Suicide*, Harvard University Press.

Jung, C. G. 1936. The concept of the collective unconscious. *Collected Works*, 9, 42.

Jung, C. G. & Hull, R. F. C. 1990. *The Basic Writings of C.G. Jung Revised Edition*, Princeton University Press.

Kalff, D. 2004. *Sandplay: A Psychotherapeutic Approach to Psyche*, Temenos Press.

Kegerreis, S. & Midgley, N. 2014. Psychodynamic Approaches. *In: The Handbook of Counselling Children and Young People*, Independent Publishers Group, 35–48.

Kevin Chien-Chang, W., Ziyi, C., Qingsong, C., Shu-Sen, C., Fai, P. S. & Y. & Ying-Yeh, C. 2022. Criminalisation of suicide and suicide rates: an ecological study of 171 countries in the world. *BMJ Open*, 12, e049425.

Kidd, I. J., Spencer, L. & Carel, H. 2022. Epistemic injustice in psychiatric research and practice. *Philosophical Psychology*, 1–29.

Kim, K. T., Jeon, J. C., Jung, C.-G., Park, J. A., Seo, J.-G. & Kwon, D. H. 2022. Etiologies of altered level of consciousness in the emergency room. *Scientific Reports*, 12, 4972.

Kim, L.-H., Lee, G.-M., Lee, W.-R. & Yoo, K.-B. 2023. The Werther effect following the suicides of three Korean celebrities (2017–2018): an ecological time-series study. *BMC Public Health*, 23, 1173.

Kivimäki, M. & Steptoe, A. 2018. Effects of stress on the development and progression of cardiovascular disease. *Nature Reviews. Cardiology*, 15, 215–229.

Klin, A. & Lemish, D. 2008. Mental disorders stigma in the media: review of studies on production, content, and influences. *Journal of Health Communication*, 13, 434–449.

Klingelschmidt, J., Milner, A., Khireddine-Medouni, I., Witt, K., Alexopoulos, E. C., Toivanen, S., Lamontagne, A. D., Chastang, J.-F. & Niedhammer, I. 2018. Suicide among agricultural, forestry, and fishery workers: a systematic literature review and meta-analysis. *Scandinavian Journal of Work, Environment & Health*, 44, 3–15.

Kohler, I. 1962. Pavlov and his dog. *The Journal of Genetic Psychology*, 100, 331–335.

Lamb, D., Lloyd-Evans, B., Fullarton, K., Kelly, K., Goater, N., Mason, O., Gray, R., Osborn, D., Nolan, F., Pilling, S., Sullivan, S. A., Henderson, C., Milton, A., Burgess, E., Churchard, A., Davidson, M., Frerichs, J., Hindle, D., Paterson, B., Brown, E., Piotrowski, J., Wheeler, C. & Johnson, S. 2020. Crisis resolution and home treatment in the UK: a survey of model fidelity using a novel review methodology. *International Journal of Mental Health Nursing*, 29, 187–201.

Langmann, C. 2021. Suicide, firearms, and legislation: a review of the Canadian evidence. *Preventive Medicine*, 152, 106471.

Leete, E. 1989. How i perceive and manage my illness. *Schizophrenia Bulletin*, 15, 197–200.

Link, B. G., Cullen, F. T., Struening, E. L., Shrout, P. E. & Dohrenwend, B. P. 1989. A modified labeling theory approach to mental disorders: an empirical assessment. *American Sociological Review*, 54, 400–423.

López-López, J. A., Davies, S. R., Caldwell, D. M., Churchill, R., Peters, T. J., Tallon, D., Dawson, S., Wu, Q., Li, J., Taylor, A., Lewis, G., Kessler, D. S., Wiles, N. & Welton, N. J. 2019. The process and delivery of CBT for depression in adults: a systematic review and network meta-analysis. *Psychological Medicine*, 49, 1937–1947.

Lowenfeld, M. 1979. *The World Technique*, George Allen & Unwin.

Marcum, J. A. 2015. Hippocrates and the Hippocratic Tradition: Impact on Development of Medical Knowledge and Practice? In: Schramme, T. & Edwards, S. (eds.) *Handbook of the Philosophy of Medicine*, Dordrecht: Springer Netherlands.

Middleton, H. & Moncrieff, J. 2019. Critical psychiatry: a brief overview. *BJPsych Advances*, 25, 47–54.

Miola, A., Dal Porto, V., Tadmor, T., Croatto, G., Scocco, P., Manchia, M., Carvalho, A. F., Maes, M., Vieta, E., Sambataro, F. & Solmi, M. 2021. Increased C-reactive protein concentration and suicidal behavior in people with psychiatric disorders: a systematic review and meta-analysis. *Acta Psychiatrica Scandinavica*, 144, 537–552.

Moncrieff, J., Cooper, R. E., Stockmann, T., Amendola, S., Hengartner, M. P. & Horowitz, M. A. 2023. The serotonin theory of depression: a systematic umbrella review of the evidence. *Molecular Psychiatry*, 28, 3243–3256.

Moradi, Y., Dowran, B. & Sepandi, M. 2021. The global prevalence of depression, suicide ideation, and attempts in the military forces: a systematic review and meta-analysis of cross sectional studies. *BMC Psychiatry*, 21, 510.

NICE. 2014. Psychosis and schizophrenia in adults: prevention and management [Online]. National Institute for Health and Care Excellence Available: https://www.nice.org.uk/guidance/cg178 [Accessed].

NICE. 2022. Depression in adults: treatment and management [Online]. National Institute for Health and Care Excellence. Available: https://www.nice.org.uk/guidance/ng222 [Accessed].

Nickum, J. & Lewis Purgason, L. 2017. Using the sand tray to facilitate client creativity: a strengths focused approach to adolescent depression. *Journal of Creativity in Mental Health*, 12, 347–359.

Okolie, C., Wood, S., Hawton, K., Kandalama, U., Glendenning, A. C., Dennis, M., Price, S. F., Lloyd, K. & John, A. 2020. Means restriction for the prevention of suicide by jumping. *Cochrane Database of Systematic Reviews*, 2, Cd013543.

Pavlo, A. J., Flanagan, E. H., Leitner, L. M. & Davidson, L. 2019. Can there be a recovery-oriented diagnostic practice? *Journal of Humanistic Psychology*, 59, 319–338.

Perkins, R. & Slade, M. 2012. Recovery in England: transforming statutory services? *International Review of Psychiatry*, 24, 29–39.

Porter, A., Franklin, M., Vocht, F. D., D'apice, K., Curtin, E., Albers, P. & Kidger, J. 2024. Estimating the effectiveness of an enhanced 'improving access to psychological therapies' (IAPT) service addressing the wider determinants of mental health: a real-world evaluation. *BMJ Open*, 14, e077220.

Rainforth, M. & Laurenson, M. 2014. A literature review of case formulation to inform mental health practice. *Journal of Psychiatric and Mental Health Nursing*, 21, 206–213.

Rapp, C. A. & Goscha, R. J. 2006. *The Strengths Model: Case Management with People with Psychiatric Disabilities*, 2nd Edition, New York, NY, US: Oxford University Press.

Rehling, J. & Moncrieff, J. 2021. The functions of an asylum: an analysis of male and female admissions to Essex County Asylum in 1904. *Psychological Medicine*, 51, 1140–1146.

Roberts, S. E., John, A., Carter, T. & Williams, J. G. 2024. Suicide rates in the UK Armed Forces, compared with the general workforce and merchant shipping during peacetime years since 1900. *BMJ Military Health*, 170(e2), e128–e133.

Roesler, C. 2019. Sandplay therapy: an overview of theory, applications and evidence base. *The Arts in Psychotherapy*, 64, 84–94.

Rogers, A. & Pilgrim, D. 2021. *A Sociology of Mental Health and Illness*, 6e Edition, McGraw-Hill Education (UK).

Rosenhan, D. L. 1973. On being sane in insane places. *Science*, 179, 250–258.

Ross, C. A. & Margolis, R. L. 2018. Research domain criteria: cutting edge neuroscience or Galen's humors revisited? *Molecular Neuropsychiatry*, 4, 158–163.

Sanghvi, H., Singh, R., Morrin, H. & Rajkumar, A. P. 2020. Systematic review of genetic association studies in people with Lewy body dementia. *International Journal of Geriatric Psychiatry*, 35, 436–448.

Scambler, G. 2009. Health-related stigma. *Sociology of Health & Illness*, 31, 441–455.

Schumann, L., Park, K., Rouse, J. & Chagigiorgis, H. 2024. The high impact of low intensity: effectiveness of the bounceback program for depression and anxiety in Ontario. *Behavior Therapy*, 55, 150–163.

Sheridan Rains, L., Zenina, T., Dias, M. C., Jones, R., Jeffreys, S., Branthonne-Foster, S., Lloyd-Evans, B. & Johnson, S. 2019. Variations in patterns of involuntary hospitalisation and in legal frameworks: an international comparative study. *Lancet Psychiatry*, 6, 403–417.

Shively, S. B. & Perl, D. P. 2012. Traumatic brain injury, shell shock, and posttraumatic stress disorder in the military--past, present, and future. *The Journal of Head Trauma Rehabilitation*, 27, 234–239.

Sugiura, K., Mahomed, F., Saxena, S. & PATEL, V. 2020. An end to coercion: rights and decision-making in mental health care. *Bulletin of the World Health Organization*, 98, 52–58.

Tan, J., Yin, H., Meng, T. & Guo, X. 2021. Effects of sandplay therapy in reducing emotional and behavioural problems in school-age children with chronic diseases: a randomized controlled trial. *Nursing Open*, 8, 3099–3110.

Tasca, C., Rapetti, M., Carta, M. G. & Fadda, B. 2012. Women and hysteria in the history of mental health. *Clinical Practice and Epidemiology in Mental Health*, 8, 110–119.

Timimi, S. 2014. No more psychiatric labels: why formal psychiatric diagnostic systems should be abolished. *International Journal of Clinical and Health Psychology*, 14, 208–215.

The Mental Capacity Act (2005). United Kingdom Government. https://www.legislation.gov.uk/ukpga/2005/9/contents.

Tulloch, A. D., Fearon, P. & David, A. S. 2011. Length of stay of general psychiatric inpatients in the United States: systematic review. *Administration and Policy in Mental Health*, 38, 155–168.

Unzicker, R. 1989. On my own: a personal journey through madness and re-emergence. *Psychosocial Rehabilitation Journal*, 13, 71–77.

Van Der Horst, H., Wahlen, S. & Reimerink, M. 2021. Snacking practices in school: othering and deviance in a health-normative context. *Critical Public Health*, 31, 595–604.

Wakefield, S., Kellett, S., Simmonds-Buckley, M., Stockton, D., Bradbury, A. & Delgadillo, J. 2021. Improving access to psychological therapies (IAPT) in the United Kingdom: a systematic review and meta-analysis of 10-years of practice-based evidence. *The British Journal of Clinical Psychology*, 60, 1–37.

Wang, K., Hu, Y., He, Q., Xu, F., Wu, Y. J., Yang, Y. & Zhang, W. 2023. Network analysis links adolescent depression with childhood, peer, and family risk environment factors. *Journal of Affective Disorders*, 330, 165–172.

Wang, N. & Xie, X. 2019. Associations of health insurance coverage, mental health problems, and drug use with mental health service use in US adults: an analysis of 2013 National Survey on Drug Use and Health. *Aging & Mental Health*, 23, 439–446.

Watson, J. 2017. *Behaviourism*, Routledge.

Wehr, G. 1987. *Jung: A biography*, Boston, MA, US: Shambhala Publications.

Zubin, J. & Spring, B. 1977. Vulnerability: a new view of schizophrenia. *Journal of Abnormal Psychology*, 86, 103–126.

CHAPTER 5

Understanding the Organisation of Health Systems and Health Economics

Chris Allen[1], Robert Slinn[2], and Sam Woodnutt[1]
[1]*School of Health Sciences, University of Southampton, Southampton, UK*
[2]*Department of Social Sciences, A Maintained Secondary and Sixth Form College, Southampton, UK*

Introduction

The distribution of healthcare resources, even in countries with little state involvement in care, is generally more complicated than the free-market transactions that typically connect consumers with sellers in other contexts. In this chapter, you will be introduced to some of the key principles in health economics and the political economy. Countries around the world are concerned with how to keep their citizens well with the available resources that they have. Health systems differ between territories and the resources available to different countries that can be invested in health and well-being differ significantly; from those with very small state provision to those with high per capita healthcare expenditure, who also invest very high percentages of their country's Gross Domestic Product (GDP) on healthcare.

Healthcare systems around the world are facing strain due to the increasing prevalence of chronic illness (see chapter 7), and chronic staff shortages (see chapter 6). A culmination of increased demand, reduced capacity and delays in elective and routine care, are forcing societies to think about how equitable and sustainable their healthcare systems are. This involves returning to important questions such as who provides healthcare, who receives healthcare and how healthcare is financed and by whom. This chapter principally serves as an overview of some of the key debates and discussions around healthcare systems that you work in and receive care from, which will help you understand their social contexts and give you a broad insight into why they are the way they are and how they might change over time.

LEARNING OUTCOMES

By the end of this chapter, you will be able to:

- Understand the basic assumptions of economics and understand the potential relevance of inputs and outputs to economic decision-making in healthcare.
- Understand some of the most common ways different treatment options are weighed against one another, to determine which options are most beneficial in terms of effectiveness and in terms of their cost.
- Consider some of the ethical and moral dilemmas that inform such decision-making about who gets what.
- Consider what the political economy is and the role of governments and society itself has on shaping the healthcare systems that we have around the world, including how care is financed and provided to populations.
- Recognise the impact that a lack of universal health coverage has on citizens across the world and how coverage might be achieved.
- Recognise the various ways that healthcare systems performance can be determined and how the performance of healthcare systems has been compared between and within nations.

Social Sciences for Healthcare Professionals, First Edition. Edited by Chris Allen.
© 2026 John Wiley & Sons Ltd. Published 2026 by John Wiley & Sons Ltd.

What Is Health Economics?

> ## Key Terms and Definitions
>
> **Healthcare systems:**   Generally, this encompasses all the activities that support health through prevention, promotion and the restoration of poor health.
>
> **Opportunity cost:**   Where there are limited resources, the opportunity cost is essentially the cost of choosing one alternative over another.
>
> **Externalities:**   These are goods and services whose consumption brings about positive or negative side effects to society (i.e. positive or negative externalities). For example, health consumption can lead to improved economic productivity (a positive externality) and tobacco consumption can lead to harms brought about by second-hand smoke (a negative externality).
>
> **Universal health coverage:**   Generally, this means that all of a countries' citizens can access the healthcare they need without facing financial hardship.
>
> **Policy:**   Generally, a position taken, or a direction set from a position of authority. This can be an individual, or more commonly an institution, or even the government (Baggot, 2015).
>
> **Gross domestic product:**   The value of all goods and services that are produced by a country within a specified period of time.

As we explored in this book's introductory chapter, economics is a social science, and is essentially the study of human behaviours and the production, distribution and consumption of scarce goods and services (Wiseman, 2011). There are a few basic assumptions in the field of economics.

These are:

- That goods and services are scarce (for society, producers and consumers).
- That the consumption of goods and services creates value.
- That available resources are best invested into those goods and services that create the most value (because we often have some choice amongst alternatives).
- That humans make rational choices (that may be guided by incentives and disincentives) about what is available to them based on availability and perceived utility or value.

(Glied and Smith, 2011, Wiseman, 2011)

Essentially, health economics is concerned with the choices people or institutions make, with the resources that they have. The choices individuals make in relation to health behaviours are unpacked more in chapters 12–14. In this chapter, we are principally concerned with the choices the governments and institutions make and how these relate to health.

Health economists are often interested in relationships between inputs and outputs (Glied and Smith, 2011, Wiseman, 2011). What we put into health (the inputs), and how these relate to benefits to health (the outputs). Inputs are generally the financial, material or human resources that we use to provide care. Outputs are essentially the benefits that are realised from these to individuals and wider society (such as increased longevity, improved health and quality of life and economic growth). A chief concern with economics, including health economics, is what options are chosen. This is because when they are chosen, other options are not. This is referred to as the 'opportunity cost' (Wiseman, 2011). When a medicine is prescribed, other alternative treatment options exist, such as other medications, surgery, psychological interventions (such as CBT) or social interventions (such as social prescribing). Each option will have their own associated expected benefits and costs. If we are going to use up resources to meet a healthcare need, we need to see some type of benefit being realised, as resources are typically perishable. They cannot be used again and again. One hour of nursing time is one hour of nursing time. We cannot get this time back and this includes the time that went into training that nurse. Likewise, consumed medicine, cannot be reused, and this includes the resources that were used to produce it. Decisions about options are complex and often involve some degree of ethical and moral debate. In chapter 3, we highlighted some of the challenges in defining health, and how such definitions are important in determining who gets what. Definitions of health and classifications of disease and epidemiological data (covered more in chapter 7), alongside finite resources, feed into the challenge of ensuring equitable access to healthcare for all and making decisions about what health is. Narrow definitions of health, such as the deficit or medical model, lead to health policy that is reactive. Wider definitions of health, on the contrary, lead to public health policy that is proactive and looks to ensure the maintenance of health across populations (Hunter, 2003). In this chapter, we principally focus on decisions about healthcare provision and in later chapters (chapter 14 in particular), we expand this to look at interventions that arise from more proactive public health policy.

How Are Decisions Made About Who Gets What?

Clearly with limited resources, decisions need to be taken about what healthcare to provide amongst multiple competing healthcare needs (Walker et al., 2012). Having some form of 'generic' outcome measure might help guide decisions about specific treatments in different health-related issues – and commonly used examples include the DALY, or Disability Adjusted Life Years, and the QALY, or Quality-Adjusted Life Years (Feng et al., 2020). These capture both the 'quantity of life' and the 'quality of life', albeit in slightly different ways (Feng et al., 2020). The DALY relates to years of perfect health lost, whereas the QALY relates to perfect health gained (Feng et al., 2020). Both aid in the comparison of the effectiveness of different interventions across conditions (Feng et al., 2020, Walker et al., 2012). As health economic outcomes, these often form the basis of Health Technology Assessment (HTA), whereby different treatment options are weighed up against cost and value in terms of health gain, and through these decisions can be taken about how to maximise population (rather than individual) health.

As with any 'catch all' measure (some others are discussed later in this chapter), these have faced criticism, particularly for reducing health experience to longevity and quality of life (ignoring many externalities that fall out of health consumption) and for its potential impact on economic decision-making (specifically cost-effectiveness) that might be seen as cold, calculated, uncaring, and even discriminatory – i.e. cost vs lives (Rand and Kesselheim, 2021). As outcomes, however, when used alongside other important information to guide decision-making, these are useful and commonly used, particularly amongst decision-makers (Walker et al., 2012). As a salient example, significant healthcare spending on treatments that have low effectiveness but are very expensive invariably prevents spending (i.e. an opportunity cost) on treatments that might be more effective and lead to greater population health gains. However, such decision-making is also tied up in a society's values, ethics and morals around health and healthcare, including what and who should be prioritised.

Stop and Think: Ethics, Costs and Benefits

What decisions would you make about who gets what?

Consider the following example. If you were in the position to decide what treatments should be made available, what would you choose and why?

Two new drugs have become available to treat the common cold. We know from epidemiological data, that the common cold is 'common'.

Drug A works some of the time (55%) but is cheap to manufacture and administer (e.g. a pill that can be swallowed at home).

Drug B works almost all the time (90%) but is expensive to manufacture and requires specialist administration (an injection by a nurse).

Based on this information, which treatment option would seem the best option for the population?

You might want to consider:

- The impact of the disease (e.g. does the disease cause massive social and economic problems?)
- Is the impact of the disease so serious that it would warrant additional spending to treat?

- Would your decision change if **Drug B** was known to have some significant and nasty side effects? In what ways might your decisions be influenced by the population experiencing the issue, as well as those who are not?

And what if the condition was different:

- How might your decision change if the two drugs were the same, but the disease was cancer or heart disease – or another disease with a high associated mortality, or high impacts on quality of life?
- What about if the condition was very rare, and only experienced by a few people?
- What about if the condition was experienced mostly by those who are very young?
- What about if the condition was experienced mostly by those who are very old?
- What impact would knowing the disease is more common in people who smoke or engage in other unhealthy behaviours that have made it more likely they would become unwell?
- How would your decision be influenced by the political climate and the culture, values and norms of your society?

Ensuring that the most appropriate treatments are available to meet a societies increasingly complex health needs in a sustainable and equitable way, generally requires a significant degree of coordination, regulation and government involvement. Governments are often concerned with health consumption because health is seen as a fundamental right and because it has positive macroeconomic consequences (i.e. externalities). Improvements in a population's health, alongside effective education and employment opportunities, can improve the health of populations, and healthy nations are generally more economically efficient nations (Meara et al., 2015, Ridhwan et al., 2022). In fact, there are measures of economic performance and development that specifically incorporate health outcomes such as life expectancy, for example, the Human Development Index (HDI)(UN, 1990) and health is prominent within the UN Sustainable Development Goals (SDG) (UN, 2016). With healthcare being recognised as a merit good, governments generally want healthcare to be consumed for reasons of equity, justice and development, and health-enhancing goods and services, as well as healthcare itself are often subsidised or paid for entirely to avoid their underconsumption.

When we access formal healthcare, such as our general practitioner (in the United Kingdom, these are generally the gatekeepers to other healthcare services), or if we go into a hospital as an inpatient requiring treatment, we are accessing a 'service'. But these services are not boundless. The people that care for those accessing these settings are often people like you – paid professionals, with years of specialist training (see chapter 6) and their supply is not limitless. In fact, globally as we unpick more in the following chapter, we are facing significant shortages in the supply of healthcare workers – with low- and middle-income countries facing the largest shortfall (Boniol et al., 2022). This, when combined with projected increases in healthcare need in relation to demographic and epidemiological transitions that we are seeing across the globe (discussed in chapter 7) is creating significant strain for most healthcare systems, which are having to consider the ongoing sustainability of how they are set up and configured.

In the context of health systems and healthcare provision, it is often governments that determine who can access what, and what must be given by its citizens (e.g. through general taxation or through insurance) in return for such provision. In this context, health economics as a scientific discipline has shaped our understanding of healthcare provision, on the development of health systems policy, on healthcare implementation and on evaluation. Governments typically have a role in all of these. And because of this, healthcare is politicised (Bambra et al., 2005).

What Is the Political Economy and How Does It Relate to Health?

Considerations of the political economy tend to focus on the political climate and how the decisions those in power make, shape the availability and distribution of economic resources (Fox, 2024, Tuohy and Glied, 2011). Decisions generally relate to the things societies care about, like economic growth, inequality, and in the context of this chapter, access to healthcare. Governments have multiple competing things they can invest in – including, for example, education which can also improve health. The political economy is often considered in the context of human culture, sociological relationships and

the ideas, ideologies, power and institutions that emerge from them (Fox, 2024, Harvey, 2021). Healthcare consumption does not occur naturally, and governments have at least some influence on the health of their nations (Tuohy and Glied, 2011), as too do a range of global healthcare institutions.

Significant Global Institutions with a Role in Health and Their Interrelations

United Nations (UN): An international diplomatic organisation whose purpose is to maintain relationships and cooperation between nations, and work towards international peace and security.

World Health Assembly (WHA): A forum that is composed of member states that governs the activities of the World Health Organisation.

World Health Organisation (WHO): Established in 1948, the WHO is an agency of the UN, that is governed by the World Health Assembly, that has specific responsibility for global public health.

Organisation for Economic Co-operation and Development (OECD): This is an intergovernmental organisation, which currently has 38 members (hence 'OECD38'). The OECD is essentially a collaboration between member states to facilitate the development of policies that may positively enhance societies.

World Bank: An international financial institution that supplies loans to low- and middle-income countries to support development. Its current loan strategy is influenced by the United Nations Sustainable Development Goals.

Governments are involved in the health of their citizens in several ways. First, healthcare is a right; it is generally seen as being determined by need (i.e. I am unwell, therefore I 'need', rather than 'want' care). In a typical market transaction, who gets what in relation to scarce resources is typically determined by pricing. Scarce resources go to those who are willing to and can pay for them. But societies often see such a mechanism as highly inappropriate in the context of healthcare, both because its consumption has positive externalities that have far-reaching benefits to a society, but also because those with the least ability to pay for healthcare, are also those who often have the largest health needs (Bartley, 2017). Despite it being a fundamental right, healthcare is still a finite resource and because of this, tensions can emerge. For example, the overconsumption of care by those not needing it uses up the resources of those who do. This is sometimes referred to as a consumer moral hazard (Koohi Rostamkalaee et al., 2022). There are only so many healthcare professionals, drugs, hospital beds, diagnostic procedures and interventions that can go around and governments often intervene to improve the equity of consumption, such as through providing 'Universal Health Coverage' (UHC) to ensure that people can access healthcare without facing economic hardship.

Whilst recognising healthcare as a fundamental right, due to its scarcity, aspects of supply and demand need to be considered with all aspects of healthcare, as is evidenced in the early days of the National Health Service (NHS). The UK health system, as with other health systems is a product of the values and beliefs of UK society at the time. That is, health is a fundamental right that should be free to all regardless of ability to pay. Launched in 1948, by 1950 it had already hit its first major funding crisis – with suggestions that healthcare that was completely free at the point of delivery for all, was overgenerous and unsustainable (Flyn, 2018). The NHS was far from the government's only spending priority and the supply of available cash for healthcare spending was quickly dwindling. As a result, an increasingly frugal NHS began to charge for some aspects of healthcare, such as health provided by dentists and opticians, and charging for prescriptions in 1952. This was in part to raise revenue, but also too to stem the unprecedented and largely unanticipated demand. These changes were abolished following the return of the Labour Party to government in 1960, but by 1968 provision had again proved to be unsustainable, and these aspects were once again taken away, albeit with some being exempt based on criteria such as age, income and health (Flyn, 2018). There is an empirical basis for this, with the now seminal RAND Health Insurance Experiment demonstrating that requiring people to pay for some care, can deter overconsumption, but crucially can also deter care that is in fact needed (Chen and Goldman, 2016, Lohr et al., 1986, Manning et al., 1988).

Aside from their role in the equitable financing and distribution of healthcare, governments also play a significant role in regulation and exactly what diagnostic and treatment options are made available to their citizens based on expected benefits, risks and costs; and who exactly they are available through (i.e. which providers) (Tuohy and Glied, 2011). Whilst patient empowerment is clearly important (and is discussed in some depth in chapter 7), unregulated choice of diagnostic and treatment options would simply be overwhelming for many people (Mol, 2008). When attending healthcare services, you are likely to not know what is wrong with you, only how you feel and what you can see. You are reliant on the healthcare professionals you are accessing to be able to make sensible decisions about what tests they might need to do to determine what is making you unwell. You also need them to make some recommendations about the treatments that might help alleviate your symptoms and help you to return to good health. Such decisions usually occur in the context of imperfect information. Unless you have had some training yourself (and arguably even if you have), you probably wouldn't be able to work this out for yourself without access to any diagnostics,

even with the instant access to the information we now have available to us online. The sheer volume of potential options (both evidence and nonevidence-based), alongside the speed of change, would make the range of possible decisions overwhelming for most people. Governments to an extent, prevent some of this overwhelm and can correct information asymmetries, by limiting the choice, and often by limiting the choice to only the options that might have some benefit. This is often done through Health Technology Assessment, for example, in the United Kingdom, the National Institute for Health and Care Excellence (NICE), provides evidence-based guidelines for healthcare professionals to follow that mean that when you are offered something to alleviate troubling signs and symptoms, there is at least some evidence that it might actually work and that it is cost-effective (NICE, 2012). This is of course sometimes seen as politically contentious, as it directs money towards interventions based on cost, at the expense of others – and this in turn, may reduce the size of the overall pot available to meet the needs of other patient groups (Claxton et al., 2013).

Government regulation works in other ways too, for example, in countries where healthcare coverage is typically gained through health insurance, governments can regulate the insurance companies and offer some protection against these companies exploiting people (Motaze et al., 2021). They can also put in place safeguards to ensure those at higher risk, such as those who have a chronic health condition already, are still able to be insured and can subsidise premiums to make them equitable (Zhao et al., 2022).

The health system is reliant on many other systems and institutions, and it is often the role of government to manage this complexity. For example, without an education system, there would be a limited pool of well-educated future healthcare professionals available to the sector, and education as we explore in chapter 8 is a known determinant of health – which governments also seek to address (Zajacova and Lawrence, 2018). As we explore later in this book, governments are also responsible for promoting public health, for example, through the provision of clean water and sanitation (as just one example), regulation and control of harmful products such as tobacco, intervening when the public are engaged in behaviours that might be deemed unhealthy (such as harmful levels of alcohol consumption), and promoting health-enhancing behaviours (Jochelson, 2006, Reich, 2019, Tuohy and Glied, 2011). Governments also have a role in promoting research and development, especially in situations where new healthcare knowledge might improve the health and well-being of their populations – both now and in the future. Whilst private companies engage in research and development too, their actions are more likely to be market-driven, and less likely to focus on future needs, or the needs of marginalised, disadvantaged and resource-constrained populations (Simpkin et al., 2019).

In summary, government and health are intertwined in even the most privatised healthcare economies. Different governments have different capacities and capabilities to provide healthcare services and have different capacities to raise money through taxation. Much of our health and the healthcare we have available to us now, and in the future, are shaped by a government's resources, capabilities and political choices, including levels of taxation to fund services, and ultimately how much they invest in healthcare as opposed to other similarly socially desirable services. Around 10% of the global GDP is spent on the provision of healthcare (WHO, 2023a). Whilst many countries spend a large amount on healthcare either directly or indirectly (through, e.g. addressing the peoples living and working conditions, and investment in prevention), the amount varies from country to country and health system funding is likely to face increasing future pressures due to the demographic and epidemiological transitions that are explored in more depth in chapter 7. Many countries have inadequate budgets, resources and logistics that make them poorly equipped to meet the health needs of their citizens and globally there is reliance on charity, community, voluntary and third-sector organisations and citizens themselves to plug often quite substantial gaps in provision, underpinning, and strengthening healthcare systems (Besançon et al., 2022, Bowles et al., 2023, Brass et al., 2018, Corbally, 2022, Taylor et al., 2021).

The United Nation's (UN) Sustainable Development Goals (SDG), specifically target 3.8 sets the ambition for states to achieve universal health coverage (UHC) by 2030. For a country to have UHC, its entire population should be able to receive high-quality healthcare without facing undue financial hardship to pay for it (WHO, 2023b). Whilst many countries, particularly high-income countries can already claim some degree of universal health coverage, other countries are, through political reforms, seeking to address issues of healthcare finance towards UHC (OECD, 2023a, Yazbeck et al., 2020).

What Is a 'Health System' and What Health Systems Are There?

We have arrived at this point without fully defining what exactly a healthcare system is. You may already have some intuitive sense of what a healthcare system is having accessed care or provided care within a healthcare system. Seminal definitions of healthcare systems point towards a system as encompassing all of the activities involved in promoting health, preventing ill health and supporting people to recover when they become unwell (WHO, 2000). Reference to a 'system' is important, as rarely can healthcare be provided **exclusively** within the confines of one particular individual or care provider such as a General Practitioner (or GP) and a single purchaser–provider relationship. As we explore in chapters 18 and 19, healthcare has simply become too complex and specialised to be delivered in this way, and increasingly

requires the complex coordinated activities of politics and policy (to set the direction), financing and provision (to fund, purchase and supply), governance and regulation (to provide care in line with policy and public expectations). These coordinated activities exist within a broad healthcare system (Mays, 2018). As an example, the care of someone who has Chronic Obstructive Pulmonary Disease (COPD), even when relatively well, requires a degree of coordination and will be provided by more than one healthcare organisation which are often separately owned and managed, but may (or may not) pull from the same sources of funding, and be governed by the same regulations.

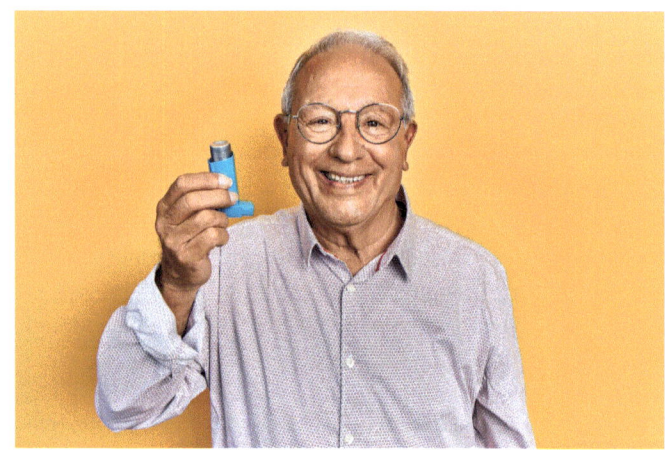

Source: Krakenimages.com/Adobe Stock Photos.

In the context of the United Kingdom, care would usually be managed by a GP but may also involve other specialists supporting other aspects of care, and medications will generally be provided by a community pharmacist. Of course, people can also become acutely unwell, and this might involve being admitted to a hospital (another separately owned and managed organisation). All of these different healthcare organisations exist within the umbrella of a healthcare 'system'. But the boundaries of any healthcare system are not clear cut, as much of societies' activities exist outside of what might be seen as 'the healthcare system' also influence health (such as education, employment and social care) (Anandaciva, 2023, Mays, 2018).

Where democratic processes exist, what aspects of health and how they should be provided are influenced by the political process, giving those in power a mandate to act and set the direction in accordance with the values and expectations of their electorate. This, alongside the impact of a country's culture, values, politics, history and needs, means that a country's health system is always a product of the society and is always continuously evolving (Anandaciva, 2023). All countries have different challenges and needs for healthcare, have citizens following different levels of health-enhancing and health-damaging behaviours, have different values relating to how individualist (concern for self) or collectivist (concern for others) they are and differing levels of resource available to meet population health needs in a fair and equitable way. How funds are raised, how care is provided and to who and how the system as a whole is regulated, differs across healthcare systems, and these differences relate to the different choices that have occurred often over many years through the directions set by policy, the political process and wider societal influences. This means that healthcare systems are often very different from country to country.

Whilst broad health system typologies do exist, and the main ones are discussed in this chapter, most healthcare systems include a range of different financing and purchasing mechanisms. This can include collecting money to pay for healthcare that is not currently needed but may be needed in the future (i.e. pooled funding) through different combinations of voluntary and compulsory insurance contributions (including through government and non-government schemes) and general taxation. It can also include personal out-of-pocket expenses at the point of healthcare need (i.e. when someone is already unwell). Alongside different funding, are different arrangements for who provides care, with a mixture of public, private (i.e. for profit) and charitable providers existing generally even within the same health economy, but with differing levels of involvement between healthcare systems (i.e. in some systems, single state-owned providers are more common, such as the NHS) (Anandaciva, 2023). There are some broad typologies that seek to capture how care is financed and then provided, and these can help us understand the core arrangements that different countries have to aid (rather rudimentary) comparisons between healthcare systems in terms of their general financing and provision arrangements.

Healthcare system models include:

- **Beveridge:** Beveridge models provide universal health coverage through general taxation to finance and provide healthcare for all citizens when they need it, generally through one state-owned provider. Examples include the UK's NHS (Or et al., 2010, van der Zee and Kroneman, 2007).
- **Bismarck:** As with Beveridge, the Bismarck model provides universal health coverage, but funding is largely through compulsory employee insurance contributions as opposed to general taxation, and citizens have more choice about who provides their care. Examples are seen in Germany and much of Europe. Comparisons are often drawn between Beveridge and Bismarck models (Or et al., 2010, van der Zee and Kroneman, 2007)

- **Mixed models:** Where multiple models of health financing and provision exist within the same healthcare system. For example, in America, some citizens are protected through private voluntary insurance schemes, and some (particularly those who are most vulnerable) are able to access care through government schemes that provide a safety net (such as Medicaid and Medicare), as well as some who are not protected at all (Anandaciva, 2023, Gotanda et al., 2020).
- **Fully out of pocket:** Care is not financed or provided by the government or compulsory insurance schemes at all and there are no pooled funds. Receiving healthcare involves out-of-pocket healthcare expenditure. When you are ill, you must finance your own healthcare. This model is still common around the world and is associated with significant economic hardship and inequality.

However, even within these broad typologies, systems can differ quite significantly both in terms of composition and performance. Health systems evolve and the boundaries of these typologies blur. For example, in the United Kingdom, out-of-pocket expenditure (as we discussed) is a feature of some aspects of care despite a Beveridge model being used. In Germany, the Bismarck model, that was originally implemented to provide healthcare coverage to workers, has been expanded to cover other citizens too, and in America's mixed model system, increasing coverage has been achieved through expansion in the protections available to societies most vulnerable members through the Affordable Care Act in 2010 (Anandaciva, 2023, Gotanda et al., 2020). The impact of this continuous evolution is that no health system truly fits with these idealised typologies– most are hybrids involving aspects of public, private and out-of-pocket provision (Anandaciva, 2023). Indeed, there is often as much difference within a typology, as between them, making it tricky to compare different healthcare systems like for like (Freeman and Frisina, 2010).

You can find some useful summaries of European countries healthcare systems, including their core features, through the European Observatories Health System Review Series (HiT series) (https://eurohealthobservatory.who.int/publications/health-systems-reviews).

Case Study: America's Mixed Model System

The United States healthcare system is one example of a mixed system with no UHC, but with some protection for their societies most vulnerable members through state-funded Medicare and Medicaid (Gotanda et al., 2020). Medicare is primarily for those over the age of 65, who during their working lives have paid into a social security pot. Younger people who have a disability, and those with some chronic conditions may also qualify (Gotanda et al., 2020, Sommers et al., 2017). Medicaid,

which has been expanded in most states through 'Obamacare', was introduced under the Affordable Care Act (2010) subsidises private health insurance for those on lower incomes (Gotanda et al., 2020).

In a recent study, expansions to Medicaid following the Affordable Care Act (2010) resulted in a reduction in out-of-pocket healthcare expenditure and a decreased risk of catastrophic financial burdens in those states that opted to expand their provision (Gotanda et al., 2020). Whilst the Affordable Care Act (2010) has resulted in more Americans being insured, issues of inadequate and inequitable health coverage remain especially in marginalised groups (Liddell and Lilly, 2022). The issue of health coverage is particularly marked for low-income households who do not qualify for Medicare or Medicaid and who do not have insurance or who are underinsured (Dickman et al., 2017). High levels of bankruptcies continue to be caused by catastrophic out-of-pocket medical expenditures arising from a lack of adequate health coverage (Laberge and Djiffa, 2023).

Whilst recent evidence suggests that the lack of uninsured people is decreasing (Tolbert and Drake, 2023), a lack of coverage, alongside out-of-pocket co-payments/deductibles can influence care decision-making about what care is sought, including preventative care, and medication adherence (Agarwal et al., 2017, Dickman et al., 2017, Hoagland and Shafer, 2021, Hughes et al., 2023, Jiang et al., 2021). For example, research has shown doctors, and their patients use strategies to lower the cost of their care based around balancing their healthcare needs with their ability to pay (Hunter et al., 2016). These conversations existed even in those with health insurance. In fact, in Hunter et al.'s (2016) study, 37% of all observed consultations involved some discussion around the cost of care, which opened opportunities for conversations that centred around cost-saving strategies for insured and uninsured patients alike. The strategies that emerged included those that fundamentally changed people's care such as switching to lower-cost interventions and drugs, reducing the dose or frequency of a drug and stopping or withholding treatment altogether (Hunter et al., 2016).

Out-of-Pocket Healthcare Expenditure

Out-of-pocket health expenditure represents a significant burden in low-income countries, with the World Bank highlighting that those living in low-income countries spend half a trillion dollars each year on out-of-pocket healthcare costs (WorldBank, 2019) and 14% of the World's population experience catastrophic out-of-pocket healthcare expenses[1] (WHO, 2023c). This rate varies from household to household though and older households more commonly experience such expenses (WHO, 2023c).

In Figure 5.1, the first image (A) shows the incidence of catastrophic health expenditure at a 10% threshold. The second image (B) shows the incidence of catastrophic health expenditure at a 25% threshold.

Whilst there is some variation, low-income, resource-constrained countries typically have low per capita (per person) spending on healthcare. Governments generally lack the capacity to generate revenue, and poor and inequitable financing generally means that expenditure on health is not at the levels required to provide efficient and high-quality healthcare services for all citizens (WorldBank, 2019). As such, out-of-pocket expenditure on health is often significant, and the typically high and increasing cost of healthcare means that what must be self-funded is generally substantial, placing individuals and their families in situations of significant material and economic hardship (WorldBank, 2019). Catastrophic healthcare expenditure, through a lack of UHC often results in the world's poorest people, who carry the greatest burden of disease, forgoing healthcare altogether and the need to fund healthcare unexpectantly can push people and their families into poverty (Sapkota et al., 2020, Yadav et al., 2021, WorldBank, 2019). If people do not have readily available access to large amounts of cash, access to credit (through legal and illegal means) or can release capital through selling personal or family assets (Kruk et al., 2009, Murphy et al., 2020), they can be forced to either forgo care or consume lower levels of care than they need. In recognition that such community's needs are poorly met, various non-government organisations, charities and religious groups have come to be associated with providing care to those living in lower-income countries in leu of adequate state provision, particularly in more impoverished areas within these countries (Bhuiyan and Haque, 2024).

The UN's SDG (3.8.2) sets a target to reduce the proportion of the world's population facing large household expenditure on health in relation to total household income or expenditure and many countries are attempting to transition away from models where healthcare costs are primarily picked up through out-of-pocket expenses towards either state pooled public health expenditure (e.g. Bolivia and Brazil) or insurance funded provision (e.g. Ethiopia and Ghana) (Gabani et al., 2023). Financing for health is undergoing various transitions, especially in countries with improving economies. However, such transitions require significant long-term investment alongside a significant administrative effort to overhaul current private and largely out-of-pocket healthcare provision (Gabani et al., 2023, Reich et al., 2016, WHO, 2019). In addition, empirical work has found that simply increasing the number of people in a population who are meant to be protected by such schemes, or increasing the percentage of GDP invested in healthcare, does not necessarily correlate to real financial protection (Wagstaff et al., 2018). Learning from the countries that have been able to achieve UHC suggests that three important processes support this transition:

1. Political processes must act as an impetus to expand access to care for all citizens in an equitable way.

2. Income levels and spending on health must increase to make more services available for more people.

---

[1] Catastrophic healthcare expenditure reflects payments made towards health that are large relative to a household's income. There are various levels for which catastrophic spending on health is set and defined including in the UN Sustainable Development Goals – for example 10%, 25% and spending that exceeds 40% of non-food consumption (Wagstaff et al., 2018).

(a)

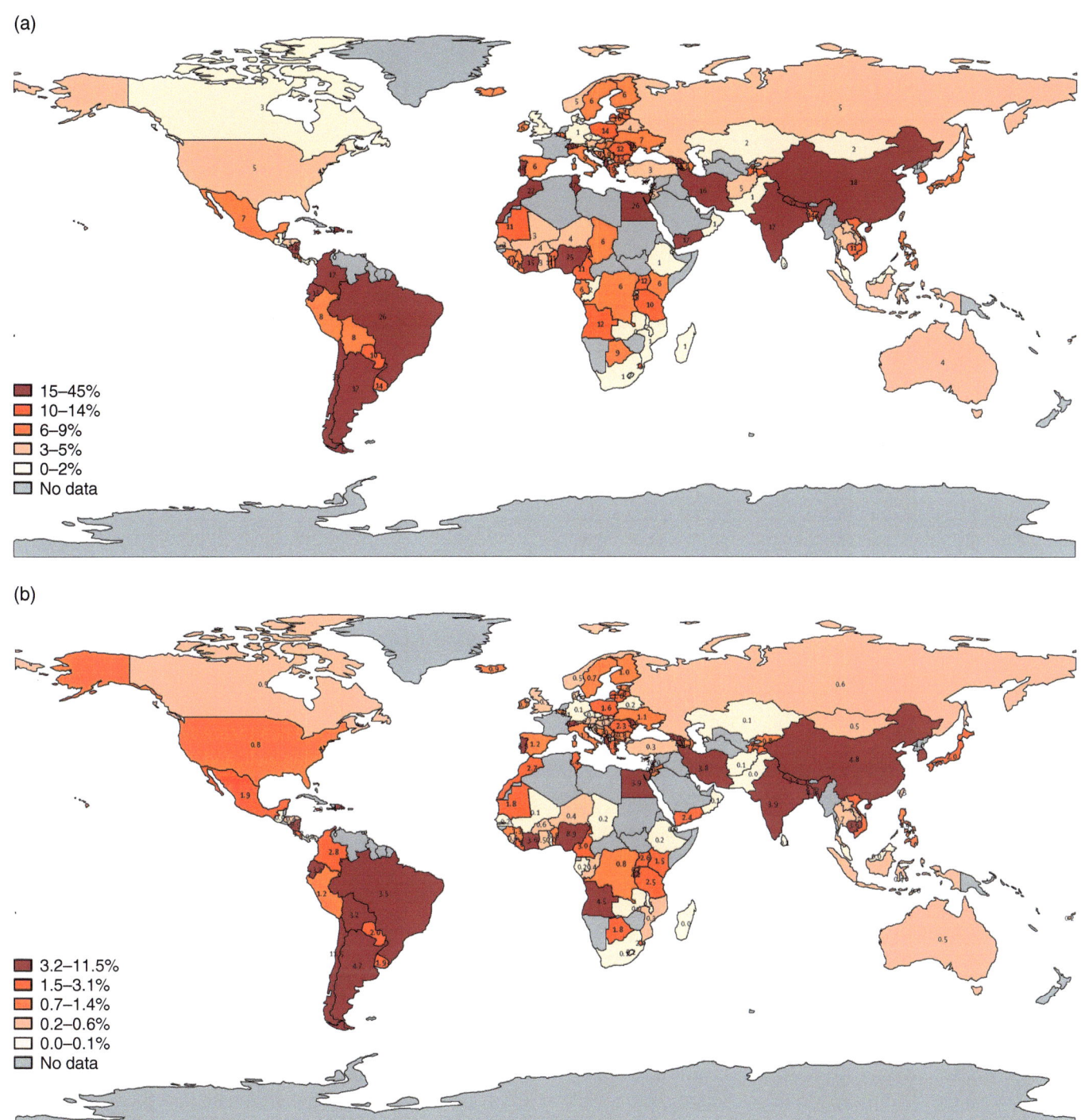

FIGURE 5.1   Global distribution of out-of-pocket expenditure on health. **Source:** Wagstaff et al. (2018)/Progress on catastrophic health spending in 113 countries: a retrospective observational study/Elsevier/CC by 4.0.

3. Increase in pooled health spending, as opposed to out-of-pocket spending.

(Savedoff et al., 2012)

Recent research looking at countries transitioning from largely out-of-pocket models to either tax-based (i.e. Beveridge) or Social Health Insurance (i.e. Bismarck) found that the greatest gains in relation to increases in life expectancy, decreases in

rates of under 5 mortality, and decreases in catastrophic healthcare-related expenditure, were seen in those adopting a primarily tax-funded (i.e. Beveridge) healthcare provision (Gabani et al., 2023). This is likely due to the increased costs associated with Social Health Insurance provision alongside its more limited health coverage (Gabani et al., 2023). However, measuring overall healthcare system effectiveness as we will now discuss, is tricky.

How Do We Measure Success and Why Should We?

There are several reasons why we might want to compare the performance of different healthcare systems. However, it is challenging to fairly compare different healthcare systems in a robust and meaningful way (Braithwaite et al., 2020, Papanicolas and Cylus, 2015). The way data is collected varies from system to system even sometimes within the same country, and can be incomplete, or not collected at all (Anandaciva, 2023, Papanicolas and Cylus, 2015, Smith et al., 2018). Outcomes that are used to judge health system performance (such as life expectancy) are often determined by things that exist wholly or largely outside of the healthcare system, such as people's general living and working conditions (Papanicolas and Cylus, 2015). Sometimes what in the United Kingdom is seen as social care is included in healthcare-related expenditure in other countries. This 'messiness' can result in data being misunderstood and then misused. Whilst acknowledging this, what follows is an overview (rather than an exhaustive list of indexes and measures) of some of the ways we can compare different healthcare systems.

Drawing comparisons with the various tools we have, can be useful because it can help countries to benchmark their performance with other comparable countries (often countries with similar resources and health-related challenges), which can help illuminate areas of a health system that work well (and that whilst acknowledging different social contexts may be useful to adopt), and those areas that may require improvement. International organisations, including many that we have already discussed, such as the WHO, the World Bank and the OECD, provide useful data and harmonisation to aid comparisons (Papanicolas and Cylus, 2015, Smith et al., 2018). We have provided some useful links in the box below.

Stop and Think: Where Can I Find This Data?

Before exploring a few examples in more depth, there are a few useful data sources to aid you in drawing comparisons of different outcomes between different healthcare systems that you might find useful.

World Health Organization and United Nations: Progress against United Nations Sustainable Development Goals (SDG)

Whilst UN SDG 3 specifically relates to health and well-being, many of the other 16 SDGs relate to social determinants of health, such as access to education (SDG 4). You can access information about the UN SDGs online (https://sdgs.un.org/goals). WHO publishes data online to show progress towards achieving these (https://www.who.int/data/gho/data/themes/sustainable-development-goals).

Comparisons are also provided in the World Health Statistics Report (WHO, 2024). In addition, you can find a range of other outcome measures, that allow you to compare health systems, on their Global Health Observatory (https://www.who.int/data/gho).

Organisation for Economic Cooperation and Development (OECD): Comparing health system performance at a glance

Provides data to help compare different aspects of performance across OECD countries. You can access this data online (https://www.oecd-ilibrary.org/social-issues-migration-health/health-at-a-glance-2023_7a7afb35-en)

Office for Health Improvement and Disparities: Public Health at Your Fingertips

Whilst you will see striking differences between countries, there are also often quite significant differences in health system performance even within countries. In England, the Office for Health Improvement and Disparities publishes data on a range of health-related outcomes. You can access this data online and use it to compare the health outcomes of different areas within England (https://fingertips.phe.org.uk).

So how can we compare healthcare systems to understand which aspects are performing well, and which aspects are performing poorly? First, we can draw comparisons in relation to what is put into **healthcare** systems. Levels of economic development in a country are generally linked to levels of spending on health (WHO, 2019). In terms of thinking about the amount that is invested in healthcare systems, two common approaches are used (Anandaciva, 2023). We can look at the amount a country spends as a percentage of its total GDP, and we can also look at the amount that is spent per person (i.e. per capita). Because GDP reflects the total value of a country's economy, 10% of GDP spent on healthcare in a high-income country looks radically different from 10% spent in a lower-income country, and therefore having access to the amount spent per person (i.e. per capita) helps to put this spending into context. What's more, there is often a lot of health-related 'work' (for example unpaid care) that sits outside of GDP and the extent of this work will vary from country to country (Pilling, 2019). As we highlighted earlier, around 10% of global GDP is spent on health, but there is a variance between countries, with lower-income countries spending less, and countries such as America spending far more (WHO, 2023a). OECD countries spend between 4% and 17% of GPD on health (OECD, 2023b). You might expect countries to spend more on health to achieve better outcomes, but this is not always consistently the case, and having UHC may be more important than spending a lot on health (Wagstaff et al., 2018, Wagstaff and Neelsen, 2020). In terms of spending and outcomes, America is a notable outlier, outspending everyone, whilst achieving worse outcomes than countries investing far less (Papanicolas et al., 2018, Scheider et al., 2021). In part, high costs can be explained by America having a particularly complex healthcare system, characterised by different financing arrangements, and a diverse market-place with a range of different buyers and providers resulting in higher prices for all (Papanicolas et al., 2018, Schneider et al., 2017, Scheider et al., 2021).

Spending also relates to what we are putting into a healthcare system in relation to resources such as people, estates and equip-ment. We might therefore be interested in how this spending relates to a system's available resources, for example, how many healthcare professionals the system employs, how many beds there are, as well as the availability of and investment in different types of technology, equipment and estate (OECD, 2023a, Anandaciva, 2023). Of course, investing lots of money into a health-care system, training and hiring appropriate levels of healthcare professionals, and investing in technology, equipment and estates does not necessarily translate into overall healthcare system performance, as these resources still need to produce **outcomes**.

Looking at outcomes allows us to consider what the healthcare system has been able to achieve. This helps us to build an understanding as to whether 'inputs' have had the desired impact on health outcomes. Healthcare system perfor-mance is multidimensional and because of this, there are many ways that performance can be considered. We can compare outcomes at micro (comparing the performance of individuals or teams), meso (comparing the performance of discrete parts of the healthcare system, such as different hospitals perfor-mance) and macro levels (comparing the performance of whole healthcare systems across countries).

In this section, we primarily focus on the macro-level comparisons that can be drawn between different healthcare systems. We can look at the performance-specific parts of a healthcare system (such as cancer screening rates, preventable COPD admissions, waiting times and inpatient length of stays), or by looking at the healthcare systems overall performance. In terms of overall performance, life expectancy, as well as treatable and preventable mortality rates are concrete outcomes that can be used to compare health system effectiveness (Anandaciva, 2023, Papanicolas and Cylus, 2015). However, whilst these may give some key indication as to a population's overall health, in the context of life expectancy and preventable ill health, it is not possible to unpick how much of this relates to healthcare system performance specifically, amongst the wider social determinants of health that mostly exist outside of the system, and for measures such as life expectancy, there is often significant variation within countries that is attributable to inequality, rather than specifically healthcare system performance (Anandaciva, 2023, Marmot et al., 2020, Papanicolas and Cylus, 2015). Mortality that is amendable to healthcare does help us focus more specifically on the healthcare system's performance, as this highlights where someone has died, but whose death could have been prevented through access to timely and effective healthcare (Anandaciva, 2023). However, most healthcare encounters do not involve much possibility of death, and most expect more

from their healthcare systems than simply helping them survive when they are critically unwell. It is therefore inappropriate to look at this outcome in isolation because countries also prioritise patient experience alongside other important things (Papanicolas and Cylus, 2015, Papanicolas et al., 2019).

Much of the data that we can use to compare different healthcare systems does require a degree of interpretation. Outcomes such as average length of stay may not be a fair way to make system-by-system comparisons. A lower-than-average length of stay may indicate a system that is providing highly effective care, but it might also reflect a healthcare system that discharges people too early, especially when these people then must be readmitted because they remain unwell, which is another health service outcome that is often looked at (Papanicolas and Cylus, 2015, Smith et al., 2018). Other considerations such as avoidable admissions, how long people wait for care and how safe care is when people can access it, are also potentially useful ways to consider the performance of different healthcare systems. However, this is not without caveats and cautions, because such data is rarely collected in a standardised way that allows for making clear comparisons. In the context of safety, high reporting levels may simply indicate health systems with good cultures around error reporting, where people are encouraged to openly talk from incidents and learn from them (we unpack this further in chapters 18 and 19), compared to systems with poorer cultures where incidents still occur, perhaps even more frequently, but are under-reported or even hidden; making safer systems look worse than unsafe systems (Howell et al., 2015).

So far, this discussion has concentrated on specific out-comes (e.g. life expectancy) and how these might be compared. But what about ranking health system performance as a whole? Already you might have some concerns about whether this is indeed possible. When Manchester City win the Premier League (or any other team, in any other league), it is because they have accumulated the highest total number of points across the sea-son, usually by winning the greatest number of games. They are being ranked on one obvious outcome- the total points they have accumulated across the season, and there is little debate about this being the most appropriate outcome to rank teams on. No one is calling for teams to be ranked on the total number of corners, or red cards in one season.

> ### Stop and Think: How Do We Measure Success?
>
> As we have shown, there are several outcomes that we can use to compare the effectiveness of different health-care systems.
>
> Take a moment to consider which outcomes you believe are most important. You can think about this in the con-text of your own healthcare system, or you might choose to think about it in the context of another healthcare system.
>
> What outcomes do you see as being most important and why?

How does this relate to your own values and norms, as well as the values and norms of your society?

How does this relate to your experience of what your own healthcare system tends to prioritise?

Do you see the need for priorities to change overtime, in response to changing population needs? If so, what changes do you anticipate?

As we have highlighted, no such outcome in health exists, and nor should it, because there are a lot of outcomes, and these are often captured in different ways, vary in importance across societies, and are affected by wider determinants that exist outside of the health system. Healthcare system performance is probably too complex to capture in this way. However, there have been attempts to compare a healthcare systems overall performance, that has sought to allow between-system comparisons. In 2000, the WHO completed its first and only global ranking of different countries' health performance, which unexpectedly placed France on top, and (at the time of war-torn) Sierre Leone on the bottom (WHO, 2000). The WHO ranking was controversial, and it was debated whether the available data could be used to create a single index to rank different healthcare system performances (Britnell, 2015). Which aspects of performance should carry the most weight? Smith et al. (2018), for example, highlight that the judgements made when making such decisions can sometimes feel very inappropriate, for example, noting that one such metric, the Euro Health Consumer Index (EHCI) places a greater value on short waiting times than survival rates.

Obviously, such an approach could allow for comparisons between overall system performance, but at the risk of losing the detail that allows us to see which aspects of a system a country does particularly well in. Whilst WHO continues to produce World Health Statistics, which includes performance against the UN SDGs, they have never repeated the activity of ranking overall healthcare system performance. However, as an exercise it prompted discourse, and others have followed with similar ranking efforts. Bloomberg, which is predominantly a financial and media outlet produces a regular ranking with more limited metrics – often related to life expectancy and absolute and relative per capita spending (Britnell, 2015, Miller and Lu, 2020). In addition, the Commonwealth Fund has produced rankings for 11 countries, with the United States of America consistently performing poorly, especially in relation to access, efficiency, equality and outcomes (Scheider et al., 2021). Whilst performing consistently poorly in other global rankings, America is rated number one in the Global Health Security Index which looks at health system preparedness (Bell and Nuzzo, 2021), highlighting that when ranking countries against one another, it really does matter what aspects of performance are used.

No one country has the perfect healthcare system. Arguably, most healthcare systems have aspects they perform well on (something to teach), as well as aspects that need to improve (something to learn) (Britnell and Edwards, 2014). Because healthcare systems are embedded within their respective societies, it is generally not appropriate, or desirable to overhaul a country's entire health system and draft an entirely new healthcare system, based on another country's 'blueprint'. However, by considering the needs of populations, through discourse and policy, health systems can evolve from their broad typologies, to provide a coverage that is equitable, effective and increasingly preventative.

Clinical Considerations

- Economics provides useful tools to think about the health gained through the consumption of different treatments, including in relation to cost. However, the decisions that fall out of Health Technology Assessments can be controversial because they shape what treatments people can access.

- Politics, the political process and societies more broadly shape the healthcare systems that we have, including what aspects of care are prioritised, how care is financed and how it is provided.

- In countries that lack universal health coverage, out-of-pocket healthcare expenditure can push people into poverty and can lead to people forgoing healthcare entirely, or receiving less healthcare than they need. This remains a problem for many people around the world. In some countries, healthcare professionals support people in making these difficult decisions.

- Assessing health system performance can be challenging, with data often being incomplete, or not collected in standardised ways that aid comparison between healthcare systems, even within the same country.

- Data that might indicate good performance (such as inpatient bed days) may actually hide poor performance (e.g. if people are discharged too early and immediately return to the hospital because they are still unwell). Data should be considered within the context it is collected, alongside other relevant outputs.

Conclusion

In this chapter, we have provided an overview of how health economics and the political economy can help us to understand the various ways governments can contribute to the health of their nations. You have also had the opportunity to consider the healthcare systems that are seen around the world, which has included consideration of the different ways healthcare is funded, who provides care and who receives care. The impact of universal health coverage has been discussed, as has the consequences to people when care is predominantly purchased through out-of-pocket expenditure. Finally, we closed this chapter by highlighting some of the ways health system performance has been measured, how these have allowed for making comparisons between different healthcare systems, and what we can learn from these comparisons alongside what we cannot.

References

Agarwal, R., Mazurenko, O. & Menachemi, N. 2017. High-deductible health plans reduce health care cost and utilization, including use of needed preventive services. *Health Affairs*, 36, 1762–1768.

Anandaciva, S. 2023. How does the NHS compare to the health care systems of other countries?

Baggot, R. 2015. *Understanding Health Policy*, Bristol: Policy Press.

Bambra, C., Fox, D. & Scott-Samuel, A. 2005. Towards a politics of health. *Health Promotion International*, 20, 187–193.

Bartley, M. 2017. *Health Inequality: An Introduction to Concepts Theories and Methods*, Cambridge Polity.

Bell, J. & Nuzzo, J. 2021. Global health security index: advancing collective action and accountability amid global crisis.

Besançon, S., Sidibé, A., Sow, D. S., Sy, O., Ambard, J., Yudkin, J. S. & Beran, D. 2022. The role of non-governmental organizations in strengthening healthcare systems in low- and middle-income countries: lessons from Santé Diabète in Mali. *Global Health Action*, 15, 2061239.

Bhuiyan, M. I. & Haque, A. 2024. Role of NGOs in providing available and affordable health care services to the slum people in Dhaka. *Clinical Epidemiology and Global Health*, 25, 101478.

Boniol, M., Kunjumen, T., Nair, T. S., Siyam, A., Campbell, J. & Diallo, K. 2022. The global health workforce stock and distribution in 2020 and 2030: a threat to equity and 'universal' health coverage? *BMJ Global Health*, 7, e009316.

Bowles, J., Clifford, D. & Mohan, J. 2023. The place of charity in a public health service: Inequality and persistence in charitable support for NHS trusts in England. *Social Science & Medicine*, 322, 115805.

Braithwaite, J., Tran, Y., Ellis, L. A. & Westbrook, J. 2020. Inside the black box of comparative national healthcare performance in 35 OECD countries: Issues of culture, systems performance and sustainability. *PLoS One*, 15, e0239776.

Brass, J. N., Longhofer, W., Robinson, R. S. & Schnable, A. 2018. NGOs and international development: a review of thirty-five years of scholarship. *World Development*, 112, 136–149.

Britnell, M. 2015. *In Search of the Perfect Health System*, Palgrave Macmillan.

Britnell, M. & Edwards, N. 2014. Something to teach, something to lead: global perspectives on healthcare.

Chen, A. & Goldman, D. 2016. Health care spending: historical trends and new directions. *Annual Review of Economics*, 8, 291–319.

Claxton, K., Martin, S., Soares, M., Rice, N., Spackman, E., Hinde, S., Devlin, N., Smith, P. & Sculpher, M. 2013. Methods for the estimation of the NICE cost effectiveness threshold.

Corbally, M. T. 2022. The role of registered charities in the delivery of global surgery in low- and middle-income countries - a personal experience. *The Surgeon*, 20, 41–47.

Dickman, S. L., Himmelstein, D. U. & Woolhandler, S. 2017. Inequality and the health-care system in the USA. *The Lancet*, 389, 1431–1441.

Feng, X., Kim, D. D., Cohen, J. T., Neumann, P. J. & Ollendorf, D. A. 2020. Using QALYs versus DALYs to measure cost-effectiveness: how much does it matter? *International Journal of Technology Assessment in Health Care*, 36, 96–103.

Flyn, C. 2018. Fees, funding and the NHS [Online]. Wellcome Collection Available: https://wellcomecollection.org/articles/WyjLYycAALyZnnTP [Accessed].

Fox, N. J. 2024. The critical (micro)political economy of health: a more-than-human approach. *Health*, 28, 22–39.

Freeman, R. & Frisina, L. 2010. Health care systems and the problem of classification. *Journal of Comparative Policy Analysis: Research and Practice*, 12, 163–178.

Gabani, J., Mazumdar, S. & Suhrcke, M. 2023. The effect of health financing systems on health system outcomes: a cross-country panel analysis. *Health Economics*, 32, 574–619.

Glied, S. & Smith, P. 2011. *The Oxford Handbook of Health Economics*, Oxford University Press.

Gotanda, H., Jha, A. K., Kominski, G. F. & Tsugawa, Y. 2020. Out-of-pocket spending and financial burden among low income adults after Medicaid expansions in the United States: quasi-experimental difference-in-difference study. *BMJ*, 368, m40.

Harvey, M. 2021. The political economy of health: revisiting its Marxian origins to address 21st-century health inequalities. *American Journal of Public Health*, 111, 293–300.

Hoagland, A. & Shafer, P. 2021. Out-of-pocket costs for preventive care persist almost a decade after the affordable care act. *Preventive Medicine*, 150, 106690.

Howell, A.-M., Burns, E. M., Bouras, G., Donaldson, L. J., Athanasiou, T. & Darzi, A. 2015. Can patient safety incident reports be used to compare hospital safety? Results from a quantitative analysis of the English national reporting and learning system data. *PLoS One*, 10, e0144107.

Hughes, D. R., Espinoza, W., Fein, S., Rula, E. Y. & Mcginty, G. 2023. Patient cost-sharing and utilization of breast cancer diagnostic imaging by patients undergoing subsequent testing after a screening mammogram. *JAMA Network Open*, 6, e234893–e234893.

Hunter, D. 2003. *Public Health Policy*, Cambridge: Polity Press.

Hunter, W. G., Zhang, C. Z., Hesson, A., Davis, J. K., Kirby, C., Williamson, L. D., Barnett, J. A. & Ubel, P. A. 2016. What strategies do physicians and patients discuss to reduce out-of-pocket costs? Analysis of cost-saving strategies in 1,755 outpatient clinic visits. *Medical Decision Making*, 36, 900–910.

Jiang, D. H., Mundell, B. F., Shah, N. D. & Mccoy, R. G. 2021. Impact of high deductible health plans on diabetes care quality and outcomes: systematic review. *Endocrine Practice*, 27, 1156–1164.

Jochelson, K. 2006. Nanny or steward? The role of government in public health. *Public Health*, 120, 1149–1155.

Koohi Rostamkalaee, Z., Jafari, M. & Gorji, H. A. 2022. A systematic review of strategies used for controlling consumer moral hazard in health systems. *BMC Health Services Research*, 22, 1260.

Kruk, M. E., Goldmann, E. & Galea, S. 2009. Borrowing and selling to pay for health care in low-and middle-income countries. *Health Affairs*, 28, 1056–1066.

Laberge, M. & Djiffa, K.-M. 2023. The effect of the affordable care act Medicaid expansion on consumer bankruptcies. *Bulletin of Economic Research*, 75, 1344–1361.

Liddell, J. L. & Lilly, J. M. 2022. Healthcare experiences of uninsured and under-insured American Indian women in the United States. *Global Health Research and Policy*, 7, 5.

Lohr, K., Brook, R., Kamberj, C., Goldberg, G., Leibowitz, A., Keesey, J., Roeboussin, D. & Newhouse, J. 1986. Use of medical care in the rand health insurance experiment RAND health insurance experiment series.

Manning, W., Newhouse, J., Duan, N., Keeler, E., Benjamin, B., Leibowitz, A., Marquis, M. & Zwanziger, J. 1988. Health insurance and the demand for medical care: evidence from a randomized experiment. RAND Health Insurance Experiment Series.

Marmot, M., Allen, J., Boyce, T., Goldblatt, P. & Morrison, J. 2020. Health equity in England: the marmot review 10 years on [Online]. The Health Foundation Available: https://www.health.org.uk/publications/reports/the-marmot-review-10-years-on [Accessed].

Mays, N. 2018. Health Care Systems. *In:* Scambler, G. (ed.) *Sociology as Applied to Health and Medicine*, Bloomsbury.

Meara, J. G., Leather, A. J., Hagander, L., Alkire, B. C., Alonso, N., Ameh, E. A., Bickler, S. W., Conteh, L., Dare, A. J. & Davies, J. 2015. Global Surgery 2030: evidence and solutions for achieving health, welfare, and economic development. *The Lancet*, 386, 569–624.

Miller, L. & Lu, W. 2020. Asia trounces U.S. in health-efficiency index amid pandemic [Online]. Bloomberg UK. Available: https://www.bloomberg.com/news/articles/2020-12-18/asia-trounces-u-s-in-health-efficiency-index-amid-pandemic [Accessed].

Mol, A. 2008. *The Logic of Care: Health and the Problem of Patient Choice*, Routledge.

Motaze, N. V., Chi, P. C., Ongolo-Zogo, P., Ndongo, J. S. & Wiysonge, C. S. 2021. Government regulation of private health insurance. *Cochrane Database of Systematic Reviews*.

Murphy, A., Palafox, B., Walli-Attaei, M., Powell-Jackson, T., Rangarajan, S., Alhabib, K. F., Avezum, A. J., Calik, K. B. T., Chifamba, J., Choudhury, T., Dagenais, G., Dans, A. L., Gupta, R., Iqbal, R., Kaur, M., Kelishadi, R., Khatib, R., Kruger, I. M., Kutty, V. R., Lear, S. A., Li, W., Lopez-Jaramillo, P., Mohan, V., Mony, P. K., Orlandini, A., Rosengren, A., Rosnah, I., Seron, P., Teo, K., Tse, L. A., Tsolekile, L., Wang, Y., Wielgosz, A., Yan, R., Yeates, K. E., Yusoff, K., Zatonska, K., Hanson, K., Yusuf, S. & Mckee, M. 2020. The household economic burden of non-communicable diseases in 18 countries. *BMJ Global Health*, 5, e002040.

NICE. 2012. The guidelines manual: assessing cost effectiveness [Online]. NICE. Available: https://www.nice.org.uk/process/pmg6/chapter/assessing-cost-effectiveness [Accessed].

OECD 2023a. *Health at a Glance 2023*, Organisation for Economic Co-operation and Development (OECD).

OECD 2023b. *Health Expenditure in Relation to GDP*, Organisation for Economic Co-operation and Development (OECD).

Or, Z., Cases, C., Lisac, M., Vrangbæk, K., Winblad, U. & Bevan, G. 2010. Are health problems systemic? Politics of access and choice under Beveridge and Bismarck systems. *Health Economics, Policy, and Law*, 5, 269–293.

Papanicolas, I. & Cylus, J. 2015. Comparison of Health Systems Performance. *In:* Kuhlmann, E., Blank, R., Bourgeault, I. & Wendt, C. (eds.) *The Palgrave International Handbook of Healthcare Policy and Governance*, Basingstoke: Palgrave Macmillan.

Papanicolas, I., Mossialos, E., Gundersen, A., Woskie, L. & Jha, A. K. 2019. Performance of UK National Health Service compared with other high income countries: observational study. *BMJ*, 367, l6326.

Papanicolas, I., Woskie, L. R. & Jha, A. K. 2018. Health care spending in the United States and other high-income countries. *JAMA*, 319, 1024–1039.

Pilling, D. 2019. *The Growth Delusion: The Wealth and Well-being of Nations*, Bloomsbury.

Rand, L. Z. & Kesselheim, A. S. 2021. Controversy over using quality-adjusted life-years in cost-effectiveness analyses: a systematic literature review. *Health Affairs*, 40, 1402–1410.

Reich, M. R. 2019. Political economy of non-communicable diseases: from unconventional to essential. *Health Systems & Reform*, 5, 250–256.

Reich, M. R., Harris, J., Ikegami, N., Maeda, A., Cashin, C., Araujo, E. C., Takemi, K. & Evans, T. G. 2016. Moving towards universal health coverage: lessons from 11 country studies. *Lancet*, 387, 811–816.

Ridhwan, M. M., Nijkamp, P., Ismail, A., Irsyad, M. & L. 2022. The effect of health on economic growth: a meta-regression analysis. *Empirical Economics*, 63, 3211–3251.

Sapkota, T., Houkes, I. & Bosma, H. 2020. Vicious cycle of chronic disease and poverty: a qualitative study in present day Nepal. *International Health*, 13, 30–38.

Savedoff, W. D., De Ferranti, D., Smith, A. L. & Fan, V. 2012. Political and economic aspects of the transition to universal health coverage. *The Lancet*, 380, 924–932.

Scheider, E., Shah, A., Doty, M., Tikkanen, R, Fields, K. & Williams, R. 2021. Mirror, mirror 2021: reflecting poorly: health care in the U.S. Compared to other high-income countries.

Schneider, E., Sarnak, D., Squires, D., Shah, A. & Doty, M. 2017. Mirror, mirror 2017: international comparison reflects flaws and opportunities for better U.S. Health care.

Simpkin, V., Namubiru-Mwaura, E., Clarke, L. & Mossialos, E. 2019. Investing in health R&D: where we are, what limits us, and how to make progress in Africa. *BMJ Global Health*, 4, e001047.

Smith, P., Karanikolos, M. & Cylus, J. 2018. Evolution of health system performance assessment: the roles of international comparisons and international institutions. *Eurohealth*, 24(2), 15–18.

Sommers, D., Maylone, B., Blendon, R., Orav, E. & Epstein, A. 2017. Three-year impacts of the affordable care act: improved medical care and health among low-income adults. *Health Affairs*, 36, 1119–1128.

Taylor, J., Forgeron, P., Vandyk, A., Finley, A. & Lightfoot, S. 2021. Pediatric health outcome evaluation in low-and middle-income countries: a scoping review of NGO practice. *Global Pediatric Health*, 8, 2333794X21991011.

Tolbert, J. & Drake, P. 2023. Key facts about the uninsured population [Online]. KFF. Available: https://www.kff.org/uninsured/issue-brief/key-facts-about-the-uninsured-population/#:~:text=The%20uninsured%20rate%20dropped%20in,to%202022%20(Figure%201). [Accessed].

Tuohy, C. H. & Glied, S. 2011. 58 The Political Economy of Health Care. *In:* Glied, S. & Smith, P. C. (eds.) *The Oxford Handbook of Health Economics*, Oxford University Press.

UN. 1990. Human development report united nations human development reports United Nations.

UN. 2016. Goal 3: ensure healthy lives and promote well-being for all at all ages [Online]. UN. Available: https://www.un.org/sustainable development/health/ [Accessed].

Van Der Zee, J. & Kroneman, M. W. 2007. Bismarck or Beveridge: a beauty contest between dinosaurs. *BMC Health Services Research*, 7, 94.

Wagstaff, A., Flores, G., Hsu, J., Smitz, M.-F., Chepynoga, K., Buisman, L. R., Van Wilgenburg, K. & Eozenou, P. 2018. Progress on catastrophic health spending in 133 countries: a retrospective observational study. *The Lancet Global Health*, 6, e169–e179.

Wagstaff, A. & Neelsen, S. 2020. A comprehensive assessment of universal health coverage in 111 countries: a retrospective observational study. *The Lancet Global Health*, 8, e39–e49.

Walker, S., Sculpher, M. & Drummond, M. 2012. The Methods of Cost-Effectiveness Analysis to Inform Decisions About the Use of Health Care Interventions and Programmes. *In:* Glied, S. & Smith, P. (eds.) *The Oxford Handbook of Health Economics*.

WHO. 2000. The world health report 2000.

WHO. 2019. Global spending on health: a world in transition [Online]. World Health Organization Available: https://iris.who.int/bitstream/handle/10665/330357/WHO-HIS-HGF-HF-WorkingPaper-19.4-eng.pdf?sequence=1 [Accessed].

WHO. 2023a. Global spending on health: coping with the pandemic.

WHO. 2023b. Tracking universal health coverage.

WHO. 2023c. Universal health coverage [Online]. World Health Organization. Available: https://www.who.int/news-room/fact-sheets/detail/universal-health-coverage-(uhc) [Accessed].

WHO. 2024. World health statistics 2024: monitoring health for the SDGs, sustainable development goals.

Wiseman, V. 2011. Key Concepts in Health Economics. *In:* Guinness, L. & Wiseman, V. (eds.) *Introduction to Health Economics*, Open University Press.

WORLDBANK. 2019. High-performance health financing for universal health coverage (Vol. 2): driving sustainable, inclusive growth in the 21st century.

Yadav, J., Menon, G. R. & John, D. 2021. Disease-specific out-of-pocket payments, catastrophic health expenditure and impoverishment effects in India: an analysis of national health survey data. *Applied Health Economics and Health Policy*, 19, 769–782.

Yazbeck, A. S., Savedoff, W. D., Hsiao, W. C., Kutzin, J., Soucat, A., Tandon, A., Wagstaff, A. & Chi-Man Yip, W. 2020. The case against labor-tax-financed social health insurance for low-and low-middle-income countries. *Health Affairs*, 39, 892–897.

Zajacova, A. & Lawrence, E. M. 2018. The relationship between education and health: reducing disparities through a contextual approach. *Annual Review of Public Health*, 39, 273–289.

Zhao, J., Zheng, Z., Nogueira, L., Yabroff, K. R. & Han, X. 2022. Preexisting condition protections under the affordable care act: changes in insurance coverage, premium contributions, and out-of-pocket spending. *Value in Health*, 25, 1360–1370.

CHAPTER 6

The Global Healthcare Workforce and the Social Science of HealthCare Professions

Assaf Givati[1] and Chris Allen[2]

[1]*Department of Population Health Sciences, King's College London, London, UK*
[2]*School of Health Sciences, University of Southampton, Southampton, UK*

Introduction

In the previous chapter, you considered healthcare systems. In this chapter, you will consider the workforce that provides healthcare within these systems and see how divisions of labour within this workforce are complex, changing and routed in history and social context. This chapter will introduce you to what it means to be a healthcare professional and what it means to be part of a healthcare profession. We will begin by considering the profile of the global healthcare workforce and building on the previous chapter, we will look at some of the challenges that the workforce is facing and the impact this has on healthcare services and delivery. With the emergence of new roles to meet increased global demand, we will look at some recent changes in healthcare professionals, and the need for specialisation, diversification and the substitution of work between roles.

We will also look at how the social sciences, and in particular sociology, studies professionals, examining some of the main sociological understandings and developments in the study of professions, specifically healthcare professions. Each professional group has a history and a context that has shaped what it is, who is able to practice and what their scope of practice is, as well as how the role fits within the overall healthcare system. This chapter is about you, and the interprofessional workforce you are either already a part of or will soon be joining. First, we will start by looking at the global healthcare workforce. A workforce that you are a part of.

LEARNING OUTCOMES

By the end of this chapter, you be able to:

- Recognise the current trends in the global healthcare workforce.
- Understand some of the challenges the current global healthcare workforce is facing.
- Recognise the impact of new healthcare professional roles on existing healthcare professional roles and how healthcare is delivered.
- Recognise the main sociological theories that have been used to understand professions, including the health professions, such as traits and functionalist approaches, neo-Weberian perspectives and new public management.
- Recognise the changing nature of professional practice and its various causes.

Social Sciences for Healthcare Professionals, First Edition. Edited by Chris Allen.
© 2026 John Wiley & Sons Ltd. Published 2026 by John Wiley & Sons Ltd.

The Global Healthcare Workforce

> ### Key Terms and Definitions
>
> **Profession:** The concept of profession is used to high-light what is distinct about different professional groups – that is, the characteristics that are unique to a 'profession'. (Evetts, 2003).
>
> **Professionalism:** This term captures the standards, practices or motivations that are associated with a profession – these are the main organising principles in service-related work (Evetts, 2003).
>
> **Professionalisation:** The concept of professionalisation refers to a process in which a certain occupation gains professional status through strategies that are used to achieve and maintain that status (Evetts, 2013).
>
> **Occupational closure:** The strategy used to obtain professional status and maintain the closure of the occupational group from external competitors in order to maintain own occupational self-interests in terms of money, power and status (Abbott, 1988, Larson, 1977).

The healthcare systems we discussed in the previous chapter are only able to function with an equitable and sustainable supply of competent healthcare workers (WHO, 2016). The global health-care workforce stock is expanding at a faster rate than the world's population (Boniol et al., 2022). However, growth relative to health need is not evenly experienced, with countries experiencing demographic transitions at different stages, resulting in different health needs experienced in different populations. With many countries' populations' growth slowing, or in fact shrinking, a key concern in wealthier countries is often not the size of the population, but the number of people in the older age categories relative to those in the younger age categories, and the increased demand for healthcare this is anticipated to bring. In contrast, some populations are still growing in number (such as many countries in Africa) but are not experiencing similar growth in their healthcare workforce to meet anticipated demand and achieve the Universal Health Coverage (UHC) that is already enjoyed by many wealthier nations (Boniol et al., 2022).

With these changing patterns of demand in mind, it is estimated that there is a current global healthcare worker shortage of 15.4 million, decreasing to around 10.2 million by 2030; though some areas are addressing this shortfall better than others (Boniol et al., 2022). The UN Sustainable Development Goals (3.c) makes a specific commitment to increasing the healthcare workforce, training and retention, especially in the least developed countries where stocks are most vulnerable (UN, 2016). The World Health Organization (WHO) maintains a list of countries with healthcare workforce vulnerabilities, in terms of UHC (WHO, 2023b). The list currently includes 55 countries, 37 of which are in Africa (WHO, 2023b), which is anticipated to experience around 50% of the total global healthcare worker shortfall by 2030 (Boniol et al., 2022). Overall, the global healthcare workforce is estimated to currently be around 65 million people (WHO, 2023a, Boniol et al., 2022). However, there is significant diversity in terms of the roles, professional status and organisation of healthcare workers from country to country and significant inequality in terms of supply (Boniol et al., 2022). For example, as shown in Figure 6.1, in high-income countries, 170 healthcare workers typically serve around 10,000 people, whereas in low-income countries, the same number of people are served by less than 30 healthcare workers (Boniol et al., 2022).

High-income countries have significantly greater availability of healthcare workers than middle- and low-income countries (Boniol et al., 2022). A map of the global distribution of healthcare workers is shown in Figure 6.2.

In contrast to the situation in Africa, within the European Union (EU), almost 7% of those in employment are employed in healthcare – with these mostly being medical doctors (13%), nurses and midwives (30%) (Eurostat, 2020). In the context of the United Kingdom, now falling outside of the EU, the healthcare workforce is unique in that healthcare is primarily provided

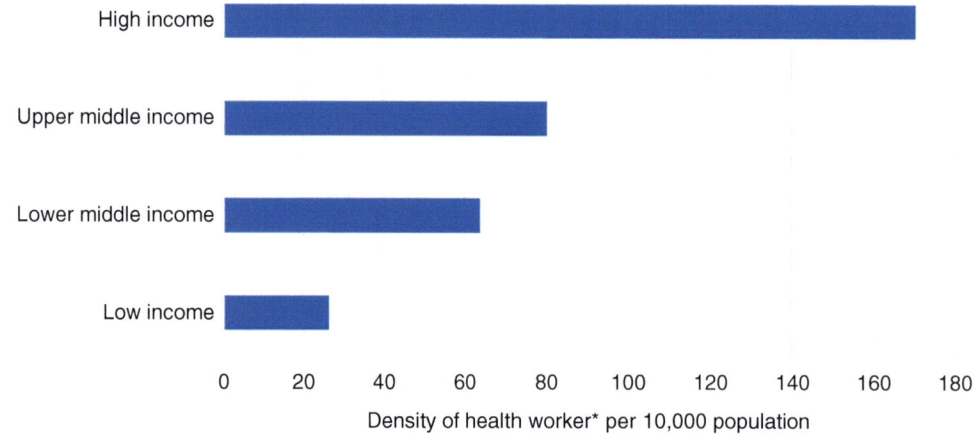

FIGURE 6.1 Density of health workers per 10,000 population in 2020 by income groups (includes medics, nurses, midwives and pharmacists).
Source: National Health Workforce Accounts Data Portal./with permission of the WHO.

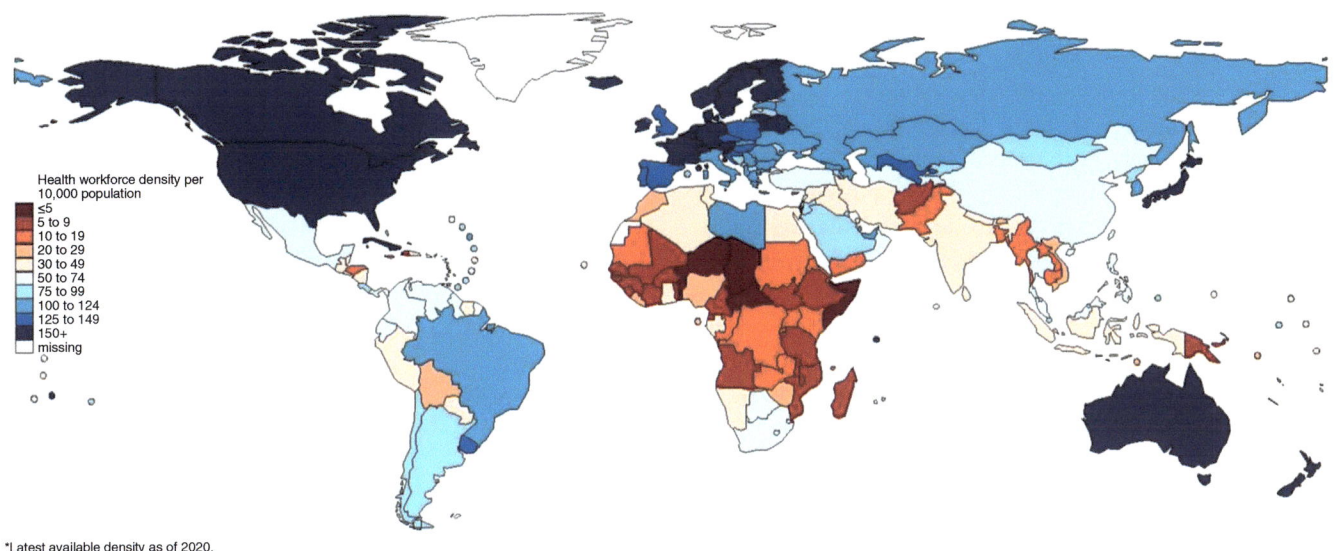

Health workforce density per 10,000 population
- ≤5
- 5 to 9
- 10 to 19
- 20 to 29
- 30 to 49
- 50 to 74
- 75 to 99
- 100 to 124
- 125 to 149
- 150+
- missing

*Latest available density as of 2020.
incl. medical doctors, nursing personnel, midwifery personnel, dentists, pharmacists

FIGURE 6.2   Map of health workers (including medical doctors, dentists, nurses, midwives and pharmacists) density per 10,000 of the population in 2020. **Source:** National Health Workforce Accounts Data Portal./with permission of the World Health Organization.

by one very large state-funded healthcare provider (the NHS), who employ most health workers, making it the largest employer in the country and one of the largest in the world (Rolewicz et al., 2024). More information about the NHS workforce is available in the House of Commons (2024) report 'The NHS workforce in England', but as a summary point, the NHS currently employs around 423,000 nurses and midwives and around 188,000 medical doctors, who combined makeup around 37% of the total NHS's workforce (Rolewicz et al., 2024). To put the NHS total workforce in a context, despite a widely documented workforce crisis (in part related to the country's aging population and the additional strain of the COVID-19 pandemic), its workforce looks relatively large (1.4 million people), when compared to the total number of healthcare workers (3.6 million) providing care to 47 countries in Africa (Ahmat et al., 2022).

But how valid is this comparison? Comparing the workforce of different countries and cultures can be challenging, not least because healthcare needs, the value and importance placed on different roles and the role of wider society in supporting and promoting health varies from place to place. The composition of healthcare workers can look very different from country to country. For example, the total number and density of healthcare workers in Africa looks comparably small – which it certainly is. However, these figures do not include practitioners of Traditional, Complementary and Alternative Medicine (TCAM), who are heavily utilised in many parts of the world, including many parts of Africa (Burki, 2023, WHO, 2013). The most recent ICD (ICD-11) covers traditional medicine in recognition that it forms the basis of the healthcare that many people are able to access in their communities, even being integrated within conventional health services in some countries, and possibly even having a role in countries working towards UHC (Burki, 2023).

Many countries have their own traditional or indigenous forms of healing, such as Chinese medicine, Ayurveda (a traditional system of Indian medicine) or Unani (also known as Tib

or Arabic medicine practices in South Asia). These 'traditional' or 'alternative' forms of medicine are themselves rooted in their countries' culture and history, much like medicine and nursing are in western societies and are often formally embedded into local healthcare systems (Bodeker et al., 2005, Burki, 2023, WHO, 2013). Many of these forms of healing have significant global popularity, including in the global north, and are joined by European and North American originating TCAM that were established between the late 1700s and late 1800s such as herbalism, chiropractic, homeopathy, naturopathy and osteopathy which are also extensively utilised worldwide (Burki, 2023, James et al., 2018, Şenel, 2019).

Globalisation and Brain Drain Amongst Healthcare Professionals

As we have highlighted, wealthier nations, including those in Europe are better supplied with healthcare professionals. Globalisation has created an increasing concern with the unequal global distribution of healthcare professionals, and overt strategies from wealthier nations, including the United Kingdom, to recruit trained healthcare professionals from other countries, typically low- and middle-income countries, who themselves have few healthcare workers, in what is often

---

Stop and Think: Would You Migrate?

Would you migrate to a different country?

What factors would contribute to you migrating to another country and how important are these to your decision?

What work-related considerations would you take into account?

referred to as a 'brain drain' (Johnson et al., 2014, Kamarulzaman et al., 2022, Misau et al., 2010, Yuksekdag, 2018).

The reasons behind the motivation to migrate are described as 'push' and 'pull' factors (Kline, 2003, Mej'ia et al., 1979). Typically, push factors are present in donor countries (i.e. pushing/encouraging people out of these countries), whilst pull factors relate to the receiving countries (i.e. luring people towards these countries). Common economic push factors include low pay, high unemployment and high taxes; whilst other push factors may be inadequate healthcare systems, high crime rate, violent conflict or famine, alongside a broader range of social factors such as gender inequalities, ethnic and racial discrimination, poor social rights, and religious conflicts (Hajian et al., 2019). Contrasting this, economic pull factors often include the high demand for labour, comparatively higher wages, a stronger economy and lower costs of living (Simpson, 2022). Non-economic pull factors include better amenities such as healthcare, family and friends already living in the receiving country, cultural and language similarities, as well as human rights and freedoms (Simpson, 2022).

Adovor et al. (2021), who analysed the brain drain of medical doctors, suggested that the sensitivity to such push and pull factors is often governed by more nuanced factors such as linguistic (i.e. speaking the same language), cultural and geographic ties between countries, immigration policies and visa restrictions, recognition of qualifications and the option of obtaining a permanent residential status in the host country. A study by Botezat and Ramos (2020) suggested that doctors from different nationalities are drawn by different pull factors – with some focussing on income, whereas others being more concerned with the quality of healthcare services, technologies and access to high-quality education for their children. So, whilst the decision to migrate is often based on individual personal circumstances and needs, macro-level factors generally also play a role in making certain countries more or less desirable to work in.

Gender Inequalities and Healthcare Professionals

One of the main sociological concepts, and central to our understanding of public health, is social stratification which explains differences between demographic groups commonly associated with socioeconomic gradients, based on factors like wealth, income, race, education, power and gender (Nancarrow and Borthwick, 2021a). This perspective is important to the profile of the healthcare workforce around the world. For example, most health workers around the world are women, and over one-third are over 50 years old (Eurostat, 2020, McIsaac et al., 2022, WHO, 2022). Whilst women account for 67% of the global waged healthcare workforce, gender inequality has been a significant issue for the sector for some time, particularly in relation to respect, pay and rank (Boniol et al., 2019, McIsaac et al., 2022). For example, it is estimated that around three-quarters of leadership roles in the sector are held by men, whilst women also earn approximately 20% less (McIsaac et al., 2022).

The Global Healthcare Professional Workforce Crisis

For various reasons, there is an increasing need for healthcare professionals. These include a combination of social, economic, political and geographical forces at global, regional and national levels. Demographic changes like aging and growing populations and growing social and health inequalities between and within countries are significant influences. As is the continued impact of global warming, which is disproportionately felt by some of the world's poorest people, the impact of COVID-19, alongside the continued threat posed by other infectious diseases, which has further exacerbated the need for healthcare workers, whilst also negatively impacting on the current workforce (Poon et al., 2022). Global economic instability, and the continued impact of wars and violent conflicts, causing mass forced displacement around the world, has also played a part (Glassman et al., 2023). These needs are significant and enduring, leading to varying degrees of workforce shortages to meet populations' needs around the world.

These challenges and ongoing workforce shortages impact negatively on current healthcare workers. Many healthcare systems are struggling to recruit and retain healthcare professionals, which significantly impacts the mental health and well-being of the existing workforce (Figueroa et al., 2019, WHO, 2020). Within the nursing workforce of around 29 million globally (Boniol et al., 2022), working conditions are often poor, toxic behaviours are common, and stress is often high, impacting negatively on job satisfaction, intention to stay, burnout and general health (Bailey, 2021, Chemali et al., 2019, Dall'Ora et al., 2020, Dubale et al., 2019, House Of Commons, 2021). During the pandemic, working conditions were particularly challenging and involved an intensification of job stress, workload and infection risks, alongside increased expectations to be 'resilient' heroes (Einboden, 2020, Ghahramani et al., 2021, Leo et al., 2021, Poon et al., 2022, Steege and Rainbow, 2017). A much-cited systematic review and meta-analysis by Galanis et al. (2021) suggests that the prevalence of emotional exhaustion amongst nurses during the pandemic was 34%, with 12% of nurses struggling with depersonalisation, and 15% feeling a lack of personal accomplishment, all signs associated with burnout, and others have noted similar trends (Dall'Ora et al., 2020).

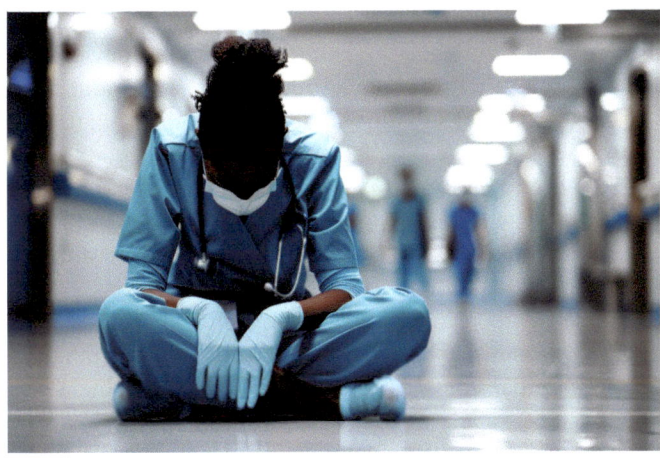

Source: id512/Adobe Stock Photos.

Who Are Healthcare Professionals?

Whilst we have been using the term 'professional', it is relevant to think about who we are referring to when we use the term 'healthcare professional', as opposed to simply someone who works in healthcare, or a 'healthcare worker'. This question has been the subject of ongoing debate amongst sociologists and other social

scientists for quite some time (Abbott, 1988, Evetts, 2013, Freidson, 1970, Johnson, 1972, Larson, 1977, Saks, 2016). As a question, its answer matters for several reasons. For example, much of what we study in the social sciences and sociology is how people interact with others, and how they interact in and with groups at all levels of society. In this context understanding the role of professions in society is important because it affects how healthcare is organised, the challenges it faces and the relationships that take place between healthcare professionals and users of health services, as well as other parts of our society.

> **Stop and Think: Which Healthcare Workers Are Healthcare Professionals?**
>
> Looking at the following list of paid healthcare workers, which of these occupations would you describe as 'healthcare professionals'?
>
> | | |
> |---|---|
> | Nurses | Caretakers |
> | Midwives | Social workers |
> | Surgeons | Cleaners |
> | Acupuncturists | Receptionists |

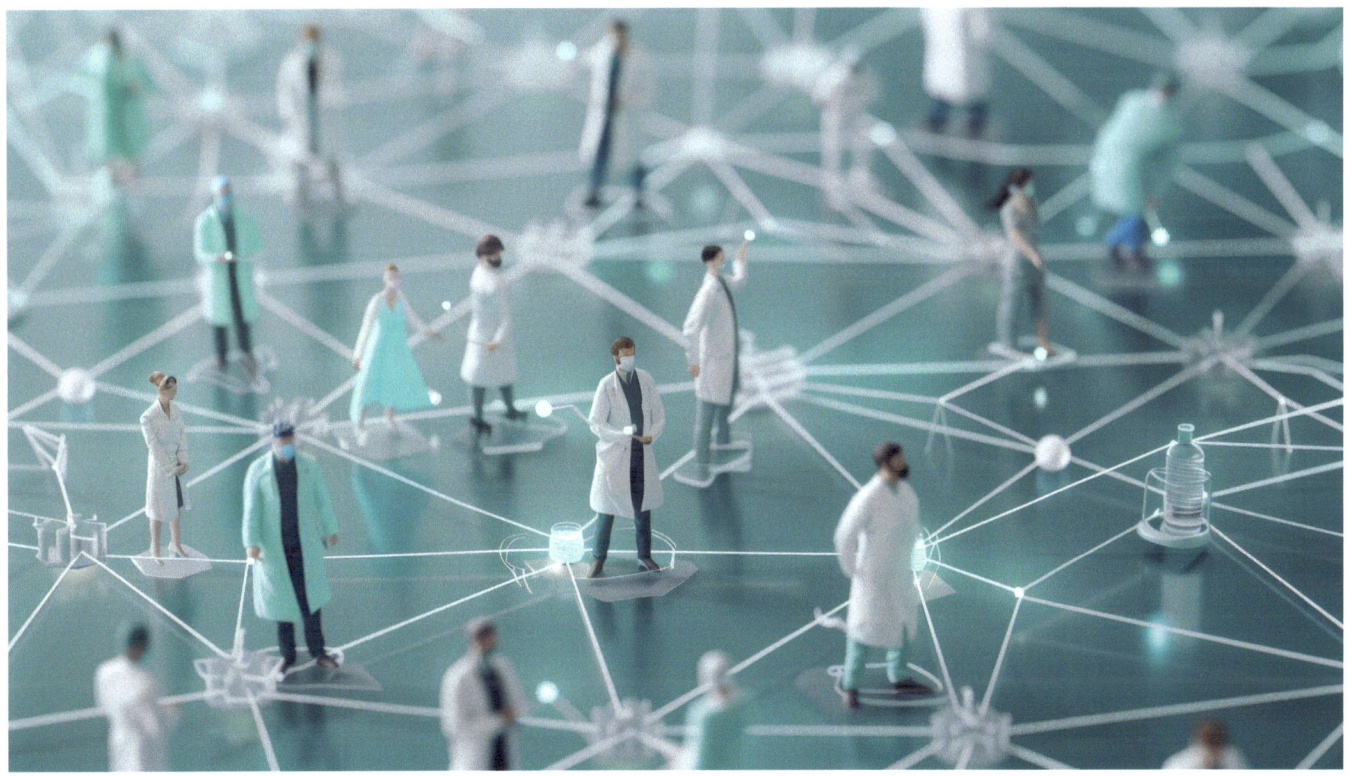

Source: Johannes/Adobe Stock Photos.

Physiotherapists	Pharmacists
Healthcare assistants	Psychologists
Podiatrists	Psychotherapists
Osteopath	Acupuncturist
Optometrists	Physician associates
Play therapists	Anaesthesia associates
Advanced care practitioners	Nursing associates
Cardiac physiologists	Chiropractor
Physio-assistant	Social prescribers

Whilst you might have identified some professionals within the above roles, there were probably also a few you were not sure of. The answer here is not straightforward.

New Healthcare Professionals

In many healthcare systems, the challenges that we have discussed have resulted in the need for increased flexibility between professional groups and their jurisdictions (WHO, 2008). Whilst not a new phenomenon, where skills shortages exist, new or sometimes existing professions are increasingly being used to plug gaps in service provision (Drennan et al., 2017, Larkin, 1983, Nancarrow and Borthwick, 2005, Timmons et al., 2023).

In western and industrialised healthcare systems in particular, and in part due to the workforce challenges we have just discussed, there has been a recent diversification of the workforce, including the emergence of several new healthcare roles, and an increase in the number of support worker roles (Drennan et al., 2017, Timmons et al., 2023, Traynor et al., 2015). In the context of the United Kingdom specifically, roles such as support workers, assistant practitioners, physician and anaesthetic associates and social prescribers (see chapter 17), have joined the healthcare workforce, alongside the shift of existing professional groups (such as nurses, pharmacists and occupational therapists) into 'Advanced Clinical Practice' roles (Timmons et al., 2023).

The emergence of new professional roles within healthcare systems with embedded existing roles is often associated with tension, role ambiguity, encroachment and challenges to professional boundaries, alongside concern around role substitution (Drennan et al., 2017, Nancarrow and Borthwick, 2005, Nancarrow and Borthwick, 2021a, Thompson and McNamara, 2022, Timmons et al., 2023). This is because healthcare professionals work within an interdependent system (Abbott, 1988), where changes to an existing occupation's remit, or the emergence of a brand-new occupation altogether, impacts on other work groups within the system (including in relation to jurisdictions, power, status, etc.). The emergence of new roles also brings about challenges in terms of identity, and understanding what new roles are, how they are defined, how they are regulated and how they relate to other established professionals (nurses, doctors, etc.) in terms of their scope of practice and relationships (Drennan et al., 2017, Thompson and McNamara, 2022, Timmons et al., 2023, Nancarrow and Borthwick, 2005, Nancarrow and Borthwick, 2021a, Traynor et al., 2015). In the case of Advanced Clinical Practice, whose members come from multiple existing professions, several interesting questions have been posed in recent work (Timmons et al., 2023), for example is Advanced Clinical Practice:

- A level of practice or a new role relating to already established professions (such as nursing, physiotherapy, etc.)?
- Or,
- A profession in its own right?

The complex challenges most healthcare systems around the world currently face, does require flexibility, either through the creation of new roles or through increased diversification and specialisation within existing roles, alongside 'vertical' and 'horizontal' substitution between professions (i.e. one profession taking on the tasks more traditionally associated with the role of another profession) (Nancarrow and Borthwick, 2005). First, diversification and specialisation involve the expansion of boundaries within a profession; with diversification reflecting that the whole professions remit has increased, whereas specialisation generally involves a subsection of the professions remit changing (i.e. becoming more narrow, and 'specialised') (Nancarrow and Borthwick, 2005).

Substitution on the other hand involves the movement of professional tasks outside of traditional boundaries. Vertical substitution allows higher-status professions to actively discard less wanted/desirable work/tasks to lower-status professions, who either have little choice but to accept these changes due to their lower status/standing or who are willing to accept these, in order to achieve a higher status themselves (Nancarrow and Borthwick, 2005). These changes are particularly visible within the new roles just discussed. For example, nurse prescribing within an Advanced Clinical Practice role is an example of vertical substitution, with nursing staff taking on tasks that were once exclusively within the domain of medicine (Kroezen et al., 2012, Timmons et al., 2023). It is 'vertical', because nursing and medicine have traditionally had very different levels of status and power. Nurses have also shredded some of their tasks, to roles that are subordinate to them, for example, nursing associates and healthcare assistants (Traynor et al., 2015). 'Horizontal substitution' in contrast, occurs when tasks are shared between occupational groups with similar status; for example, when an occupational therapist takes on some tasks that were once performed by a nurse. A summary of these different ways the work tasks of the healthcare workforce can shift and move around different groups is shown in Figure 6.3.

Sociological Explanations in the Study of Healthcare Professionals

The sociology of professions, sometimes called the theory of professions, has a long and nuanced history (Pekkola et al., 2018, Saks, 2016). Within the scope of this chapter, we cannot explore all the debates and theories that relate to professions. A useful overview tracking how key debates and theories have evolved over time is provided by Saks (2016). Many of these are underpinned by many of sociologies grand theories, including those that were introduced in chapter 2, such as functionalism, conflict theory and symbolic interactionism (Pekkola et al., 2018, Saks, 2016). In this section, we will outline the main sociological explanations of the nature and development of professions from an Anglo-American viewpoint, where much of the sociology of professions work has occurred, with concrete reference to the *healthcare professions*. We start first with trait and functionalist ways of thinking, before then moving onto neo-Weberian contributions. We will then briefly consider later discussions around *de-professionalisation* and *new public management*.

According to the sociologist of the professions, Julia Evetts, three central concepts to the study of professions are *profession*, *professionalism* and *professionalisation* (Evetts, 2013). The concept of *profession* relates to the distinct characteristics of one profession compared to others. For example, a nurse has distinct characteristics that set them apart from an occupational therapist. The term *professionalism* captures the standards, practices or motivations associated with a particular profession (Evetts, 2003) and is rather complex to define. Evetts (2013) suggests that an 'optimistic view' of professionalism reflects the way professions create and maintain distinct professional values and moral obligations that encourage cooperation as well as practitioner pride and satisfaction in their work. This serves as internal self-regulation within a profession and is unique to that profession. Finally, the concept *professionalisation* refers to the processes that enable an occupation to gain the status of a '*profession*'. This includes, for example, the strategies that are used by those within the profession to achieve and maintain professional status; as well as the relationships between professionals and their clients, other occupational groups, the government and other institutions (Abbott, 1988, Freidson, 1970, Johnson, 1972, Larson, 1977).

Early sociological interest in healthcare professionals mainly related to the medical profession, reflecting concern about biomedicine (introduced in chapter 3) and the way the medical profession was perceived to have asserted its dominance and authority, both over populations, but also over other therapies and practices (Saks and Lee-Treweek, 2020). Over time, work examining the medical profession was joined by work on health and care occupations, and the recognition that many of these were becoming more organised, regulated and formal and hence 'professionalised', such as nurses and midwives, social workers, dietitians, pharmacists, radiographers, physiotherapists, paramedics, optometrists and speech and language therapists (Abrahams et al., 2019, Cant and Sharma, 1998, Givati and Hatton, 2015, Givati et al., 2018, Kunnemann, 2005,

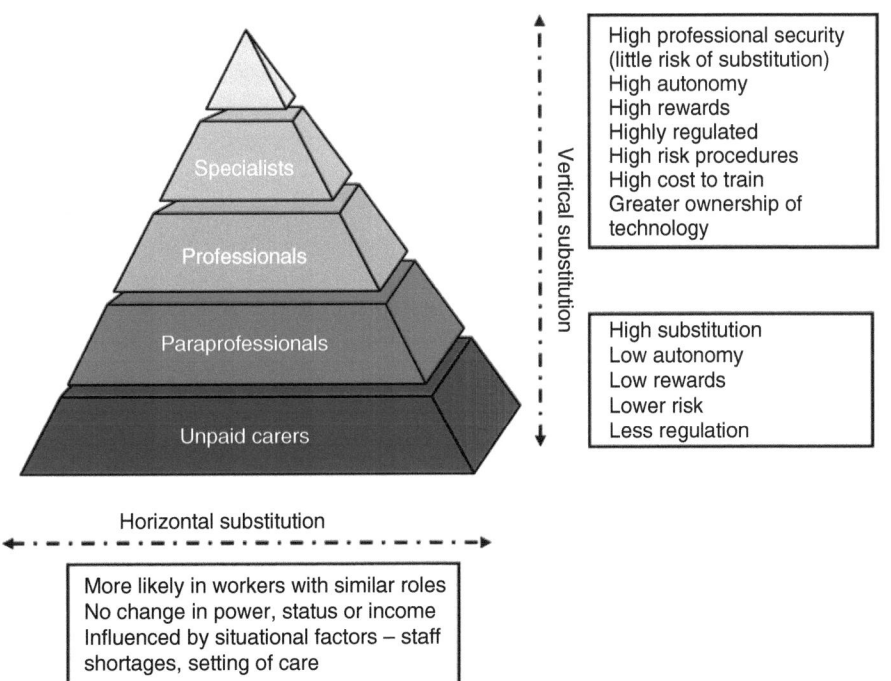

FIGURE 6.3   The influence of vertical and horizontal task substitution between healthcare workers. **Source:** Nancarrow, SA., and Borthwick, AM (2005)/Dynamic professional boundaries in healthcare workforce./with permission of John Wiley & Sons.

Nancarrow and Borthwick, 2021b, Saks, 1995, Snell et al., 2020, Timmons, 2011, Witz, 1990).

The Functionalist Perspective and the Traits Approach

Early studies into the professions, tended to focus on the way 'elite' professions such as medicine and law were perceived as being different from other occupations based on their unique functions within society. Traits theorists essentially sought to distinguish 'professional work' from 'work', and 'professions', from 'workers', etc., based on a list of traits (Barber, 1963, Goode, 1957, Greenwood, 1957, Millerson, 1964). Whilst there's a lack of consensus as to which traits are most important, common ones have included:

- **Altruistic orientation to work:** Wanting 'to do good' and 'make a difference' within a society.
- **Shared ethical codes, morals and values:** Such as having an ethical code of practice/conduct, or a shared set of values with others in the profession (as healthcare professions do).
- **Specialised knowledge:** Having knowledge that is not available to others in a society, such as the knowledge that is gained through your professional healthcare education.
- **Formal, lengthy training:** Similar to the educational programmes you are currently taking, or have already taken. Often within these programmes, there are assessments that are used to test if you have acquired the necessary knowledge to enter the profession. Credentials also provide the public with assurance that you have met a required standard and are safe to practice.
- **Internal organisation:** Having some type of regulatory organisation that oversees a profession, its activities and often who controls entry into the profession (such as the Nursing and Midwifery Council, General Medical Council or Health and Care Professions Council in the United Kingdom).

The traits and functions approach was developed in the context of the functionalist theoretical paradigm, which was largely influenced by the seminal work of Talcott Parsons (1951), who we introduced to you in chapter 2. At the centre of the functionalist perspective was the question of how society achieves social stability and, as part of it, functionalists assumed that professions such as medicine, law and engineering, alongside their associated institutions, played a vital and irreplaceable role in meeting the functional needs of society. Because of this, societies granted these professions significant status, economic rewards and privileges, in return for their highly specialised and much-needed knowledge, skills and high moral values (Saks, 2016).

Trait and functionalist perspectives generally adopted a positive take on professions, specifically in seeing 'elite' professions, as vital to the smooth functioning of society.

However, we know that different professions hold different positions of power and status in society, and it is important to understand the social and political contexts that saw professions like medicine, obtain such significant power in the first place (Evetts, 2013, Saks, 1995), which was the essence of the work of neo-Weberian scholars, discussed next.

Neo-Weberian Perspectives: The Monopoly and Power of the Professions

Considerable attention has been paid to the different societal and professional status obtained by health professions (Adams, 2015, Saks, 2015). Saks (2015) for example, highlights that professions can be:

- **Dominant:** Where they hold significant status, alongside power over other professional groups. An example of a traditionally dominant group is medicine.
- **Marginalised:** Where they have less status and are subordinated to higher-status professional groups, but still maintain state-protected titles. An example of a traditionally marginalised group is nursing.
- **Marginal:** These are typically unregulated groups, with no state-protected title, such as those from traditional and complementary medicine, who may be sidelined from mainstream healthcare provision entirely.

Medicine is a well-cited example of a dominant profession within healthcare. As the first formally regulated healthcare profession and one that has historically enjoyed lots of status and power, it gets a lot of critique from the neo-Weberian perspective. Whilst other forms of healing have existed for centuries (including traditional and complimentary healing), in the 19th century, medicine was able to secure its monopoly as a formally recognised healthcare profession, and through its new power, was able to determine who was sick, and who was not, through its main technology – *medical diagnosis*. Following on from the influential work of Max Weber (1864–1920), Neo-Weberian perspectives take a more critical view of professions than that offered by the traits and functionalist perspectives (Saks, 2016), but do offer valuable insights into how professions are able to gain power, and gain exclusive access to aspects of health and healthcare, through social *closure*. In this process, an aspiring occupational group can use its status and influence to obtain and then sustain its privileged position in society, whilst excluding others from gaining similar status and power (Macdonald, 1995). The impact of this closure is essentially state-sanctioned occupational monopolies that arise through a process of social closure, which is a social process of closing the profession to those not meeting the conditions imposed by the professions members (Saks, 2016). The main features of social closure are:

- **A formal university education system, or credentialism:** These give those who attend knowledge that is difficult for others to obtain.

- **Monopoly and maintaining an exclusive pool of clients:** This is gained through practices that make other occupational groups inferior, or even taking action to remove competing occupations altogether. This process often involves some degree of state legislation, mandating who can/cannot join certain professional groups and who can do what within different professions.
- **Maintaining control and autonomy:** Discretion over the nature of work and how work is conducted and carried out.

(Freidson, 1984, Larson, 1977, Larson, 1980)

The neo-Weberian perspective, rather than assuming that elite professions like medicine are driven by altruism and selfless concern for the well-being of others, instead sees professional traits as an occupational closure technique (Macdonald, 1995, Saks, 2016, Turner, 1995). This approach, therefore, assumes that professionalisation is a process related to self-interest, that involves restricting access to the occupational group whilst creating a clear delineation between 'insiders' (members of the group) and 'outsiders'. This ensures that those already within the group can maintain the status, political power and financial advantages that they enjoy through credentialism and protected title (Abbott, 1988, Larson, 1977), thus ensuring market conditions continue to favour the profession. For example, if everyone was able to enter the profession of medicine, there would be less need for medics. A more limited supply of medics, on the other hand, increases the

economic rewards and status of those medics. This neo-Weberian perspective has become a dominant way to think about professions, allowing professions to be considered within the societies in which they are embedded, and often provides a very tangible lens through which we can make inferences about whether a workgroup is a profession in its own right (Saks, 2016).

Occupational Closure and the Medical Profession

We will now expand on some of the criticism that has been directed at the profession of medicine. This discussion aims to get you to think critically about medicine as a profession, amongst the other healthcare professions, and consider the historical context, political power and dominance that have shaped its status and its position over time; allowing it significant impact over other healthcare professions and patients. Eliot Freidson (1923–2005) suggested that we can understand the medical profession through occupational closure (Freidson, 1970, Freidson, 1984). In other words, he argued that the medical profession controls and defines medical knowledge, as well as who can obtain this knowledge, using the strategies we have just discussed, to gain a monopoly over medical knowledge and medical practice. In addition, Freidson argued that medicine was able to place other professions such as nursing, midwifery, pharmacy, physiotherapy and other healthcare occupations into *subordinate* positions, whereby these professions primarily fulfilled roles and tasks delegated to them by the medical profession (Crinson, 2018, Saks, 1995). In the context of the United Kingdom, in particular, the medical profession has traditionally had a lot of power to determine the remit and scope of practice of other groups (Larkin, 1983). Medical dominance has been quite influential in shaping not only the profession of medicine but also other professions within the UK healthcare system.

The history of medicine as a profession gives some clues as to how this power and status was obtained. For example, whilst being far from the only type of healing at the time (e.g. traditional and complementary forms also existed), through the state-supported formation of the American Medical Association (AMA) in 1847, and the passing of the Medical Act in the United Kingdom in 1858, medical doctors obtained monopoly over medical practice (Saks and Lee-Treweek, 2020). Through this, the profession established a unified medical profession which won exclusive rights to the title 'doctor', and held a register of the professions' practitioners, which provided the basis for self-regulation (Saks and Lee-Treweek, 2020). The boundary placed around the profession through social closure techniques, especially prior to the formalisation of other healthcare professions, led to the upward social mobility of the medical profession, increasing medicines market control and position, and

---

A Professional Ecology: How This All Fits Together

Let's take nursing as one example. A student nurse in the United Kingdom, will be enrolled in an education programme, and because of government policy changes (i.e. project 2000), this programme will be a degree at a higher education institution (Le Var, 1997). The quality of the programme, and what is being taught as part of it are overseen by a professional regulator, in this case the Nursing & Midwifery Council (NMC, 2023), which gains its power and status from the government (in this case through the Nursing and Midwifery Order 2001) (UK Government, 2019). Students, as part of their programme, need to work in clinical settings, and many students will also belong to a learning society, or workers union such as in the United Kingdom the Royal College of Nursing (RCN) that is attached to that profession, and often carries significant influence over policies relating to the profession. Most professions, especially in the context of health, have their own internal ecology like this, which involve many institutions involved in shaping who is in the profession, the knowledge and skills those in the profession have and what their scope of practice (or jurisdiction) is. All of this highlights a profession that is formal, organised and regulated.

enhancing the income, status, power and prestige of those carrying the title of doctor (Parry and Parry, 1977). From this privileged position, the medical profession was able to regulate and bring under their control other areas of healthcare, including influencing the regulation of other healthcare groups (Saks and Lee-Treweek, 2020). The professionalisation of allied health occupations that followed has been argued to be characterised by *subordination* and *limitation* (Turner, 1995). In the United Kingdom for example, this meant, that midwifery, through the Midwives Act in 1902, and nursing, through the Nursing Registration Act, 1919 and later during 1960 (through the Professions Supplementary to Medicine Act), other groups such as Physiotherapists, were able to obtain formal, legally protected professional standing, albeit whilst being subordinated to medicine (Larkin, 1995).

The current climate of healthcare professions is very different from that critiqued by neo-Weberian perspectives. Medicine, whilst still a dominant profession within healthcare in most contexts, carries less influence over the professional registration and regulation of other groups. In addition, whilst hierarchies still exist, with some professions carrying greater status than others, previously subordinated roles such as nursing, and many allied health professional roles have been introducing their own subordinate roles (such as associates and assistant roles) for some time.

Gender and Dual Closure – The Profession of Nursing

We have previously highlighted that nursing shares many of the traits that professions such as medicine have. They are both well organised, they are both regulated in many countries; they have formal codes of practice and codes of ethics; and they have developed a body of specialised knowledge that is often taught as academic degrees in higher education institutions (Hoeve et al., 2014). At the same time, whilst gaining increasing autonomy in recent years, nursing is an example of an occupation that has been 'subjugated' to medicine in that historically, nursing has been practiced under medical supervision and direction (Hoeve et al., 2014).

Witz (1992) and Jones (1994) argued that it is not coincidental that professions like nursing and midwifery are placed in the position of subordinate to medicine, and that occupational closure is based, in part, on enduring gender inequalities. Witz (1992) pointed out that in the context of professional power and inclusion, men have greater economic, political and societal resources available to them, and that women were traditionally limited from entering elite professions such as medicine, through two strategies: *exclusion,* for example, by preventing them from obtaining the required qualifications,

and *demarcation* of their practice under the control of male doctors, as in the case of nursing and midwifery (Moore, 2013).

However, that nurses and midwives have been subordinate to medicine, whilst developing their own professional traits can be viewed as nurses' deliberate *professionalisation* strategy. Some have argued that nurses and midwives have deployed 'dual closure' strategies in response to being separated from and subordinated to the medical professional (Witz, 1992). By resisting separation, nurses and midwives utilised the same closure strategies as medicine, establishing new areas of professional knowledge and competency, creating a professional register and adopting codes of ethics and practice to create a boundary around the profession and exclude competing professions (Witz, 1992). Essentially, this represents a 'professional compromise'. Nurses and midwives through such strategies are able to obtain professional status and monopoly over their practice, but historically this has largely been under medical supervision.

Deprofessionalisation

One other insightful perspective on the way medicine obtained its high status compared to other occupations was that of the French Sociologists Jamous and Peloille (1970), who discussed the nature of medical knowledge. This also provides a useful starting point for thinking about deprofessionalisation. Their work has been used to discuss the nature of medical power, as well as its relation to nursing (Traynor, 2009) and complementary and alternative medicine (Givati and Hatton, 2015, Hirschkorn, 2006). Jamous and Peloille (1970) suggested that what gives a profession like medicine its social prestige is the extent of the social distance between professionals and their clients, and this they argued is influenced by the degree to which the public can themselves access specialised knowledge and skills. Where knowledge is very *unique, closed, mystified* and *inaccessible* to patients, the social distance between the public and the professional increases, resulting in greater professional prestige (Jamous and Peloille, 1970). In contrast, if the professional knowledge is accessible, easy to understand and use, then it becomes 'de-mystified'. Anyone can use it, which invariably lowers the prestige enjoyed by those professionals who previously enjoyed exclusive access (Jamous and Peloille, 1970).

Think about when something in your house breaks, let's say your toilet (or any other household utility). Now with the internet, and access to hundreds of online tutorials giving lay people the knowledge and skills they need to fix things in their own homes like this, such knowledge has become 'de-mystified'. People are empowered to do more home repairs, rather than relying on someone else. In the case of fixing toilets though, being able to access online tutorials and do this yourself, does somewhat lower reliance on plumbers, at least for basic repairs. However, in the contemporary knowledge economy, far from a close-guarded secret used to maintain the importance of work groups, it is often those within these groups who have specific knowledge and skills that are sharing this with others, often freely.

Of course, even within the home, there are exemptions to what you can and cannot do, and this is often supported by legislation. This legislation often exists to maintain public safety. For example, whilst you can fix your own toilet with minimal risk, attempting to fix your own boiler involves significant risk (to yourself, and possibly your entire street) and, therefore, those able to fix boilers enjoy a protective monopoly over this. Likewise, for many professions, regulation exists to maintain public trust in the profession and safety. The public would likely not want the surgeon who is carrying out their surgery, to have gained their knowledge exclusively online. That is not to say that the internet has not demystified medical knowledge. Now, what might previously have involved going to a library, and searching through many books and other written resources to find the relevant information, largely just involves a Google search. This increased lay access to medical knowledge is reducing medicines dominance, and promoting patients to be less passive in decisions about their care (Timmermans, 2020).

However, the increasing access to information is not the only feature of contemporary society that is now seen to be eroding the power of professions, such as medicine. Other trends have been highly significant here too. Technology (as we explore in chapter 20) has the potential to change professional roles, and what professionals do (Petrakaki et al., 2012). In addition, as healthcare systems have over time expanded and as they have become more complex and sophisticated, governments have become increasingly involved in regulating healthcare professionals, which has included introducing new regulatory frameworks to ensure greater public accountability and safety (Crinson, 2018, Saks and Lee-Treweek, 2020). The emergence of new public management, alongside public-sector reforms (many of which are driven by market-orientated neo-liberalism), and increased bureaucracy and managerialism within healthcare, have resulted in a loss of exclusive access to knowledge, increasingly regulated working conditions and erosion of professions (particularly medicines) autonomy and authority over their own practice (Crinson, 2018).

However, healthcare professional roles are also changing, and their scope expanding to include many new tasks, many of which are more aligned to managerialism. Professionals like doctors, nurses, etc. now no longer just care for patients, they now organise care, collaborate and share with other healthcare professionals and a range of stakeholders, often across very complex multi-team systems, as well as

set up and implement improvement projects to ensure sustainability amongst increasing shortages and financial strain (Noordegraaf, 2015). Managerial and professional authorities have arguably combined within many settings (i.e. 'professional-managerial hybridity') (Noordegraaf, 2015), with the conduct of the professions being influenced by organisations, and vice versa. Other examples of professional-managerial hybridity are the increasing emphasis on interdisciplinarity and integrated care pathways, and designing healthcare around patients' increasingly complex needs (that will generally involve the input of multiple different healthcare professionals working together), rather than according to traditional specialties (Liberati et al., 2016). Because of this, sociological analysis has shifted to the examination of the relationships between healthcare professionals (discussed more in chapter 19) (Liberati et al., 2016), and leadership and managerial values and practices (discussed more in chapter 18) and its impact on professionalism, for example, in nursing (Beardwood et al., 1999, Carvalho, 2014, Traynor, 1999), paramedics (Givati et al., 2018, McCann et al., 2013), social workers (Harlow et al., 2013), physiotherapists and pharmacists (Germov, 2005), maternity services in the NHS (Deery and Fisher, 2017) and medical practice (McGivern et al., 2015).

Clinical Considerations

- The composition and density of the healthcare workforce are different from country to country. Some countries, notably many countries in Africa, are more vulnerable to healthcare worker shortages.

- Healthcare professionals around the world are facing many work-related challenges that amount to significant work-related stress and burnout.

- New professional roles have emerged to meet increased demand and reduce worker supply in many countries.

- The emergence of new professions and roles can create tension, role ambiguity and uncertainties about boundaries and responsibilities.

- Different roles within healthcare attract different status. Some professions have considerably higher status than others (such as medicine). The hierarchies that exist have a historical and social context.

- The increased complexity of healthcare is changing how professions are seen and understood, with less of a focus on protecting jurisdictions, and a greater focus on collaboration and interprofessional work.

Conclusion

In this chapter, the current global healthcare workforce has been considered alongside some of its current challenges. We have examined how new roles and the increased flexibility of work between different healthcare professions allow healthcare systems to be responsive to changing population needs, amidst healthcare worker shortages. As part of this, we also explored some of the tensions this can create, especially where new roles emerge (such as Physician Associates and Advanced Clinical Practitioners), alongside existing healthcare professional roles.

We have also provided a summary of some of the ways professions have been seen and understood within societies, drawing on seminal approaches such as traits, functionalist and neo-Weberian perspectives. In the context of neo-Weberian perspectives, we have highlighted how some professional groups (such as medicine) have been able to obtain their high-status over time, and the impact this has on other healthcare professional groups. Finally, we have drawn this chapter to a close by considering the increasing roles of organisations and increasing complexity in shaping healthcare professional practice, and the increasing focus on integrated care systems, and interprofessional work.

References

Abbott, A. 1988. *The System of Professions: An Essay on the Division of Expert Labor*, University of Chicago Press.

Abrahams, K., Kathard, H., Harty, M. & Pillay, M. 2019. Inequity and the Professionalisation of Speech-Language Pathology. *Professions and Professionalism*, 9.

Adams, T. L. 2015. Sociology of professions: international divergences and research directions. *Work, Employment and Society*, 29, 154–165.

Adovor, E., Czaika, M., Docquier, F. & Moullan, Y. 2021. Medical brain drain: how many, where and why? *Journal of Health Economics*, 76, 102409.

Ahmat, A., Okoroafor, S. C., Kazanga, I., Asamani, J. A., Millogo, J. J. S., Illou, M. M. A., Mwinga, K. & Nyoni, J. 2022. The health workforce status in the WHO African region: findings of a cross-sectional study. *BMJ Global Health*, 7, e008317.

Bailey, S. 2021. Parliamentary report on workforce burnout and resilience. *BMJ*, 373, n1603.

Barber, B. 1963. Some problems in the sociology of the professions. *Daedalus*, 92, 669–688.

Beardwood, B., Walters, V., Eyles, J. & French, S. 1999. Complaints against nurses: a reflection of 'the new managerialism' and consumerism in health care? *Social Science & Medicine*, 48, 363–374.

Bodeker, G., Ong, C.-K., Grundy, C., Burford, G., Shein, K. & World Health Organization. Programme on Traditional, M. & DEVELOPMENT, W. H. O. C. F. H 2005. *WHO Global Atlas of Traditional, Complementary and Alternative Medicine*, Kobe, Japan: WHO Centre for Health Development.

Boniol, M., Kunjumen, T., Nair, T. S., Siyam, A., Campbell, J. & Diallo, K. 2022. The global health workforce stock and distribution in 2020 and 2030: a threat to equity and 'universal' health coverage? *BMJ Global Health*, 7.

Boniol, M., Mcisaac, M., Xu, L., Wuliji, T., Diallo, K. & Campbell, J. 2019. *Gender Equity in the Health Workforce: Analysis of 104 Countries*, World Health Organization.

Botezat, A. & Ramos, R. 2020. Physicians' brain drain - a gravity model of migration flows. *Globalization and Health*, 16, 7.

Burki, T. 2023. WHO's new vision for traditional medicine. *The Lancet*, 402, 763–764.

Cant, S. & Sharma, U. 1998. *A New Medical Pluralism: Complementary Medicine, Doctors, Patients and the State*, Routledge.

Carvalho, T. 2014. Changing connections between professionalism and managerialism: a case study of nursing in Portugal. *Journal of Professions and Organization*, 1, 176–190.

Chemali, Z., Ezzeddine, F. L., Gelaye, B., Dossett, M. L., Salameh, J., Bizri, M., Dubale, B. & Fricchione, G. 2019. Burnout among healthcare providers in the complex environment of the Middle East: a systematic review. *BMC Public Health*, 19, 1337.

House of Commons. 2024. The NHS workforce in England [Online]. House of Commons Library House of Commons. Available: https://researchbriefings.files.parliament.uk/documents/CBP-9731/CBP-9731.pdf [Accessed].

Crinson, I. 2018. The Health Professions and Professional Practice. *In*: Scambler, G. (ed.) *Sociology as Applied to Health and Medicine*, Bloomsbury.

Dall'ora, C., Ball, J., Reinius, M. & Griffiths, P. 2020. Burnout in nursing: a theoretical review. *Human Resources for Health*, 18, 41.

Deery, R. & Fisher, P. 2017. Professionalism and person-centredness: developing a practice-based approach to leadership within NHS maternity services in the UK. *Health Sociology Review*, 26, 143–159.

Drennan, V. M., Gabe, J., Halter, M., De Lusignan, S. & Levenson, R. 2017. Physician associates in primary health care in England: a challenge to professional boundaries? *Social Science & Medicine*, 181, 9–16.

Dubale, B. W., Friedman, L. E., Chemali, Z., Denninger, J. W., Mehta, D. H., Alem, A., Fricchione, G. L., Dossett, M. L. & Gelaye, B. 2019. Systematic review of burnout among healthcare providers in sub-Saharan Africa. *BMC Public Health*, 19, 1247.

Einboden, R. 2020. SuperNurse? Troubling the hero discourse in COVID Times. *Health*, 24, 343–347.

Eurostat. 2020. Majority of health jobs held by women [Online]. Eurostat. Available: https://ec.europa.eu/eurostat/web/products-eurostat-news/-/ddn-20200409-2 [Accessed].

Evetts, J. 2003. The sociological analysis of professionalism: occupational change in the modern world. *International Sociology*, 18, 395–415.

Evetts, J. 2013. Professionalism: value and ideology. *Current Sociology*, 61, 778–796.

Figueroa, C. A., Harrison, R., Chauhan, A. & Meyer, L. 2019. Priorities and challenges for health leadership and workforce management globally: a rapid review. *BMC Health Services Research*, 19, 239.

Freidson, E. 1970. *Profession of Medicine: A Study of the Sociology of Allied KNowledge*, New York: Harper & Row.

Freidson, E. 1984. The changing nature of professional control. *Annual Review of Sociology*, 10, 1–20.

Galanis, P., Vraka, I., Fragkou, D., Bilali, A. & Kaitelidou, D. 2021. Nurses' burnout and associated risk factors during the COVID-19 pandemic: a systematic review and meta-analysis. *Journal of Advanced Nursing*, 77, 3286–3302.

Germov, J. 2005. Managerialism in the Australian public health sector: towards the hyper-rationalisation of professional bureaucracies. *Sociology of Health & Illness*, 27, 738–758.

Ghahramani, S., Lankarani, K. B., Yousefi, M., Heydari, K., Shahabi, S. & Azmand, S. 2021. A systematic review and meta-analysis of burnout among healthcare workers during covid-19. *Frontiers in Psychiatry*, 12, 758849.

Givati, A. & Hatton, K. 2015. Traditional acupuncturists and higher education in Britain: the dual, paradoxical impact of biomedical alignment on the holistic view. *Social Science & Medicine*, 131, 173–180.

Givati, A., Markham, C. & Street, K. 2018. The bargaining of professionalism in emergency care practice: NHS paramedics and higher education. *Advances in Health Sciences Education: Theory and Practice*, 23, 353–369.

Glassman, A., Keller, J. & Smitham, E. 2023. The Future of Global Health Spending Amidst Multiple Crises. CGD Note, Center for Global Development, Washington, DC.

Goode, W. J. 1957. Community within a community: the professions. *American Sociological Review*, 22, 194–200.

Greenwood, E. 1957. Attributes of a profession. *Social Work*, 2, 45–55.

Hajian, S., Khoshnevisan, M. H., Yazdani, S. H. & Jadidfard, M. P. 2019. Factors influencing the migration intention of dental and medical graduates in developing countries. *European Journal of Public Health*, 29.

Harlow, E., Berg, E., Barry, J. & Chandler, J. 2013. Neoliberalism, managerialism and the reconfiguring of social work in Sweden and the United Kingdom. *Organization*, 20, 534–550.

Hirschkorn, K. A. 2006. Exclusive versus everyday forms of professional knowledge: legitimacy claims in conventional and alternative medicine. *Sociology of Health & Illness*, 28, 533–557.

Hoeve, Y. T., Jansen, G. & Roodbol, P. 2014. The nursing profession: public image, self-concept and professional identity. A discussion paper. *Journal of Advanced Nursing*, 70, 295–309.

House of Commons. 2021. Workforce burnout and resilience in the NHS and social care: second report of session 2021–22 [Online]. Available: https://committees.parliament.uk/publications/6158/documents/68766/default/ [Accessed].

James, P. B., Wardle, J., Steel, A. & Adams, J. 2018. Traditional, complementary and alternative medicine use in Sub-Saharan Africa: a systematic review. *BMJ Global Health*, 3, e000895.

Jamous, H. & Peloille, B. 1970. *Professions or Self-Perpetuating System; Changes in the French University-Hospital System*, Cambridge: Cambridge University Press.

Johnson, S. E., Green, J. & Maben, J. 2014. A suitable job?: A qualitative study of becoming a nurse in the context of a globalizing profession in India. *International Journal of Nursing Studies*, 51, 734–743.

Johnson, T. 1972. *Professions and Power*, London: Macmillan.

Jones, L. 1994. *The Social Context of Health and Health Work*, Bloomsbury Publishing.

Kamarulzaman, A., Ramnarayan, K. & Mocumbi, A. O. 2022. Plugging the medical brain drain. *The Lancet*, 400, 1492–1494.

Kline, D. S. 2003. Push and pull factors in international nurse migration. *Journal of Nursing Scholarship*, 35, 107–111.

Kroezen, M., Francke, A. L., Groenewegen, P. P. & Van Dijk, L. 2012. Nurse prescribing of medicines in Western European and Anglo-Saxon countries: a survey on forces, conditions and jurisdictional control. *International Journal of Nursing Studies*, 49, 1002–1012.

Kunnemann, H. 2005. Social work as laboratory for normative professionalisation. *Social Work and Society*, 3, 191–200.

Larkin, G. 1983. *Occupational Monopoly and Modern Medicine*, London: Taverstock.

Larkin, G. 1995. *Health Professions and the State in Europe*, Taylor & Francis.

Larson, M. 1977. *The Rise of Professionalism*, Berkeley: University of California Press.

Larson, M. S. 1980. Proletarianization and educated labor. *Theory and Society*, 9, 131–175.

Leo, C. G., Sabina, S., Tumolo, M. R., Bodini, A., Ponzini, G., Sabato, E. & Mincarone, P. 2021. Burnout among healthcare workers in the covid 19 Era: a review of the existing literature. *Frontiers in Public Health*, 9, 750529.

Le Var, R. M. 1997. Project 2000: a new preperation for practice- has policy been realized? *Nurse Education Today*, 17(3).

Liberati, E. G., Gorli, M. & Scaratti, G. 2016. Invisible walls within multidisciplinary teams: disciplinary boundaries and their effects on integrated care. *Social Science & Medicine*, 150, 31–39.

Macdonald, K. 1995. *The Sociology of the Professions*, Sage Publications.

Mccann, L., Granter, E., Hyde, P. & Hassard, J. 2013. Still blue-collar after all these years? An ethnography of the professionalization of emergency ambulance work. *Journal of Management Studies*, 50, 750–776.

Mcgivern, G., Currie, G., Ferlie, E., Fitzgeraldi, L. & Waring, J. 2015. Hybrid manager-professionals' identity work: the maintenance and hybridization of medical professionalism in managerial contexts. *Public Administration*, 93, 412–432.

Mcisaac, M., Vazquez-Alvarez, R. & Amo-Agyei, S. 2022. The gender pay gap in the health and care sector: a global analysis in the time of the COVID-19. [Online]. Available: https://policycommons.net/artifacts/2654493/the-gender-pay-gap-in-the-health-and-care-sector/ [Accessed].

Mej'ia, A., Pizurki, H. & Royston, E. 1979. *Physician and Nurse Migration: Analysis and Policy Implications, Report on a WHO Study*, World Health Organization.

Millerson, G. 1964. *The Qualifying Associations: A Study in Professionalization*, Taylor & Francis.

Misau, Y. A., Al-Sadat, N. & Gerei, A. B. 2010. Brain-drain and health care delivery in developing countries. *Journal of Public Health in Africa*, 1, e6.

Moore, S. 2013. Health, Medicine and the Body. *In:* Haralambos, M. & Holborn, M. (eds.) *Sociology: Themes and Perspectives*, 8th Edition, Collins.

Nancarrow, S. & Borthwick, A. 2021a. *The Allied Health Professions: A Sociological Perspective*, Policy Press.

Nancarrow, S. & Borthwick, A. 2021b. Emerging Allied Health Professions. *In:* Nancarrow, S. & Borthwick, A. (eds.) *The Allied Health Professions*, Policy Press.

Nancarrow, S. A. & Borthwick, A. M. 2005. Dynamic professional boundaries in the healthcare workforce. *Sociology of Health & Illness*, 27, 897–919.

Noordegraaf, M. 2015. Hybrid professionalism and beyond: (new) forms of public professionalism in changing organizational and societal contexts. *Journal of Professions and Organization*, 2, 187–206.

Nursing & Midwifery Council. 2023. Part 1: standards framework for nursing and midwifery education. Available online at: https://www.nmc.org.uk/globalassets/sitedocuments/standards/2024/standards-framework-for-nursing-and-midwifery-education.pdf.

Parry, N. & Parry, J. 1977. *Social Closure and Collective Social Mobility*, Routledge.

Parsons, T. 1951. *The Social System*, England: Routledge.

Pekkola, E., Carvalho, T., Siekkinen, T. & Johansson, J.-E. 2018. The Sociology of Professions and the Study of the Academic Profession. *In:* Pekkola, E., Kivistö, J., Kohtamäki, V., Yuzhuo, C. & Lyytinen, A. (eds.) *Theoretical and Methodological Perspectives on Higher Education Management and Transformation: An Advanced Reader for PhD Students*, Tampere University Press.

Petrakaki, D., Barber, N. & Waring, J. 2012. The possibilities of technology in shaping healthcare professionals: (Re/De-) professionalisation of pharmacists in England. *Social Science & Medicine*, 75, 429–437.

Poon, Y. R., Lin, Y. P., Griffiths, P., Yong, K. K., Seah, B. & Liaw, S. Y. 2022. A global overview of healthcare workers' turnover intention amid COVID-19 pandemic: a systematic review with future directions. *Human Resources for Health*, 20, 70.

Rolewicz, L., Palmer, B. & Lobont, C. 2024. The NHS workforce in numbers [Online]. Nuffield Trust: Evidence for Better Health Care. Available: https://www.nuffieldtrust.org.uk/resource/the-nhs-workforce-in-numbers#:~:text=Across%20NHS%20hospital%2C%20community%20and,%25)%20of%20the%20total%20workforce. [Accessed].

Saks, M. 1995. *Professions and the Public Interest: Medical Power, Altruism and Alternative Medicine*, Psychology Press.

Saks, M. 2015. Inequalities, marginality and the professions. *Current Sociology*, 63, 850–868.

Saks, M. 2016. A review of theories of professions, organizations and society: the case for neo-weberianism, neo-institutionalism and eclecticism. *Journal of Professions and Organization*, 3, 170–187.

Saks, M. & Lee-Treweek, G. 2020. *Political Power and Professionalisation*, Routledge.

Şenel, E. 2019. Evolution of homeopathy: a scientometric analysis of global homeopathy literature between 1975 and 2017. *Complementary Therapies in Clinical Practice*, 34, 165–173.

Simpson, N. B. 2022. Demographic and economic determinants of migration. *IZA World of Labor*.

Snell, R., Fyfe, S., Fyfe, G., Blackwood, D. & Itsiopoulos, C. 2020. Development of professional identity and professional socialisation in allied health students: a scoping review. *Focus on Health Professional Education: A Multi-Professional Journal*, 21, 29–56.

Steege, L. M. & Rainbow, J. G. 2017. Fatigue in hospital nurses — 'supernurse' culture is a barrier to addressing problems: a qualitative interview study. *International Journal of Nursing Studies*, 67, 20–28.

Thompson, W. & Mcnamara, M. 2022. Constructing the advanced nurse practitioner identity in the healthcare system: a discourse analysis. *Journal of Advanced Nursing*, 78, 834–846.

Timmermans, S. 2020. The engaged patient: the relevance of patient–physician communication for twenty-first-century health. *Journal of Health and Social Behavior*, 61, 259–273.

Timmons, S. 2011. Professionalization and its discontents. *Health (London, England)*, 15, 337–352.

Timmons, S., Mann, C., Evans, C., Pearce, R., Overton, C. & Hinsliff-Smith, K. 2023. The advanced clinical practitioner (ACP) in UK healthcare: dichotomies in a new 'multi-professional' profession. *SSM - Qualitative Research in Health*, 3, 100211.

Traynor, M. 1999. *Managerialism and Nursing: Beyond Opppression and Profession*, Psychology Press.

Traynor, M. 2009. Indeterminacy and technicality revisited: how medicine and nursing have responded to the evidence based movement. *Sociology of Health & Illness*, 31, 494–507.

Traynor, M., Nissen, N., Lincoln, C. & Buus, N. 2015. Occupational closure in nursing work reconsidered: UK health care support workers and assistant practitioners: a focus group study. *Social Science & Medicine*, 136-137, 81–88.

Turner, B. 1995. *Medical Power and Social Knowledge*, London: Sage.

UK Government. 2019. The nursing and midwifery order 2001. Available online at: https://www.legislation.gov.uk/uksi/2002/253/article/5.

UN. 2016. Goal 3: ensure healthy lives and promote well-being for all at all ages [Online]. UN. Available: https://www.un.org/sustainable development/health/ [Accessed].

WHO. 2008. Task shifting: global recommendations and guidelines. [Online]. The World Health Organization. Available: https://iris.who.int/bitstream/handle/10665/43821/9789241596312_eng.pdf [Accessed].

WHO. 2013. WHO traditional medicine strategy: 2014–2023.

WHO. 2016. Global strategy on human resources for health: workforce 2030 [Online]. World Health Organization Available: https://iris.who.int/bitstream/handle/10665/250368/9789241511131-eng.pdf?sequence=1 [Accessed].

WHO. 2020. Urgent health challenges for the next decade [Online]. The World Health Organization. Available: https://www.who.int/news-room/photo-story/photo-story-detail/urgent-health-challenges-for-the-next-decade [Accessed].

WHO. 2022. The gender pay gap in the health and care sector: a global analysis in the time of COVID-19. [Online]. World Health Oganization. Available: https://www.who.int/publications/i/item/9789240052895 [Accessed].

WHO. 2023a. Global health workforce statistics database [Online]. Available: https://www.who.int/data/gho/data/themes/topics/health-workforce [Accessed].

WHO. 2023b. WHO health workforce support and safeguards list 2023 [Online]. The World Health Organization Available: https://www.who.int/publications/i/item/9789240069787 [Accessed].

Witz, A. 1990. Patriarchy and professions: the gendered politics of occupational closure. *Sociology*, 24, 675–690.

Witz, A. 1992. *Professions and Patriarchy*, Routledge.

Yuksekdag, Y. 2018. Health without care? Vulnerability, medical brain drain, and health worker responsibilities in underserved contexts. *Health Care Analysis*, 26, 17–32.

PART 2

Meeting Population Health Needs and Health Inequalities

CHAPTER 7

Population Health Needs: Understanding the Care Transition

Chris Allen[1], Lindsay Welch[2], and Lynn Calman[1]

[1]*School of Health Sciences, University of Southampton, Southampton, UK*
[2]*Faculty of Health and Social Sciences, Bournemouth University, Bournemouth, UK*

Introduction

This chapter will consider the global demographic and epidemiological transitions that have typically led to people living longer, healthier lives. We will critically reflect on how such changes have fundamentally changed the needs and focus of population health and will introduce you to the public health science of Epidemiology. Health needs have changed over time in response to changes in societies and knowledge about health and disease. This chapter's contents largely reflect the health needs of the period that this book was written in – and largely from a wealthy and developed society viewpoint; the United Kingdom, where universal personalised care has become an increasing focus in policy and practice. Had it been written at a different point in time or in a different population, its focus would have been very different. However, the tools that we have provided in this chapter should help you move with the times as patterns of disease change nationally or even locally – helping you to identify the health needs of your own populations and what might be able to be done to improve them.

Through our discussion of these transitions, you will have the opportunity within this chapter to consider long-term conditions, multi-morbidity and how people can be supported to live fulfilling lives with these conditions. We will also consider the ways healthcare systems that were largely set up to meet the needs of acute illness can be reorientated to the needs of chronic illness and multi-morbidity – specifically through recognising the increasing importance of self-management support and personalised care in meeting people's needs. During this chapter, we will consider the broader social and economic changes that have occurred alongside these shifts and the impact that these changes have had on the delivery of care for an increasingly aged population as well as society more generally, and how these are shaping future expectations about health with people living longer and with increased multi-morbidity and complexity.

LEARNING OUTCOMES

By the end of this chapter, you will be able to:

- Understand the demographic and epidemiological transitions that have occurred within western industrialised societies and how these impact health and healthcare provision.
- Recognise the importance of demography and epidemiology to understanding populations and patterns of disease within a society, including the significance of population aging.
- Understand some of the key tools of epidemiology and how these can help us understand the health needs of populations.
- Recognise the increased focus on self-management and personalised care in the context of long-term conditions.
- Recognise the impact of the burden of treatment and patient activation on people's self-management and how likely self-management will be engaged with.

Social Sciences for Healthcare Professionals, First Edition. Edited by Chris Allen.
© 2026 John Wiley & Sons Ltd. Published 2026 by John Wiley & Sons Ltd.

A Changing Society, with Changing Health Needs

> **Key Terms and Definitions**
>
> **Population aging:** A shift in a country's age profile with more being in the older age categories compared to younger age categories.
>
> **Long-term condition:** A condition that cannot be cured now but can be controlled through medication or therapy.
>
> **Demography:** The study of human populations, using statistics to determine size and composition, as well as the factors that cause these to change, such as births, deaths and migration.
>
> **Epidemiology:** The study of patterns of a disease within a population.

In the years prior to now, the nature of threats to health has differed across the globe and was largely shaped by society – the knowledge of disease, living and working conditions, and general progress and development. What makes us ill now is not the same as what made us ill 150 years ago and health-related treatments look very different too (Omran, 2005, ONS, 2017, Santosa et al., 2014, Weisz and Olszynko-Gryn, 2010). Likewise, our health 150 years ago was radically different from what was experienced when humans were primarily hunter-gatherers or during agricultural society; further highlighting the impact of societies and behaviour on health (Berbesque et al., 2014, Milner, 2019). Indeed, even now, the hunter-gatherer societies that remain have been highlighted as an example of public health due to their radically different health compared to sedentism (living in one place) in industrialised societies (Page et al., 2018, Pontzer et al., 2018). Agricultural society presented many opportunities for human flourishing and importantly led to significant population expansion, but this new type of society brought with it new health-related challenges and changes to health-related behaviours. Our diets for example changed in line with the food we were able to access more consistently, through the domestication of plants and animals for farming (Diamond, 2002, Milner, 2019, Richards, 2002); and with humans having to labour more, living in closer proximity to one another, and typically staying in the same place – work, sanitation, proximity to others and associated infectious disease became more significant determinants of health (Barrett et al., 1998, Larsen, 2006). Population health remained poor during the Industrial Revolution, especially in relation to infant mortality, though some people did enjoy significant longevity (Crane-Kramer and Buckberry, 2020, Davenport, 2021). Poor living and working conditions, especially amongst society's poorest members (Davenport, 2021), child labour (Humphries, 2013), unsanitary urban living (Sullivan et al., 2022) and the increasing use of machinery in the absence of adequate health and safety provision (Western and Bekvalac, 2020), all contributed to poor population health. As with now, significant differences existed in terms of life expectancy, particularly between richer and poorer areas (Davenport, 2021). Despite this, it is recognised that the Industrial Revolution brought about significant human development, and largely alongside this development came some highly significant breakthroughs in our understanding of health and disease that would go on to have a significant impact on population health, including increased sanitation (Morley, 2007).

> ## John Snow (1813–1858): King Cholera
>
> In tracing the care transition through the ages as we have begun to do in this chapter, it is worth highlighting some of the key thinkers that have shaped our understanding of what causes disease, and how we can monitor these causes of disease across populations and over time. We cannot do this without talking about John Snow. John Snow set the stage for the discipline of epidemiology (Tulchinsky, 2018).
>
> In 1854, Cholera, an infectious disease characterised by severe watery diarrhoea, took hold of London. In just a few weeks, several hundred people had died following infection, particularly those living in tightly packed tenements. People typically lived in close proximity (even a matter of meters) to cesspools where human waste was discharged. These cesspools were also located nearby to water supplies. This unsurprisingly was very smelly and created some horrid living conditions. Outbreaks of disease, such as Cholera, were common. The prevailing theory at the time was that disease was caused by miasma, or "bad air" (Halliday, 2001). The volume of people stricken with Cholera in Soho, allowed Snow to study the possible causes of the disease. In doing so, he identified that most people who had fallen ill had consumed water from one specific pump, the now infamous 'Broad Street Pump'.
>
> Snow also had two accidental control groups (Tulchinsky, 2018). Nearby there was a brewery. The brewery workers, living near the pump, had all the same exposures as those stricken with Cholera with one important difference. They more typically drank beer, and the clean water serving the brewery, than water from the pump. In addition, the workers of the nearby workhouses (who were some of societies poorest members) seemingly avoided contracting the virus too. This is because the workhouses had their own uninfected water supplies. Snow was able to gather evidence using methods not dissimilar to that used in modern-day epidemiology, to demonstrate that the water from the Broad Street Pump was causing the Cholera outbreak. As a result, he infamously removed the pump's handle to prevent its further use, and London's water and sewage systems were overhauled. Snow's work also cleared a path for germ theory which states that disease can be caused by microorganisms or germs (Tulchinsky, 2018). A controversial theory at the time, but a scientifically accepted theory now for many diseases.

The role of economic development in relation to 'health' is debated, because the concept of health is itself contested (Patterson, 2023). Certainly, modern-day hunter-gather groups whose lives have remained disconnected from much of what economic development has brought societies can still lead healthy lives – even being held up as an example for public health due to low rates of non-communicable disease (Pontzer et al., 2018). However, it is generally recognised that rapid economic development has led to improved living standards for many in sedentism societies, for example, in relation to access to food, warmth, shelter, work and improved working conditions, and sanitation, alongside an increasingly improved understanding of health and disease (Birchenall, 2007, Patterson, 2023). Whilst infectious diseases have maintained their hold on more disadvantaged populations, alongside chronic disease, commonly referred to as a 'dual burden of disease' (Kushitor and Boatemaa, 2018), the most significant changes in the patterning of disease relate to degenerative, and chronic disease, largely brought about through increasing longevity, modern lifestyles and behaviours (Dai et al., 2020, Griswold et al., 2018, He et al., 2022, Katzmarzyk et al., 2021). As we have begun to demonstrate, population health needs change over time in response to the changes observed in society. In the United Kingdom, as with much of the planet, there have been dramatic changes in the death rates and causes of death over the last 100–150 years (ONS, 2017), and as a result, much of the world's population is now aging – albeit at quite different rates (UN, 2024). These changes can be tracked in the following interactive activity.

Stop and Think: An Aging World

You can track increased life expectancy across the world using some fantastic free resources at https://www.gapminder.org/tools/#$chart-type=bubbles&url=v1.

Using Gapminders free tools, you can visually track changes in life expectancy over the last 200 years.

Take some time to use the available interactive tools. Each country is represented in a bubble. The larger the country's bubble, the larger its population is. India and China jump straight off the page as they are countries with very large populations. If you click play, you can track changes in life expectancy and wealth (measured in Gross Domestic Product (GDP)) over the last 200 years.

What trends did you observe over the past 200 years?

You will likely have noticed that in 1800 most of the world's countries had poor life expectancy, and were also relatively poor in relation to their GDP per capita (per person).

You will likely see that since then, most countries have experienced increased longevity (albeit to different extents) as well as an improvement in their GDP per capita (i.e. as nations, they have got richer).

You will likely also see that there are some quite significant differences between poorer and richer countries – which we will explore in more depth in the following chapters.

One last thing to do here – change the vertical axis to 'Child Mortality'.

What trends did you observe over the last 200 years?

You will have likely noticed that 200 years ago child mortality was staggeringly high – with around 400 deaths per 1,000 live births. Since then, rates of childhood mortality have improved dramatically in every country though there is a wealth gradient – with poorer countries improving at a slower rate.

There is a key relationship with reduced fertility rates here – fewer children are planned in part not only because of improved education and opportunities for women, but also because of an increased expectation that children will survive into adulthood.

Demographic Transition

For the age composition of a country to change, there needs to either be a change in the birth or death rate (Bongaarts, 2009), or there needs to be changes in the number of people leaving/arriving in a country (i.e. through inward and outward migration) (Marois et al., 2023). If everything else remains stable, a reduction in fertility rates (i.e. the total births per woman) reduces the size of younger birth cohorts. As a result, the number of younger people relative to older people changes. Likewise, a population can age even where fertility rates are stable if a decrease in later-life mortality results in an increasing number of people within a population surviving into later life (Bongaarts, 2009). Various social factors result in decreased fertility rates, and reduced mortality, meaning that demographic transition occurs at different times and in different contexts across different countries; but some trends are particularly common and can be broken down into the following broad phases:

Pre-transition: This period is characterised by both high fertility rates and high mortality rates. The overall population size remains relatively stable in its size and composition as new births are offset by new deaths.

Demographic transition: This happens when something disrupts fertility and mortality rates. For example, falling fertility rates, alongside falling mortality rates, result in a larger cohort of older people relative to younger people. Less people being born shrinks the bottom end of the population pyramid and less people dying enlarges the older end of the population pyramid. You can see this in the interactive 'Stop and Think: Population Pyramids' activity.

Stop and Think: Population Pyramids

Using Gapminders free tools, we can also visualise a country's age composition through their interactive population pyramids. Population pyramids are one way to visualise the age structure of a country – how many people are older, how many people are working age and how many people are younger. This is generally in the form of stacked histogram bars, which resemble a pyramid (of sorts) by displaying male and female sexes on either side. A typical population pyramid is shown in figure 7.1 for the world and shows projected demographic changes and their impact on the shape and size of the global population over time.

an increasing proportion of people in the older age categories relative to the number of people in the younger working age categories. It is worth looking at a few different countries to draw comparisons. For example, Nigeria has a very young population (UNDP, 2018), but Japan has a very old population. In Japan, deaths currently exceed births and it is in fact the 'oldest' country in the world (Nakatani, 2019). The dependency ratios in most countries are worsening in response to demographic transitions. Such changes have micro (e.g. family structures, size and caring arrangements) and macro (e.g. work, employment, pensions, health and

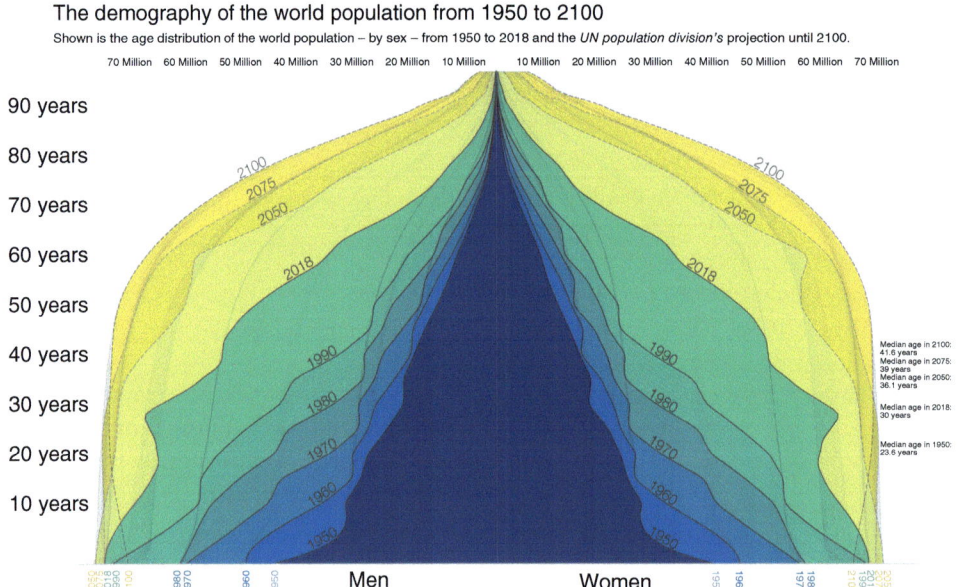

FIGURE 7.1   The global population pyramid. **Source:** Roser (2019) / The global population pyramid: How global demography has changed and what we can expect for the 21st century / 'https://ourworldindata.org/global-population-pyramid / OurWorldinData.org. / CC by 4.0.

It is important to highlight that the resources on Gapminder do not break down age by sex (as per figure 7.1) and therefore their illustrations of age composition are not pyramid-shaped.

You can access this resource at: https://www.gapminder.org/tools/#$chart-type=popbyage&url=v1

By clicking 'play' on the resource, you should see that the world is anticipated to get older over the next 75 years with

social care provision) implications (UK Government, 2016).

You can see a more typical population pyramid for areas in the United Kingdom through this interactive ONS resource:

https://www.ons.gov.uk/visualisations/dvc418/pyramids_projections/index.html#0/0/2/null/null/false/false/na/0.

You might want to consider looking at the UK population pyramids and considering their relevance to the provision of health and care.

So, excluding inward and outward migration, for the age composition of a country to change something needs to happen to mortality or fertility. In wealthier societies, as well as increasingly elsewhere, positive social and cultural changes to women's social and economic prospects, including access to opportunities such as education outside of the home, have occurred alongside reductions in childhood mortality and access to

contraception (Reher, 2021, Upadhyay et al., 2014). Such changes have resulted in decreased fertility rates, and medical advances have resulted in decreased child and infant mortality, resulting in more of those children who are born, surviving into adulthood (Aksan and Chakraborty, 2014, Dyson, 2010).

In addittition, mortality has shifted towards later life through the societal advances that we will go on to consider more fully.

Through advancements in science and overall living and working conditions, an increasing number of people are now more likely to have increasingly long lives (Santosa et al., 2014).

What Can a Bath Tell Us About Population Health?

Before diving into explore further how population health is changing across the globe, we must first introduce you to some important terms in the field of epidemiology that help us understand patterns of disease across populations.

Key Terms and Definitions

Incidence: The proportion of new cases of people who develop the disease during a specified period. It is a **rate** "how fast" at which new cases occur in a given period.

$$\text{Incidence} = \frac{\text{Number of new cases}}{\text{at risk population in a given time frame}}$$

To allow comparison the incidence rate is often reported as a fraction of the population at risk (e.g. per 100,000 or per million population)*.

Prevalence: The proportion of a population that are cases at a point in time (current burden)

$$\text{Prevalence} = \text{Number of cases/Population at risk}$$

Prevalence is usually expressed as a fraction, as a percentage (proportion), or as the number of cases per 10,000 or 100,000 people*.

Commonly two types of prevalence are reported.

- Point prevalence is the proportion of a population that has the condition at a specific point in time.
- Period prevalence is the proportion of a population that has the condition at some time during a given period (e.g. 12-month prevalence).

Mortality: This is presented as a rate. The incidence of death from a disease over a period of time, or the number of deaths in a population over a period of time. Mortality is typically expressed in units of deaths, for example, 5 deaths per 1,000 individuals per year.

Morbidity: You might also see this term – it simply means, having a condition.

* This is so that we don't accidentally make one country look sicker, simply because they have a larger population. You would expect a country the size of China to record more deaths than a country the size of the United Kingdom just because of the significant differences in terms of the size of the population – so by comparing rates, you are comparing 'like with like'.

Epidemiology is a public health science that helps us to understand the occurrence and frequency of a disease in a given population (Webb et al., 2017) as John Snow (1813–1858) did. Epidemiology is important not only so we can understand how much of a disease there is, who is affected and where poor health is occurring, but this information can also be used to distribute resources and target areas for health intervention. It is incredibly important to help us to understand the social patterning of disease. In fact, many of the social determinants – the things that we know determine health – are known through the science of epidemiology.

Epidemiology like other sciences has its own language that is used in a precise way. So, we must get to know this language and some underpinning concepts before we can apply them – we have provided some key terms and definitions in the box.

It can be helpful to use an analogy to help to understand a new topic. For epidemiology, a useful analogy is a bathtub as it makes it easier to see how these terms are interrelated. We do not know exactly who came up with the bath first; certainly, a lot of people use it. It is a particularly useful analogy to help us explain, and for you to understand, some of the key terms that will be referred to throughout this book and set the scene for some of our current challenges.

In figure 7.2, the bathtub represents the 'at risk' population. Analysis in epidemiology is always carried out with reference to a specific population. This population is the group of individuals that are 'at risk'.

New cases enter the bathtub as '*incidence*'. (see figure 7.3) **Incidence** therefore reflects the total number of **new** people who have the condition. Over time these cases fill the bathtub. Like a tap incidence is a rate, so it can change. It can in some cases be turned on and off, or the rate can change, faster or slower. For example, a new screening program might identify new people with a condition and increase incidence rates[1], or in the winter season, incidence rates of flu may increase, as just two examples.

The number of total cases within the bathtub is the '**prevalence**' of a condition (see figure 7.4). As more people enter the bathtub through incidence, the prevalence also increases, provided people do not either die from the condition (known as **mortality**), or are cured (see figure 7.5).

As treatments have changed and improved for many diseases, prevalence can reduce as more people get cured. However, for conditions that can only be controlled, rather than cured – such as many long-term conditions, we can see the prevalence increase. In the context of chronic illness, preventing people from becoming unwell in the first place, remains a key priority, but increasing prevalence is not always bad, as it can simply mean people are being supported to live with the disease. Whilst they are not able to be cured, they are not dying from it.

HIV is a good example. In the 1980s and 1990s before we understood the condition and had treatments that prevented

---

[1] This doesn't mean that more people have the condition, merely that we are better at detecting those with it.

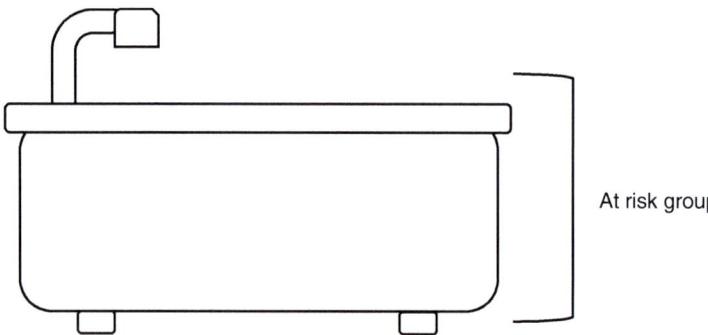

FIGURE 7.2 Bathtub representing the 'at risk' population.

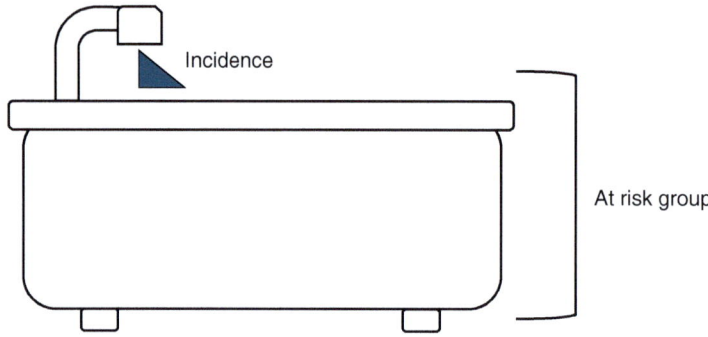

FIGURE 7.3 New cases filling the bathtub as 'incidence'.

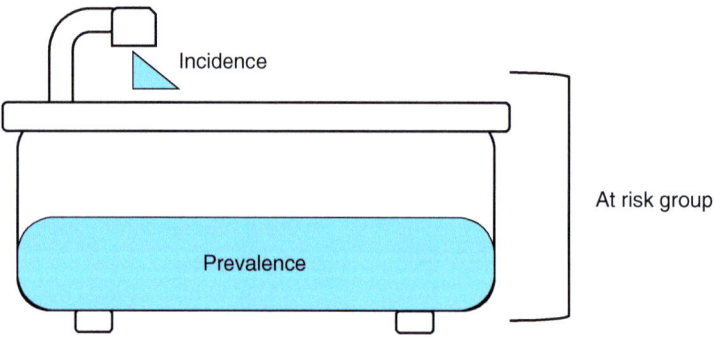

FIGURE 7.4 'Prevalence' representing the total number of cases.

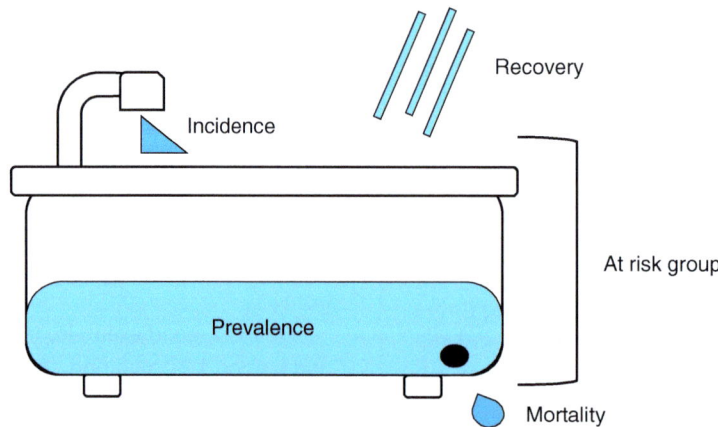

FIGURE 7.5 'Prevalence', mortality and recovery.

the condition from getting worse, those recently contracting the virus would be represented in the incidence, but they would join the total number of people with the virus (the prevalence). As a new condition, which we knew little about, many people left the prevalence group quickly through mortality (Trickey et al., 2024, Wang et al., 2016). Because we have a test for HIV we can measure incidence and prevalence – provided people are able to be tested. This can help us understand the impact of interventions and changing health needs. For example, in many areas incidence has changed (i.e. the number of new people contracting the condition) due to the availability of prophylactic treatments (specifically pre-exposure prophylaxis) for at-risk groups that is becoming increasingly available in some populations, albeit unequally (Bavinton and Grulich, 2021), alongside an increased lay understanding of risks.

Additionally, fewer people are now leaving the pool of prevalence (through mortality), because more people with the condition have access to new treatments and can now go on to live a more complete life course with good health (Trickey et al., 2023, 2024). So, whilst rates of new infections might decrease in response to prophylactic treatment, because fewer people are dying (and therefore leaving the tub), the prevalence might continue to increase. As with other long-term conditions, there is currently no definitive cure for HIV, meaning prevalence continues to rise. In this context, higher prevalence, whilst still concerning, is related to social and scientific progress. Because more people can successfully live with the condition and enjoy longer lives with it than what was previously possible.

Stop and Think: How Are Incidence, Prevalence, Mortality and Cure Linked?

We have demonstrated how incidence, prevalence and mortality relate to one another.

1. Think of a condition that you encounter frequently in your clinical practice. What could change the incidence and mortality associated with that condition?

2. What impact does this have on the condition's prevalence?

3. You might want to consider if this is a condition where incidence is easily identifiable or if there might be a lot of people out there with the condition who have never been diagnosed.

4. How is the condition identified? Is there a specific test or is it identified and diagnosed through clinical judgement alone – like most mental health conditions?

5. How do you think knowing about incidence and prevalence could help us to allocate resources or point us to new interventions to support people?

Demographic and Epidemiological Transitions: Why Increasing Chronic Illness, Multi-morbidity and Complexity Necessitates a Change in Care Paradigm

Bringing this together, changing demographic and epidemiological profiles have largely been the result of the rapid economic developments that have improved general living and working conditions for many (Birchenall, 2007, Patterson, 2023). These have occurred alongside further improvements in our knowledge of health and the spread and control of disease, such as access to new curative and risk reduction approaches, advances in medicines and therapeutic treatments, increased prevention of disease (e.g. through public health interventions such as improved access to clean water and sanitation), as well as campaigns and laws directed at reducing harmful health behaviours such as smoking (Kuipers et al., 2019). Risk reduction and curative approaches have reduced early mortality, resulting in more mortality occurring later in life (Santosa et al., 2014).

Many of these advances are interrelated, with improvements to population health being related to advancements across society generally. Take cancer as one example (though you could pick many). In the United Kingdom, cancer survival has increased substantially – due to improved treatments and access to care (Quaresma et al., 2015). During this time, there has been more understanding of the causes of cancer, such as smoking, alcohol, obesity and genetic factors (Byrne et al., 2023, Latino-Martel et al., 2016). This has led to, for example, tobacco control legislation and an increased focus on the role of behaviour change in cancer prevention and management (Byrne et al., 2023, Gredner et al., 2021). In addition, there has been an increased awareness of cancer symptoms through public health campaigns and the introduction of national screening programmes for some cancers (Hughes-Hallett et al., 2016, Lai et al., 2021, Plackett et al., 2020). This is leading to earlier diagnosis and improved survival (Jansen et al., 2020). In addition, there is a growing understanding of the social determinants of cancer – this allows for more targeted intervention for those most at risk. For example, deaths from cancer are more common in deprived areas (Exarchakou et al., 2018).

As we have highlighted, significant developments have reduced the impacts of many causes of poor health – not just cancer. This has led to significant improvements in care and treatment, resulting in people living longer in most countries. However, alongside this has also been a trend towards increased morbidity – largely through increased longevity, but also through poor health behaviours throughout the life course such as smoking, alcohol excess, inactivity and obesity (Dai et al., 2020, Griswold et al., 2018, He et al., 2022, Katzmarzyk et al., 2021). The impact of this, as we highlighted earlier, is that chronic disease now reflects a greater burden on health in affluent countries and is becoming a more significant burden alongside acute disease in poorer nations too (Kushitor and Boatemaa, 2018). The nature of chronic disease makes it necessary to think about how care is delivered. Chronic conditions, such as diabetes and Chronic Obstructive Pulmonary Disease (COPD), differ from acute illness, in that they typically require management across the life course and cannot be cured (Bernell and Howard, 2016). Because of this, these conditions are associated with greater healthcare utilisation and higher associated costs than acute illness (Soley-Bori et al., 2021, van Oostrom et al., 2014). Of those with chronic illness, an increasing number have more than one condition (i.e. multi-morbidity) (Barnett et al., 2012, Chowdhury et al., 2023, Mangin et al., 2012, van Blarikom et al., 2023). The increasing prevalence of multi-morbidity creates complex challenges for healthcare providers, patients and those providing care (both formally and informally). This is because there is often a complex set of interactions between different physical and mental health conditions that can negatively impact their management, a person's quality of life and their daily symptoms and functional ability (Calderón-Larrañaga et al., 2019), including in the context of managing cancer (Corbett et al., 2022, Cummings et al., 2018).

As we highlighted in Chapter 5, most healthcare systems will need to adapt to increasing demand and changing healthcare needs to remain sustainable over time (Britnell, 2015). Considering these changes, increasing attention is now being paid to ensuring we have sustainable models of care that better reflect the more chronic care needs of our populations. The relatively high cost of chronic illness, both now and in the future, has seen policy increasingly stating a need for patients to take on a greater role in the management of their own health conditions. Drivers for patients taking on a greater role in their own health have largely been led by concerns of service demand and the recognition that people's quality of life can be improved, and their healthcare-related burdens reduced if they can manage aspects of their health and their condition themselves, in partnership with healthcare professionals when they are needed (Brand and Timmons, 2021, NHS, 2019a).

Not a Bath, but an Ocean

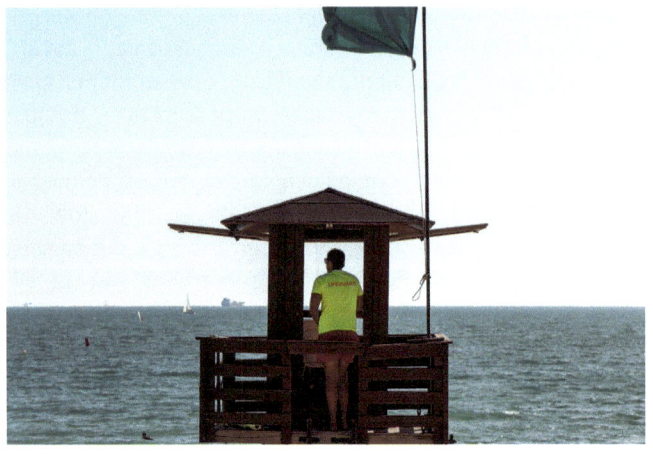

Source: ADDICTIVE STOCK/Adobe Stock Photos.

In considering how this all relates to the need to change the way we think about care, we are returning to the bathtub analogy. With more and more people now having at least one condition, and with an increasing number now experiencing multi-morbidity, the bathtub is becoming full and it is perhaps more appropriate to look at this using the analogy of the sea and rising sea levels.

In the sea, our role as healthcare professionals can be both swim teacher and lifeguard. As swim teachers, we can equip people with the necessary tools to stay afloat (i.e. to manage their conditions successfully in everyday life, without needing to access healthcare or other forms of aid to do so). However, from time to time, even the most competent swimmer can face conditions that become overwhelming and result in the need for support, for example, when their condition becomes too challenging to manage independently. At these times, they might need to be supported by other swimmers such as their friends and family sunbathing on the beach. For those who have received an adequate number of swimming lessons, very occasionally, conditions might be so challenging that they need to be rescued by the lifeguard (e.g. when they need to access formal healthcare). If people are taught to swim well, using approaches that we know work, then this shouldn't happen very often. For the most part, people should just be able to enjoy spending time in the sea with their friends and family.

Most importantly, not everyone with a long-term condition enters the sea in the same way. Some enter the sea very slowly over a period of many years allowing them a period to adjust to learn to swim in the currents and adjust to the challenges the sea poses. Others fall straight in. Some will need more swimming lessons than others. Likewise, some will enter the sea with various supportive tools, for example, buoyancy aids such as various forms of social capital (the resources that are gained from other people, some of which are relevant to health), and health literacy (the ability to read, interpret and make use of health-related information), and education that makes it easier for them to stay afloat (Welch et al., 2021).

Stop and Think: What Types of Things Are People with a Long-Term Condition Increasingly Expected to Be Able to "Do"? What Impact Do You Think These Things Have on Their Everyday Life?

Managing a long-term condition such as diabetes, COPD, Crohn's disease, etc., might involve:

Monitoring: Including monitoring biomedical variables, for example, measuring and recording peak flow, and measuring and recording blood sugar levels.

Self-medication: Including having the knowledge to adjust doses according to measurements and symptoms, etc.

Healthy behaviour: Following dietary and lifestyle advice.

Seeking medical expertise: Knowing when the condition is bad enough to warrant professional help, and attending appointments (which might involve travel, cost and organisation).

Stop and Think: What Factors Might Affect the Extent to Which Professionals Are Involved in Management?

- The risk of the condition variability (such as exacerbations).
- The impact of the condition and symptoms on daily life.
- The extent to which complications can be reduced through effective self-monitoring.
- The potential for the disease course to be modified.
- Multi-morbidity and complexity.
- And an individual's capacity to cope with both the condition and the work of the condition, on top of daily work.

(Conley and Redeker, 2016, Powers et al., 2016, Welch et al., 2021, Zwerink et al., 2014)

Increased Responsibilities and the Burden of Treatment and Disease

Making people more responsible for their own health is a fundamentally new way of thinking about care. Such changes increasingly place value on the patient voice and user experience, meaning that increasingly people should be able to shape the care they receive (Greenhalgh, 2009). However, the shift in responsibility to patients and the public that has occurred around chronic illness management may not be for everyone and may disadvantage those whose needs are very complex and who have less resources to take on an increased role in the management of their own health that policy and practice increasingly demands (Ellis et al., 2017, Jones, 2018). There are several factors that impact the extent to which patients can and will be willing to 'self-manage' their own health and conditions (Krein et al., 2007, Taylor et al., 2014, Welch et al., 2020). Important factors include how complex the condition is, what is involved and how easy it is to do, whether there are other conditions (i.e. multi-morbidity), how well a person feels, how well the person knows what is required, as well as how confident and motivated they are to manage their condition themselves (Johnson et al., 2016). With the increasing individual responsibility of managing a long-term condition falling onto those with a long-term condition themselves (Ellis et al., 2017, Ong et al., 2014), academics and those in practice have begun to consider the importance of minimally disruptive healthcare (May et al., 2009) and the increasing burden of treatment that goes alongside the burden of illness (May et al., 2014). The burden of treatment associated with managing chronic illness is not insignificant. For example, a systematic analysis using US condition-specific

guidelines for those with multi-morbidity found if a patient were to fully comply with the recommendations, they would take around 13 medications a day and spend around 50–70 hours per month accessing healthcare professionals (and in America, this can come with a significant financial cost!) (Buffel du Vaure et al., 2016).

Obviously being acutely unwell is burdensome too – we have all had the experience of having an unpleasant cold. A cold can disrupt our daily lives, reducing our ability to participate fully in our work and our personal lives. But these disruptions are short-lived. Whilst treatment might be unpleasant, and burdensome, it is not likely to be needed for very long, meaning that acute illness rarely has the same ongoing disruptive impact that a chronic illness has. The burden of treatment theory helps us to think about how much is being expected from patients themselves and whether they have the resources to be able to cope with these new demands from them. Being unwell can be very demanding, especially when our own internal reserves are depleted. The extent of the burden of illness and treatment will vary by condition and between different people who are all equipped with different capabilities, health literacies and resources (Lippiett et al., 2022).

With the changes we have noted throughout this chapter, patients and their personal networks (more on this in Chapter 15) are being expected to do more. This increasing burden of treatment has the potential to overwhelm people and may lead to situations in which people can no longer take on this increased role and responsibility, resulting in them no longer being able to manage their condition themselves, or choosing not to. Alongside the condition itself, those with chronic illness, especially where they have multi-morbidity, often face significant challenges brought around by social disadvantage in other aspects of their lives (Bisquera et al., 2022).

Self-Management to Support Individuals

In creating minimally disruptive models of care, it is relevant to consider the importance of treatment and care that is tailored specifically to the needs of those with a long-term condition, rather than to the needs of the healthcare system more generally – to make it easier for people to access healthcare support that is suitable to their needs when they need it, as well as follow recommended treatments and behaviours to prevent their condition from getting worse.

Taking on the tasks associated with self-management invariably involves learning new skills and being able to adopt and embed these within daily routines. It can also involve changing how you live and changing some of your habits, particularly those that might be harmful to your health – for example, it is common for people to be encouraged to make changes such as giving up smoking and monitoring dietary intake more precisely, or for example, in the context of diabetes counting carbohydrates, or taking new medications. Making changes such as these requires being motivated to do so, as well as having the appropriate knowledge, skills and confidence (Johnson et al., 2016).

Currently in the United Kingdom and elsewhere, the Patient Activation Measure (PAM) has become a popular and validated way to identify whether someone has the appropriate motivation, knowledge, skills and confidence to take on a more enhanced role in the management of their own health and conditions (Hibbard et al., 2004). Research has highlighted that those scoring low in the measure (i.e. those who are 'poorly activated') can become overwhelmed by their conditions and their management and are less likely to take on an active role in the management of their own health and conditions. Because of this, they will likely seek and require more professional involvement in their care (Bu and Fancourt, 2021). Those with poor levels of activation access care more frequently and are more likely to access urgent unscheduled care than those with higher levels of activation (Bu and Fancourt, 2021, Hibbard and Greene, 2013).

The increasing focus on patients to be able to better manage their own health and conditions has occurred largely alongside the increasing focus on people being able to access personalised care when they need it (Entwistle and Watt, 2013, Epstein et al., 2010, NHS, 2019b). Traditionally conditions have been treated according to disease-specific approaches – largely through the dominance of medicine and medicalisation (see Chapter 3). Personalised care instead focusses more on the thoughts, feelings and wishes of those with a chronic health issue (Entwistle and Watt, 2013, Epstein et al., 2010). It has the potential to open opportunities for people to have more choice and control over their mental and physical health, or to manage a condition more independently, which may reduce overall healthcare utilisation and in turn reduce the cost of providing care to those with a long-term condition (Coulter et al., 2015).

Most healthcare professionals are professionally bound to deliver personalised care. At the level of policy in the United Kingdom, the NHS long-term plan (NHS, 2019a) set out a commitment to roll out a comprehensive model of personalised care. The NHS's current vision is for relationships between health providers and patients to be reconfigured towards what those accessing care want – with consideration of overall well-being, and the social determinants of health (Mello, 2020). The notion of personalised care is not new, but the NHS's commitment to reconfigure care around shared decision-making, self-management support, social prescribing and community-based support (see Chapter 17) and personalised care and budgets, highlight a very different orientation to healthcare provision, that focusses on peoples broader needs, and capabilities to live lives that are valued, despite having a chronic illness (Mello, 2020, NHS, 2019b).

Clinical Considerations

- Epidemiology can help us to identify health needs within a population and target those areas most at risk of poor health.
- Those with a chronic health condition must be able to carry out multiple health-related tasks in order to successfully manage their condition in everyday life.
- Having more than one condition increases the complexity of a person's care.
- Care should be tailored to the specific needs of those individuals with a long-term condition, focussing on their needs and what they value most.

- In chronic illness, it is important to consider someone's burden of treatment, alongside their burden of illness, ensuring care is minimally disruptive.
- Those with good health literacy, and supportive personal networks are more likely to be able to self-manage their own long-term condition, in collaboration with healthcare professionals.
- There are various ways that we can identify how likely someone is to be able to engage with self-management. The PAM has become one commonly used tool.

Conclusion

In this chapter, we have provided a broad overview of changing population health needs by considering the relevant demographic and epidemiological transitions that have occurred. We have highlighted the relevance of the public health science of epidemiology to better understand patterns of illness and disease in our populations and how these change over time in response to demographic transitions and advancements in our knowledge and understanding of health and disease.

We have been able to demonstrate how care is increasingly being orientated around the needs of those with a long-term condition, or who have complex multi-morbidity and highlighted the relevance of the different needs that have arisen from such epidemiological transitions to how care is thought about, understood and configured now and in the future.

We have also highlighted how managing a chronic condition can impact on people's everyday lives, and the differential burdens posed by chronic illness compared to acute illness. This has allowed us to consider and understand how best to meet the needs of people who might have very different motivations, confidence, knowledge and skills to be able to take on an increased role in the management of their own health and conditions – alongside the relevance of increasingly personalised care and support, much of which we will continue to expand upon in the rest of this book.

References

Aksan, A. M. & Chakraborty, S. 2014. Mortality versus morbidity in the demographic transition. *European Economic Review*, 70, 470–492.

Barnett, K., Mercer, S. W., Norbury, M., Watt, G., Wyke, S. & Guthrie, B. 2012. Epidemiology of multimorbidity and implications for health care, research, and medical education: a cross-sectional study. *The Lancet*, 380, 37–43.

Barrett, R., Kuzawa, C. W., Mcdade, T. & Armelagos, G. J. 1998. Emerging and re-emerging infectious diseases: the third epidemiologic transition. *Annual Review of Anthropology*, 27, 247–271.

Bavinton, B. R. & Grulich, A. E. 2021. HIV pre-exposure prophylaxis: scaling up for impact now and in the future. *The Lancet Public Health*, 6, e528–e533.

Berbesque, J. C., Marlowe, F. W., Shaw, P. & Thompson, P. 2014. Hunter-gatherers have less famine than agriculturalists. *Biology Letters*, 10, 20130853.

Bernell, S. & Howard, S. W. 2016. Use your words carefully: what is a chronic disease? *Frontiers in Public Health*, 4, 159.

Birchenall, J. A. 2007. Economic development and the escape from high mortality. *World Development*, 35, 543–568.

Bisquera, A., Turner, E. B., Ledwaba-Chapman, L., Dunbar-Rees, R., Hafezparast, N., Gulliford, M., Durbaba, S., Soley-Bori, M., Fox-Rushby, J., Dodhia, H., Ashworth, M. & Wang, Y. 2022. Inequalities in developing multimorbidity over time: a population-based cohort study from an urban, multi-ethnic borough in the United Kingdom. *Lancet Regional Health Europe*, 12, 100247.

Bongaarts, J. 2009. Human population growth and the demographic transition. *Philosophical Transactions of the Royal Society of London. Series B, Biological Sciences*, 364, 2985–2990.

Brand, S. & Timmons, S. 2021. Knowledge sharing to support long-term condition self-management—patient and health-care professional perspectives. *Health Expectations*, 24, 628–637.

Britnell, M. 2015. *In Search of the Perfect Health System*, Palgrave Macmillan.

Bu, F. & Fancourt, D. 2021. How is patient activation related to health-care service utilisation? evidence from electronic patient records in England. *BMC Health Services Research*, 21, 1196.

Buffel du Vaure, C., Ravaud, P., Baron, G., Barnes, C., Gilberg, S. & Boutron, I. 2016. Potential workload in applying clinical practice guidelines for patients with chronic conditions and multimorbidity: a systematic analysis. *BMJ Open*, 6, e010119.

Byrne, S., Boyle, T., Ahmed, M., Lee, S. H., Benyamin, B. & Hyppönen, E. 2023. Lifestyle, genetic risk and incidence of cancer: a prospective cohort study of 13 cancer types. *International Journal of Epidemiology*, 52, 817–826.

Calderón-Larrañaga, A., Vetrano, D. L., Ferrucci, L., Mercer, S. W., Marengoni, A., Onder, G., Eriksdotter, M. & Fratiglioni, L. 2019. Multimorbidity and functional impairment–bidirectional interplay, synergistic effects and common pathways. *Journal of Internal Medicine*, 285, 255–271.

Chowdhury, S. R., Chandra Das, D., Sunna, T. C., Beyene, J. & Hossain, A. 2023. Global and regional prevalence of multimorbidity in the adult population in community settings: a systematic review and meta-analysis. *eClinicalMedicine*, 57, 101860.

Conley, S. & Redeker, N. 2016. A systematic review of self-management interventions for inflammatory bowel disease. *Journal of Nursing Scholarship*, 48, 118–127.

Corbett, T., Lee, K., Cummings, A., Calman, L., Farrington, N., Lewis, L., Young, A., Richardson, A., Foster, C. & Bridges, J. 2022. Self-management by older people living with cancer and multi-morbidity: a qualitative study. *Supportive Care in Cancer*, 30, 4823–4833.

Coulter, A., Entwistle, V. A., Eccles, A., Ryan, S., Shepperd, S. & Perera, R. 2015. Personalised care planning for adults with chronic or long-term health conditions. *Cochrane Database Syst Rev*, 3, Cd010523.

Crane-Kramer, G. M. & Buckberry, J. 2020. Is the Pen Mightier than the Sword? Exploring Urban and Rural Health in Victorian England and Wales Using the Registrar General Reports. *In:* Betsinger, T. K. & DeWitte, S. N. (eds.) *The Bioarchaeology of Urbanization: The Biological, Demographic, and Social Consequences of Living in Cities*, Life Sciences, 403–433.

Cummings, A., Grimmett, C., Calman, L., Patel, M., Permyakova, N. V., Winter, J., Corner, J., Din, A., Fenlon, D., Richardson, A., Smith, P. W. & Foster, C. 2018. Comorbidities are associated with poorer quality of life and functioning and worse symptoms in the 5 years following colorectal cancer surgery: results from the ColoREctal Well-being (CREW) cohort study. *Psychooncology*, 27, 2427–2435.

Dai, H., Alsalhe, T. A., Chalghaf, N., Riccò, M., Bragazzi, N. L. & Wu, J. 2020. The global burden of disease attributable to high body mass index in 195 countries and territories, 1990-2017: an analysis of the Global Burden of Disease Study. *PLoS Medicine*, 17, e1003198.

Davenport, R. J. 2021. Mortality, migration and epidemiological change in English cities, 1600–1870. *International Journal of Paleopathology*, 34, 37–49.

Diamond, J. 2002. Evolution, consequences and future of plant and animal domestication. *Nature*, 418, 700–707.

Dyson, T. 2010. *Population and Development: The Demographic Transition*, Bloomsbury Publishing.

Ellis, J., Boger, E., Latter, S., Kennedy, A., Jones, F., Foster, C. & Demain, S. 2017. Conceptualisation of the 'good' self-manager: a qualitative investigation of stakeholder views on the self-management of long-term health conditions. *Social Science & Medicine*, 176, 25–33.

Entwistle, V. A. & Watt, I. S. 2013. Treating patients as persons: a capabilities approach to support delivery of person-centered care. *The American Journal of Bioethics*, 13, 29–39.

Epstein, R. M., Fiscella, K., Lesser, C. S. & Stange, K. C. 2010. Why the nation needs a policy push on patient-centered health care. *Health Aff (Millwood)*, 29, 1489–1495.

Exarchakou, A., Rachet, B., Belot, A., Maringe, C. & Coleman, M. P. 2018. Impact of national cancer policies on cancer survival trends and socioeconomic inequalities in England, 1996-2013: population based study. *BMJ*, 360, k764.

Gredner, T., Mons, U., Niedermaier, T., Brenner, H. & Soerjomataram, I. 2021. Impact of tobacco control policies implementation on future lung cancer incidence in Europe: an international, population-based modeling study. *The Lancet Regional Health Europe*, 4, 100074.

Greenhalgh, T. 2009. Patient and public involvement in chronic illness: beyond the expert patient. *BMJ*, 338, b49.

Griswold, M. G., Fullman, N., Hawley, C., Arian, N., Zimsen, S. R. M., Tymeson, H. D., Venkateswaran, V., Tapp, A. D., Forouzanfar, M. H., Salama, J. S., Abate, K. H., Abate, D., Abay, S. M., Abbafati, C., Abdulkader, R. S., Abebe, Z., Aboyans, V., Abrar, M. M., Acharya, P., Adetokunboh, O. O., Adhikari, T. B., Adsuar, J. C., Afarideh, M., Agardh, E. E., Agarwal, G., Aghayan, S. A., Agrawal, S., Ahmed, M. B., Akibu, M., Akinyemiju, T., Akseer, N., Asfoor, D. H. A., Al-Aly, Z., Alahdab, F., Alam, K., Albujeer, A., Alene, K. A., Ali, R., Ali, S. D., Alijanzadeh, M., Aljunid, S. M., Alkerwi, A. A., Allebeck, P., Alvis-Guzman, N., Amare, A. T., Aminde, L. N., Ammar, W., Amoako, Y. A., Amul, G. G. H., Andrei, C. L., Angus, C., Ansha, M. G., Antonio, C. A. T., Aremu, O., Ärnlöv, J., Artaman, A., Aryal, K. K., Assadi, R., Ausloos, M., Avila-Burgos, L., Avokpaho, E. F., Awasthi, A., Ayele, H. T., Ayer, R., Ayuk, T. B., Azzopardi, P. S., Badali, H., Badawi, A., Banach, M., Barker-Collo, S. L., Barrero, L. H., Basaleem, H., Baye, E., Bazargan-Hejazi, S., Bedi, N., Béjot, Y., Belachew, A. B., Belay, S. A., Bennett, D. A., Bensenor, I. M., Bernabe, E., Bernstein, R. S., Beyene, A. S., Beyranvand, T., Bhaumik, S., Bhutta, Z. A., Biadgo, B., Bijani, A., Bililign, N., Birlik, S. M., Birungi, C., Bizuneh, H., Bjerregaard, P., Bjørge, T., Borges, G., Bosetti, C., Boufous, S., Bragazzi, N. L., Brenner, H., Butt, Z. A., et al. 2018. Alcohol use and burden for 195 countries and territories, 1990– 2016: a systematic analysis for the Global Burden of Disease Study 2016. *The Lancet*, 392, 1015–1035.

Halliday, S. 2001. Death and miasma in Victorian London: an obstinate belief. *BMJ*, 323, 1469–1471.

He, H., Pan, Z., Wu, J., Hu, C., Bai, L. & Lyu, J. 2022. Health effects of tobacco at the global, regional, and national levels: results from the 2019 global burden of disease study. *Nicotine & Tobacco Research*, 24, 864–870.

Hibbard, J. H. & Greene, J. 2013. What the evidence shows about patient activation: better health outcomes and care experiences; fewer data on costs. *Health Aff (Millwood)*, 32, 207–214.

Hibbard, J. H., Stockard, J., Mahoney, E. R. & Tusler, M. 2004. Development of the Patient Activation Measure (PAM): conceptualizing and measuring activation in patients and consumers. *Health Services Research*, 39, 1005–1026.

Hughes-Hallett, A., Browne, D., Mensah, E., Vale, J. & Mayer, E. 2016. Assessing the impact of mass media public health campaigns. Be Clear on Cancer 'blood in pee': a case in point. *BJU International*, 117, 570–575.

Humphries, J. 2013. Childhood and child labour in the British industrial revolution 1. *The Economic History Review*, 66, 395–418.

Jansen, E. E. L., Zielonke, N., Gini, A., Anttila, A., Segnan, N., Vokó, Z., Ivanuš, U., Mckee, M., de Koning, H. J., de Kok, I. M. C. M., Veerus, P., Anttila, A., Heinävaara, S., Sarkeala, T., Csanádi, M., Pitter, J., Széles, G., Vokó, Z., Minozzi, S., Segnan, N., Senore, C., Van Ballegooijen, M.,

de Kok, I., Gini, A., Heijnsdijk, E., Jansen, E., de Koning, H., Vogelaar, I., van Ravesteyn, N., Zielonke, N., Ivanus, U., Jarm, K., Mlakar, D. N., Primic-Žakelj, M., Mckee, M. & Priaulx, J. 2020. Effect of organised cervical cancer screening on cervical cancer mortality in Europe: a systematic review. *European Journal of Cancer*, 127, 207–223.

Johnson, M. L., Zimmerman, L., Welch, J. L., Hertzog, M., Pozehl, B. & Plumb, T. 2016. Patient activation with knowledge, self-management and confidence in chronic kidney disease. *Journal of Renal Care*, 42, 15–22.

Jones, L. 2018. Pastoral power and the promotion of self-care. *Sociology of Health & Illness*, 40, 988–1004.

Katzmarzyk, P. T., Friedenreich, C., Shiroma, E. J. & Lee, I.-M. 2021. Physical inactivity and non-communicable disease burden in low-income, middle-income and high-income countries. *British journal of sports medicine*, 2, 101–106.

Krein, S. L., Heisler, M., Piette, J. D., Butchart, A. & Kerr, E. A. 2007. Overcoming the influence of chronic pain on older patients' difficulty with recommended self-management activities. *The Gerontologist*, 47, 61–68.

Kuipers, M. A. G., West, R., Beard, E. V. & Brown, J. 2019. Impact of the "Stoptober" smoking cessation campaign in England From 2012 to 2017: a quasiexperimental repeat cross-sectional study. *Nicotine & Tobacco Research*, 22, 1453–1459.

Kushitor, M. K. & Boatemaa, S. 2018. The double burden of disease and the challenge of health access: evidence from access, bottlenecks, cost and equity facility survey in Ghana. *PLoS One*, 13, e0194677.

Lai, J., Mak, V., Bright, C. J., Lyratzopoulos, G., Elliss-Brookes, L. & Gildea, C. 2021. Reviewing the impact of 11 national be clear on cancer public awareness campaigns, England, 2012 to 2016: a synthesis of published evaluation results. *International Journal of Cancer*, 148, 1172–1182.

Larsen, C. S. 2006. The agricultural revolution as environmental catastrophe: implications for health and lifestyle in the Holocene. *Quaternary International*, 150, 12–20.

Latino-Martel, P., Cottet, V., Druesne-Pecollo, N., Pierre, F. H. F., Touillaud, M., Touvier, M., Vasson, M.-P., Deschasaux, M., Le Merdy, J., Barrandon, E. & Ancellin, R. 2016. Alcoholic beverages, obesity, physical activity and other nutritional factors, and cancer risk: a review of the evidence. *Critical Reviews in Oncology/Hematology*, 99, 308–323.

Lippiett, K., Richardson, A. & May, C. R. 2022. How do illness identity, patient workload and agentic capacity interact to shape patient and caregiver experience? Comparative analysis of lung cancer and chronic obstructive pulmonary disease. *Health & Social Care in the Community*, 30, e4545–e4555.

Mangin, D., Heath, I. & Jamoulle, M. 2012. Beyond diagnosis: rising to the multimorbidity challenge. *BMJ*, 344, e3526.

Marois, G., Potancokova, M. & Gonzalez-Leonardo, M. 2023. Demographic and labor force impacts of future immigration flows into Europe: does an immigrant's region of origin matter? *Humanities and Social Sciences Communications*, 10, 957.

May, C., Montori, V. & Mair, F. 2009. We need minimally disruptive medicine. *BMJ*, 339, b2803.

May, C. R., Eton, D. T., Boehmer, K., Gallacher, K., Hunt, K., Macdonald, S., Mair, F. S., May, C. M., Montori, V. M., Richardson, A., Rogers, A. E. & Shippee, N. 2014. Rethinking the patient: using Burden of Treatment Theory to understand the changing dynamics of illness. *BMC Health Services Research*, 14, 281.

Mello, M. 2020. Practising personalised care. *British Journal of Nursing*, 29, 82–82.

Milner, G. R. 2019. Early agriculture's toll on human health. *Proceedings of the National Academy of Sciences of the United States of America*, 116, 13721–13723.

Morley, I. 2007. City chaos, contagion, Chadwick, and social justice. *The Yale Journal of Biology and Medicine*, 80, 61–72.

Nakatani, H. 2019. Population aging in Japan: policy transformation, sustainable development goals, universal health coverage, and social determinates of health. *Glob Health Med*, 1, 3–10.

NHS. 2019a. The NHS long term plan [Online]. NHS. Available online at: https://www.longtermplan.nhs.uk/publication/nhs-long-term-plan/ [Accessed].

NHS. 2019b. Universal personalised care: implementing the comprehensive model NHS England.

Omran, A. R. 2005. The epidemiologic transition: a theory of the epidemiology of population change. 1971. *The Milbank Quarterly*, 83, 731–757.

Ong, B. N., Rogers, A., Kennedy, A., Bower, P., Sanders, T., Morden, A., Cheraghi-Sohi, S., Richardson, J. C. & Stevenson, F. 2014. Behaviour change and social blinkers? The role of sociology in trials of self-management behaviour in chronic conditions. *Sociology of Health & Illness*, 36, 226–238.

ONS. 2017. *Causes of death over 100 years* [Online]. Office for National Statistics. Available online at: https://www.ons.gov.uk/peoplepopulationandcommunity/birthsdeathsandmarriages/deaths/articles/causesofdeathover100years/2017-09-18 [Accessed].

Page, A. E., Minter, T., Viguier, S. & Migliano, A. B. 2018. Hunter-gatherer health and development policy: how the promotion of sedentism worsens the Agta's health outcomes. *Social Science & Medicine*, 197, 39–48.

Patterson, A. C. 2023. Is economic growth good for population health? a critical review. *Canadian Studies in Population*, 50, 1.

Plackett, R., Kaushal, A., Kassianos, A. P., Cross, A., Lewins, D., Sheringham, J., Waller, J. & von Wagner, C. 2020. Use of social media to promote cancer screening and early diagnosis: scoping review. *Journal of Medical Internet Research*, 22, e21582.

Pontzer, H., Wood, B. M. & Raichlen, D. A. 2018. Hunter-gatherers as models in public health. *Obesity Reviews*, 19(1), 24–35.

Powers, M. A., Bardsley, J., Cypress, M., Duker, P., Funnell, M. M., Fischl, A. H., Maryniuk, M. D., Siminerio, L. & Vivian, E. 2016. Diabetes self-management education and support in type 2 diabetes: a joint position statement of the American Diabetes Association, the American Association of Diabetes Educators, and the Academy of Nutrition and Dietetics. *Clinical Diabetes*, 34, 70–80.

Quaresma, M., Coleman, M. P. & Rachet, B. 2015. 40-year trends in an index of survival for all cancers combined and survival adjusted for age and sex for each cancer in England and Wales, 1971–2011: a population-based study. *The Lancet*, 385, 1206–1218.

Reher, D. S. 2021. The aftermath of the demographic transition in the developed world: interpreting enduring disparities in reproductive behavior. *Population and Development Review*, 47, 475–503.

Richards, M. P. 2002. A brief review of the archaeological evidence for Palaeolithic and Neolithic subsistence. *European Journal of Clinical Nutrition*, 56, 1270–1278.

Roser, M. 2019. *The global population pyramid: how global demography has changed and what we can expect from the 21st century*. [Online]. Our World in Data Available online at: https://ourworldindata.org/global-population-pyramid [Accessed].

Santosa, A., Wall, S., Fottrell, E., Högberg, U. & Byass, P. 2014. The development and experience of epidemiological transition theory over four decades: a systematic review. *Global Health Action*, 7, 23574.

Soley-Bori, M., Ashworth, M., Bisquera, A., Dodhia, H., Lynch, R., Wang, Y. & Fox-Rushby, J. 2021. Impact of multimorbidity on healthcare costs and utilisation: a systematic review of the UK literature. *The British Journal of General Practice*, 71, e39–e46.

Sullivan, N., Hincha, N., Resler, S. & Dougherty, S. 2022. And as things have been they remain: enteric disease and differential mortality among ethnic groups in early twentieth century Milwaukee. *International Journal of Paleopathology*, 37, 1–5.

Taylor, S. J. C., Pinnock, H., Epiphaniou, E., Pearce, G., Parke, H. L., Schwappach, A., Purushotham, N., Jacob, S., Griffiths, C. J., Greenhalgh, T. & Sheikh, A. 2014. Health Services and Delivery Research. A rapid synthesis of the evidence on interventions supporting self-management for people with long-term conditions: PRISMS – Practical systematic Review of Self-Management Support for long-term conditions.;2(53) Southampton (UK): NIHR Journals Library

Trickey, A., Mcginnis, K., Gill, M. J., Abgrall, S., Berenguer, J., Wyen, C., Hessamfar, M., Reiss, P., Kusejko, K., Silverberg, M. J., Imaz, A., Teira, R., D'arminio Monforte, A., Zangerle, R., Guest, J. L., Papastamopoulos, V., Crane, H., Sterling, T. R., Grabar, S., Ingle, S. M. & Sterne, J. A. C. 2024. Longitudinal trends in causes of death among adults with HIV on antiretroviral therapy in Europe and North America from 1996 to 2020: a collaboration of cohort studies. *The Lancet HIV*, 11, e176–e185.

Trickey, A., Sabin, C. A., Burkholder, G., Crane, H., D'arminio Monforte, A., Egger, M., Gill, M. J., Grabar, S., Guest, J. L., Jarrin, I., Lampe, F. C., Obel, N., Reyes, J. M., Stephan, C., Sterling, T. R., Teira, R., Touloumi, G., Wasmuth, J.-C., Wit, F., Wittkop, L., Zangerle, R., Silverberg, M. J., Justice, A. & Sterne, J. A. C. 2023. Life expectancy after 2015 of adults with HIV on long-term antiretroviral therapy in Europe and North America: a collaborative analysis of cohort studies. *The Lancet HIV*, 10, e295–e307.

Tulchinsky, T. H. 2018. John Snow, Cholera, the Broad Street Pump; Waterborne Diseases Then and Now. *In:* Tulchinsky, T. H. (ed.) *Case Studies in Public Health*, Elsevier, Academic Press An imprint of Elsevier, 77–99.

UKGOVERNMENT. 2016. Future of an Ageing Population.

UN. 2024. World Population Prospects United Nations: Department of Economic and Social Affairs.

UNDP. 2018. Policy Brief: Nigeria's Youth Bulge- From potential 'demographic bomb' to 'demographic dividend'.

Upadhyay, U. D., Gipson, J. D., Withers, M., Lewis, S., Ciaraldi, E. J., Fraser, A., Huchko, M. J. & Prata, N. 2014. Women's empowerment and fertility: a review of the literature. *Social Science & Medicine*, 115, 111–120.

van Blarikom, E., Fudge, N. & Swinglehurst, D. 2023. The emergence of multimorbidity as a matter of concern: a critical review. *BioSocieties*, 18, 614–631.

Van Oostrom, S. H., Picavet, H. S. J., De Bruin, S. R., Stirbu, I., Korevaar, J. C., Schellevis, F. G. & Baan, C. A. 2014. Multimorbidity of chronic diseases and health care utilization in general practice. *BMC Family Practice*, 15, 61.

Wang, H., Wolock, T. M., Carter, A., Nguyen, G., Kyu, H. H., Gakidou, E., Hay, S. I., Mills, E. J., Trickey, A., Msemburi, W., Coates, M. M., Mooney, M. D., Fraser, M. S., Sligar, A., Salomon, J., Larson, H. J., Friedman, J., Abajobir, A. A., Abate, K. H., Abbas, K. M., Razek, M. M. A. E., Abd-Allah, F., Abdulle, A. M., Abera, S. F., Abubakar, I., Abu-Raddad, L. J., Abu-Rmeileh, N. M. E., Abyu, G. Y., Adebiyi, A. O., Adedeji, I. A., Adelekan, A. L., Adofo, K., Adou, A. K., Ajala, O. N., Akinyemiju, T. F., Akseer, N., Lami, F. H. A., Al-Aly, Z., Alam, K., Alam, N. K. M., Alasfoor, D.,

Aldhahri, S. F. S., Aldridge, R. W., Alegretti, M. A., Aleman, A. V., Alemu, Z. A., Alfonso-Cristancho, R., Ali, R., Alkerwi, A. A., Alla, F., Mohammad, R., Al-Raddadi, S., Alsharif, U., Alvarez, E., Alvis-Guzman, N., Amare, A. T., Amberbir, A., Amegah, A. K., Ammar, W., Amrock, S. M., Antonio, C. A. T., Anwari, P., Ärnlöv, J., Artaman, A., Asayesh, H., Asghar, R. J., Assadi, R., Atique, S., Atkins, L. S., Avokpaho, E. F. G. A., Awasthi, A., Quintanilla, B. P. A., Bacha, U., Badawi, A., Barac, A., Bärnighausen, T., Basu, A., Bayou, T. A., Bayou, Y. T., Bazargan-Hejazi, S., Beardsley, J., Bedi, N., Bennett, D. A., Bensenor, I. M., Betsu, B. D., Beyene, A. S., Bhatia, E., Bhutta, Z. A., Biadgilign, S., Bikbov, B., Birlik, S. M., Bisanzio, D., Brainin, M., Brazinova, A., Breitborde, N. J. K., Brown, A., Burch, M., Butt, Z. A., Campuzano, J. C., Cárdenas, R., et al. 2016. Estimates of global, regional, and national incidence, prevalence, and mortality of HIV, 1980–2015: the global burden of disease study 2015. *The Lancet HIV*, 3, e361–e387.

Webb, P., Bain, C. & Page, A. 2017. *Essential Epidemiology: An Introduction for Students and Healthcare Professionals*, Cambridge university press.

Weisz, G. & Olszynko-Gryn, J. 2010. The theory of epidemiologic transition: the origins of a citation classic. *Journal of the History of Medicine and Allied Sciences*, 65, 287–326.

Welch, L., Orlando, R., Lin, S. X., Vassilev, I. & Rogers, A. 2020. Findings from a pilot randomised trial of a social network self-management intervention in COPD. *BMC Pulmonary Medicine*, 20, 162.

Welch, L., Sadler, E., Austin, A. & Rogers, A. 2021. Social network participation towards enactment of self-care in people with chronic obstructive pulmonary disease: a qualitative meta-ethnography. *Health Expectations*, 24, 1995–2012.

Western, G. & Bekvalac, J. 2020. Manufactured Bodies: The Impact of Industrialisation on London Health.

Zwerink, M., Brusse-Keizer, M., van der Valk, P. D., Zielhuis, G. A., Monninkhof, E. M., van der Palen, J., Frith, P. A. & Effing, T. 2014. Self management for patients with chronic obstructive pulmonary disease. *Cochrane Database Syst Rev*, 2014, Cd002990.

CHAPTER 8

Social Determinants of Health and Inequality

Chris Allen[1] and Lindsay Welch[2]

[1] *School of Health Sciences, University of Southampton, Southampton, UK*
[2] *Faculty of Health and Social Sciences, Bournemouth University, Bournemouth, UK*

Introduction

In this chapter, you will have the opportunity to consider the social influences that work to shape the patterns of health and illness across different groups. Looking at these is useful in explaining why some face better health outcomes than others. This chapter will offer you the opportunity to critically consider how these things *determine* our health (the 'cause of causes') and in doing so will provide an overview of how these determinants are shaped by our social context. One of the main focusses of social science is the study of inequalities; how they are created, what the implications of these are, how people experience differences in outcomes and opportunities and what can be done to alleviate their harmful effects on society (because most evidence suggests inequality is bad for everyone, not just those who are most disadvantaged by it). As this has been such an important focus for social sciences, this chapter serves as an overview and is best read in combination with other chapters in this book that explain different social processes and determinants, and how they can be addressed in more detail. Particularly relevant are the following two chapters covering stigma and social exclusion, as well as later chapters on understanding unhealthy behaviour, public health, social networks and social prescribing.

Inequalities and the resultant health inequalities exist across societies, but some societies fare significantly better than others. In some countries, the distance between the very rich and the very poor is huge – whereas other countries are more equal. We will explore the social basis for why some live longer, healthier and happier lives than others – by further unpicking some of the 'cause of causes' or social determinants, to help explain why we often see such large differences between people from different countries, within countries and even within neighbourhoods, towns and cities. For a while now, there has been a recognition that our health and illness are defined by more than simply our biology. Even where healthcare is free at point of access (such as in the United Kingdom), people still experience significantly different health outcomes, suggesting that what determines our health is far more than simply being able to access healthcare when we need it (though this is one factor). In fact, a range and diversity of social and economic conditions have a bearing on our opportunities, our health and our well-being, often in varied

LEARNING OUTCOMES

By the end of this chapter, you will be able to:

- Recognise the social determinants of health, including the impact of individual constitutional factors such as age, sex, gender, race and ethnicity on health and healthcare access.

- Recognise the impact of wider determinants of health and how these are interconnected, such as people's health behaviours, their social networks and their living and working conditions.

- Understand the impact of these determinants on health outcomes within populations, including how they manifest in health inequalities leading to societies poorest experiencing poorer health and shorter lives.

- Consider some of the different explanations for health inequalities, including material, psycho-social, cultural behavioural and life course explanations.

Social Sciences for Healthcare Professionals, First Edition. Edited by Chris Allen.
© 2026 John Wiley & Sons Ltd. Published 2026 by John Wiley & Sons Ltd.

and interconnected ways. Such contexts often lead to unequal health outcomes in those living in different places, and those with different social characteristics, such as gender, race and class. Because of this, healthcare professionals have a growing role in addressing health inequalities, in collaboration with the societies and people they care for, and a range of other stakeholders.

What Determines Health?

> ### Key Terms and Definitions
>
> **Socio-economic status (SES):** Generally relates to a person's work, their access to economic resources and their social position in relation to others.
>
> **Social stratification:** Ranks people in a society according to their SES.
>
> **Gender:** The socially constructed characteristics of women, men, girls and boys. Gender encapsulates the norms and behaviours, as well as often the roles (such as being a father) associated with, for example, being a man or being a woman. Some of the gendered norms around behaviour are harmful, for example, toxic notions of masculinity. Sex is a biological construct, whereas gender is a sociologically defined construct.
>
> **Race:** When people share similar physical characteristics, such as skin colour, they may be placed into a group based on these characteristics. It is important to note that race and ethnicity are related concepts, but they are not the same thing.
>
> **Ethnicity:** Essentially the culture of a group of people. A group of people who identify with one another on the basis of perceived similar or shared attributes that set them apart from other groups. These attributes can include religions and customs, birth nation, language, etc. These shared characteristics can relate to race.

It is now widely acknowledged that many factors combine to affect the health of individuals and populations (Braveman and Gottlieb, 2014). As we will unpack throughout this chapter, these include the person's social and economic environment, their physical environment and their own habits and behaviours – with some degree of influence and interconnectedness between all of these (Braveman and Gottlieb, 2014). Each of these is shaped by powerful social processes that often lie outside of the control of individuals and their own choices and behaviours (Townshend and Lake, 2017).

Models of Health Determinants

In the over 30 years since its inception[1], the Dahlgren and Whitehead model (or 'Rainbow Model') has become the most widely used model to illustrate determinants of health (Dahlgren and Whitehead, 2021, Whitehead and Dahlgren, 1991). The model is particularly useful in getting us to look past simply the provision of healthcare, and instead consider the broader factors that may contribute to a person's health. In fact, one of the most important findings from the now seminal UK Black Report was that differences in health outcomes actually got worse following the introduction of the NHS – highlighting that our health is determined by far more than simply being able to access healthcare when we are unwell (Department of Health and Social Security, 1980). Even now, our knowledge of things such as new technologies and innovations (e.g. digital) that influence our health, continues to expand and has been incorporated into new models considering digital divides in the context of the rainbow (e.g. Jahnel et al., 2022). But, sticking with the original model, even a cursory look highlights just how many things determine our health. In our discussion below, we begin to explore how many of these impact and influence one another.

The model shown in Figure 8.1 includes not only things that are positive to health but also things that may negatively impact health (Dahlgren and Whitehead, 2021). Whilst this section necessarily begins to demonstrate how these determinants create inequalities in health, the model does not explain health inequalities – this will be explored in greater detail later in this chapter. The model has become widely used as a heuristic because it provides such a simple and illustrative overview of how multifactorial health determinants are, and how they cover micro, meso and macro aspects of our society. Looking at the model, you can choose to dissect it either by starting at the outermost layer (i.e. the general, socio-economic, cultural and environmental conditions layer) which are largely macro considerations. Alternatively, you can start at the innermost layer, at the level of the individual. To step you through the model with some concrete examples, we have chosen to start with the innermost circle – looking at the individual. The model covers such a diversity of determinants, that we cannot cover every aspect in depth, and some aspects particularly those relating to social and community networks, and health behaviours are covered more fully in their own chapters (e.g. Chapters 12–17).

---

[1] For some interesting reflections on the models creation and eventual widespread use against a backdrop of pioneering research into the social determinants of health, you may wish to read Dahlgren and Whitehead (2021), which is provided in the reference list.

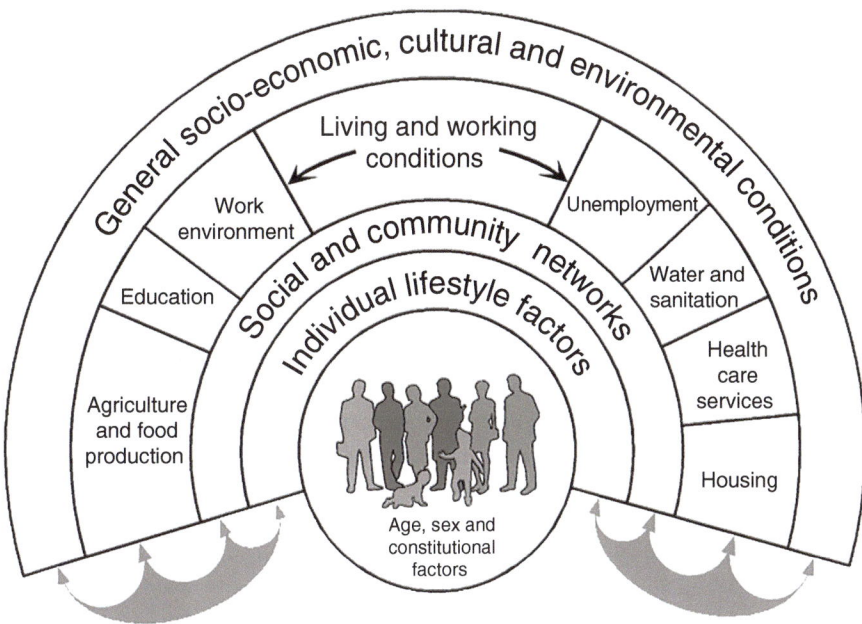

FIGURE 8.1   Dahlgren and Whitehead's model of health determinants. **Source:** Dahlgren and Whitehead (2021)/with permission of Elsevier.

Constitutional Factors – Modifiable or Unmodifiable?

Age, sex and other constitutional factors such as gender, race, ethnicity and disability can determine someone's health (Lund and Burgess, 2021, Niccoli and Partridge, 2012, Robertson et al., 2019). These are often called 'unmodifiable' determinants, or risk factors (NICE, 2023). They are not things we can change, like much of the other determinants we will discuss, as they fundamentally make up the person and who they are. This is not to say that the social processes that exist around these characteristics cannot be influenced to change behaviour, or to widen access and it is often highly important that we do this. For example, we cannot change a person's race or gender, or that they have a learning disability, but we can change how responsive care is to the needs of people from different groups (Doherty et al., 2020, Lund and Burgess, 2021, Purnell et al., 2016).

As we discussed in the previous chapter, advancing age is strongly associated with many chronic physical and mental health conditions and multi-morbidity (Kingston et al., 2018, Niccoli and Partridge, 2012). Whilst it is hard to ignore this risk, other factors influence how we age, including many of the social determinants that are discussed throughout this chapter. Poor diet, stressful living and working conditions, alcohol excess and levels of physical can all influence the aging process (Daskalopoulou et al., 2017, Leitão et al., 2022, Yegorov et al., 2020). Even a lack of meaningful social contact, especially

where it causes an individual to feel lonely (as discussed in Chapter 16), has been shown to accelerate the process of aging (Wilson et al., 2018). Whilst we all age, our age can influence how people respond to us, and the care that we can access (Nemiroff, 2022). Therefore, whilst we cannot change people's age, we can change the social processes that accelerate aging, and society's response to aging, is also amenable to change (Burnes et al., 2019).

Our biological sex is also something that we cannot modify (Muehlenhard and Peterson, 2011). Men are more predisposed to some conditions than women and vice versa. Some of this is related to biology – sex greatly determines some conditions for biological reasons. For example, whilst male breast cancer is not as uncommon as some would believe, prevalence is far higher in women (Co et al., 2020, Jackson et al., 2022). Other cancers, such as cancers of the blood, are more common in men than women (Amini et al., 2023). Alongside the different health outcomes that relate to anatomy and the different outcomes experienced by biological sex, there are also gendered norms in how and whether people present to healthcare at all, and if they do, how early they present (Finneran et al., 2023). For example, in western societies, women may consult primary care doctors more than men (Thompson et al., 2016, Wang et al., 2013), but often receive discriminatory care across settings including in relation to pain and prescription (Bingefors et al., 2017, Chen et al., 2008). Globally, women and girls face many disadvantages in relation to access to care across the life course and have a more limited voice in shaping the availability of, and provision of care around their needs (Kennedy et al., 2020).

The healthcare system, including in the United Kingdom, has traditionally been created by men, for men, with women's health issues being sidelined (Department of Health and Social Care, 2022). In addition, because women have historically had less opportunities to participate in research than men, interventions including pharmacological interventions are often designed through datasets and analysis that do not adequately take into account gender differences (Holdcroft, 2007, Merone et al., 2022). One widely discussed disparity relates to myocardial infarction. It is not uncommon for women to present with different symptoms to men (such as palpitations, nausea and vomiting), which may lead to poorer recognition and subsequently reduced rates of survival (Gopal et al., 2021). Studies have also highlighted gendered differences in out-of-hospital bystander cardiac pulmonary resuscitation and defibrillation, with recent research highlighting women are less likely to receive defibrillation, due to concerns about inappropriately exposing women during pad placement (Paratz et al., 2024).

Men face a different set of health challenges. Men tend to die younger than women for a variety of biological and social reasons (Baker, 2020). Gendered beliefs and norms around masculinity may result in men delaying presentation to healthcare, especially in relation to mental health, and being more likely to ignore pain, or downplay the severity of symptoms (Farrimond, 2011, Galdas et al., 2005, Sagar-Ouriaghli et al., 2020, Seidler et al., 2016). Men are also less likely to look up health-related information online, and when they do, the quality of information that they access is generally poorer (Alvarez-Galvez et al., 2020).

Transgender people face significant barriers to care and receive poor care when they are able to. This can include staff lacking cultural competence and poorly understanding their health needs, insurance issues and discrimination (Bakko and Kattari, 2020, Korpaisarn and Safer, 2018). So, as with age, whilst we cannot change someone's biological sex or gender, we can look at addressing norms, issues of access and how care is provided by looking closer at why sex and gender results in care being experienced in such different ways, to reduce some of the risks experienced by different genders (Gupta et al., 2019). Such awareness is driving calls for gendered considerations in the design and delivery of healthcare services (Gupta et al., 2019) and has resulted in calls for a men's health strategy to be implemented (Baker, 2020, White and Tod, 2022), alongside the United Kingdom's existing women's health strategy (Department of Health and Social Care, 2022, Hamoda and Moger, 2022), with an increasing focus on gendered care being seen globally (Weber et al., 2019).

As with age and sex, our race and ethnicity are not modifiable. Race and ethnicity determine our health in many complex ways (Stronks et al., 2013). Studies consistently highlight that some races and ethnicities face increased risks of some conditions, but the explanations for these differences more frequently than not can be explained by social inequality (Lee et al., 2023, White et al., 2021). Even as far back as 1899, there has been an empirical basis for arguments that the disparities in health and well-being (in this case, Tuberculosis) seen by black people are generally not related to biology, but are instead the product of racial disparities relating to living and working conditions such

as access to education, and higher rates of service sector jobs (White et al., 2021). This relationship was identified in the important seminal work of sociologist W.E.B. Du Bois (1868–1963) in 'The Philadelphia Negro' (White et al., 2021).

Even as recently as the COVID-19 pandemic, those from global majority groups faced poorer outcomes though these were also largely socially determined, such as through increased exposure to the virus through the nature of employment, poverty, access to care and pre-existing poorer health (Abedi et al., 2021, Irizar et al., 2023, Khazanchi et al., 2020, Mude et al., 2021). Problematic biological explanations fail to identify the true social causes for differences in health outcomes by race for most health issues. This is complicated and arguably a harmful artifact of eugenics (Mold, 2022). In addition, research consistently highlights unequal care and discriminatory provision based on race and ethnicity across the full range of care settings (Ajayi Sotubo, 2021, Barnett et al., 2019, Knight et al., 2018). Even where a person's race does potentially biologically pre-dispose them to certain conditions, for example, Sickle Cell Anemia, the care provided for these conditions can end up being significantly poorer than that provided for other health needs (Redhead, 2021). Whilst a person's race and ethnicity are obviously not modifiable, the social processes that result in an increased likelihood of poor health, differing access to care and poorer care, are amenable to change. As too are the influences of culture on health behaviour such as diet, and one's living and working conditions.

Individual Lifestyle Factors

Moving out from beyond the personal characteristics that lay at the centre of the model, the other social determinants of health can broadly be considered modifiable at the micro, meso and macro levels (moving from the centre to the outside of the rainbow). Individual lifestyle behaviours such as diet, activity levels, smoking and alcohol consumption can have a significant impact on mortality and morbidity (GBD2019 Risk Factor Collaborators, 2020). Culture means that sometimes these relate to the constitutional factors we have just discussed, and they can also relate to SES as well as the influence of people's personal social networks (Christakis and Fowler, 2007, 2008, 2013, Smith and Christakis, 2008, Gurung, 2019, Rosenquist et al., 2010). For now, it is worth unpicking just how relevant these modifiable (i.e. they can be changed) behaviours are to our health and wellbeing. Whilst the 'Rainbow Model' is not a medicalised model (i.e. it does not seek to explain the causes of a specific disease), there are a range of health behaviours that global burden of disease studies consistently highlight as relating to the aetiology of many common chronic health conditions contributing to global morbidity and mortality. In particular tobacco smoking, excessive alcohol consumption, physical inactivity and obesity are known to contribute to morbidity and mortality internationally (Dai et al., 2020, Griswold et al., 2018, He et al., 2022, Katzmarzyk et al., 2021).

Of course, there are many healthy and unhealthy behaviours that people may choose to follow. We will expand more fully on some of those that studies have demonstrated as being most impactful in later chapters that consider unhealthy behaviour and evidence-based behaviour change strategies (Chapters 12–13). The extent to which people should be held responsible for their own unhealthy or healthy behaviours is contested. Certainly, people can control what they consume and how they behave, to an extent. However, these behaviours are generally influenced by many social processes that exist outside of any one individual. At this point, it is relevant to point out that there is a 'policy preoccupation' around behaviour change as a panacea for addressing health inequalities, rather than committed efforts to address the upstream issues through other interventions that may lead to such behaviours in the first place (Williams and Fullagar, 2019). This will be unpacked further when we consider evidence-based public health interventions later in this book (Chapter 14).

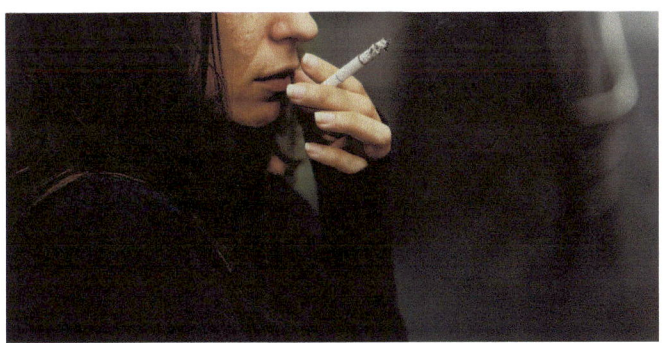

Source: Rawpixel.com/Adobe Stock Photos. With permission from 'The Health Foundation'.

Social and Community Networks

Our social and community networks influence the norms of the community in which we live. Well-known seminal studies, such as the Framingham heart study, have highlighted that health behaviours and health and well-being-related outcomes spread across social networks (Christakis and Fowler, 2008, Fowler and Christakis, 2008, van den Ende et al., 2024). Networks set the boundaries for what is, and what is not acceptable health behaviours. Normative behaviours can influence whether people follow health-promoting behaviours such as attending screening programmes (Manjer et al., 2015), breastfeeding (Baño-Piñero et al., 2018), regular physical exercise (Montgomery et al., 2020) and consuming a healthy diet (Harmon et al., 2016). Networks can also influence people's engagement in unhealthy behaviours, such as alcohol and substance misuse (Knox et al., 2019, Rosenquist et al., 2010), and overeating (Christakis and Fowler, 2007). Networks may also provide a stress-buffering effect, increasing our resilience and making it less likely we will engage in unhealthy behaviours to cope with stressful life

situations (Thoits, 2011). We will dive deeper into the role of social networks in health behaviours, and the relevance of social capital and various types of instrumental (i.e. practical support), emotional and informational support in Chapter 15.

Living and Working Conditions

The living and working conditions that determine health are particularly numerous and diverse. Here, we have focussed on some of the most significant aspects as illustrative examples of their impact on our health and our well-being.

Housing

Understanding housing as a social determinant of health is complex. The quality of housing, in terms of the impact of construction defects (leading to safety concerns and exposure to toxins) and poor ventilation (leading to dampness and mould), alongside inadequate heating and insulation, are known causes of morbidity and other health-related issues (Rolfe et al., 2020). There are also less tangible impacts of housing on health and well-being more generally – such as their impact on status, identity and ontological security (meaning simply stability and a sense of continuity) (Clapham et al., 2018, Rolfe et al., 2020), through which social and community assets can be accessed.

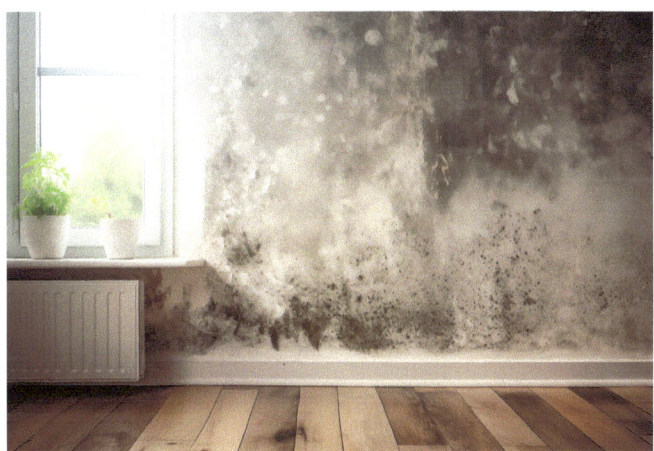

Source: EdNurg/Adobe Stock Photos. With permission from 'The Health Foundation'.

Work Environment and Unemployment

Generally, we need access to money to live happy healthy lives. In some countries, particularly wealthier ones, people's income is protected to at least some extent by social welfare policies (O'Campo et al., 2015). These provide money to secure needed resources to help people meet their material needs, as well as provide some degree of assurance that at least some basic level of sustenance can continue despite unemployment. Because of this, such protection is important in maintaining people's health and well-being during times of increased personal and economic uncertainty (O'Campo et al., 2015). Even in countries where citizens enjoy at least some access to social welfare provision, the impact of losing employment is often significant, not just in terms of income, but also in terms of esteem, stigma and how people are seen by themselves and by others (Krug et al., 2019, Smith and Anderson, 2018). In particular, the sudden withdrawal of large employers or whole industries from certain areas can have a large impact on the available opportunities, broader social support (such as work ties) and attendant facilities and infrastructure for people living in these areas (Smith and Anderson, 2018). Associated with this, research has consistently highlighted the health risk posed by unemployment (Norström et al., 2019, Pratap et al., 2021, Tapia Granados et al., 2014), with much of this risk arising from the increased stress and in part associated changes in health behaviours as a coping mechanism (Kivimäki et al., 2012, Monsivais et al., 2015, Nyberg et al., 2014). Those who have lost their job face additional psychological stress and are more likely to suffer from depression and low self-esteem (Brand, 2015). In addition, they are also significantly more likely to attempt or complete suicide, than their securely employed counterparts (Choi et al., 2022).

The nature of someone's work also has a profound impact on someone's health and well-being both in terms of ascribed status which is now recognised to have psycho-social impacts on health (Marmot, 2015), but also too in relation to occupational exposures of particular types of work (Armenti et al., 2023). In wealthier nations, through regulation and better overall working conditions, including safety, the health risks posed by most forms of employment are very closely monitored. Even in these countries though, some jobs and working conditions (e.g. shift work especially at night) carry greater occupational risk than others (Okechukwu et al., 2023). As one example, during COVID-19, many frontline workers experienced significantly greater levels of exposure to the virus, leading to increased mortality (Green and Semple, 2023). Those with low autonomy at work, especially where the work is demanding, and with low reward (both in terms of monetary reward, but also in terms of status and meaning) typically experience poorer health outcomes including increased cardiovascular risk (Kivimäki et al., 2012, Marmot, 2015, Niedhammer et al., 2021). Insecure jobs in particular, such as those within the 'gig economy'[2] (a model of employment that a large number of your delivery drivers work under), are increasingly being seen as harmful to health (Julià et al., 2017).

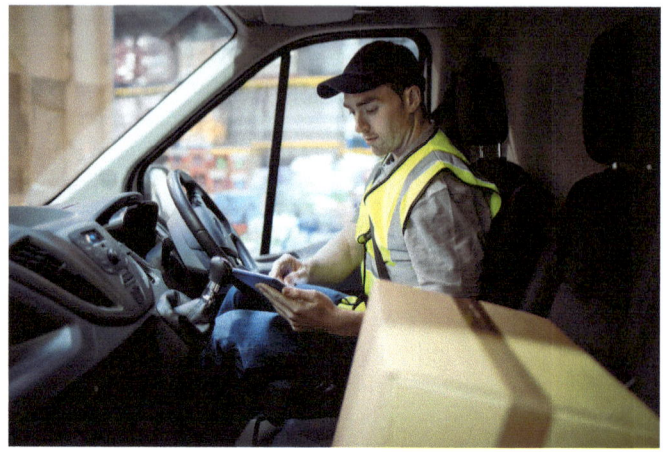

Source: WavebreakMediaMicro/Adobe Stock Photos.

Education

It is widely recognised that educational attainment is linked to mortality and morbidity (Zajacova and Lawrence, 2018). The reasons for this are complex and interrelated. Educational attainment is linked to health literacy, which is basically a measure of how well someone can obtain, interpret and apply health-related information to make decisions about and manage their own health (Clouston et al., 2016). We have discussed the importance of employment already – but it is worth highlighting its relationship with education – good education can also help people into well-paid, meaningful employment (Raghupathi and Raghupathi, 2020). The nature of someone's employment and their levels of education are central aspects of someone's social status – and we know that SES, a concept we explore later in this chapter, is related to health outcomes (Kivimäki et al., 2020, Laine et al., 2019). Well-educated adults live healthier and longer lives than their less-educated peers with the differences in health outcomes relating to education expanding (Zajacova and Lawrence, 2018).

Health Services

In Chapter 5, we highlighted that much of the world does not enjoy universal health coverage (Wagstaff and Neelsen, 2020). The provision of health services in a society affects health in several ways, from public health provision (i.e. primary prevention) that intends to prevent ill health in the first place, through to the provision of screening programmes, and where necessary, access to treatment. How such services are financed, differs from country to country. In countries lacking universal coverage, people need to fund care through out-of-pocket expenditures. This can be catastrophic and can involve selling important family assets and resources (Dickman et al., 2017, Getachew et al., 2023).

---

[2]A relatively new model of employment relations (considered below when discussing class) that typically involves consumers being able to directly connect with workers usually through some type of digitally mediated technology.

Social Position, Social Class and Social Status

Before exploring health inequalities, it is important to first consider social inequality briefly as a related concept. There has been a historic lack of consensus in our approach to social inequalities. This lack of consensus has made drawing comparisons between different groups and nations challenging with a high reliance being placed on looking at income, class and status differences. For clarity, before diving in to consider how health inequalities manifest, it is important to outline social stratification, and the role of class, social status and social positions in how different groups are seen, as well as how these social processes shape and influence our health. The terms social class and social status are often used interchangeably, yet they are different but related concepts. By understanding these, and what they mean, you should be able to start to see how they might impact on someone's health and well-being.

In Marx's early work (some of which is explored in Chapter 2), people were primarily put into one of two broad categories. People either owned the means of production (i.e. the capital), or did not, and therefore had to labour (i.e. the workers or the proletariat, as Marx called them). These categories broadly defined someone's social standing, or class. Essentially, does a person need to work, and if they do need to work, what is the nature of that work and their general employment conditions?

This binary starting point provides something of a conceptual framework through which we can explore class relations. For those having to work, what they do and how this relates to those they work for (i.e. levels of seniority, autonomy and control) are important to determining their class. UK readers will be very familiar with the concept of the upper, middle and working class. The usefulness of thinking about class along these three strata has arguably waned, owing to there being much more variety in the nature of work, culture and the role of people's social connections (Manstead, 2018). As a result, such largely work-related classifications have evolved over time, and now one of the most common systems in the United Kingdom, where it is used in the census, is the NS-SEC, which is a validated classification scheme for social class that principally aims to capture and categorise occupations with similar employment relations and conditions (Goldthorpe, 2000, ONS, 2021). Within the NS-SEC occupations are 'clumped together', due to members of these occupations sharing similar levels of income, security (often based on the nature of their employment contract), mobility (i.e. opportunities to advance), authority and autonomy, knowledge and skills, and levels of manual labour (ONS, 2021). Whilst this system is not intended to infer a hierarchy, higher status is afforded to those in higher managerial roles, compared to those in routine occupations, as we will go on to explore.

> ## The National Statistics Socio-Economic Classification System (NS-SEC)
>
> 1. **Higher managerial, and professional occupations**, including employers in large firms, higher managers and professionals, whether they are employees or self-employed.
> 2. **Lower managerial and professional occupations** and higher technical occupations.
> 3. **Intermediate occupations** (clerical, administrative, sales workers with no involvement in general planning or supervision but high levels of job security, some career prospects and some autonomy over their own work schedule).
> 4. **Small employers and self-employed workers.**
> 5. **Lower technical occupations** (with little responsibility for planning own work), lower supervisory occupations (with supervisory responsibility but no overall planning role and less autonomy over work schedule).
> 6. **Semi-routine occupations** (moderate levels of job security; little career prospects; no pay increments; some degree of autonomy over their own work).
> 7. **Routine occupations** (low job security; no career prospects; closely supervised routine work).
>
> (ONS, 2021)

Importantly, the structure of many countries' class systems is subject to change, in line with changing occupational profiles, for example, the rapid emergence of jobs in technology, may require more detailed consideration of the underlying characteristics of new forms of employment as they emerge (Williams, 2017). One other notable attempt to capture this, is the findings put forward by the Great British Class Survey (Savage et al., 2013). When considering the various forms of capital that sociologist Pierre Bourdieu (1930–2002) identified as important to class, notably economic (i.e. money), cultural (ability to recognise and engage with culture) and social (having important social contacts), seven classes were identified. These were: elite (such as CEOs), established middle class (such as midwives), technical middle class (such as pharmacists), new affluent workers (such as electricians), traditional working class (such as cleaners), emergent service sector (such as bar staff) and finally precariat (such as van drivers and retail workers – precariat highlighting the precarious nature of this type of employment) (Savage et al., 2013).

Where social class essentially refers to someone's occupational relations and conditions (i.e. all clerical workers make up the same 'intermediate' class), social status relates to individuals and their perceived status in each society (i.e. what personal characteristics are valued in a given social context). A society's belief about the importance of different characteristics is ultimately what leads to social stratification. Because the process of social status ranks people based on the characteristics that are valued in that particular social context, the people who are advantaged and disadvantaged will differ between societies. Even in more socially mobile countries, status is generally stubbornly persistent across generations. Higher-status parents raise kids who themselves reflect the status of their parents, and so on.

Capturing social status is complex but attempts to measure social status have typically focussed on understanding the ascribed value or prestige attached to different occupations, which is often derived from the income of that job, alongside the length of education needed to do it. Income, education and occupation being used together in an attempt to describe someone's status is often termed 'socio-economic status' (SES) (income, education, occupation) (Pollack et al., 2007). For some time, there have been calls for some kind of standardisation in terms of how SES should be measured – as this would allow for comparisons across populations and studies (Oakes and Rossi, 2003), and there are several different tools being used for its measurement, with some recently validated objective tools existing that consider access to material and social resources (Sacre et al., 2023) alongside subjective 'ladder' measurements that capture a person's perceived social standing (as a rung on a ladder) relative to others in their community. There is some suggestion that these might in fact better predict health outcomes (Zhao et al., 2023). Indeed, as we will explore later, your perception of where you rank within your society can have a significant impact on your health and well-being.

Intersectionality

The concept of intersectionality was originally developed within feminism. Black feminist academics, alongside activists, highlighted that they experienced disadvantages relating to more than one characteristic. For example, a black woman, in a low-status profession, faces disadvantages that are different from that typically experienced by a black woman in a higher-status profession. Intersectionality essentially highlights that people can be disadvantaged, and advantaged in several ways – with people's own unique set of characteristics, including their cognitive, mental and physical abilities contributing to their experiences and how societies respond to them. There is an increased focus on incorporating this into health inequalities research (Bambra, 2022).

What Are Health Inequalities?

Having now explored the determinants of health, defined and considered the concepts of class, social status and socioeconomic position, we are now in a position to begin to consider how these concepts create situations whereby individuals and societies have unequal health outcomes. To start this section,

we must first consider a fundamental question – what do we mean when we refer to 'inequalities of health?' Spoilers are laden throughout the early sections of this chapter, but inequalities of health are essentially the:

'Systematic differences in the health status of different population groups. These inequities have significant social and economic costs both to individuals and to societies' (WHO, 2018).

These systematic variations between social groups are largely socially produced and are thus considered avoidable and socially unjust (Whitehead, 2007). As you will see in this chapter, these differences can have a significant impact on health; those with poor objective and subjective SES tend to experience poorer health and shorter lives (Lago-Peñas et al., 2021, Laine et al., 2019). Whilst the 'Rainbow Model' is not a model of health inequalities, as a model of health determinants, we can look towards it to start to consider how different groups of people have unequal access to things that are health enhancing, as well as exposure to things that have a negative impact on health and well-being (Dahlgren and Whitehead, 2021). Some examples have already been provided to get us to this point. It is important to highlight that most of the determinants in the model do not relate to an individual's choice – they lie outside an individual's control, and therefore, it is inappropriate to make moral judgements relating to a person's health, and their decisions. Even individual health behaviours are shaped by the social environment in which people find themselves in, and who they interact with in that environment – as we have highlighted already (and will explore in more depth in Chapter 12).

The now seminal Marmot review (2010) and the further review 10 years on (Marmot et al., 2020) highlighted a clear health gradient within England (shown in Figures 8.2 and 8.3). Looking at these, as just one source of evidence, of just two outcomes (life expectancy and disability-free life expectancy), it is hard to argue that such differences in outcomes exist, even in a country with free healthcare at the point of need, such as in England.

In Figures 8.2 and 8.3, you can see several grey dots and several green dots. Each dot is a neighbourhood. The grey dots represent a neighbourhoods life expectancy (how long people in that area typically live on average). The green dots represent a neighbourhood's disability-free life expectancy (this is a complicated calculation, but is essentially how long people in that neighbourhood can expect to live in good health, on average). The line through these dots represents the relationship between a neighbourhood's level of deprivation and the life expectancy (grey) or disability-free life expectancy (green) for those living in that area. As you can see, this relationship is grim. Those living in the most affluent areas within England can often expect to enjoy over 10 years of life more than those living in the least affluent areas. There are some stark differences in the disability-free life expectancy of different neighbourhoods too. In the context of the United Kingdom, recent work has further highlighted that those from more deprived areas are significantly more likely to have at least one diagnosed illness, as well as having an increased risk of multi-morbidity (Barnett et al., 2012, Knies and Kumari, 2022, Watt et al., 2022).

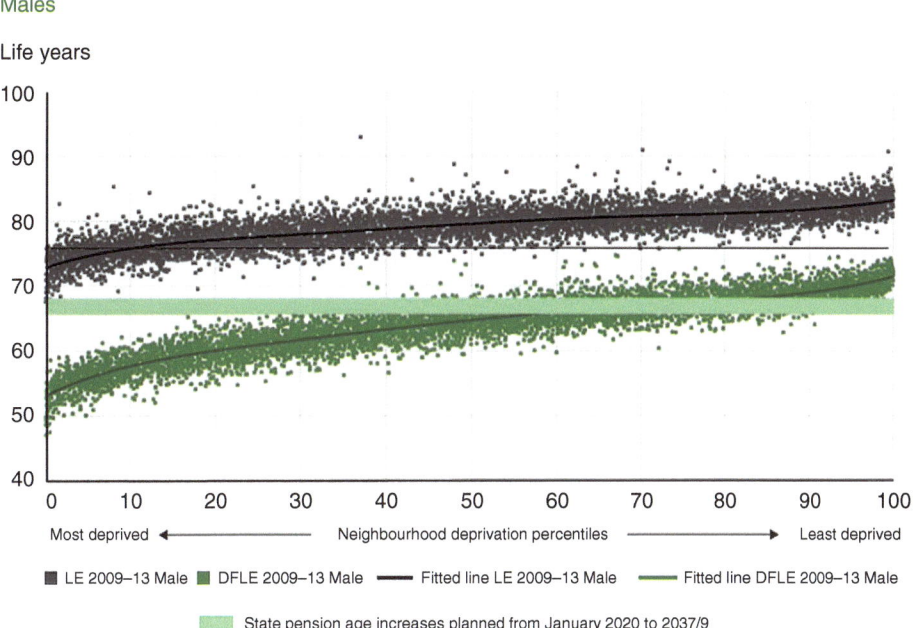

FIGURE 8.2 Male life expectancy and disability-free life expectancy at birth by neighbourhood deprivation, 2009–2013. **Source:** Reproduced with permission from Marmot et al (2020) / The Health Foundation/ https://www.instituteofhealthequity.org/resources-reports/marmot-review-10-years-on/the-marmot-review-10-years-on-full-report.pdf/ Last accessed on Feb 10, 2025.

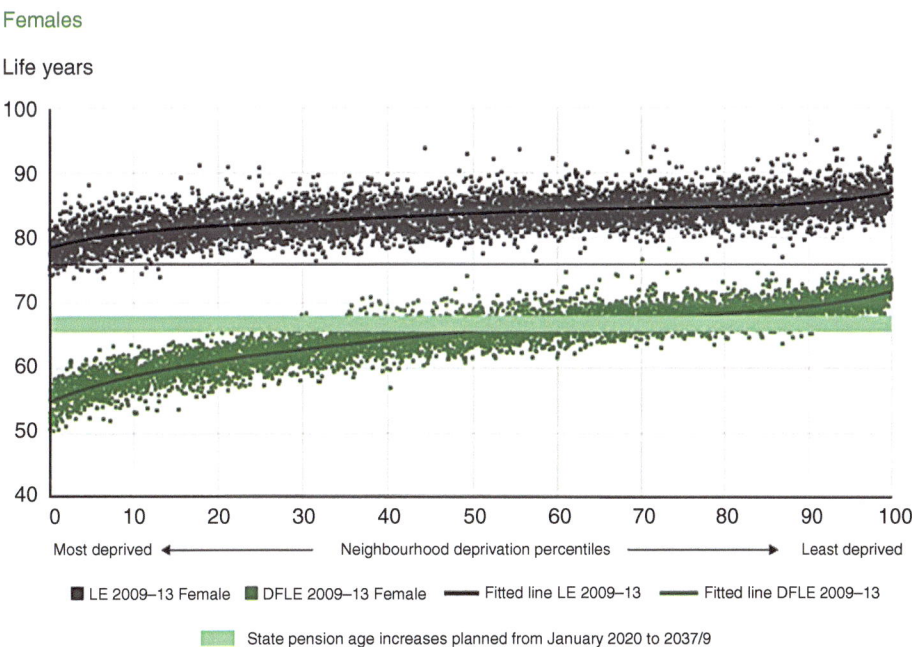

FIGURE 8.3 Female life expectancy and disability-free life expectancy at birth by neighbourhood deprivation, 2009–2013. **Source:** Reproduced with permission from Marmot et al (2020) / The Health Foundation/ https://www.instituteofhealthequity.org/resources-reports/marmot-review-10-years-on/the-marmot-review-10-years-on-full-report.pdf/ Last accessed on Feb 10, 2025.

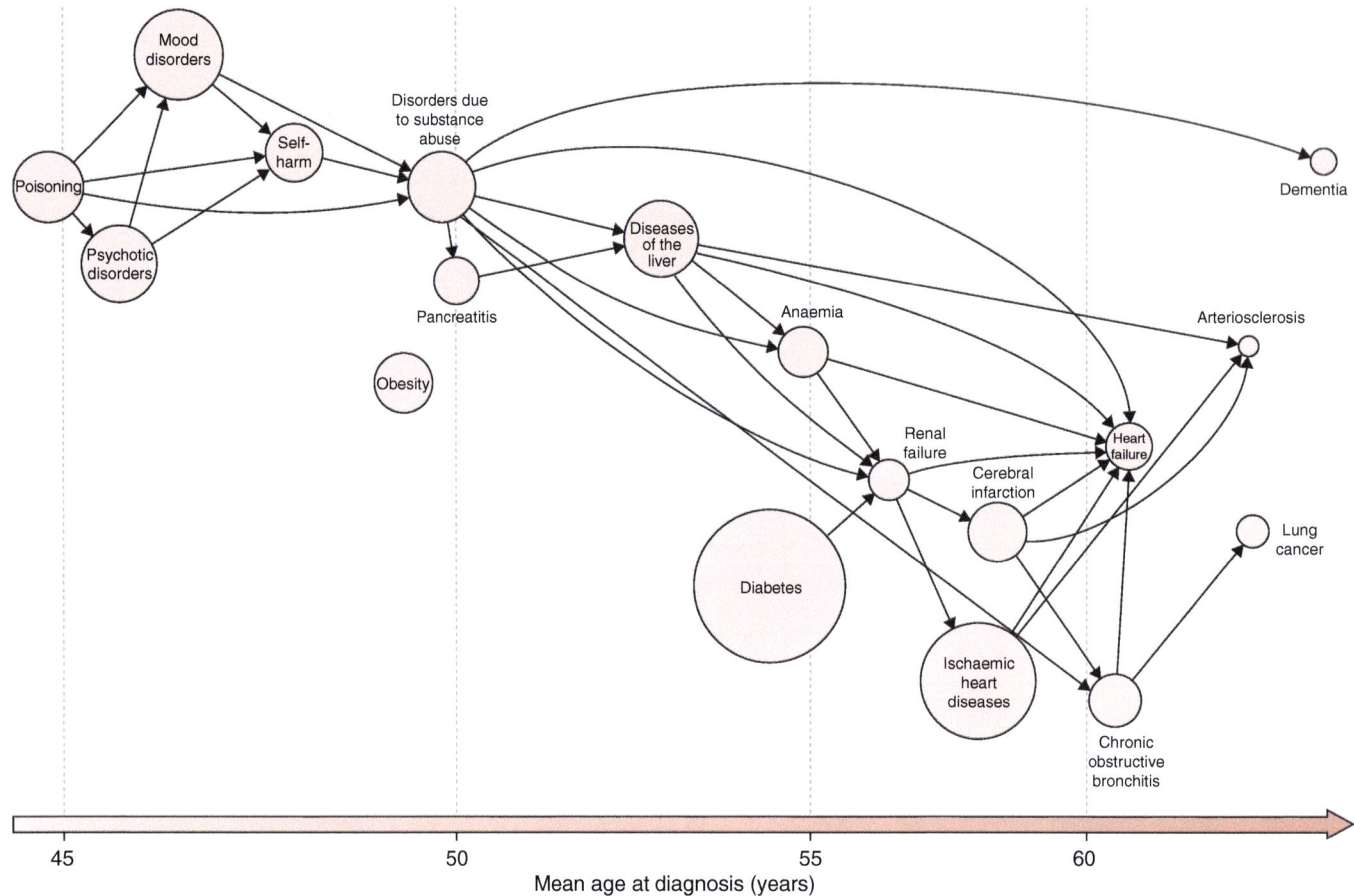

FIGURE 8.4   Cascade of disease and health status in socio-economically disadvantaged populations. **Source:** Kivimäki et al. (2020)/ Association between socio-economic status and the development of mental and physical health conditions in adulthood: a multi-cohort study/ Elsevier/CC by 4.0.(3).

As we will explore, having a diagnosed illness, be it mental or physical, can create a cascade that leads to further health conditions, creating an accumulation of further disadvantages that reveal themselves across the life course (Kivimäki et al., 2020). This is shown in Figure 8.4, which highlights a cascade of disease in socio-economically disadvantaged populations that generally involves the accumulation of mental health and behavioural disorders, followed by the development of chronic health conditions such as liver disease and pancreatitis.

The relationship between wealth and health is observed within communities, within towns, within cities, within nations and between countries (Health Foundation, 2021). Over many years, despite efforts, this relationship has been remarkably resistant to change. Because we all fit on the graph somewhere (and nearly all of us are not at the very top!), this issue negatively impacts on us all. However, the impacts of health inequalities are especially felt by society's poorest members. There is no one explanation for why these significant differences exist. The reasons behind this are complex and multifactorial, and there are a few interrelated explanations that are useful in understanding why such differences exist. Some of which, we will now explore.

Explanations for Health Inequalities

Material Explanations

Material explanations essentially highlight the damage caused by poverty and suggest that those with lower incomes may experience poorer health because of more limited access to health-enhancing resources (Smith and Anderson, 2018). Lacking cash reduces people's opportunities to access the range of resources that are needed to live healthy and fulfilled lives and this can include access to even basic resources and needs such as adequate housing, fuel to heat these homes, sanitation, food and clean water, transport and access to healthcare when it is needed. Across the globe, people experience unequal access to the material resources they need to live healthy lives, and even in rich countries such as the United Kingdom, societies' poorest members can experience food, fuel and transportation poverty (Jenkins et al., 2021, Sovacool et al., 2023). Not being able to acquire needed resources, both for themselves and for their families and those they care about, can be a source of shame for those experiencing material disadvantage (Smith and Anderson, 2018).

A lack of cash can also limit our choices, including restricting our access to healthier alternatives. Healthy food can be expensive and rising food prices and insecurity in those with lower incomes who are especially vulnerable, might lead to the adoption of unhealthy, and disordered patterns of consumption within families (Penne and Goedemé, 2021, Pilgrim et al., 2012). For families on the lowest income centile, following the UK NHS Eatwell Guide would involve spending almost 75% of their disposable income on food (Scott et al., 2018). Research has highlighted that whilst people recognise the importance of following a healthy diet, dietary choices are primarily guided by cost which invariably leads to the consumption of unhealthier options (Puddephatt et al., 2020). As one further example, those with COPD are often advised to eat a diet high in protein (Bernardes et al., 2022). However, high-protein diets are expensive (Brooks et al., 2010), and there is a socio-economic pattern to COPD, meaning it is more common in those less likely to be able to afford such a diet (Gershon et al., 2012).

Psycho-social Explanations

Where material explanations highlight the damage done through people lacking the means to secure basic needed resources, psycho-social explanations focus more on the inequality between people with different statuses and different incomes (Marmot and Wilkinson, 2001) alongside the social processes and mechanisms linking social inequality to health inequality (Pickett and Wilkinson, 2015, Wilkinson and Pickett, 2019). This is relevant, because as we have shown, those who are very rich, still have better health outcomes than those who are above the poverty threshold and do have enough money to secure needed and essential resources – generally, we all have worse health than the people in the top centile. This means that differential health outcomes cannot be explained solely based on whether or not people can shelter, stay warm, eat, drink and eliminate safely. Instead, we can look to some psycho-social explanations for such differences that may actually trigger biological changes in the body that explain poorer health (Bartley, 2017). These can include, for example, how stressful one's life is, how in control one feels (both in relation to work and life in general), how much social support one has and how fair one feels life is (especially when comparing their situation with others) (Bartley, 2017, Pickett and Wilkinson, 2015, Wilkinson and Pickett, 2019). Bartley (2017) highlights that research examining psycho-social explanations has typically considered the influence of home, work and community contexts. We cover the relevance of social and community support in Chapters 15–17, but it is relevant to discuss work strain here.

The now seminal and ongoing Whitehall studies, particularly Whitehall II, highlighted differences between people's occupational class and their health. Whitehall II, a very large longitudinal study of around 10,000 British civil servants, showed an inverse relationship between class and early mortality from a range of health conditions, particularly cardiovascular disease (Bosma et al., 1997, Marmot et al., 1991). Those from lower occupational classes had worse health and were also more likely to engage in unhealthy behaviour (Marmot et al., 1991). The materially different resources that people can access, as well as their status, especially when this is compounded by feelings of inequity and unfairness, plays a role in how people evaluate themselves in relation to others and can amount to strain and stress that can be harmful to our health (Marmot, 2015). It has been suggested that this can result in biological changes to a person's body, which can explain why low autonomy and low-status roles may harm people's health (Bartley, 2017, Pickett and Wilkinson, 2015).

Cultural Explanations

There is a known relationship between several unhealthy behaviours and class and lower SES (Katainen and Gronow, 2024, Pampel et al., 2010). Several health behaviours are seemingly paradoxical. For example, harmful health behaviours such as smoking are relatively expensive – but smoking is now more common in those with less financial means (Chen et al., 2019). In contrast, going for a walk and lots of other outdoor well-being-related activities, are either free or relatively cheap, but a more likely pursuit of those with more financial means for several reasons (Rigby et al., 2020). Pierre Bourdieu's (1930–2002) concept of habitus is useful here and has been used by medical sociologists to view the role of social class in determining people's behaviours (Rogers and Pilgrim, 2024). Our tastes, choices and behaviours are generated through our social circumstances, as well as through our social networks; therefore, largely determining what we do – the food we eat, whether we drink and how much, whether we smoke, whether we exercise and what exercise we do (Rogers and Pilgrim, 2024). Essentially, the concept of habitus is used to highlight the role of class in shaping health behaviours: salutogenic ones (such as walks in nature) as well as harmful ones (such as smoking) (McCartney et al., 2019, Rogers and Pilgrim, 2024, Wami et al., 2020). Habitus as a theory, is not without its critics, and it is relevant to highlight that people do have their own agency to choose which behaviours they follow. But it is also unwise to dismiss the relevance of people's social contexts to the patterning of their behaviours altogether. In attempting to move beyond simply identifying class-based differences in health outcomes, recent work has incorporated habitus into a wider theory-driven analysis of social class and health to examine the underlying mechanisms that determine why such class-based differences exist in the first place, using longitudinal methods (we unpack this further in Chapter 12) (McCartney et al., 2019, Wami et al., 2020). This is important, because many of these behaviours are set in early life, but have implications for later life well-being, as we will now briefly explore.

Life Course Explanations

The life course perspectives of health are discussed extensively in Chapter 15. Essentially, the life course approach considers the accumulated advantages and disadvantages that people experience throughout their life course. The various opportunities and exposures that people face and how these impact on their health and well-being in the future (Bartley, 2017). To an extent, it can capture all of the other explanations for inequality we have already discussed.

All the explanations that we have considered here, taken together, go some way to explaining why those in lower socio-economic status groups experience worse health outcomes. Inequalities in health are complex and multi-causal, and it is unlikely there will ever be one unifying explanation for their existence.

How Are Health Inequalities Experienced?

Despite the interest in health inequalities within the academic literature, there have been surprisingly few studies that have sought to understand how health inequalities are experienced by those who are disadvantaged, with the underlying assumption being that lay people, particularly those most affected, do not fully recognise the role of their SES on their health. One nice example of how the impact of health inequalities has been communicated to lay people is Clare Bambra's health inequalities football tables (Bambra, 2016). Recent work has drawn together examples of the different ways inequalities are experienced (Rogers and Pilgrim, 2024). In an interesting recent study, Smith and Anderson (2018) used 17 existing qualitative studies in a meta-ethnography and highlighted that whilst people were aware of the connections between SES and their health, people are often reluctant to acknowledge the impact these relationships have on them personally (Smith and Anderson, 2018). This is possibly due to stigmatising processes (covered in the following chapter) around deprivation, and a lack of autonomy and control (Smith and Anderson, 2018). The authors found factors, such as material, psycho-social and lifestyle behavioural factors, that contributed to socio-economic health-related inequalities, and factors that then linked these to negative health impacts (Smith and Anderson, 2018). They also found that people identified a whole series of amplifying (i.e. things that people felt made their situation worse), alongside factors that built up resilience against the deleterious impacts of inequalities on their health, such as their local community having nice places to go, having supportive social networks and positive experiences of education.

> ### Clinical Considerations
>
> - People's age, sex, gender, race and ethnicity can impact on their health in many ways. Many of these are social in nature, such as access to healthcare and the quality of healthcare provision.
> - People's health is determined by many things beyond this, much of which lies outside of an individual's control.
> - People's social, economic and material resources impact on their health in several ways. Those from lower SES groups are more likely to experience poor health and shorter lives.
> - A lack of material and financial resources can mean that some in society do not have the means to secure the things they and their families need to live a healthy and fulfilled life.
> - Certain living and working conditions are associated with poor health and poor health outcomes.
> - Advantages and disadvantages accumulate across the life course, and poor health can create a cascade of health problems that extend across the life course.

Conclusion

Life has ups and downs for all of us. The impact of these ups and downs can be influenced by a myriad number of factors including who we are, what resources we have, what our cultural norms and behaviours are and what are living and working conditions are like – amongst many other things. Generally, health inequalities mirror social inequalities such that those with lower SES typically face poorer health. This is experienced between countries, within countries and even within relatively small geographical areas such as within towns.

There are various explanations for why those with lower SES have poorer health. These include material, psycho-social and cultural-behavioural explanations. No explanation can adequately explain the complexity of health inequalities, but together, these explanations can go some way to helping us understand the underlying causes, and from this, we can look at how differences in outcomes can be addressed by interventions that target individuals, but most importantly in interventions that target upstream issues that cause people to experience poor health in the first place.

References

Abedi, V., Olulana, O., Avula, V., Chaudhary, D., Khan, A., Shahjouei, S. & LI, J. & Zand, R. 2021. Racial, economic, and health inequality and COVID-19 infection in the United States. *Journal of Racial and Ethnic Health Disparities*, 8, 732–742.

Ajayi Sotubo, O. 2021. A perspective on health inequalities in BAME communities and how to improve access to primary care. *Future Healthc J*, 8, 36–39.

Alvarez-Galvez, J., Salinas-Perez, J. A., Montagni, I. & Salvador-Carulla, L. 2020. The persistence of digital divides in the use of health information: a comparative study in 28 European countries. *International Journal of Public Health*, 65, 325–333.

Amini, M., Sharma, R. & Jani, C. 2023. Gender differences in leukemia outcomes based on health care expenditures using estimates from the GLOBOCAN 2020. *Archives of Public Health*, 81, 151.

Armenti, K., Sweeney, M. H., Lingwall, C. & Yang, L. 2023. Work: a social determinant of health worth capturing. *International Journal of Environmental Research and Public Health*, 20.

Baker, P. 2020. *From the Margins to the Mainstream: Advocating the Inclusion of Men's Health in Policy. A Scoping Study*, London: Global Action on Men's Health.

Bakko, M. & Kattari, S. K. 2020. Transgender-related insurance denials as barriers to transgender healthcare: differences in experience by insurance type. *Journal of General Internal Medicine*, 35, 1693–1700.

Bambra, C. 2016. *Health Divides: Where You Live Can Kill You*, Polity Press.

Bambra, C. 2022. Placing intersectional inequalities in health. *Health & Place*, 75, 102761.

Baño-Piñero, I., Martínez-Roche, M. E., Canteras-Jordana, M., Carrillo-García, C. & Orenes-Piñero, E. 2018. Impact of support networks for breastfeeding: a multicentre study. *Women and Birth*, 31, e239–e244.

Barnett, K., Mercer, S. W., Norbury, M., Watt, G., Wyke, S. & Guthrie, B. 2012. Epidemiology of multimorbidity and implications for health care, research, and medical education: a cross-sectional study. *The Lancet*, 380, 37–43.

Barnett, P., Mackay, E., Matthews, H., Gate, R., Greenwood, H., Ariyo, K., Bhui, K., Halvorsrud, K., Pilling, S. & smith, S. 2019. Ethnic variations in compulsory detention under the Mental Health Act: a systematic review and meta-analysis of international data. *The Lancet Psychiatry*, 6, 305–317.

Bartley, M. 2017. *Health Inequality: An Introduction to Concepts Theories and Methods*, Cambridge Polity.

Bernardes, S., Eckert, I. D. C., Burgel, C. F., Teixeira, P. J. Z. & Silva, F. M. 2022. Increased energy and/or protein intake improves anthropometry and muscle strength in chronic obstructive pulmonary disease patients: a systematic review with meta-analysis on randomised controlled clinical trials. *The British Journal of Nutrition*, 129(8), 1332–1349.

Bingefors, K., Hedborg, K., Isacson, D. & Sundbom, L. T. 2017. Are men under-treated and women over-treated with antidepressants? Findings from a cross-sectional survey in Sweden. *BJPsych Bulletin*, 41, 145–150.

Bosma, H., Marmot, M. G., Hemingway, H., Nicholson, A. C., Brunner, E. & Stansfeld, S. A. 1997. Low job control and risk of coronary heart disease in Whitehall II (prospective cohort) study. *BMJ*, 314, 558–565.

Brand, J. E. 2015. The far-reaching impact of job loss and unemployment. *Annual Review of Sociology*, 41, 359–375.

Braveman, P. & Gottlieb, L. 2014. The social determinants of health: it's time to consider the causes of the causes. *Public Health Reports*, 129(Suppl 2), 19–31.

Brooks, R. C., Simpson, S. J. & RAUBENHEIMER, D. 2010. The price of protein: combining evolutionary and economic analysis to understand excessive energy consumption. *Obesity Reviews*, 11, 887–894.

Burnes, D., Sheppard, C., Henderson, C. R., Jr., Wassel, M., Cope, R., Barber, C. & Pillemer, K. 2019. Interventions to reduce ageism against older adults: a systematic review and meta-analysis. *American Journal of Public Health*, 109, e1–e9.

Chen, A., Machiorlatti, M., Krebs, N. M. & Muscat, J. E. 2019. Socioeconomic differences in nicotine exposure and dependence in adult daily smokers. *BMC Public Health*, 19, 375.

Chen, E. H., Shofer, F. S., Dean, A. J., Hollander, J. E., Baxt, W. G., Robey, J. L. & sease, K. L. & Mills, A. M. 2008. Gender disparity in analgesic treatment of emergency department patients with acute abdominal pain. *Academic Emergency Medicine*, 15, 414–418.

Choi, N. G., Marti, C. N. & Choi, B. Y. 2022. Job loss, financial strain, and housing problems as suicide precipitants: Associations with other life stressors. *SSM Popul Health*, 19, 101243.

Christakis, N. A. & Fowler, J. H. 2007. The spread of obesity in a large social network over 32 years. *The New England Journal of Medicine*, 357, 370–379.

Christakis, N. A. & Fowler, J. H. 2008. The collective dynamics of smoking in a large social network. *New England Journal of Medicine*, 358, 2249–2258.

Christakis, N. A. & Fowler, J. H. 2013. Social contagion theory: examining dynamic social networks and human behavior. *Statistics in Medicine*, 32, 556–577.

Clapham, D., Foye, C. & Christian, J. 2018. The concept of subjective well-being in housing research. *Housing, Theory and Society*, 35, 261–280.

Clouston, S. A. P., Manganello, J. A. & Richards, M. 2016. A life course approach to health literacy: the role of gender, educational attainment and lifetime cognitive capability. *Age and Ageing*, 46, 493–499.

Co, M., Lee, A. & Kwong, A. 2020. Delayed presentation, diagnosis, and psychosocial aspects of male breast cancer. *Cancer Medicine*, 9, 3305–3309.

Dahlgren, G. & Whitehead, M. 2021. The Dahlgren-Whitehead model of health determinants: 30 years on and still chasing rainbows. *Public Health*, 199, 20–24.

Dai, H., Alsalhe, T. A., Chalghaf, N., Riccò, M., Bragazzi, N. L. & Wu, J. 2020. The global burden of disease attributable to high body mass index in 195 countries and territories, 1990–2017: an analysis of the Global Burden of Disease Study. *PLoS Medicine*, 17, e1003198.

Daskalopoulou, C., Stubbs, B., Kralj, C., Koukounari, A., Prince, M. & Prina, A. M. 2017. Physical activity and healthy ageing: a systematic review and meta-analysis of longitudinal cohort studies. *Ageing Research Reviews*, 38, 6–17.

Department of Health and Social Care. 2022. Policy paper: Women's Health Strategy for England. Available online at: https://www.gov.uk/government/publications/womens-health-strategy-for-england/womens-health-strategy-for-england.

Department of Health and Social Security. 1980. Inequalities in health: Report of a Working Group (The Black Report).

Dickman, S. L., Himmelstein, D. U. & Woolhandler, S. 2017. Inequality and the health-care system in the USA. *The Lancet*, 389, 1431–1441.

Doherty, A. J., Atherton, H., Boland, P., Hastings, R., Hives, L., Hood, K., James-Jenkinson, L., Leavey, R., Randell, E., Reed, J., Taggart, L., Wilson, N. & Chauhan, U. 2020. Barriers and facilitators to primary health care for people with intellectual disabilities and/or autism: an integrative review. *BJGP Open*, 4(3).

Farrimond, H. 2011. Beyond the caveman: rethinking masculinity in relation to men's help-seeking. *Health*, 16, 208–225.

Finneran, P., Toribio, M. P., Natarajan, P. & Honigberg, M. C. 2023. Delays in accessing healthcare across the gender spectrum in the all of us research program. *Journal of General Internal Medicine*, 39, 1156–1163.

Fowler, J. H. & Christakis, N. A. 2008. Dynamic spread of happiness in a large social network: longitudinal analysis over 20 years in the Framingham Heart Study. *BMJ*, 337.

Galdas, P. M., Cheater, F. & Marshall, P. 2005. Men and health help-seeking behaviour: literature review. *Journal of Advanced Nursing*, 49, 616–623.

GBD2019 Risk factor Collaborators 2020. Global burden of 87 risk factors in 204 countries and territories, 1990–2019: a systematic analysis for the Global Burden of Disease Study 2019. *The Lancet*, 396, 1223–1249.

Gershon, A. S., Dolmage, T. E., Stephenson, A. & Jackson, B. 2012. Chronic obstructive pulmonary disease and socioeconomic status: a systematic review. *COPD: Journal of Chronic Obstructive Pulmonary Disease*, 9, 216–226.

Getachew, N., Shigut, H., Jeldu Edessa, G. & Yesuf, E. A. 2023. Catastrophic health expenditure and associated factors among households of non community based health insurance districts, Illubabor zone, Oromia regional state, southwest Ethiopia. *International Journal for Equity in Health*, 22, 40.

Goldthorpe, J. H. 2000. Social class and the differentiation of employment contracts. *In: On Sociology: Numbers, Narratives, and the Integration of Research and Theory*, Oxford.

Gopal, D. P., Chetty, U., O'donnell, P., Gajria, C. & Blackadder-Weinstein, J. 2021. Implicit bias in healthcare: clinical practice, research and decision making. *Future Healthcare Journal*, 8, 40–48.

Green, M. A. & Semple, M. G. 2023. Occupational inequalities in the prevalence of COVID-19: a longitudinal observational study of England, August 2020 to January 2021. *Public Library of Science One*, 18, e0283119.

Griswold, M. G., Fullman, N., Hawley, C., Arian, N., Zimsen, S. R. M., Tymeson, H. D., Venkateswaran, V., Tapp, A. D., Forouzanfar, M. H., Salama, J. S., Abate, K. H., Abate, D., Abay, S. M., Abbafati, C., Abdulkader, R. S., Abebe, Z., Aboyans, V., Abrar, M. M., Acharya, P., Adetokunboh, O. O., Adhikari, T. B., Adsuar, J. C., Afarideh, M., Agardh, E. E., Agarwal, G., Aghayan, S. A., Agrawal, S., Ahmed, M. B., Akibu, M., Akinyemiju, T., Akseer, N., Asfoor, D. H. A., Al-Aly, Z., Alahdab, F., Alam, K., Albujeer, A., Alene, K. A., Ali, R., Ali, S. D., Alijanzadeh, M., Aljunid, S. M.,

Alkerwi, A. A., Allebeck, P., Alvis-Guzman, N., Amare, A. T., Aminde, L. N., Ammar, W., Amoako, Y. A., Amul, G. G. H., Andrei, C. L., Angus, C., Ansha, M. G., Antonio, C. A. T., Aremu, O., Ärnlöv, J., Artaman, A., Aryal, K. K., Assadi, R., Ausloos, M., Avila-Burgos, L., Avokpaho, E. F., Awasthi, A., Ayele, H. T., Ayer, R., Ayuk, T. B., Azzopardi, P. S., Badali, H., Badawi, A., Banach, M., Barker-Collo, S. L., Barrero, L. H., Basaleem, H., Baye, E., Bazargan-Hejazi, S., Bedi, N., Béjot, Y., Belachew, A. B., Belay, S. A., Bennett, D. A., Bensenor, I. M., Bernabe, E., Bernstein, R. S., Beyene, A. S., Beyranvand, T., Bhaumik, S., Bhutta, Z. A., Biadgo, B., Bijani, A., Bililign, N., Birlik, S. M., Birungi, C., Bizuneh, H., Bjerregaard, P., Bjørge, T., Borges, G., Bosetti, C., Boufous, S., Bragazzi, N. L., Brenner, H., Butt, Z. A., et al. 2018. Alcohol use and burden for 195 countries and territories, 1990–2016: a systematic analysis for the Global Burden of Disease Study 2016. *The Lancet*, 392, 1015–1035.

Gupta, G. R., Oomman, N., Grown, C., Conn, K., Hawkes, S., Shawar, Y. R., Shiffman, J., Buse, K., Mehra, R., Bah, C. A., Heise, L., Greene, M. E., Weber, A. M., Heymann, J., Hay, K., Raj, A., Henry, S., Klugman, J. & Darmstadt, G. L. 2019. Gender equality and gender norms: framing the opportunities for health. *The Lancet*, 393, 2550–2562.

Gurung, R. A. R. 2019. *Cultural Influences on Health*, Cross-Cultural Psychology.

Hamoda, H. & Moger, S. 2022. Women's Health Strategy: Time to have women's voices at the top of the agenda. *Post Reproductive Health*, 28, 5–7.

Harmon, B. E., Forthofer, M., Bantum, E. O. & Nigg, C. R. 2016. Perceived influence and college students' diet and physical activity behaviors: an examination of ego-centric social networks. *BMC Public Health*, 16, 473.

He, H., Pan, Z., Wu, J., Hu, C., Bai, L. & Lyu, J. 2022. Health effects of tobacco at the global, regional, and national levels: results from the 2019 global burden of disease study. *Nicotine & Tobacco Research*, 24, 864–870.

Health Foundation. 2021. Relationship between income and healthy life expectancy by local authority [Online]. The Health Foundation Available: https://www.health.org.uk/evidence-hub/money-and-resources/income/relationship-between-income-and-healthy-life-expectancy-by-local-authority [Accessed].

Holdcroft, A. 2007. Gender bias in research: how does it affect evidence based medicine? *Journal of the Royal Society of Medicine*, 100, 2–3.

Irizar, P., Kapadia, D., Amele, S., Bécares, L., Divall, P., Katikireddi, S. V., Kibuchi, E., Kneale, D., Mccabe, R., Nazroo, J., Nellums, L. B., Taylor, H., Sze, S., Pan, D. & Pareek, M. 2023. Pathways to ethnic inequalities in COVID-19 health outcomes in the United Kingdom: a systematic map. *Social Science & Medicine*, 329, 116044.

Jackson, S. S., Marks, M. A., Katki, H. A., Cook, M. B., Hyun, N., Freedman, N. D., Kahle, L. L., Castle, P. E., Graubard, B. I. & Chaturvedi, A. K. 2022. Sex disparities in the incidence of 21 cancer types: quantification of the contribution of risk factors. *Cancer*, 128, 3531–3540.

Jahnel, T., Dassow, H. H., Gerhardus, A. & Schüz, B. 2022. The digital rainbow: digital determinants of health inequities. *Digit Health*, 8, 20552076221129093.

Jenkins, R. H., Aliabadi, S., Vamos, E. P., Taylor-Robinson, D., Wickham, S., Millett, C. & Laverty, A. A. 2021. The relationship between austerity and food insecurity in the UK: a systematic review. *EClinicalMedicine*, 33.

Julià, M., Vanroelen, C., Bosmans, K., Van Aerden, K. & Benach, J. 2017. Precarious employment and quality of employment in relation to health and well-being in Europe. *International Journal of Health Services*, 47, 389–409.

Katainen, A. & Gronow, A. 2024. Habits and the socioeconomic patterning of health-related behaviour: a pragmatist perspective. *Social Theory & Health*, 22, 36–52.

Katzmarzyk, P. T., Friedenreich, C., Shiroma, E. J. & Lee, I.-M. 2021. Physical inactivity and non-communicable disease burden in low-income, middle-income and high-income countries. *British Journal of Sports Medicine*, 56, 101–106.

Kennedy, E., Binder, G., Humphries-Waa, K., Tidhar, T., Cini, K., Comrie-Thomson, L., Vaughan, C., Francis, K., Scott, N., Wulan, N., Patton, G. & Azzopardi, P. 2020. Gender inequalities in health and wellbeing across the first two decades of life: an analysis of 40 low-income and middle-income countries in the Asia-Pacific region. *The Lancet Global Health*, 8, e1473–e1488.

Khazanchi, R., Evans, C. T. & Marcelin, J. R. 2020. Racism, not race, drives inequity across the COVID-19 continuum. *JAMA Network Open*, 3, e2019933.

Kingston, A., Robinson, L., Booth, H., Knapp, M., Jagger, C. & Project, M. 2018. Projections of multi-morbidity in the older population in England to 2035: estimates from the Population Ageing and Care Simulation (PACSim) model. *Age and Ageing*, 47, 374–380.

Kivimäki, M., Batty, G. D., Pentti, J., Shipley, M. J., Sipilä, P. N., Nyberg, S. T., Suominen, S. B., Oksanen, T., Stenholm, S., Virtanen, M., Marmot, M. G., Singh-Manoux, A., Brunner, E. J., Lindbohm, J. V., Ferrie, J. E. & Vahtera, J. 2020. Association between socioeconomic status and the development of mental and physical health conditions in adulthood: a multi-cohort study. *The Lancet Public Health*, 5, e140–e149.

Kivimäki, M., Nyberg, S. T., Batty, G. D., Fransson, E. I., Heikkilä, K., Alfredsson, L., Bjorner, J. B., Borritz, M., Burr, H., Casini, A., Clays, E., de Bacquer, D., Dragano, N., Ferrie, J. E., Geuskens, G. A., Goldberg, M., Hamer, M., Hooftman, W. E., Houtman, I. L., Joensuu, M., Jokela, M., Kittel, F., Knutsson, A., Koskenvuo, M., Koskinen, A., Kouvonen, A., Kumari, M., Madsen, I. E., Marmot, M. G., Nielsen, M. L., Nordin, M., Oksanen, T., Pentti, J., Rugulies, R., Salo, P., Siegrist, J., Singh-Manoux, A., Suominen, S. B., Väänänen, A., Vahtera, J., Virtanen, M., Westerholm, P. J., Westerlund, H., Zins, M., Steptoe, A. & Theorell, T. 2012. Job strain as a risk factor for coronary heart disease: a collaborative meta-analysis of individual participant data. *Lancet*, 380, 1491–1497.

Knies, G. & Kumari, M. 2022. Multimorbidity is associated with the income, education, employment and health domains of area-level deprivation in adult residents in the UK. *Scientific Reports*, 12, 7280.

Knight, M., Bunch, K., Tuffnell, D., Jayakody, H., Shakespeare, J., Kotnis, R., Kenyon, S. & Kurinczuk, J. 2018. Saving Lives, Improving Mothers' Care-Lessons learned to inform maternity care from the UK and Ireland Confidential Enquiries into Maternal Deaths and Morbidity 2014-16. MBRACE-UK. Available online at: https://www.npeu.ox.ac.uk/assets/downloads/mbrrace-uk/reports/maternal-report-2023/MBRRACE-UK_Maternal_Compiled_Report_2023.pdf.

Knox, J., Schneider, J., Greene, E., Nicholson, J., Hasin, D. & Sandfort, T. 2019. Using social network analysis to examine alcohol use among adults: a systematic review. *PLoS One*, 14, e0221360.

Korpaisarn, S. & Safer, J. D. 2018. Gaps in transgender medical education among healthcare providers: a major barrier to care for transgender persons. *Reviews in Endocrine and Metabolic Disorders*, 19, 271–275.

Krug, G., Drasch, K. & Jungbauer-Gans, M. 2019. The social stigma of unemployment: consequences of stigma consciousness on job search attitudes, behaviour and success. *Journal for Labour Market Research*, 53, 11.

Lago-Peñas, S., Rivera, B., Cantarero, D., Casal, B., Pascual, M., Blázquez-Fernández, C. & Reyes, F. 2021. The impact of socioeconomic position on non-communicable diseases: what do we know about it? *Perspectives in Public Health*, 141, 158–176.

Laine, J. E., Baltar, V. T., Stringhini, S., Gandini, M., Chadeau-Hyam, M., Kivimaki, M., Severi, G., Perduca, V., Hodge, A. M., Dugué, P.-A., Giles, G. G., Milne, R. L., Barros, H., Sacerdote, C., Krogh, V., Panico, S., Tumino, R., Goldberg, M., Zins, M., Delpierre, C., Consortium, L. & Vineis, P. 2019. Reducing socio-economic inequalities in all-cause mortality: a counterfactual mediation approach. *International Journal of Epidemiology*, 49, 497–510.

Lee, K. K., Norris, E. T., Rishishwar, L., Conley, A. B., Mariño-Ramírez, L., Mcdonald, J. F. & Jordan, I. K. 2023. Ethnic disparities in mortality and group-specific risk factors in the UK Biobank. *PLOS Global Public Health*, 3, e0001560.

Leitão, C., Mignano, A., Estrela, M., Fardilha, M., Figueiras, A., Roque, F. & Herdeiro, M. T. 2022. The effect of nutrition on aging-A systematic review focusing on aging-related biomarkers. *Nutrients*, 14.

Lund, E. M. & Burgess, C. M. 2021. Sexual and gender minority health care disparities: Barriers to care and strategies to bridge the gap. *Primary Care; Clinics in Office Practice*, 48, 179–189.

Manjer, Å. R., Emilsson, U. M. & Zackrisson, S. 2015. Non-attendance in mammography screening and women's social network: a cohort study on the influence of family composition, social support, attitudes and cancer in close relations. *World Journal of Surgical Oncology*, 13, 1–7.

Manstead, A. S. R. 2018. The psychology of social class: How socioeconomic status impacts thought, feelings, and behaviour. *British Journal of Social Psychology*, 57, 267–291.

Marmot, M. 2015. *Status Syndrome: How Your Place on the Social Gradient Directly Affects Your Health London*, Bloomsbury.

Marmot, M., Allen, J., Boyce, T., Goldblatt, P. & Morrison, J. 2020. Health Equity in England: The Marmot Review 10 Years On [Online]. The Health Foundation. Available: https://www.health.org.uk/publications/reports/the-marmot-review-10-years-on [Accessed].

Marmot, M. & Wilkinson, R. G. 2001. Psychosocial and material pathways in the relation between income and health: a response to Lynch et al. BMJ, 322, 1233–6.

Marmot, M. G. 2010. Fair society, healthy lives: the Marmot Review: strategic review of health inequalities in England post. Institute of Health Equity.

Marmot, M. G., Smith, G. D., Stansfeld, S., Patel, C., North, F., Head, J., White, I., Brunner, E. & Feeney, A. 1991. Health inequalities among British civil servants: the Whitehall II study. *Lancet*, 337, 1387–1393.

McCartney, G., Bartley, M., Dundas, R., Katikireddi, S. V., Mitchell, R., Popham, F., Walsh, D. & Wami, W. 2019. Theorising social class and its application to the study of health inequalities. *SSM – Population Health*, 7, 100315.

Merone, L., Tsey, K., Russell, D. & Nagle, C. 2022. Sex inequalities in medical research: a systematic scoping review of the literature. *Womens Health Rep (New Rochelle)*, 3, 49–59.

Mold, A. 2022. Publics and their health: 50 years of continuity and change. *Journal of Public Health*, 44, i17–i22.

Monsivais, P., Martin, A., Suhrcke, M., Forouhi, N. G. & Wareham, N. J. 2015. Job-loss and weight gain in British adults: evidence from two longitudinal studies. *Social Science & Medicine*, 143, 223–231.

Montgomery, S. C., Donnelly, M., Bhatnagar, P., Carlin, A., Kee, F. & Hunter, R. F. 2020. Peer social network processes and adolescent health behaviors: a systematic review. *Preventive Medicine*, 130, 105900.

Mude, W., Oguoma, V. M., Nyanhanda, T., Mwanri, L. & Njue, C. 2021. Racial disparities in COVID-19 pandemic cases, hospitalisations, and deaths: a systematic review and meta-analysis. *Journal of Global Health*, 11, 05015.

Muehlenhard, C. L. & Peterson, Z. D. 2011. Distinguishing between sex and gender: history, current conceptualizations, and implications. *Sex Roles*, 64, 791–803.

Nemiroff, L. 2022. We can do better: addressing ageism against older adults in healthcare. *Healthcare Management Forum*, 35, 118–122.

Niccoli, T. & Partridge, L. 2012. Ageing as a risk factor for disease. *Current Biology*, 22, R741–R752.

NICE. 2023. CVD risk assessment and management: What are the risk factors? [Online]. NICE: National Institute for Health and Care Excellence. Available: https://cks.nice.org.uk/topics/cvd-risk-assessment-management/background-information/risk-factors-for-cvd/ [Accessed].

Niedhammer, I., Bertrais, S. & Witt, K. 2021. Psychosocial work exposures and health outcomes: a meta-review of 72 literature reviews with meta-analysis. *Scandinavian Journal of Work, Environment & Health*, 47, 489–508.

Norström, F., Waenerlund, A.-K., Lindholm, L., Nygren, R., Sahlén, K.-G. & Brydsten, A. 2019. Does unemployment contribute to poorer health-related quality of life among Swedish adults? *BMC Public Health*, 19, 457.

Nyberg, S. T., Fransson, E. I., Heikkilä, K., Ahola, K., Alfredsson, L., Bjorner, J. B., Borritz, M., Burr, H., Dragano, N., Goldberg, M., Hamer, M., Jokela, M., Knutsson, A., Koskenvuo, M., Koskinen, A., Kouvonen, A., Leineweber, C., Madsen, I. E., Magnusson Hanson, L. L., Marmot, M. G., Nielsen, M. L., Nordin, M., Oksanen, T., Pejtersen, J. H., Pentti, J., Rugulies, R., Salo, P., Siegrist, J., Steptoe, A., Suominen, S., Theorell, T., Väänänen, A., Vahtera, J., Virtanen, M., Westerholm, P. J., Westerlund, H., Zins, M., Batty, G. D., Brunner, E. J., Ferrie, J. E., Singh-Manoux, A. & Kivimäki, M. 2014. Job strain as a risk factor for type 2 diabetes: a pooled analysis of 124,808 men and women. *Diabetes Care*, 37, 2268–2275.

O'Campo, P., Molnar, A., Ng, E., Renahy, E., Mitchell, C., Shankardass, K., John, S. T. & A., Bambra, C. & Muntaner, C. 2015. Social welfare matters: a realist review of when, how, and why unemployment insurance impacts poverty and health. *Social Science & Medicine*, 132, 88–94.

Oakes, J. M. & Rossi, P. H. 2003. The measurement of SES in health research: current practice and steps toward a new approach. *Social Science & Medicine*, 56, 769–784.

Okechukwu, C. E., Colaprico, C., Di Mario, S., Oko-Oboh, A. G., Shaholli, D., Manai, M. V., Torre, L. A. & G. 2023. The relationship between working night shifts and depression among nurses: a systematic review and meta-analysis. *Healthcare (Basel)*, 11.

ONS. 2015. Inequality in Helath and Life Expectancies within Upper Tier Local Authorities Statistical bulletins [Online]. Office of National Statistics Available: https://www.ons.gov.uk/peoplepopulationandcommunity/healthandsocialcare/healthandlifeexpectancies/bulletins/inequalityinhealthandlifeexpectancieswithinuppertierlocalauthorities/previousReleases [Accessed].

ONS.2021. The National Statistics Socio-Economic Classification (NS-SEC) [Online]. Available: https://www.ons.gov.uk/methodology/classificationsandstandards/otherclassifications/thenationalstatisticssocioeconomicclassificationnssecrebasedonsoc2010 [Accessed].

Pampel, F. C., Krueger, P. M. & Denney, J. T. 2010. Socioeconomic disparities in health behaviors. *Annual Review of Sociology*, 36, 349–370.

Paratz, E. D., Nehme, E., Heriot, N., Sundararajan, V., Page, G., Fahy, L., Rowe, S., Anderson, D., Stub, D., La Gerche, A. & Nehme, Z. 2024. Sex disparities in bystander defibrillation for out-of-hospital cardiac arrest. *Resusc Plus*, 17, 100532.

Penne, T. & Goedemé, T. 2021. Can low-income households afford a healthy diet? Insufficient income as a driver of food insecurity in Europe. *Food Policy*, 99, 101978.

Pickett, K. E. & Wilkinson, R. G. 2015. Income inequality and health: a causal review. *Social Science & Medicine*, 128, 316–326.

Pilgrim, A., Barker, M., Jackson, A., Ntani, G., Crozier, S., Inskip, H., Godfrey, K., Cooper, C. & Robinson, S. 2012. Does living in a food insecure household impact on the diets and body composition of young children? Findings from the Southampton Women's Survey. *Journal of Epidemiology and Community Health*, 66, e6–e6.

Pollack, C. E., Chideya, S., Cubbin, C., Williams, B., Dekker, M. & Braveman, P. 2007. Should health studies measure wealth?: a systematic review. *American Journal of Preventive Medicine*, 33, 250–264.

Pratap, P., Dickson, A., Love, M., Zanoni, J., Donato, C., Flynn, M. A. & Schulte, P. A. 2021. Public health impacts of underemployment and unemployment in the United States: exploring perceptions, gaps and opportunities. *International Journal of Environmental Research and Public Health*, 18.

Puddephatt, J.-A., Keenan, G. S., Fielden, A., Reaves, D. L., Halford, J. C. G. & Hardman, C. A. 2020. 'Eating to survive': a qualitative analysis of factors influencing food choice and eating behaviour in a food-insecure population. *Appetite*, 147, 104547.

Purnell, T. S., Calhoun, E. A., Golden, S. H., Halladay, J. R., Krok-Schoen, J. L., Appelhans, B. M. & Cooper, L. A. 2016. Achieving health equity: closing the gaps in health care disparities, interventions, and research. *Health Affairs*, 35, 1410–1415.

Raghupathi, V. & Raghupathi, W. 2020. The influence of education on health: an empirical assessment of OECD countries for the period 1995–2015. *Archives of Public Health*, 78, 20.

Redhead, G. 2021. 'A British Problem affecting British people': Sickle cell anaemia, medical activism and race in the National Health Service, 1975–1993. *Twentieth Century British History*, 32, 189–211.

Rigby, B. P., Dodd-Reynolds, C. J. & Oliver, E. J. 2020. Inequities and inequalities in outdoor walking groups: a scoping review. *Public Health Reviews*, 41, 4.

Robertson, J., Raghavan, R., Emerson, E., Baines, S. & Hatton, C. 2019. What do we know about the health and health care of people with intellectual disabilities from minority ethnic groups in the United Kingdom? A systematic review. *Journal of Applied Research in Intellectual Disabilities*, 32, 1310–1334.

Rogers, A. & Pilgrim, D. 2024. *Living with Health Inequalities*, Routledge.

Rolfe, S., Garnham, L., Godwin, J., Anderson, I., Seaman, P. & Donaldson, C. 2020. Housing as a social determinant of health and wellbeing: developing an empirically-informed realist theoretical framework. *BBMC Public Health*, 20, 1138.

Rosenquist, J. N., Murabito, J., Fowler, J. H. & Christakis, N. A. 2010. The spread of alcohol consumption behavior in a large social network. *Annals of Internal Medicine*, 152, 426–433.

Sacre, H., Haddad, C., Hajj, A., Zeenny, R. M., Akel, M. & Salameh, P. 2023. Development and validation of the socioeconomic status composite scale (SES-C). *BMC Public Health*, 23, 1619.

Sagar-Ouriaghli, I., Godfrey, E., Graham, S. & Brown, J. S. 2020. Improving mental health help-seeking behaviours for male students: a framework for developing a complex intervention. *International Journal of Environmental Research and Public Health*, 17, 4965.

Savage, M., Devine, F., Cunningham, N., Taylor, M., Li, Y., Hjellbrekke, J., Le Roux, B., Friedman, S. & Miles, A. 2013. A new model of social class? Findings from the BBC's Great British Class Survey experiment. *Sociology*, 47, 219–250.

Scott, C., Sutherland, J. & Taylor, A. 2018. Affordability of the UK's Eatwell Guide. *The Food Foundation*, 17.

Seidler, Z. E., Dawes, A. J., Rice, S. M., Oliffe, J. L. & Dhillon, H. M. 2016. The role of masculinity in men's help-seeking for depression: a systematic review. *Clinical Psychology Review*, 49, 106–118.

Smith, K. E. & Anderson, R. 2018. Understanding lay perspectives on socioeconomic health inequalities in Britain: a meta-ethnography. *Sociology of Health & Illness*, 40, 146–170.

Smith, K. P. & Christakis, N. A. 2008. Social Networks and Health. *Annual Review of Sociology*, 34, 405–429.

Sovacool, B. K., Upham, P., Martiskainen, M., Jenkins, K. E. H., Torres Contreras, G. A. & Simcock, N. 2023. Policy prescriptions to address energy and transport poverty in the United Kingdom. *Nature Energy*, 8, 273–283.

Stronks, K., Snijder, M. B., Peters, R. J. G., Prins, M., Schene, A. H. & Zwinderman, A. H. 2013. Unravelling the impact of ethnicity on health in Europe: the HELIUS study. *BMC Public Health*, 13, 402.

Tapia Granados, J. A., House, J. S., Ionides, E. L., Burgard, S. & Schoeni, R. S. 2014. Individual joblessness, contextual unemployment, and mortality risk. *American Journal of Epidemiology*, 180, 280–287.

Thoits, P. A. 2011. Mechanisms linking social ties and support to physical and mental health. *Journal of Health and Social Behavior*, 52, 145–161.

Thompson, A. E., Anisimowicz, Y., Miedema, B., Hogg, W., Wodchis, W. P. & Aubrey-Bassler, K. 2016. The influence of gender and other patient characteristics on health care-seeking behaviour: a QUALICOPC study. *BMC Family Practice*, 17, 38.

Townshend, T. & Lake, A. 2017. Obesogenic environments: current evidence of the built and food environments. *Perspectives in Public Health*, 137, 38–44.

Van den Ende, M. W. J., Van der Maas, H. L. J., Epskamp, S. & Lees, M. H. 2024. Alcohol consumption as a socially contagious phenomenon in the Framingham Heart Study social network. *Scientific Reports*, 14, 4499.

Wagstaff, A. & Neelsen, S. 2020. A comprehensive assessment of universal health coverage in 111 countries: a retrospective observational study. *The Lancet Global Health*, 8, e39–e49.

Wami, W., McCartney, G., Bartley, M., Buchanan, D., Dundas, R., Katikireddi, S. V., Mitchell, R. & Walsh, D. 2020. Theory driven analysis of social class and health outcomes using UK nationally representative longitudinal data. *International Journal for Equity in Health*, 19, 193.

Wang, Y., Hunt, K., Nazareth, I., Freemantle, N. & Petersen, I. 2013. Do men consult less than women? An analysis of routinely collected UK general practice data. *BMJ Open*, 3, e003320.

Watt, T., Raymond, A. & Rachet-Jacquet, L. 2022. Quantifying health inequalities in the UK [Online]. The Health Foundation. Available: https://www.health.org.uk/news-and-comment/charts-and-infographics/quantifying-health-inequalities [Accessed].

Weber, A. M., Cislaghi, B., Meausoone, V., Abdalla, S., Mejía-Guevara, I., Loftus, P., Hallgren, E., Seff, I., Stark, L., Victora, C. G., Buffarini, R., Barros, A. J. D., Domingue, B. W., Bhushan, D., Gupta, R., Nagata, J. M., Shakya, H. B., Richter, L. M., Norris, S. A., Ngo, T. D., Chae, S., Haberland, N., Mccarthy, K., Cullen, M. R., Darmstadt, G. L., Darmstadt, G. L., Greene, M. E., Hawkes, S., Heise, L., Henry, S., Heymann, J., Klugman, J., Levine, R., Raj, A. & Rao Gupta, G. 2019. Gender norms and health: insights from global survey data. *The Lancet*, 393, 2455–2468.

White, A., Thornton, R. L. J. & Greene, J. A. 2021. Remembering past lessons about structural racism - recentering black theorists of health and society. *The New England Journal of Medicine*, 385, 850–855.

White, A. & Tod, M. 2022. The need for a strategy on men's health. *Trends in Urology & Men's Health*, 13, 2–8.

Whitehead, M. 2007. A typology of actions to tackle social inequalities in health. *Journal of Epidemiology and Community Health*, 61, 473–478.

Whitehead, M. & Dahlgren, G. 1991. What can be done about inequalities in health? *The Lancet*, 338, 1059–1063.

WHO. 2018. Health inequities and their causes [Online]. World Health Organization. Available: https://www.who.int/news-room/facts-in-pictures/detail/health-inequities-and-their-causes [Accessed].

Wilkinson, R. & Pickett, K. 2019. *The Inner Level: How More Equal Societies Reduce Stress, Restore Sanity and Improve Everyone's Well-Being*, Penguin.

Williams, M. 2017. An old model of social class? Job characteristics and the NS-SEC schema. *Work, Employment and Society*, 31, 153–165.

Williams, O. & Fullagar, S. 2019. Lifestyle drift and the phenomenon of 'citizen shift' in contemporary UK health policy. *Sociology of Health & Illness*, 41, 20–35.

Wilson, S. J., Woody, A., Padin, A. C., Lin, J., Malarkey, W. B. & Kiecolt-GLASER, J. K. 2018. Loneliness and telomere length: immune and parasympathetic function in associations with accelerated aging. *Annals of Behavioral Medicine*, 53, 541–550.

Yegorov, Y. E., Poznyak, A. V., Nikiforov, N. G., Sobenin, I. A. & Orekhov, A. N. 2020. The link between chronic stress and accelerated aging. *Biomedicines*, 8.

Zajacova, A. & Lawrence, E. M. 2018. The relationship between education and health: reducing disparities through a contextual approach. *Annual Review of Public Health*, 39, 273–289.

Zhao, M., Huang, C.-C., Mendoza, M., Tovar, X., Lecca, L. & Murray, M. 2023. Subjective socioeconomic status: an alternative to objective socioeconomic status. *BMC Medical Research Methodology*, 23, 73.

CHAPTER 9

Stereotyping, Bias and Health-Related Stigma

Chris Allen
School of Health Sciences, University of Southampton, Southampton, UK

Introduction

At some point in our lives, we will all need healthcare. For those who are in some way perceived as 'different' – either by themselves or by others, this can be more challenging for a variety of reasons. This chapter will review the key social processes that work to make such access more challenging as well as influencing the experiences of people when they do access healthcare – specifically stereotyping, bias and health-related stigma.

This chapter builds on some of the discussion in Chapter 4, particularly around the concept of deviance. In that chapter, we outlined the importance of social and cultural norms, and how presenting or conducting ourselves in a way that does not fit within these norms can be a form of 'deviance'. What is

deemed normal changes over time. In any given society there are situations that people might find themselves in that others may see as being different, perhaps even shameful. When we find ourselves in these situations, we are likely to also feel shame. Many health-related conditions, presentations and behaviours can lead to people being negatively evaluated by themselves and by others. This chapter will examine some of these and consider what can be done to support people in these situations.

Understanding Our Bias: Stereotyping and Unconscious Bias

LEARNING OUTCOMES

By the end of this chapter, you will be able to:

- Consider a range of harmful stereotypes alongside the social processes that underpin them.
- Recognise how the content of stereotypes can influence how we respond to people from different groups.
- Recognise the harmful impact of stigma and stigmatising processes on health and help-seeking, including health-related stigma.
- Recognise bias, including the various types of bias and how they influence and impact on care.
- Identify some evidence-based interventions that attempt to address stigma and bias in healthcare settings.

Key Terms and Definitions

Stereotype: An over-generalised belief about a person or group.

Prejudice: Holding a negative view or responding negatively towards someone based on one or more of their characteristics.

Stigma: Something that sets someone apart from others and allows them to be discredited either by themselves or by others.

Bias: Negatively evaluating one group over another, leading to differences in care and caring interactions. This can be deliberate (i.e. conscious bias) or accidental (i.e. unconscious bias).

Social Sciences for Healthcare Professionals, First Edition. Edited by Chris Allen.
© 2026 John Wiley & Sons Ltd. Published 2026 by John Wiley & Sons Ltd.

What Is a Stereotype?

The term 'stereotype' was first used as far back as 1798, when it was used to describe a printing plate that duplicated typography (i.e. a font) (Beeghly, 2015, Hinton, 2017). The duplication of typography serves as a useful metaphor for what a stereotype is. The plate revolutionised the publishing industry as it allowed work to be mass-produced quickly; likewise, stereotypes help us to make quick judgements about people and situations. In social psychology, a stereotype is simply a schema, something that allows us to organise and interpret information and make generalisations about how those from a particular social group might be or behave (Beeghly, 2015). We are hardwired to do this, and at one stage in our history, this would have been particularly useful in helping us to identify friends from foes (Banaji and Greenwald, 2016). Even now, cognitive shortcuts such as this can help us quickly make sense of a complex world (Dovidio et al., 2010). As academics have highlighted, medical training often involves consideration of group-level risk factors, for example, those who are homeless are objectively more likely to have certain health needs and conditions, and healthcare professionals, it has been argued, do need to be responsive to this (Puddifoot, 2019). The basis for this is more social than biological, but nonetheless, when decisions are often made during time-sensitive critical situations, generalisations may not only be useful but are often relied upon to support clinical decision-making and diagnosis (Chapman et al., 2013).

We can think of stereotypes as an over-generalised belief about how a person might be based on their membership of a group, or shared characteristics with members of that group: for example, 'all older people are frail' (Ng et al., 2015, Nicholson et al., 2016). Stereotypes assign people with traits, based on their personal characteristics with the assumption being that all people with these characteristics are broadly similar (Beeghly, 2015). For example, making assumptions about the type of music a lecturer enjoys, or the car that they drive – a Volvo and classical music, seems a better fit than a Ferrari and drum and bass. There can be some fit with these assumptions based on class, status and other social processes that shape and restrict people's choices and behaviours. Most lecturers do not drive around in a Ferrari, but some surely do. Those born in certain parts of Manchester are more likely to support Manchester United, but not everyone born in that part of Manchester does. In similarity to the printing plate, a stereotype creates assumptions about a person, or about a social group and their attributes and behaviours and applies this to *all* of the people from this group. Assuming someone could never afford a Ferrari, based on a trait, could be quite offensive. Aside from this, in most contexts, these are relatively inoffensive examples of stereotypes. However, many stereotypes are much more harmful than these examples that have been provided, to illustrate just how ubiquitous stereotyping is, for all manner of things. It is important to note briefly that because stereotypes offer us a shortcut to understanding how someone might be, the beliefs that are gained about someone do not necessarily need to be negative, or unkind – in some cases, stereotypes can lead to very positive evaluations of people – known as 'positive stereotyping' (however, these are often also unhelpful) (Czopp et al., 2015, Kay et al., 2013).

The cognitive shortcuts that we make through stereotypes can be incredibly powerful, enduring, unfair and harmful to individuals and groups who we are making judgements about. Prejudicial attitudes and behaviours can follow such evaluations, leading us to assume things about people that are unfair and unkind, and leading to us change our behaviour around people and treating them in a different way to others based on how we believe them to be. This can include judgements as to their traits, character and competence and this can influence how we respond to people. This isn't always hostile but can be. For example, we might overhelp if we *perceive* (perceive being a crucial word here) an older person to be incompetent, or we might avoid certain groups altogether because we *perceive* them to be a threat, such as those who are homeless, or those who have committed an offence (Cuddy et al., 2008, Fiske, 2018, Fiske et al., 2002).

Stereotypes are often reinforced by society itself and its structures (Durante and Fiske, 2017). These can influence the content of stereotypes, and in turn, these stereotypes can influence a societies structures (Durante and Fiske, 2017). For example, we might view someone with lower socio-economic status as being less competent based on their social status, which ignores most of the structural and material features of society such as reduced access to material resources and opportunities (covered in the previous chapter), that led to them being in that socio-economically disadvantaged position in the first place (Durante and Fiske, 2017).

One useful way to think about how stereotypes alter our response to people is the stereotype content model (Cuddy et al., 2008, Fiske et al., 2002). This model suggests that we perceive individuals and groups based on whether we warm to them, and how competent we believe them to be, which is often derived from a person or group's social status (Cuddy et al., 2007, Fiske et al., 2019). The balance between warmth and competence relates to how we respond to people and has been seen as broadly consistent across cultures (Cuddy et al., 2009). When we see people as warm, but incompetent, we might respond with unwanted pity and overhelping behaviours. This is commonly experienced by older people and those with some form of disability (Canton et al., 2023, Shepherd and Brochu, 2021). We may avoid people altogether who we perceive as cold and incompetent, such as those with severe mental illness, those misusing drugs and alcohol or those who are homeless (Allstadt Torras et al., 2023, Canton et al., 2023, Fiske, 2018).

A summary of how you may respond based on perceived warmth and competence is shown in an adapted version of the stereotype content model in Table 9.1.

The content of stereotypes impacts on how we respond to people, in some cases deliberately through overt prejudice, but often we do this unconsciously (i.e. without even thinking about it).

TABLE 9.1	Stereotype content – the relevance of perceived warmth and competence.	
	Competence	
Warmth	**Low**	**High**
High	May react to in an overly paternalistic way – examples include older people, those with a disability, children.	May act with admiration – examples include the middle and upper classes. Societies 'reference groups'
Low	May avoid, or treat with contempt – examples include homeless people, immigrants, those misusing drugs and alcohol.	May act with envy – examples include rich, professional, technical experts, as well as the discriminatory and prejudicial attitudes held towards Jewish and Asian groups.

Source: Fiske (2018) Stereotype Content: Warmth and Competence Endure. Current Directions in Psychological Science/with permission of Sage Publications.

What Is Stigma?

Stigma, as we will explore, is a social process and exists outside of any one individual. In Chapter 4, we highlighted that those who are perceived as in some way different to society's 'reference groups', can be labelled as 'deviant'. 'Deviant' is a harsh word, and most would not want to be labelled as such. Labelling can be thought of as an interpersonal (i.e. between people) response to deviance that considers perceived differences between individuals and groups (Hatzenbuehler et al., 2013, Richman and Hatzenbuehler, 2014). Deviance and labelling can relate to social power (Scambler, 2018). Those who are seen as 'deviant' more typically have less power, with norms and laws in a given society generally favouring those outside of deviant groups, who are often those in a position to set the norms and laws in the first place (Friedman et al., 2022).

Labelling and the resultant stigma can significantly reduce people's power and status and have been seen as a social function or control that keeps those with a stigmatised status away and out of sight (Hatzenbuehler et al., 2013, Link and Phelan, 2001, Phelan et al., 2008). Labelling in the context of health remains largely the domain of medicine, through the application of diagnostic labels, which for some, can become a form of master status. Unfortunately, you have probably seen this in your practice. The 'fractured neck of femur (NOF) patient in bed 10' for example, rather than 'the engineer, husband, and father of two, who happens to have a fractured NOF and happens to be being cared for in bed 10'.

But what is stigma? The origins of the term stigma relate to a marking or tattoo that was burned or cut onto the skin of someone who society believed needed to be marked as different in some way; generally based on perceived moral shortcomings, or to maintain ownership over someone (e.g. this was generally done to criminals, traitors and slaves) (Rössler, 2016, Scambler, 2009, 2018). In current times, stigma has been described as an attribute or characteristic that is devalued in a given social context (Scambler, 2009). Something that sets someone apart as being 'different'. It is a social process and is typically characterised by labelling and stereotyping that leads to status loss and discrimination (Phelan et al., 2008). Erving Goffman (1922–1982), whose 'Stigma: Notes on the Management of a Spoiled Identity' is considered a seminal text in the conceptualisation of stigma, highlighted that it is a social process that has the potential to reduce an individual from a 'whole and usual person to a tainted, discounted one' (Goffman, 1963, p. 3). Goffman argued that stigma is something that significantly discredits an individual, to the extent that they are 'devalued in a particular social context' (p. 505) based on a real, or perceived unwanted difference.

Stigma is something that sets us apart from other people in our society, and to varying degrees, it is something that we will all experience in our lives. In his original thesis, Goffman noted that it is: 'not whether a person has experience with stigma of his own, because he has, but rather how many varieties he has had his own experience with' (Goffman, 1963, p. 129). Such a remark does not intend to trivialise the very real damage stigma creates for people, especially those with conditions or behaviours that are very stigmatised, such as human immunodeficiency virus (HIV), schizophrenia, substance use disorders, highly infectious conditions, etc. It does however highlight that most of us will at points in our lives be devalued by others and by ourselves. For example, most of us will live long enough to be seen as 'old' and other stigmatised personal attributes such as depression and obesity are very common in most western industrialised societies (Pachankis et al., 2018). Stigma can occur in relation to health conditions and behaviours, for example, a specific health condition, or an unwanted health behaviour, and in relation to personal characteristics, for example, our gender identity, our sexual orientation and our migration status; and these may intersect (Agnew et al., 2023, Bockting et al., 2013, Cabieses et al., 2024). Health-related stigma, the main focus of this chapter, is simply the stigma related to living with a specific condition and or health-related behaviour (Scambler, 2009).

Stigmatising processes are entangled with society's attitudes towards deviant behaviours and can change over time (Earnshaw et al., 2022). Attitudes towards health conditions are in part guided through medicalisation, which may change how behaviours are seen by individuals and by the public. Whether medicalisation helps or hinders is debated – with suggestions that it may help, as well as suggestions that it may make people's situations worse (Kvaale et al., 2013). For example, harmful alcohol use has historically been seen as a personal moral failing but is now seen as a disease, which frees people, at least in part, from some of the moral judgements that exist around harmful alcohol consumption. There has been a recent suggestion that the reduction in the stigma of alcohol use disorder has resulted in younger generations seeking support sooner than previous generations (Bourdon et al., 2020). Whilst biomedical explanations for conditions may reduce blame, those suffering from medicalised psychological conditions continue to experience stigma, have a label suggesting there is something wrong with them, and may have a poorer expectation for recovery due to their conditions being highlighted as long-term, chronic and relating to biomedical processes that may be outside of their control (Kvaale et al., 2013).

At a structural level, work has highlighted that the presence of public stigma (i.e. the extent to which a society as a whole discredits a personal trait or behaviour, and thus sees those with these as having less status) can create a cascade of personal (how an individual sees themselves), interpersonal (how people see each other) and sociocultural or structural processes that induce negative health behaviours, stress and biological changes in the body, which can in turn worsen inequalities relating to physical and mental health (Chaudoir et al., 2013, Flentje et al., 2020, Frost et al., 2015, Frost and Meyer, 2023). Such a cascade highlights how the social process of stigma can get under people's skin and negatively influence their health and well-being (Hatzenbuehler, 2009). Research has highlighted, for example, in the context of LGBTQ+, that areas with less protective legislation (e.g. where same-sex relationships are illegal), result in significant sexual orientation-related disparities in physical and mental health and differences in access to care (Falck and Bränström, 2023, Hatzenbuehler et al., 2010, 2012).

At the same time, due in part to its impact on status, it can have a significant impact on the opportunities that are available to people, with those who are stigmatised facing poorer outcomes in relation to educational attainment, secure housing, employment, social relationships, emotional well-being, health and healthcare (Hatzenbuehler et al., 2013).

There are various mechanisms through which stigma places those with a stigmatised status at a disadvantage. For example, as highlighted above, for various reasons stigma reduces people's access to resources, including those that we highlighted in the previous chapter as being essential to living healthy and fulfilling lives such as housing, employment and education (Hatzenbuehler et al., 2013). In addition, through shame, people's help-seeking may reduce and they may seek solitude and social isolation due to their stigmatised status, which has an impact on their ability to build and maintain social contacts, which as we show in Chapter 15 are vitally important across the life course. Finally, the psychological impact of stigma can lead to the adoption or worsening of unhealthy behaviours as a coping mechanism. For these reasons, those experiencing stigma often say it has a greater impact on their lives than the condition, attribute or behaviour that caused them to be stigmatised in the first place (Thornicroft et al., 2022).

Goffman's seminal work highlighted that stigmatising conditions can be either discredited or discreditable depending on how visible they are (Goffman, 1963). For example, a condition that is potentially concealable in everyday social interactions (such as HIV) leads to very different social interactions than do conditions that are not concealable, such as many physical disabilities, or other ailments or states that can be seen, such as obesity (Puhl and Heuer, 2010). Stigma impacts on people even with a concealable stigmatised status, influencing interactions with others through anticipatory stigma and concern and fear that they might be discovered and thus discredited in some way (Quinn and Chaudoir, 2009, Reinka et al., 2020, Scambler, 2009).

Felt and self-stigma are related, but distinct experiences. Felt stigma relates to the perception that others may treat you differently based on a visible or concealable stigmatised status (Scambler, 2009). Essentially it relates to the anticipation that others may treat you less favourably. Self-stigma, on the other hand, has been described as a 'second misfortune', whereby those with a characteristic or behaviour that is devalued, discredited or discreditable by others, might begin to accept society's stereotypes of them – impacting on their own self-evaluations of themselves, their self-esteem, self-efficacy and may also impact on the nature and frequency of their interactions with others, their communities and healthcare (Clement et al., 2015, Corrigan et al., 2006, 2011, Livingston and Boyd, 2010, Mojtabai, 2010, Treves-Kagan et al., 2015). Even where the individual does not personally believe the stereotype that has been assigned to them (i.e. it is not internalised), the recognition that others might see them in that way is likely to have a significant impact on how someone lives their life and the opportunities that they seek and have available to them, further exacerbating inequalities by further marginalising those already facing disadvantage. In fact, concealed stigmatised status can result in more negative psychological outcomes, more negative affect and lower self-esteem (Chaudoir et al., 2013), and people may withdraw and isolate themselves from their communities and possible forms of support (Link et al., 2015, Quinn and Chaudoir, 2009).

Symbolic interactionism (covered in Chapter 2) provides one useful lens through which to examine the concept of stigma. Symbolic interactionists highlight that we anticipate how others might respond to us, what might happen when we interact with certain people or groups and how we might rehearse the encounter to achieve a desired outcome or appraisal. Put simply, we take steps to manage how other people might see us – such as in the clothes we wear and other status markers. What is anticipated will be shaped by who the interaction is with. People care about how they are seen by society as a whole, but also often more importantly how they are seen by those they are close to and who they rely on such as friends, family and employers (Allen et al., 2020, Markowitz et al., 2011).

Several dimensions have been suggested and tested across different stigmas that dictate how stigma is experienced, relating to the condition's concealability (something Goffman also suggested in his early thesis), its course (i.e. how the condition is likely to progress), its disruptiveness, the conditions aesthetics, the conditions origin and whether the condition is likely to bring about early mortality (Pachankis et al., 2018). How does this relate to people's experiences of stigma? This all relates to the nature of the condition and how it is seen and understood by society. For example, conditions whose origins relate in part to a person's own behaviour (such as drinking) are often judged more harshly than those with an origin that was outside of an individual's control (Pachankis et al., 2018). Head injuries occurring in those who were intoxicated before the accident, for example, are judged more harshly, and may therefore receive poorer care, than those who were not (Linden et al., 2007, Redpath et al., 2010). As such, perceived origins can elicit different responses from people ranging from pity and unwanted over helping, through to hostility and avoidance (Pachankis et al., 2018).

Enacted stigma represents the point at which stigmatising beliefs about someone result in targeted negative or discriminatory behaviour being directed at a person with a stigmatised status (Scambler, 2009). The issues stigma presents to access to healthcare are now widely documented. Those with a stigmatised status can be denied care, might be made to wait longer for their care or face other barriers to accessing care (Nyblade et al., 2009, 2019). When they do access care, the quality of care they receive is likely to be poorer and they are more likely to be the subjects of physical and emotional abuse (Nyblade et al., 2009, 2019).

Implicit and Unconscious Bias

Before moving on to consider stigma in the context of health, it is relevant to first consider how stereotypes influence our care. The now seminal work of Professor Patricia Devine highlighted two main pathways through which bias occurs – these are conscious and unconscious bias (Devine, 1989). Bias can be described broadly as a negative evaluation of an individual, or group, relative to another leading to differences in how we interact with people (Blair et al., 2011, Devine, 1989). It often refers to implicit stereotypes and prejudice. In the context of healthcare, as we will explore, such bias can significantly alter people's experiences of care. Unconscious bias differs from conscious bias. Conscious bias occurs when someone's discriminatory values and beliefs lead them to see and respond to people from different groups inequitably as a conscious and targeted act (Devine, 1989, Green et al., 2023, Nosek and Riskind, 2012). Conscious bias is formed of explicit thoughts that a person is aware of. Where someone knowingly acts in a prejudicial or discriminatory way against a person or a group who has a trait or characteristic they dislike. Policy and regulatory bodies often specifically highlight conscious bias and the need to treat people fairly and healthcare professionals such as you, necessarily follow professional standards that stipulate that people should be treated fairly – regardless of their characteristics or their behaviours (NMC, 2019, Nosek and Riskind, 2012). In western industrialised societies, conscious forms of overt prejudice,

whilst still present and of concern, have waned (Marcelin et al., 2019). However unconscious bias is still very common, particularly in healthcare settings, leading to people responding to people and making decisions about care that do not align with their explicitly held values and beliefs (FitzGerald and Hurst, 2017, Gopal et al., 2021, Marcelin et al., 2019).

Both conscious and unconscious bias affect the quality and fairness of the healthcare that we provide. Unconscious bias happens automatically – without us even thinking or being aware of it. These biases are believed to develop in our early childhood and are believed to be reinforced by social stereotypes that shape how people in different groups are perceived (Chapman et al., 2013, Newheiser and Olson, 2012). Think about the most recent care setting you worked in. Were there any patients or service users that you particularly warmed to? What were they like? Were they pretty similar to yourself – in relation to their age, gender or social class? Did they end up getting maybe even just that little bit more attention from you than others did? Potentially. Even if you did not do this deliberately – the evidence suggests you may have (FitzGerald and Hurst, 2017, Puddifoot, 2019).

You will often care for those you have less similarities with and whilst not deliberate, you may unconsciously give them poorer care as a result (FitzGerald and Hurst, 2017). Healthcare professionals such as you, are recognised as being as predisposed to unconscious bias as the general population (FitzGerald and Hurst, 2017, Hall et al., 2015, VanPuymbrouck et al., 2020). You may even change the way you speak to people, and what you speak to them about. Even the care and treatments that people are offered, how person-centred the care is, how much choice they are given about that care, and the level and type of information that is offered may be based on unconscious bias (Cooper et al., 2012, FitzGerald and Hurst, 2017, Green et al., 2007, Hull et al., 2021, Mathur et al., 2014, Penner et al., 2010). The impact of this on care is quite significant – leading to differences in a person's access, questioning, diagnosis, how their condition is managed (including access to needed pain relief) and how much they can be involved in decision-making, as well as care outcomes (Centola et al., 2021, Dijksterhuis et al., 2021, Eneanya et al., 2022, Fiscella et al., 2021, FitzGerald and Hurst, 2017, Gopal et al., 2021, Greenwood et al., 2020, Meghani et al., 2012, Wisniewski and Walker, 2020). Implicit or unconscious bias can explain the difference in how someone wants to and believes they are caring for someone (i.e. fairly), and how they care for someone, which is influenced by hidden negative implicit (i.e. unconscious) associations that might lead to them seeing a group or individual as less warm, or competent than someone from a different group. This can then create a mismatch between what you believe and want to do and what you actually do. Research has highlighted that when you are under increased pressure and cognitive load, you are more likely to let your implicit bias influence your care and decision-making (Burgess et al., 2014, Byrne and Tanesini, 2015, Johnson et al., 2016). Of course, the public are prone to unconscious bias too. Research has highlighted for example that female doctors are more likely to be mistaken for nurses than men (Boge et al., 2019, Cooke, 2017).

Whilst we are all able to make biased decisions, how biased we are may be down to the society we live in more generally, as well as our own personal characteristics, experiences and exposures. Those who end up providing paid care and their levels of influence within the healthcare system are also subject to biases. For example, those with a disability are less likely to be accepted into nursing programs, resulting in a nursing workforce that may be unconsciously biased towards those with disabilities, and might be less able to relate to the challenges those with a disability experience (Aaberg Vicki, 2012, Jamal-Eddine et al., 2024). Within healthcare, minoritised groups are also less likely to progress into leadership and management roles where they can positively influence how care is delivered (Iheduru-Anderson, 2020, Wilbur et al., 2020). It is possible that a lack of diversity in the healthcare workforce, especially in positions associated with greater prestige and power, might increase levels of explicit and implicit bias.

Even when we work hard to consciously correct any negative ideas or images that we might automatically generate for individuals or groups, our culture immerses us in negative stereotypes and negative evaluations of people and groups, for example, those with mental ill health are frequently portrayed as being unstable and aggressive in films (Riles et al., 2021). Whilst we do not currently know the extent to which such immersion relates to implicit negative stereotypes, the widespread existence of these ideas and images in most societies suggests that there are significant cultural influences on how people are seen (such as migrants, those with a disability, or those with a substance use disorder) that are hard to shake off. We know these are hard to shake off, as implicit bias exists even in those who explicitly state their values of fairness and equality. This can further negatively impact on the care of those who are already disadvantaged (some of whom are considered in the following chapter) through material and structural features of our society. Even when not intentional, the nature of care can look very different depending on a person's age, gender, race and ethnicity, current health status and engagement with unhealthy behaviours (Attanasio and Hardeman, 2019, Wisniewski and Walker, 2020). In short, disparities in care and poor care-related decision-making can be the result of implicit bias – especially in healthcare environments where decision-making is often necessarily quick (Thirsk et al., 2022). Whilst the extent to which individuals and groups face disadvantage varies across societies and cultures, those who may face disadvantage through implicit bias in relation to both healthcare access and quality include many of those who face disadvantage in other aspects of life, such as those from lower socioeconomic groups, sexually and ethnically minoritised groups, older people and those with long-term physical and mental health conditions (Martin et al., 2014). Bias that leads to poor care experiences is likely to reduce further healthcare utilisation through fear of similar future treatment.

Health-Related Stigma

Most health conditions and health-related behaviours involve stigmatising processes. We cannot cover all within the confines of this chapter – but instead focus on two.

First, we will broadly consider the stigma that follows mental ill health (in its broadest sense, though with some specific examples), and then we will consider stigma in relation to HIV.

Mental Health-Related Stigma

Mental health, as with physical health, is broad. It is not possible to cover the full diversity of stigma relating to specific mental health conditions here. Whilst stigma is experienced in different ways across different mental health presentations, it is widely recognised that significant stigmatising beliefs endure around mental illness (Pescosolido et al., 2021, Tyler and Slater, 2018). Much of this is attributable to society's historically poor knowledge, perceptions and attitudes towards those experiencing mental health issues (Mehta et al., 2009, Pescosolido et al., 2010, 2013, Schomerus et al., 2012), often leading to those with mental health-related issues experiencing higher rates of 'felt' or 'self' stigma (Evans-Lacko et al., 2012, Link et al., 2015), which can lead to delayed help-seeking, leading to poorer physical and mental health outcomes (Clement et al., 2015), and even increased suicidal ideation, especially in those who are socially isolated (Xu et al., 2016) and where people anticipate stigma (Oexle et al., 2018).

Research has highlighted that whilst poor mental health is increasingly seen and understood as a health condition, this does not necessarily translate into increasing acceptance of those with mental health conditions (Pescosolido et al., 2010, 2021, Schomerus et al., 2012). As a more severe mental health issue, schizophrenia is accompanied by significant stigma including perceived threat and incompetency, and avoidance or distancing, including within healthcare contexts (Mannarini et al., 2022, Valery and Prouteau, 2020). The extent to which these stigmatising beliefs occur relates to healthcare professional characteristics and practice settings (Mannarini et al., 2022, Valery and Prouteau, 2020). Even for less severe mental health presentations, an often unnecessary degree of cautiousness still exists around those with mental health issues – for example, research has highlighted that people are less likely to want their children looked after by someone with mental health issues, or have someone with poor mental health married into their family (Pescosolido et al., 2013). In addition, the stigmatised status of mental health has a recognised impact on the opportunities that those with a mental health condition have available to them. For example, those with a mental health condition face disadvantages relating to employment (Evans-Lacko et al., 2012). Whilst stigmatising beliefs still exist that place those with mental ill health at a significant disadvantage, recent work has highlighted that whilst other mental health-related stigmas have remained relatively static, or in the case of schizophrenia and alcohol use disorders potentially increased, there is a trend towards decreasing public stigma directed towards those with depression (Pescosolido et al., 2021).

Human Immunodeficiency Virus (HIV)/Acquired Immune Deficiency Syndrome (AIDS)

The care and treatment of HIV now looks very different to what it did in 1981 when it was first recognised (Fauci et al., 2019). Early in the pandemic, HIV attracted significant levels of fear amongst the non-infected population, resulting in significant stigma for those with the condition. Many of these were members of intersecting stigmatised groups, such as men who have sex with men, intravenous drug users and sex workers (Purcell, 2021). An early lack of action was compounded by society's negative evaluations and views of these groups at the time. In the case of America, during the early days of the epidemic, sex between members of the same sex was illegal in many states and homosexuality had only been removed from the American Psychiatric Association's (APA) Diagnostic and Statistical Manual (DSM) a decade earlier (Drescher, 2015). In the United Kingdom, public health messaging was deliberately dramatic and fear-inducing. The now infamous 'Don't Die of Ignorance' advertisement featured the word 'AIDS' being literally chiselled onto a black tombstone to a dramatic background score (Flint et al., 2023).

Now though, HIV care and people's prognosis are significantly different from what it was when the condition was first identified and the decades that followed. The current life expectancy for those with HIV in wealthy and industrialised societies, provided they are diagnosed early and can access treatment, is not that dissimilar to those without the condition (Trickey et al., 2023). Despite such changes, it is widely recognised that stigma continues to be one of the largest challenges facing people with HIV and is not dissimilar to that experienced at the start of the epidemic (Rzeszutek et al., 2021). It has been suggested that the levels of co-morbid post-traumatic stress disorder (PTSD) that continue to be high in those with HIV, are likely to be related in part to the severity of stigmatising processes (Tang et al., 2020).

Through stigmatising processes, those with HIV have higher rates of depression, increased suicidal ideation, lower social support, poor adherence to medication regimes including those relevant to managing their condition such as antiretroviral medications, lower well-being, and overall poorer access and use of healthcare services (Armoon et al., 2022, Rueda et al., 2016, Rzeszutek et al., 2021). As the respondents' narratives in a recent study highlight, social responses to HIV largely remain stuck in a bygone era and have failed to keep up

with the rapid advances in medical science that have significantly changed the prognosis for those with the condition (Flint et al., 2023). As with other stigmatised statuses, the extent to which people with HIV are stigmatised relates to intersecting forms of disadvantage, such as age, gender and race (Dada et al., 2024, Rice et al., 2018, Rzeszutek et al., 2021).

Addressing Stigma and Reducing Implicit Bias in Healthcare

Addressing stigma and reducing implicit bias in healthcare is a huge interest and concern. We cannot cover every current approach, but in this final section, a few recent approaches are discussed.

Addressing Stigma

Because stigma is a multi-level social process that exists at individual, interpersonal and broader societal levels, this makes it challenging to overcome and as such, stigmatising beliefs tend to endure without broader societal level changes happening (Cook et al., 2014). As we have discussed, stigma and bias are inherently tied up in the social structures, institutions and cultures that propagate them in the first place. Because stigma is complex, the importance of mapping proposed interventions has been emphasised to ensure the impacts are measurable and intended (Stutterheim et al., 2023). Recent work has argued that there has historically been too great a focus on educating people, or on supporting those who are stigmatised to better manage, at the expense of addressing the broader structural issues that allow such differences in power to exist in the first place (Tyler and Slater, 2018) and recent work has highlighted that there is a paucity of work seeking to address structural causes of stigma and implicit bias (Rao et al., 2019).

There are some examples of interventions applied at macro, meso and micro levels that have demonstrated some impact. However, these often only look at specific contexts and micro-level interactions, whereas stigmatising beliefs and biases exist across societies' multiple layers and systems. For example, we can provide education and training that hopes to ensure that healthcare professionals treat those presenting with stigmatised conditions sympathetically, and fairly, but without addressing the broader social and cultural judgements that are applied to stigmatised groups, people may be more likely to need support due to the stigmatisation and resultant inequality they face, but are also more unlikely to seek it – either professionally or from their personal networks.

Recent work has highlighted the challenges of designing well-thought-through interventions that might reduce stigma and its impacts through targeted actions at all levels (Rao et al., 2019). Interventions tend to target individual and inter-personal levels and there has been a relative paucity of measuring stigma at a broader societal level – hindering intervention development (Rao et al., 2019). A systematic review by Rao and colleagues (2019) highlighted that interventions tend to focus on education and training, as well as 'social contact'.

Alongside education and training interventions, social contact interventions are commonly deployed. These seek to breakdown 'in group' and 'outgroup differences' through exposure to a range of different people, which may be effective in reducing and sustaining reductions in stigmatising processes (Corrigan et al., 2012, Kohrt et al., 2020, Nyblade et al., 2019). One notable example, where people can gain insight from those most affected through contact is the Human Library Initiative, which allows people to access 'human book' volunteers. Essentially people who share their experiences of their stigmatised status. Such an approach may be effective in reducing stigma and increasing inclusion (Chung and Tse, 2022, Kwan, 2020, Paul et al., 2024).

One example of a macro level intervention for reducing stigma – in this case, mental health-related stigma was England's 'Time to Change' campaign. This was England's largest mental health-related stigma reduction campaign and was shown to be effective in changing public attitudes towards those with mental ill health (Evans-Lacko et al., 2014). Reportedly, following the campaign public attitudes changed such that people were more willing to live with, live near too, work with or be in a relationship with someone with poor mental health, with changing attitudes being more significant in areas of the country with highest levels of exposure to the campaign (Evans-Lacko et al., 2014). In addition, the 'Heads Together' campaign, fronted by members of the UK Royal Family, looked to end stigma as a barrier to help seeking in mental ill health, through role-modelling conversations about personal experiences with poor mental health (Tyler and Slater, 2018). The campaign involved a range of celebrities and well-known public figures talking about their experiences of mental ill health (Tyler and Slater, 2018). Other campaigns to normalise mental health communication include England's football 'Heads up campaign' – though evaluations of this suggest challenges in terms of implementation, delivery and evaluation (Elsey et al., 2024).

Addressing Unconscious Bias

As with stigma reduction, unconscious bias interventions have examined the use of education. There are numerous examples of education and training across the literature that suggest they may reduce bias in healthcare settings (Burgess et al., 2007, Gill et al., 2022, Morris et al., 2019, Stone and Moskowitz, 2011). Education may be effective in combating conscious bias. However, it is likely to be more limited in addressing unconscious bias – which typically requires longer-term reflective and supportive approaches (Corrigan and Penn, 1999, Webster et al., 2022). To date, some of these approaches have involved asking healthcare professionals to take an Implicit Association Test (IAT) (a commonly used method to test for unconscious bias), followed by a facilitated discussion (Zeidan et al., 2019). Cultural competence training is another commonly used approach, which essentially instructs participants about the needs of different groups. In a Cochrane review, cultural competence training was shown to potentially increase service users' perceptions of treating healthcare professionals, increase levels of attendance and lead to greater levels of involvement in care (Horvat et al., 2014). However, recent work has emphasised that cultural competence training may in fact have unintended consequences in terms of stereotyping and 'othering' patients from different groups, and putting people into distinct groups of need, risks healthcare professionals losing sight of the intersecting forms of disadvantage that people typically face (Lekas et al., 2020).

What is needed is for healthcare professionals to be able to reflect on, and recognise their own biases, and through this, be able to challenge themselves to overcome them (Hughes et al., 2020). Because of this, what has instead been emphasised in recent literature is the need for cultural humility – for healthcare professionals to be supported to reflect and critique their own practice, bias and assumptions, appreciate and draw on the experiences of those they provide care for, and to share power with those accessing care (Lekas et al., 2020). Examples of coaching tools for promoting cultural humility exist, for example, Masters et al.'s (2019) 5 Rs – reflection, respect, regard, relevance and resiliency – which aim to reduce biases. Similarly, approaches such as mindfulness have been suggested as one way in which healthcare professionals might be able to gain non-judgemental awareness of their practice and its impacts so that they can challenge their implicit prejudicial beliefs (Burgess et al., 2017). Other work has highlighted the relevance of healthcare professional peer networks that may be useful in helping them to have their biases challenged and decision-making checked and suggest that digital platforms could promote peer involvement in decision-making in practice (Centola et al., 2021).

As with stigma reduction approaches, social contact may have some impact on explicit and implicit bias through more frequent and more favourable exposure to different groups (Onyeador et al., 2020). In your programs, you will likely have exposure to Simulation-Based Education (SBE) and recent work has highlighted that poorly thought-through SBE can exacerbate stereotypes (Vora et al., 2021), but that when well-planned and co-developed, may provide an opportunity to address unconscious bias in future healthcare professionals (Tjia et al., 2023, Vora et al., 2021). Much like the social contact approaches seen in stigma reduction interventions, those looking at simulation-based education to reduce bias aim to mitigate it in patient-healthcare professional interactions, through providing simulated opportunities that provide inter-group contact that allow people to reflect, challenge their assumptions and provide person-centred care (Tjia et al., 2023).

Clinical Considerations
• Stigma and stigmatising processes can impact on people's health in many ways.
• It can limit opportunities to participate in many aspects of society and should be considered a social determinant of health.
• It can also influence people's help-seeking behaviours and their access to healthcare.
• It is important to monitor our own biases and consider how these may be influencing the care we are providing. This allows us to work on them and improve the care we give to all.
• We are particularly prone to unconscious bias when we are working quickly, and in high-pressure situations.
• When caring for those whose needs you do not understand, be curious. Find out more about them and what they want, need and value.

Conclusion

This chapter has introduced the concepts of stereotypes, bias and stigma and has highlighted their relevance to the delivery of healthcare. In relation to stereotypes, we have highlighted why stereotypes might exist, and how inferring what someone is like based on perceived group-level characteristics can be unfair and harmful. This chapter has also explored the relationships between stereotypes and stigma and highlighted how stigma as a social process can negatively affect people in several ways that are the product of how individuals see themselves, how others may see them and how society in general relates to whatever it is that marks them as different. Mental health and HIV have been explored in a little bit more depth, to allow for some of the historical and social context of stigma to be further unpacked. In this chapter, you were also introduced to the concept of unconscious bias and had the opportunity to consider how this might be impacting on your own care. At the end of this chapter, you were also able to look at some different approaches to reducing the impacts of stigma and unconscious bias in healthcare.

References

Aaberg Vicki, A. 2012. A path to greater inclusivity through implicit attitudes toward disability. *Journal of Nursing Education*, 51, 505–510.

Agnew, E. R., Mcaloney-Kocaman, K. & Wiseman-Gregg, K. 2023. Variations in stigma by sexual orientation and substance use: an investigation of double stigma. *Journal of Gay & Lesbian Social Services*, 35, 1–12.

Allen, C., Vassilev, I., Kennedy, A. & Rogers, A. 2020. The work and relatedness of ties mediated online in supporting long-term condition self-management. *Sociology of Health & Illness*, 42, 579–595.

Allstadt Torras, R. C., Scheel, C. & Dorrough, A. R. 2023. The stereotype content model and mental disorders: Distinct perceptions of warmth and competence. *Frontiers in Psychology*, 14, 1069226.

Armoon, B., Fleury, M.-J., Bayat, A.-H., Fakhri, Y., Higgs, P., Moghaddam, L. F. & Gonabadi-Nezhad, L. 2022. HIV related stigma associated with social support, alcohol use disorders, depression, anxiety, and suicidal ideation among people living with HIV: a systematic review and meta-analysis. *International Journal of Mental Health Systems*, 16, 17.

Attanasio, L. B. & Hardeman, R. R. 2019. Declined care and discrimination during the childbirth hospitalization. *Social Science & Medicine*, 232, 270–277.

Banaji, M. R. & Greenwald, A. G. 2016. *Blindspot: Hidden Biases of Good People*, Bantam.

Beeghly, E. 2015. What is a Stereotype? what is stereotyping? *Hypatia*, 30, 675–691.

Blair, I. V., Steiner, J. F. & Havranek, E. P. 2011. Unconscious (implicit) bias and health disparities: where do we go from here? *The Permanente Journal*, 15, 71–78.

Bockting, W. O., Miner, M. H., Swinburne Romine, R. E., Hamilton, A. & Coleman, E. 2013. Stigma, mental health, and resilience in an online sample of the US transgender population. *American Journal of Public Health*, 103, 943–951.

Boge, L. A., Dos Santos, C., Moreno-Walton, L. A., Cubeddu, L. X. & Farcy, D. A. 2019. The relationship between physician/nurse gender and patients' correct identification of health care professional roles in the emergency department. *Journal of Women's Health (2002)*, 28, 961–964.

Bourdon, J. L., Tillman, R., Francis, M. W., Dick, D. M., Stephenson, M., Kamarajan, C., Edenberg, H. J., Kramer, J., Kuperman, S. & Bucholz, K. K. 2020. Characterization of service use for alcohol problems across generations and sex in adults with alcohol use disorder. *Alcoholism: Clinical and Experimental Research*, 44, 746–757.

Burgess, D., Van Ryn, M., Dovidio, J. & Saha, S. 2007. Reducing racial bias among health care providers: lessons from social-cognitive psychology. *Journal of General Internal Medicine*, 22, 882–887.

Burgess, D. J., Beach, M. C. & Saha, S. 2017. Mindfulness practice: a promising approach to reducing the effects of clinician implicit bias on patients. *Patient Education and Counseling*, 100, 372–376.

Burgess, D. J., Phelan, S., Workman, M., Hagel, E., Nelson, D. B., Fu, S. S., Widome, R. & Van Ryn, M. 2014. The effect of cognitive load and patient race on physicians' decisions to prescribe opioids for chronic low back pain: a randomized trial. *Pain Medicine*, 15, 965–974.

Byrne, A. & Tanesini, A. 2015. Instilling new habits: addressing implicit bias in healthcare professionals. *Advances in Health Sciences Education: Theory and Practice*, 20, 1255–1262.

Cabieses, B., Belo, K., Calderón, A. C., Rada, I., Rojas, K., Araoz, C. & Knipper, M. 2024. The impact of stigma and discrimination-based narratives in the health of migrants in Latin America and the Caribbean: a scoping review. *The Lancet Regional Health – Americas*, 40.

Canton, E., Hedley, D. & Spoor, J. R. 2023. The stereotype content model and disabilities. *The Journal of Social Psychology*, 163, 480–500.

Centola, D., Guilbeault, D., Sarkar, U., Khoong, E. & Zhang, J. 2021. The reduction of race and gender bias in clinical treatment recommendations using clinician peer networks in an experimental setting. *Nature Communications*, 12, 6585.

Chapman, E. N., Kaatz, A. & Carnes, M. 2013. Physicians and implicit bias: how doctors may unwittingly perpetuate health care disparities. *Journal of General Internal Medicine*, 28, 1504–1510.

Chaudoir, S. R., Earnshaw, V. A. & Andel, S. 2013. "Discredited" versus "discreditable": understanding how shared and unique stigma mechanisms affect psychological and physical health disparities. *Basic and Applied Social Psychology*, 35, 75–87.

Chung, E. Y.-H. & Tse, T. T.-O. 2022. Effect of human library intervention on mental health literacy: a multigroup pretest–posttest study. *BMC Psychiatry*, 22, 73.

Clement, S., Schauman, O., Graham, T., Maggioni, F., Evans-Lacko, S., Bezborodovs, N., Morgan, C., Rüsch, N., Brown, J. S. & Thornicroft, G. 2015. What is the impact of mental health-related stigma on help-seeking? A systematic review of quantitative and qualitative studies. *Psychological Medicine*, 45, 11–27.

Cook, J. E., Purdie-Vaughns, V., Meyer, I. H. & Busch, J. T. 2014. Intervening within and across levels: a multilevel approach to stigma and public health. *Social Science & Medicine*, 103, 101–109.

Cooke, M. 2017. Implicit bias in academic medicine:# WhatADoctorLooksLike. *JAMA Internal Medicine*, 177, 657–658.

Cooper, L. A., Roter, D. L., Carson, K. A., Beach, M. C., Sabin, J. A., Greenwald, A. G. & Inui, T. S. 2012. The associations of clinicians' implicit attitudes about race with medical visit communication and patient ratings of interpersonal care. *American Journal of Public Health*, 102, 979–987.

Corrigan, P. W., Morris, S. B., Michaels, P. J., Rafacz, J. D. & Rüsch, N. 2012. Challenging the public stigma of mental illness: a meta-analysis of outcome studies. *Psychiatric Services*, 63, 963–973.

Corrigan, P. W. & Penn, D. L. 1999. Lessons from social psychology on discrediting psychiatric stigma. *The American Psychologist*, 54, 765–776.

Corrigan, P. W., Rafacz, J. & Rüsch, N. 2011. Examining a progressive model of self-stigma and its impact on people with serious mental illness. *Psychiatry Research*, 189, 339–343.

Corrigan, P. W., Watson, A. C. & BARR, L. 2006. The self-stigma of mental illness: implications for self-esteem and self-efficacy. *Journal of Social and Clinical Psychology*, 25, 875–884.

Cuddy, A. J., Fiske, S. T. & Glick, P. 2007. The BIAS map: behaviors from intergroup affect and stereotypes. *Journal of Personality and Social Psychology*, 92, 631–648.

Cuddy, A. J., Fiske, S. T. & Glick, P. 2008. Warmth and competence as universal dimensions of social perception: the stereotype content model and the BIAS map. *Advances in Experimental Social Psychology*, 40, 61–149.

Cuddy, A. J., Fiske, S. T., Kwan, V. S., Glick, P., Demoulin, S., Leyens, J. P., Bond, M. H., Croizet, J. C., Ellemers, N., Sleebos, E., Htun, T. T., Kim, H. J., Maio, G., Perry, J., Petkova, K., Todorov, V., Rodríguez-Bailón, R., Morales, E., Moya, M., Palacios, M., Smith, V., Perez, R., Vala, J. & Ziegler, R. 2009. Stereotype content model across cultures: towards universal similarities and some differences. *The British Journal of Social Psychology*, 48, 1–33.

Czopp, A. M., Kay, A. C. & Cheryan, S. 2015. Positive stereotypes are pervasive and powerful. *Perspectives on Psychological Science*, 10, 451–463.

Dada, D., Abu-Ba'are, G. R., Turner, D., Mashoud, I. W., Owusu-Dampare, F., Apreku, A., NI, Z., Djiadeu, P., Aidoo-Frimpong, G., Zigah, E. Y., Nyhan, K., Nyblade, L. & Nelson, L. E. 2024. Scoping review of HIV-related intersectional stigma among sexual and gender minorities in sub-Saharan Africa. *BMJ Open*, 14, e078794.

Devine, P. G. 1989. Stereotypes and prejudice: Their automatic and controlled components. *Journal of Personality and Social Psychology*, 56, 5.

Dijksterhuis, W. P. M., Kalff, M. C., Wagner, A. D., Verhoeven, R. H. A., Lemmens, V. E. P. P., Van Oijen, M. G. H., Gisbertz, S. S., Van Berge Henegouwen, M. I. & Van Laarhoven, H. W. M. 2021. Gender differences in treatment allocation and survival of advanced gastroesophageal cancer: a population-based study. *Journal of the National Cancer Institute*, 113, 1551–1560.

Dovidio, J. F., Hewstone, M., Glick, P. & Esses, V. M. 2010. *The SAGE Handbook of Prejudice, Stereotyping and Discrimination*, London: SAGE Publications Ltd.

Drescher, J. 2015. Out of DSM: Depathologizing Homosexuality. *Behavioral Sciences (Basel)*, 5, 565–575.

Durante, F. & Fiske, S. T. 2017. How social-class stereotypes maintain inequality. *Current Opinion in Psychology*, 18, 43–48.

Earnshaw, V. A., Watson, R. J., Eaton, L. A., Brousseau, N. M., Laurenceau, J.-P. & Fox, A. B. 2022. Integrating time into stigma and health research. *Nature Reviews Psychology*, 1, 236–247.

Elsey, C., Southwood, J., Winter, P., Thomas, G., Litchfield, S. J., Ogweno, S. & Billington, L. 2024. Assessment of the delivery and implementation of the Football Association's Heads Up mental health promotion campaign. *Sport in Society*, 1–25.

Eneanya, N. D., Boulware, L. E., Tsai, J., Bruce, M. A., Ford, C. L., Harris, C., Morales, L. S., Ryan, M. J., Reese, P. P., Thorpe, R. J., Morse, M., Walker, V., Arogundade, F. A., Lopes, A. A. & Norris, K. C. 2022. Health inequities and the inappropriate use of race in nephrology. *Nature Reviews Nephrology*, 18, 84–94.

Evans-Lacko, S., Brohan, E., Mojtabai, R. & Thornicroft, G. 2012. Association between public views of mental illness and self-stigma among individuals with mental illness in 14 European countries. *Psychological Medicine*, 42, 1741–1752.

Evans-Lacko, S., Corker, E., Williams, P., Henderson, C. & Thornicroft, G. 2014. Effect of the time to change anti-stigma campaign on trends in mental-illness-related public stigma among the English population in 2003-13: an analysis of survey data. *Lancet Psychiatry*, 1, 121–128.

Falck, F. & Bränström, R. 2023. The significance of structural stigma towards transgender people in health care encounters across Europe: Health care access, gender identity disclosure, and discrimination in health care as a function of national legislation and public attitudes. *BMC Public Health*, 23, 1031.

Fauci, A. S., Redfield, R. R., Sigounas, G., Weahkee, M. D. & Giroir, B. P. 2019. Ending the HIV epidemic: a plan for the United States. *JAMA*, 321, 844–845.

Fiscella, K., Epstein, R. M., Griggs, J. J., Marshall, M. M. & Shields, C. G. 2021. Is physician implicit bias associated with differences in care by patient race for metastatic cancer-related pain? *PLoS One*, 16, e0257794.

Fiske, S. T. 2018. Stereotype content: warmth and competence endure. *Current Directions in Psychological Science*, 27, 67–73.

Fiske, S. T., Cuddy, A. J., Glick, P. & Xu, J. 2002. A model of (often mixed) stereotype content: competence and warmth respectively follow from perceived status and competition. *Journal of Personality and Social Psychology*, 82, 878–902.

Fiske, S. T., Cuddy, A. J., Peter, G. & Xu, J. 2019. "A model of (often mixed) stereotype content: Competence and warmth respectively follow from perceived status and competition": Correction to Fiske et al. (2002). *J Pers Soc Psychol*, 82, 878–902.

FitzGerald, C. & Hurst, S. 2017. Implicit bias in healthcare professionals: a systematic review. *BMC Medical Ethics*, 18, 19.

Flentje, A., Heck, N. C., Brennan, J. M. & Meyer, I. H. 2020. The relationship between minority stress and biological outcomes: A systematic review. *Journal of Behavioral Medicine*, 43, 673–694.

Flint, A., Günsche, M. & Burns, M. 2023. We Are Still Here: Living with HIV in the UK. *Medical Anthropology*, 42, 35–47.

Friedman, S. R., Williams, L. D., Guarino, H., Mateu-Gelabert, P., Krawczyk, N., Hamilton, L., Walters, S. M., Ezell, J. M., Khan, M., Di Iorio, J., Yang, L. H. & Earnshaw, V. A. 2022. The stigma system: How sociopolitical domination, scapegoating, and stigma shape public health. *Journal of Community Psychology*, 50, 385–408.

Frost, D. M., Lehavot, K. & Meyer, I. H. 2015. Minority stress and physical health among sexual minority individuals. *Journal of Behavioral Medicine*, 38, 1–8.

Frost, D. M. & Meyer, I. H. 2023. Minority stress theory: Application, critique, and continued relevance. *Current Opinion in Psychology*, 51, 101579.

Gill, A. C., Zhou, Y., Greely, J. T., Beasley, A. D., Purkiss, J. & Juneja, M. 2022. Longitudinal outcomes one year following implicit bias training in medical students. *Medical Teacher*, 44, 744–751.

Goffman, E. 1963. *Stigma: Notes on the Management of a Spoiled Identity*, Prentice Hall.

Gopal, D. P., Chetty, U. & O'donnell, Gajria, Blackadder-Weinstein, P., C., J. 2021. Implicit bias in healthcare: clinical practice, research and decision making. *Future Healthcare Journal*, 8, 40–48.

Green, A. R., Carney, D. R., Pallin, D. J., Ngo, L. H., Raymond, K. L., Iezzoni, L. I. & Banaji, M. R. 2007. Implicit bias among physicians and its prediction of thrombolysis decisions for black and white patients. *Journal of General Internal Medicine*, 22, 1231–1238.

Green, T. L., Vu, H., Swan, L. E. T., Luo, D., Hickman, E., Plaisime, M. & Hagiwara, N. 2023. Implicit and explicit racial prejudice among medical professionals: updated estimates from a population-based study. *The Lancet Regional Health – The Americas*, 21.

Greenwood, B. N., Hardeman, R. R., Huang, L. & Sojourner, A. 2020. Physician-patient racial concordance and disparities in birthing mortality for newborns. *Proceedings of the National Academy of Sciences of the United States of America*, 117, 21194–21200.

Hall, W. J., Chapman, M. V., Lee, K. M., Merino, Y. M., Thomas, T. W., Payne, B. K., Eng, E., Day, S. H. & Coyne-Beasley, T. 2015. Implicit racial/ethnic bias among health care professionals and its influence on health care outcomes: a systematic review. *American Journal of Public Health*, 105, e60–e76.

Hatzenbuehler, M. L. 2009. How does sexual minority stigma "get under the skin"? A psychological mediation framework. *Psychological Bulletin*, 135, 707–730.

Hatzenbuehler, M. L., Mclaughlin, K. A., Keyes, K. M. & Hasin, D. S. 2010. The impact of institutional discrimination on psychiatric disorders in lesbian, gay, and bisexual populations: a prospective study. *American Journal of Public Health*, 100, 452–459.

Hatzenbuehler, M. L., O'cleirigh, C., Grasso, C., Mayer, K., Safren, S. & Bradford, J. 2012. Effect of same-sex marriage laws on health care use and expenditures in sexual minority men: a quasi-natural experiment. *American Journal of Public Health*, 102, 285–291.

Hatzenbuehler, M. L., Phelan, J. C. & Link, B. G. 2013. Stigma as a fundamental cause of population health inequalities. *American Journal of Public Health*, 103, 813–821.

Hinton, P. 2017. Implicit stereotypes and the predictive brain: cognition and culture in "biased" person perception. *Palgrave Communications*, 3, 17086.

Horvat, L., Horey, D., Romios, P. & Kis-Rigo, J. 2014. Cultural competence education for health professionals. *Cochrane Database of Systematic Reviews*, (5), CD009405. DOI: 10.1002/14651858.CD009405.pub2.

Hughes, V., Delva, S., Nkimbeng, M., Spaulding, E., Turkson-Ocran, R.-A., Cudjoe, J., Ford, A., Rushton, C., D'aoust, R. & Han, H.-R. 2020. Not missing the opportunity: strategies to promote cultural humility among future nursing faculty. *Journal of Professional Nursing*, 36, 28–33.

Hull, S. J., Tessema, H., Thuku, J. & Scott, R. K. 2021. Providers PrEP: identifying primary health care providers' biases as barriers to provision of equitable PrEP services. *Journal of Acquired Immune Deficiency Syndromes*, 88, 165–172.

Iheduru-Anderson, K. 2020. Accent bias: a barrier to Black African-born nurses seeking managerial and faculty positions in the United States. *Nursing Inquiry*, 27, e12355.

Jamal-Eddine, S., Savage, T. & Gill, C. 2024. Assets, not burdens: disabled students in nursing education. *International Journal of Nursing Studies*, 154, 104775.

Johnson, T. J., Hickey, R. W., Switzer, G. E., Miller, E., Winger, D. G., Nguyen, M., Saladino, R. A. & Hausmann, L. R. 2016. The impact of cognitive stressors in the emergency department on physician implicit racial bias. *Academic Emergency Medicine*, 23, 297–305.

Kay, A. C., Day, M. V., Zanna, M. P. & Nussbaum, A. D. 2013. The insidious (and ironic) effects of positive stereotypes. *Journal of Experimental Social Psychology*, 49, 287–291.

Kohrt, B. A., Turner, E. L., Rai, S., Bhardwaj, A., Sikkema, K. J., Adelekun, A., Dhakal, M., Luitel, N. P., Lund, C., Patel, V. & Jordans, M. J. D. 2020. Reducing mental illness stigma in healthcare settings: Proof of concept for a social contact intervention to address what matters most for primary care providers. *Social Science & Medicine*, 250, 112852.

Kvaale, E. P., Haslam, N. & Gottdiener, W. H. 2013. The 'side effects' of medicalization: a meta-analytic review of how biogenetic explanations affect stigma. *Clinical Psychology Review*, 33, 782–794.

Kwan, C. K. 2020. A qualitative inquiry into the human library approach: facilitating social inclusion and promoting recovery. *International Journal of Environmental Research and Public Health*, 17.

Lekas, H. M., Pahl, K. & fuller Lewis, C. 2020. Rethinking cultural competence: shifting to cultural humility. *Health Services Insights*, 13, 1178632920970580.

Linden, M. A., Hanna, D. & Redpath, S. 2007. The influence of aetiology and blame on prejudice towards survivors of brain injury. *Archives of Clinical Neuropsychology*, 22, 665–673.

Link, B. G. & Phelan, J. C. 2001. Conceptualizing Stigma. *Annual Review of Sociology*, 27, 363–385.

Link, B. G., Wells, J., Phelan, J. C. & Yang, L. 2015. Understanding the importance of "symbolic interaction stigma": how expectations about the reactions of others adds to the burden of mental illness stigma. *Psychiatric Rehabilitation Journal*, 38, 117–124.

Livingston, J. D. & Boyd, J. E. 2010. Correlates and consequences of internalized stigma for people living with mental illness: a systematic review and meta-analysis. *Social Science & Medicine*, 71, 2150–2161.

Mannarini, S., Taccini, F., Sato, I. & Rossi, A. A. 2022. Understanding stigma toward schizophrenia. *Psychiatry Research*, 318, 114970.

Marcelin, J. R., Siraj, D. S., Victor, R., Kotadia, S. & Maldonado, Y. A. 2019. The impact of unconscious bias in healthcare: how to recognize and mitigate it. *The Journal of Infectious Diseases*, 220, S62–S73.

Markowitz, F. E., Angell, B. & Greenberg, J. S. 2011. Stigma, reflected appraisals, and recovery outcomes in mental illness. *Social Psychology Quarterly*, 74, 144–165.

Martin, A. K., Tavaglione, N. & Hurst, S. 2014. Resolving the conflict: clarifying 'vulnerability' in health care ethics. *Kennedy Institute of Ethics Journal*, 24, 51–72.

Masters, C., Robinson, D., Faulkner, S., Patterson, E., Mcilraith, T. & Ansari, A. 2019. Addressing biases in patient care with the 5Rs of cultural humility, a clinician coaching tool. *Journal of General Internal Medicine*, 34, 627–630.

Mathur, V. A., Richeson, J. A., Paice, J. A., Muzyka, M. & Chiao, J. Y. 2014. Racial bias in pain perception and response: experimental examination of automatic and deliberate processes. *The Journal of Pain*, 15, 476–484.

Meghani, S. H., Byun, E. & Gallagher, R. M. 2012. Time to take stock: a meta-analysis and systematic review of analgesic treatment disparities for pain in the United States. *Pain Medicine*, 13, 150–174.

Mehta, N., Kassam, A., Leese, M., Butler, G. & Thornicroft, G. 2009. Public attitudes towards people with mental illness in England and Scotland, 1994–2003. *The British Journal of Psychiatry*, 194, 278–284.

Mojtabai, R. 2010. Mental illness stigma and willingness to seek mental health care in the European Union. *Social Psychiatry and Psychiatric Epidemiology*, 45, 705–712.

Morris, M., Cooper, R. L., Ramesh, A., Tabatabai, M., Arcury, T. A., Shinn, M., Im, W., Juarez, P. & Matthews-Juarez, P. 2019. Training to reduce LGBTQ-related bias among medical, nursing, and dental students and providers: a systematic review. *BMC Medical Education*, 19, 325.

Newheiser, A.-K. & Olson, K. R. 2012. White and Black American children's implicit intergroup bias. *Journal of Experimental Social Psychology*, 48, 264–270.

Ng, R., Allore, H. G., Trentalange, M., Monin, J. K. & Levy, B. R. 2015. Increasing negativity of age stereotypes across 200 years: Evidence from a database of 400 million words. *PLoS One*, 10, e0117086.

Nicholson, C., Gordon, A. L. & Tinker, A. 2016. Changing the way "we" view and talk about frailty. . . . *Age and Ageing*, 46, 349–351.

NMC. 2019. *The Code: Professional standards of practice and behaviour for nurses, midwives and nursing associates* [Online]. Available: https://www.nmc.org.uk/standards/code/ [Accessed].

Nosek, B. A. & Riskind, R. G. 2012. Policy implications of implicit social cognition. *Social Issues and Policy Review*, 6, 113–147.

Nyblade, L., Stangl, A., Weiss, E. & Ashburn, K. 2009. Combating HIV stigma in health care settings: what works? *Journal of the International AIDS Society*, 12, 15–15.

Nyblade, L., Stockton, M. A., Giger, K., Bond, V., Ekstrand, M. L., Lean, R. M., Mitchell, E. M., Nelson, L. R. E., Sapag, J. C. & Siraprapasiri, T. 2019. Stigma in health facilities: why it matters and how we can change it. *BMC Medicine*, 17, 1–15.

Oexle, N., Waldmann, T., Staiger, T., Xu, Z. & Rüsch, N. 2018. Mental illness stigma and suicidality: the role of public and individual stigma. *Epidemiology and Psychiatric Sciences*, 27, 169–175.

Onyeador, I. N., Wittlin, N. M., Burke, S. E., Dovidio, J. F., Perry, S. P., Hardeman, R. R., Dyrbye, L. N., Herrin, J., Phelan, S. M. & Van Ryn, M. 2020. The value of interracial contact for reducing anti-black bias among non-black physicians: a cognitive habits and growth evaluation (CHANGE) study report. *Psychological Science*, 31, 18–30.

Pachankis, J. E., Hatzenbuehler, M. L., Wang, K., Burton, C. L., Crawford, F. W., Phelan, J. C. & Link, B. G. 2018. The burden of stigma on health and well-being: a taxonomy of concealment, course, disruptiveness, aesthetics, origin, and peril across 93 stigmas. *Personality and Social Psychology Bulletin*, 44, 451–474.

Paul, M., John, B., Grace, C., Sheena, F., Zoe, G., Clare, I., Paul, J., Rose, J., Steven, H. J., Hameed, K., Christopher, L., Karen, M., Erin, M., Sarah, P., Samantha, R., Jo, R.-M., Mike, S., Lesley, W. & Fiona, L. 2024. Designing a library of lived experience for mental health: integrated realist synthesis and experience-based co-design study in UK mental health services. *BMJ Open*, 14, e081188.

Penner, L. A., Dovidio, J. F., West, T. V., Gaertner, S. L., Albrecht, T. L., Dailey, R. K. & Markova, T. 2010. Aversive racism and medical interactions with black patients: a field study. *Journal of Experimental Social Psychology*, 46, 436–440.

Pescosolido, B. A., Halpern-Manners, A., Luo, L. & Perry, B. 2021. Trends in public stigma of mental illness in the US, 1996–2018. *JAMA Network Open*, 4, e2140202–e2140202.

Pescosolido, B. A., Martin, J. K., Long, J. S., Medina, T. R., Phelan, J. C. & Link, B. G. 2010. "A disease like any other"? a decade of change in public reactions to schizophrenia, depression, and alcohol dependence. *The American Journal of Psychiatry*, 167, 1321–1330.

Pescosolido, B. A., Medina, T. R., Martin, J. K. & Long, J. S. 2013. The "backbone" of stigma: identifying the global core of public prejudice associated with mental illness. *American Journal of Public Health*, 103, 853–860.

Phelan, J. C., Link, B. G. & Dovidio, J. F. 2008. Stigma and prejudice: one animal or two? *Social Science & Medicine*, 67, 358–367.

Puddifoot, K. 2019. Stereotyping patients. *Journal of Social Philosophy*, 50, 69–90.

Puhl, R. M. & Heuer, C. A. 2010. Obesity stigma: important considerations for public health. *American Journal of Public Health*, 100, 1019–1028.

Purcell, D. W. 2021. Forty years of HIV: the intersection of laws, stigma, and sexual behavior and identity. *American Journal of Public Health*, 111, 1231–1233.

Quinn, D. M. & Chaudoir, S. R. 2009. Living with a concealable stigmatized identity: the impact of anticipated stigma, centrality, salience, and cultural stigma on psychological distress and health. *Journal of Personality and Social Psychology*, 97, 634–651.

Rao, D., Elshafei, A., Nguyen, M., Hatzenbuehler, M. L., Frey, S. & Go, V. F. 2019. A systematic review of multi-level stigma interventions: state of the science and future directions. *BMC Medicine*, 17, 41.

Redpath, S. J., Williams, W. H., Hanna, D., Linden, M. A., Yates, P. & Harris, A. 2010. Healthcare professionals' attitudes towards traumatic brain injury (TBI): the influence of profession, experience, aetiology and blame on prejudice towards survivors of brain injury. *Brain Injury*, 24, 802–811.

Reinka, M. A., Pan-Weisz, B., Lawner, E. K. & Quinn, D. M. 2020. Cumulative consequences of stigma: Possessing multiple concealable stigmatized identities is associated with worse quality of life. *Journal of Applied Social Psychology*, 50, 253–261.

Rice, W. S., Logie, C. H., Napoles, T. M., Walcott, M., Batchelder, A. W., Kempf, M.-C., Wingood, G. M., Konkle-Parker, D. J., Turan, B., Wilson, T. E., Johnson, M. O., Weiser, S. D. & Turan, J. M. 2018. Perceptions of intersectional stigma among diverse women living with HIV in the United States. *Social Science & Medicine*, 208, 9–17.

Richman, L. S. & Hatzenbuehler, M. L. 2014. A multilevel analysis of stigma and health: implications for research and policy. *Policy Insights From the Behavioral and Brain Sciences*, 1, 213–221.

Riles, J. M., Miller, B., Funk, M. & Morrow, E. 2021. The modern character of mental health stigma: a 30-year examination of popular film. *Communication Studies*, 72, 668–683.

Rössler, W. 2016. The stigma of mental disorders: a millennia-long history of social exclusion and prejudices. *EMBO Reports*, 17, 1250–1253.

Rueda, S., Mitra, S., Chen, S., Gogolishvili, D., Globerman, J., Chambers, L., Wilson, M., Logie, C. H., Shi, Q., Morassaei, S. & Rourke, S. B. 2016. Examining the associations between HIV-related stigma and health outcomes in people living with HIV/AIDS: a series of meta-analyses. *BMJ Open*, 6, e011453.

Rzeszutek, M., Gruszczyńska, E., Pięta, M. & Malinowska, P. 2021. HIV/AIDS stigma and psychological well-being after 40 years of HIV/AIDS: a systematic review and meta-analysis. *European Journal of Psychotraumatology*, 12, 1990527.

Scambler, G. 2009. Health-related stigma. *Sociology of Health & Illness*, 31, 441–455.

Scambler, G. 2018. Heaping blame on shame: 'Weaponising stigma' for neoliberal times. *The Sociological Review*, 66, 766–782.

Schomerus, G., Schwahn, C., Holzinger, A., Corrigan, P. W., Grabe, H. J., Carta, M. G. & Angermeyer, M. C. 2012. Evolution of public attitudes about mental illness: a systematic review and meta-analysis. *Acta Psychiatrica Scandinavica*, 125, 440–452.

Shepherd, B. F. & Brochu, P. M. 2021. How do stereotypes harm older adults? a theoretical explanation for the perpetration of elder abuse and its rise. *Aggression and Violent Behavior*, 57, 101435.

Stone, J. & Moskowitz, G. B. 2011. Non-conscious bias in medical decision making: what can be done to reduce it? *Medical Education*, 45, 768–776.

Stutterheim, S. E., Van Der Kooij, Y. L., Crutzen, R., Ruiter, R. A. C., Bos, A. E. R. & Kok, G. 2023. Intervention mapping as a guide to developing, implementing, and evaluating stigma reduction interventions. *Stigma and Health*, 10, 3–20. No Pagination Specified-No Pagination Specified.

Tang, C., Goldsamt, L., Meng, J., Xiao, X., Zhang, L., Williams, A. B. & Wang, H. 2020. Global estimate of the prevalence of post-traumatic stress disorder among adults living with HIV: a systematic review and meta-analysis. *BMJ Open*, 10, e032435.

Thirsk, L. M., Panchuk, J. T., Stahlke, S. & Hagtvedt, R. 2022. Cognitive and implicit biases in nurses' judgment and decision-making: a scoping review. *International Journal of Nursing Studies*, 133, 104284.

Thornicroft, G., Sunkel, C., Alikhon Aliev, A., Baker, S., Brohan, E., El Chammay, R., Davies, K., Demissie, M., Duncan, J., Fekadu, W., Gronholm, P. C., Guerrero, Z., Gurung, D., Habtamu, K., Hanlon, C., Heim, E., Henderson, C., Hijazi, Z., Hoffman, C., Hosny, N., Huang, F.-X., Kline, S., Kohrt, B. A., Lempp, H., Li, J., London, E., Ma, N., Mak, W. W. S., Makhmud, A., Maulik, P. K., Milenova, M., Morales Cano, G., Ouali, U., Parry, S., Rangaswamy, T., Rüsch, N., Sabri, T.,

Sartorius, N., Schulze, M., Stuart, H., Taylor Salisbury, T., Juan, V. S. & Votruba, Winkler, N., N., P. 2022. The Lancet commission on ending stigma and discrimination in mental health. *The Lancet*, 400, 1438–1480.

Tjia, J., Pugnaire, M., Calista, J., Eisdorfer, E., Hale, J., Terrien, J., Valdman, O., Potts, S., Garcia, M., Yazdani, M., Puerto, G., Okero, M., Duodu, V. & Sabin, J. 2023. Using simulation-based learning with standardized patients (SP) in an implicit bias mitigation clinician training program. *Journal of Medical Education and Curricular Development*, 10, 23821205231175033.

Treves-Kagan, S., Steward, W. T., Ntswane, L., Haller, R., Gilvydis, J. M., Gulati, H., Barnhart, S. & Lippman, S. A. 2015. Why increasing availability of ART is not enough: a rapid, community-based study on how HIV-related stigma impacts engagement to care in rural South Africa. *BMC Public Health*, 16, 1–13.

Trickey, A., Sabin, C. A., Burkholder, G., Crane, H., D'arminio Monforte, A., Egger, M., Gill, M. J., Grabar, S., Guest, J. L., Jarrin, I., Lampe, F. C., Obel, N., Reyes, J. M., Stephan, C., Sterling, T. R., Teira, R., Touloumi, G., Wasmuth, J.-C., Wit, F., Wittkop, L., Zangerle, R., Silverberg, M. J., Justice, A. & Sterne, J. A. C. 2023. Life expectancy after 2015 of adults with HIV on long-term antiretroviral therapy in Europe and North America: a collaborative analysis of cohort studies. *The Lancet HIV*, 10, e295–e307.

Tyler, I. & Slater, T. 2018. Rethinking the sociology of stigma. *The Sociological Review*, 66, 721–743.

Valery, K.-M. & Prouteau, A. 2020. Schizophrenia stigma in mental health professionals and associated factors: a systematic review. *Psychiatry Research*, 290, 113068.

VanPuymbrouck, L., Friedman, C. & Feldner, H. 2020. Explicit and implicit disability attitudes of healthcare providers. *Rehabilitation Psychology*, 65, 101–112.

Vora, S., Dahlen, B., Adler, M., Kessler, D. O., Jones, V. F., Kimble, S. & Calhoun, A. 2021. Recommendations and guidelines for the use of simulation to address structural racism and implicit bias. *Simulation in Healthcare*, 16, 275–284.

Webster, C. S., Taylor, S., Thomas, C. & Weller, J. M. 2022. Social bias, discrimination and inequity in healthcare: mechanisms, implications and recommendations. *BJA Education*, 22, 131–137.

Wilbur, K., Snyder, C., Essary, A. C., Reddy, S., Will, K. K. & Mary, S. 2020. Developing workforce diversity in the health professions: a social justice perspective. *Health Professions Education*, 6, 222–229.

Wisniewski, J. M. & Walker, B. 2020. Association of simulated patient race/ethnicity with scheduling of primary care appointments. *JAMA Network Open*, 3, e1920010–e1920010.

Xu, Z., Müller, M., Heekeren, K., Theodoridou, A., Metzler, S., Dvorsky, D., Oexle, N., Walitza, S., Rössler, W. & Rüsch, N. 2016. Pathways between stigma and suicidal ideation among people at risk of psychosis. *Schizophrenia Research*, 172, 184–188.

Zeidan, A. J., Khatri, U. G., Aysola, J., Shofer, F. S., Mamtani, M., Scott, K. R., Conlon, L. W. & Lopez, B. L. 2019. Implicit bias education and emergency medicine training: step one? awareness. *AEM Education and Training*, 3, 81–85.

CHAPTER 10

Meeting the Needs of Those Experiencing Social Exclusion and Significant Inequality

Lindsay Welch[1], Jasmine Snowden[2], and Chris Allen[2]

[1] *Faculty of Health and Social Sciences, Bournemouth University, Bournemouth, UK*
[2] *School of Health Sciences, University of Southampton, Southampton, UK*

Introduction

In previous chapters, we considered the social determinants of health and the role of stigma in influencing attitudes and behaviours, and in turn, reducing access to support and impacting health-related outcomes. The communities we live in are increasingly 'super diverse'. Whilst diversity is positive, where power relations exist within society, including through many of its institutions, the needs of vulnerable groups (who often themselves carry the greater health burdens) can be sidelined. Such power relations can influence and shape health and opportunities, resulting in poor quality, culturally insensitive and potentially unsafe care for those who find themselves socially excluded. Personal characteristics and behaviours can set people apart from the communities in which they live, and these differences can lead to barriers and various negative experiences with health and well-being. There is an increasing policy, research and practice focus on inclusion health, and supporting the health needs of those who have historically been socially excluded. In this chapter, we will have the opportunity to consider some of the inclusion health needs of people from socially excluded groups, as well as those facing disadvantaged access to care.

To help readers consider social exclusion, and the impact this has on the care people access, we have provided three applied case studies (two specifically relating to inclusion health, and one relating to racial inequality in screening programmes), alongside consideration of how the health of those who are socially excluded can be supported. There are though, many ways through which people can be socially excluded. We cannot explore all of these within the pages of this chapter. As such, this is a starting point for you to consider some of the concepts explored in Chapters 8 and 9 specifically, and how these relate to the health and social exclusion of people by individuals, by organisations and by wider society. We can use this knowledge, to begin to consider how those who are socially excluded can be better included in healthcare.

LEARNING OUTCOMES

By the end of this chapter, you will be able to:

- Understand what social exclusion and marginalisation are and consider some of the common causes.
- Consider the health inequalities that are commonly faced by those targeted by inclusion health programmes and how these occur.
- Consider how those experiencing social exclusion can be better included in health research, and the design of healthcare systems to better meet their needs.

Social Sciences for Healthcare Professionals, First Edition. Edited by Chris Allen.
© 2026 John Wiley & Sons Ltd. Published 2026 by John Wiley & Sons Ltd.

What Is Social Exclusion and Marginalisation?

> ### Key Terms and Definitions
>
> **Social exclusion:**   Reflects a lack of opportunity or difficulty using available opportunities, thus preventing full participation, or exclusion from society (O'Donnell et al., 2021).
>
> **Marginalisation:**   Involves the treatment of an individual, or a group in a way that places them outside of mainstream society, that is, their needs are placed at the periphery, margins or fringe (Cheraghi-Sohi et al., 2020).
>
> **Intersectionality:**   People can be excluded based on more than one characteristic. These characteristics can combine (or intersect) to create unique experiences with advantages and disadvantages (Bambra, 2022).
>
> **Global majority:**   Is increasingly a term used to describe non-white people, reflecting the important observation that whilst in some countries white people constitute the cultural majority, globally they are in fact the numerical minority, with most of the world's population being non-white (Campbell-Stephens, 2021).
>
> **Cultural competence/cultural humility:**   Reflects the capacity, or competence of a person, or a system to respond appropriately to people from all races, ethnicities and identities (Lekas et al., 2020).

'Social exclusion' and 'marginalisation' as terms are often used interchangeably. Marginalisation describes the casting aside, or 'othering' of people or groups within a society, in a way that places them at society's fringes (Cheraghi-Sohi et al., 2020). Similarly, whilst there is a lack of unified definition, social exclusion generally refers to a lack of opportunity or difficulty utilising the opportunities that there are, thereby limiting an individual or group's full participation in society (Cuesta et al., 2024, O'Donnell et al., 2021). Whilst we highlighted the challenges presented by poverty in Chapter 8, social exclusion is a multi-dimensional concept and is about more than simply lacking material resources, as it also involves disadvantages stemming from political, social and cultural influences (Cuesta et al., 2024; O'Donnell et al., 2021). In fact, whilst disadvantaged in other ways, socially excluded people are not always poor (Cuesta et al., 2024). Whilst people may be able to intuitively identify those who are excluded, it is difficult to precisely define the experience of social exclusion and who is/who is not socially excluded (O'Donnell et al., 2021). Recent work has estimated that through identity, circumstances and socio-economic conditions, around 30% of the world's population is at risk of social exclusion (Cuesta et al., 2024), with the following dimensions of exclusion being emphasised:

- **Identity:** Such as someone's age, gender, race and ethnicity. This is not to say that, for example, being a woman or being black means you are automatically socially excluded, but in certain contexts, gender and race can certainly lead to exclusion (Cuesta et al., 2024).
- **Circumstances:** Such as being forcibly displaced through violent conflict, or engaging in employment that others within a society might disapprove of (such as sex work).
- **Socio-economic position:** Such as income, education and employment status.

The social exclusion of individuals or groups invariably ends up in their needs being sidelined. Societies are generally not set up to include those who are perceived (being a keyword) as being 'different' or 'challenging', instead they focus on meeting the needs of the 'mainstream', in turn neglecting the needs of those falling outside of this (Hui et al., 2020, O'Donnell et al., 2021). This puts some at a significant disadvantage when it comes to accessing needed resources and opportunities, with societies' various institutions, such as legal, education and health, often providing discriminatory, inadequate or culturally incompetent provisions (Bradby et al., 2020, Cuesta et al., 2023, O'Donnell et al., 2021). Social exclusion can influence people's experiences of care at the micro (through disparaging treatment from healthcare professionals, social and cultural differences between healthcare professionals and patients, or through communication difficulties/language barriers, etc.), meso (i.e. through local services poorly meeting their needs) and macro levels (i.e. through health systems being poorly designed to meet excluded group's needs and through exclusion from decision making about how services operate) (Hui et al., 2020, Shulman et al., 2018, Siddiqui, 2014, Van Rosse et al., 2016).

There are also several routes to social exclusion and they are often relational. For example, stigma, a social process explored in the previous chapter, can lead to individuals and groups becoming excluded and facing inequality, based on their real or perceived differences being viewed negatively by others or by themselves (Hatzenbuehler et al., 2013). People's identities, circumstances, unconventional lifestyles and histories, cultural differences and undesirable behaviours, as well as a person's health, can result in people being judged, or feeling judged; and as a result, being socially excluded (Cuesta et al., 2024). As we explored in the previous chapter, it is not just people's personal characteristics and their health that can lead to stigmatisation. People's behaviour, especially where it deviates from society's expectations about how people should be and how they should behave, can essentially mark people out as being different in some way (Goffman, 1963, Link and Phelan, 2001, Phelan et al., 2008). The extent to which these behaviours are accepted by society can have a significant impact on a person's life in general, as well as their access to care and supportive services. This is especially the case where people feel they may be judged for their engagement in them (such as taking harmful drugs, working in the sex industry or engaging in other unsafe, or socially undesirable behaviours) (Benoit et al., 2015, Muncan et al., 2020). Societies' exclusionary practices and stigma can lead to people feeling like they are in some way responsible for their exclusion, and research has suggested that this can lead to those experiencing exclusion to perceive attempts to overcome the obstacles they face as futile (O'Donnell et al., 2021).

Exclusionary processes differ between groups and change over time. In terms of marginalisation, as this largely relates to power, status, cultures, norms and judgements, exactly who experiences marginalisation and the consequences of marginalisation will vary across different societies. How this is actually experienced, and the resultant impact on someone's life, will differ based on a number of intersecting factors such as gender, ethnicity, sexual orientation and socio-economic status (Crenshaw, 1989, Ruiz et al., 2021). Intersectionality helps us to consider how aspects of disadvantage may interact and combine; for example, a less affluent black woman with a disabled child seeking help and support, and a white wealthy family seeking help for a disabled child, will experience stigma and its resultant marginalisation very differently, due to intersecting class, ethnicity and disability. Through considering social exclusion and marginalisation through the lens of intersectionality, we can see how disadvantage can be further exacerbated, through different aspects of disadvantages combining and accumulating.

Healthcare systems can also exacerbate exclusion, especially where significant barriers to access and participation exist and where provision poorly accounts for the needs of historically underserved groups. Those creating public services are often far removed from the challenges that those in socially excluded groups face (O'Donnell et al., 2021), and as we explore later in this chapter, health research more commonly includes those with higher socio-economic status and this can further exacerbate the inequitable design of healthcare systems, which are already largely designed around the needs of advantaged groups, over more seldom heard voices (Islam et al., 2021). This ends up resulting in services that are inflexible, and complex, which may discourage engagement from those with challenging lives who are experiencing social exclusion (O'Donnell et al., 2021). Exclusionary practices can extend to societies and other institutions too, and research has suggested that those experiencing social exclusion are either denied or provided only limited access to finance, housing, employment and education, alongside healthcare (O'Donnell et al., 2021). As we outlined in Chapter 8, these also have an important role in shaping the health and opportunities that people have.

Inclusion Health

Those experiencing social exclusion are also often those carrying the greatest health-related burdens. This has been coined the 'inverse care law' (Hart, 1971, Mercer et al., 2021, Watt, 2018), which typically sees those with the greatest healthcare needs having to navigate services that are poorly designed to meet them and having more limited say in how these services are run

(Hui et al., 2020). Remember the Marmot curves from Chapter 8? In those curves, you would have seen that some in society have especially good health and longevity, and some have especially bad health and longevity. Social exclusion and social inclusion can be thought of as two ends of a continuum (O'Donnell et al., 2021). Efforts to address social exclusion tend to focus on increasing social inclusion (O'Donnell et al., 2021). Recently, there has been an increasing interest (in policy, in practice and in academic research) in those doing especially badly, often through addressing the needs of socially excluded groups through the targeted activities of 'inclusion health' (Aldridge et al., 2018, Luchenski et al., 2018, Marmot, 2018, Tweed et al., 2022). Inclusion health is an approach and umbrella term that seeks to address society's most socially excluded individuals and groups, who experience significant social disadvantage, marginalisation and very poor health (Aldridge et al., 2018, Luchenski et al., 2018, Marmot, 2018).

In the UK NHS (2023), the target of inclusion health initiatives typically include:

- Those experiencing homelessness, or who are vulnerably housed.
- Those who are dependent on drugs and alcohol.
- Migrants and refugees, especially those who are at risk of harm and exploitation.
- Travelling communities including Gypsy and Roma communities.
- Those who are in some way in contact with the justice system, such as those who have previously committed an offence.
- Those who are victims of modern slavery.
- Those working in the sex industry.
- As well as any other marginalised group.

Many of those inclusion health provision seeks to support, fit more than one of the above groups (Aldridge et al., 2018, Filia et al., 2022, McVicar et al., 2015). For example, substance misuse is common in homelessness (McVicar et al., 2015, Stablein et al., 2021). The importance of focussing on these groups is emphasised by the extremely poor health outcomes they typically face (Aldridge et al., 2018, NHS, 2023). In one recent review, inclusion health groups were found to have significantly higher mortality rates compared to even the poorest neighbourhoods (Aldridge et al., 2018). For example, in inclusion health groups, men experienced 7.9 times higher mortality, and women 11.9 times higher mortality, in contrast to those in the most deprived areas experiencing 2.8 times higher mortality when compared to the least deprived areas (Aldridge et al., 2018). These significant differences in mortality arise through almost all health conditions, and whilst this is not one large homogenous group with identical health risks and outcomes, mortality rates are most influenced by injury, poisoning and external causes (Aldridge et al., 2018). This significant inequality is particularly visible in Figure 10.1, when comparing these groups with even the most deprived populations.

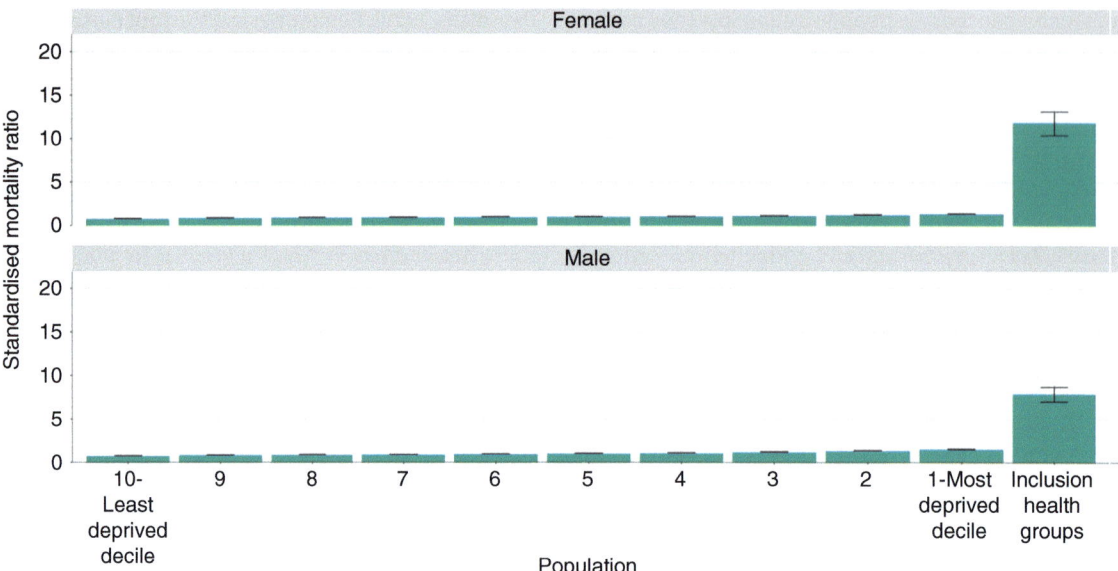

FIGURE 10.1 Inclusion health groups have higher mortality ratios than even those in the most deprived groups. **Source:** Office for Health Improvement and Disparities (2022)/Crown Copyright/CC by 3.0. **Source data:** Office for National Statistics Deaths by underlying cause, deprivation decile areas, 5-year age groups and sex, England and Wales, 1981 to 2015. Office for National Statistics Populations by deprivation decile areas, 5-year age groups and sex, England and Wales, 2001 to 2015. Aldridge et al. 2017.

However, some have argued that the identification of these groups within targeted inclusion health activities may further stigmatise people with these identities, circumstances or socio-economic positions (Tweed et al., 2022). Whilst inclusion health has led to communities of practice forming (academic and clinical) around significant unmet healthcare needs, there continues to be a need to focus also on the broader social influences and exclusionary practices that cause those within these groups to be so disadvantaged in the first place (Tweed et al., 2022). Another challenge is that the inclusion health groups mentioned above, are not one single homogenous group, with similar needs, health risks, health outcomes and pathways into and out of social exclusion. Often, needs and pathways to exclusion are very different. Some of these aspects will be considered within the case studies below.

international law (Amnesty International, 2024, European Parliament, 2015, Zimmerman et al., 2011).

Asylum seeker: An asylum seeker is also leaving their country through fear of their safety and life, but they have not yet legally been recognised as a refugee (Amnesty International, 2024, Zimmerman et al., 2011).

Irregular migrant: Someone staying outside of their country of origin, who is not a refugee or asylum seeker, and does not have a legal right to remain (Cuibus and Walsh, 2025).

In the context of health, these terms are important, as they often relate to what services people can access, how they access them, and in many countries, whether they are eligible for care.

Forced Displacement, Migration and Health

Key Terms and Definitions

Refugee: A refugee is someone who is fleeing their country because if they remained, they would be at a serious risk of having their human rights violated, or of being persecuted. These people leave their country because its institutions cannot or will not protect them, and because the risk to their safety and life means they have no choice. Refugees are protected by

In recent years involuntary or forced displacement, through conflict, war and political instability is becoming increasingly common (UNHCR, 2020). In 2020, before the outbreak of the war in Ukraine, and before the escalation of tensions between Israel and Palestine, 82.4 million people were forcibly displaced worldwide (UNHCR, 2020), rising to 108.4 million at the end of 2022 (UNHCR, 2023a). With new conflicts emerging through increasing geo-political tensions between and within countries, alongside climate change and overall worsening planetary health increasing the risk of natural disasters and food insecurity, the number of people being forcibly displaced is likely to only continue rising (UNHCR, 2023b). Those who are forcibly displaced, and who do cross a border into another country, can find themselves in situations with little rights, resources, personal contacts or safety. Generally, for quite some time, they will lack safe and stable living conditions, have limited access to employment and limited access to many of society's institutions including education and health (UNHCR, 2023a).

Whilst not a homogenous group, those who are forcibly displaced face numerous complex health needs relating to their previous situation, travel between countries and the associated risks this brings, and barriers to health access in receiving countries (Bendavid et al., 2021, BMA, 2024, Cuadrado et al., 2023, Head et al., 2022, Jawad et al., 2020, Kang et al., 2024, Lebano et al., 2020, Matlin et al., 2018). It is common for people to have no access to care, or other forms of social support for extended periods of time, exacerbating pre-existing disease, whilst increasing the risk of further chronic and acute morbidity (BMA, 2024, Cuadrado et al., 2023, Head et al., 2022, Jawad et al., 2020, Matlin et al., 2018).

In the context of the United Kingdom, refugees, asylum seekers and irregular migrants face various challenges when trying to access healthcare support (Asif and Kienzler, 2022). Anyone, at least in principle, can register with a GP[1], even without identification. However, there remains significant confusion amongst healthcare workers about who can and who cannot register and receive NHS treatment (Asif and Kienzler, 2022, Hodson et al., 2019) even in designated cities of sanctuary[2] (Scott et al., 2022). Undocumented migrants, who often live in limbo, and fear due to legacy 'hostile environment' policies, may have concerns about accessing care through their GP (Webber, 2019, Woodward et al., 2014), despite their details no longer ordinarily being shared with the Home Office[3] (Asif and Kienzler, 2022, Webber, 2019).

As we explored in Chapter 5, the United Kingdom enjoys relatively privileged Universal Health Coverage. Whilst barriers certainly still exist that place those who have been involuntarily displaced in the United Kingdom at a disadvantage in relation to accessing health, the situation is better than that which is experienced in countries lacking this coverage, often even for its own citizens (Haque et al., 2020).

Case Study: Fleeing Conflict

Sylvia arrived in the United Kingdom with their son, Jordan, following the outbreak of war in their home country. With the situation simply becoming too unsafe to remain, Sylvia, a teacher in her home country, made the difficult decision to leave her husband and seek asylum in the United Kingdom. She has since lost contact with her husband and believes he has died in conflict. Like others who find themselves forcibly displaced, Sylvia's journey to the United Kingdom was not straightforward. Arriving in the United Kingdom with limited personal possessions combined with having limited access to people she knows, or who are like her, made her feel very isolated, alone and vulnerable. Sylvia and her son were fortunate to be able to locate a friend's brother, and he put them up in his front room in a small one-bedroom flat on an estate in the outskirts of the city. Her friend's brother is a largely solitary man, who is poorly connected with others in the local community, and who mostly just works long hours in various jobs to keep up with his rent.

Lacking what she believed to be the necessary documentation (passport or other forms of identification, proof of address, etc.), she did not really know where to even begin with regards to getting a secure, safe and permanent place to live, gaining secure and legal employment, and accessing formal education and healthcare services. The estate where she is staying has poor access to primary care. A new build estate, which sprung up relatively quickly with little consideration for providing vital services for its residents who either find themselves having to drive everywhere, or where they don't have access to a car, relying on expensive public transport to access the services they need. Her brother's friend had signposted her to the nearest doctor's surgery that was accepting new patients, several miles away.

The only way she can get there is by bus service, which runs infrequently and is expensive. Whilst waiting for her migration status to be approved, she is unable to work, and as a result, has to manage on a very small state provision, that is provided to people who find themselves involuntarily displaced, and seeking refuge. Her weekly money through this allowance barely covers essentials, placing her in poverty, and she is reluctant to use some of this to get the bus to register for the surgery. However, being aware of her and her son's current and likely future healthcare needs, decided to do so. At the surgery, she was given a new patient registration form in a format she could not interpret, and her broken English conversation with a receptionist led her to incorrectly believe that she needed

---

[1] Currently in the United Kingdom, NHS guidance clearly states that a person cannot be refused access to GP services because they cannot identify themselves, or because they cannot confirm their migration status. GP services, along with other primary care services are free to all (UK Government, 2023). However, there are misconceptions from both providers and those seeking treatments, as well as other barriers that reduce people's access to these essential services when they need them (Asif and Kienzler, 2022).

[2] In the United Kingdom, City of Sanctuary is a charity whose aims are to build communities that are welcoming and inclusive to refugees and those seeking asylum.

[3] A UK Government Institution charged with responsibility for immigration, amongst other things.

to be a resident to register, and would require some form of identification. Being in a new situation, with a healthcare system she did not know or understand, and with no access to the internet, she had little opportunity to find out if this was in fact correct, nor did she have much power or voice to challenge this. She asked her brother's friend what she needed to register, but he didn't know either – he did so several years ago, but he rarely visits the GP, even when he is unwell.

Since arriving in the United Kingdom, and as a direct consequence of the horrors his family witnessed, Jordan has been struggling with symptoms of Post-Traumatic Stress Disorder (PTSD), and his mother has significantly increased her alcohol consumption to help manage her emotions, pass the time and adjust to the stress of what has happened – as well as the new situation she now finds herself in. Before fleeing, Sylvia and her husband had been trying for another baby, and it has now been a few months since she had her last period, which alongside other bodily changes indicated that she may be pregnant. She was able to confirm this by taking a home test. She has since struggled to access any formal sexual or reproductive healthcare and went on to experience new bleeding and abdominal pain which indicated that the pregnancy may be at risk. Her continued lack of a fixed abode, and formal identification continued to make it challenging to access formal care in a timely way; but through fear for the health of her baby, she managed to get to a local accident and emergency department to be assessed, alongside her son. Having been assessed, the pregnancy was deemed to still be viable, and she was given advice about her drinking and the potential impact this was having on herself, and on her baby. Not being able to speak English, all her care in the department and the health advice that she received was delivered through a trained interpreter. However, the interpreter was not available for quite a while, and until they were available, one of the department nurses had used Google to translate, which she appreciated, but felt that many of her symptoms and concerns were either incorrectly translated or simply dismissed altogether. She felt staff lacked warmth towards her, and that they viewed her with contempt and a lack of sympathy, through their disproval of her decision to drink heavily whilst pregnant, despite knowing the risks to herself and her baby. No one actually said they disproved, but she wasn't treated in the same way she could see other patients being treated, who she saw generally being treated with warmth and kindness. The staff spent as little time with her as they could, and explained very little, even when the interpreter was available. She felt devalued and judged.

Following discharge with minimal support, and significant safeguarding concerns being raised about her family, her heavy drinking has continued, and having attended the appointment with her, Jordan's PTSD has worsened, having been triggered through flashbacks caused by the department's loud noises, including that of distressed people screaming. They have since been referred to children's services, and placed on a child protection plan, but despite this they continue to find it challenging to access any support

from the general practitioner (an example of primary care, which in the United Kingdom is the main gatekeeper to wider healthcare services) and then in turn struggling to access child and adolescent mental health services. She is deeply dissatisfied with her care experience, but is hesitant and lacks the confidence to voice these concerns, as she now feels she and her family are now 'marked'. In essence, she has found herself further stigmatised, yet no closer to the support and resources she actually needs, through healthcare she is now increasingly reluctant to access.

You may wish to consider the following points:

- What specific barriers did this family face in relation to accessing healthcare services?

- Were there any opportunities for the family to have been better supported? Which needs in particular were poorly addressed?

- What barriers to accessing healthcare services were there and what needs to be considered in order for people from displaced communities to be able to access care in a timely, equitable and safe manner?

Clinical Considerations

- Those caring for diverse communities should adopt a human rights-based approach to care (Vanderpyl et al., 2024).

- As a healthcare professional, it is vital that you understand the impact of someone's migration status, what services they can access and how they can be supported to access these services. This will differ from country to country.

- Poor mental health is common in displaced communities, especially in conflict-affected populations (Charlson et al., 2019, Grasser, 2022, Kang et al., 2024).

- Sexual health and antenatal care are known health disparities experienced by displaced populations (Cuadrado et al., 2023, Davidson et al., 2022, Logie et al., 2024, Saunders et al., 2022).

- Access to care depends on a person's individual capacity, as well as how the healthcare system is set up and funded (O'Donnell et al., 2016).

- There are several factors at the micro, meso and macro levels of society that can make care more difficult to access for some people reducing their opportunities to be seen and heard.

- Translation services are important and it is also important to consider who the translator is, and whether there are any specific cultural needs (Brandenberger et al., 2019).

- It is important that we treat everyone fairly, because it is the right thing to do, and can build up trust and confidence (Brandenberger et al., 2019). We may find it more challenging to do this, when we perceive that people are very different from us, or that their behaviour is perceived to have in some way contributed to their situation (Duveau et al., 2022, Fitzgerald and Hurst, 2017). It is important to acknowledge this, as we have the capacity to act in biased ways, even without intending to (i.e. implicitly). Only by acknowledging this, can we begin to focus on ensuring that our care is fair and equitable to all we see.

- The experiences of migrants will differ from place to place and will depend on several factors (Platts-Fowler and Robinson, 2015).

- To promote positive, and culturally acceptable healthcare encounters, work on cultural competence, education and understanding that goes further than equality and diversity training, is necessary to deliver safe and effective care to underserved individuals and groups (Flynn et al., 2020).

- Various initiatives are looking at addressing the treatment of people in this situation, such as the City of Sanctuary, a UK charity whose aim is to provide support through community groups and other institutions, including local government, to those seeking refuge (City of Sanctuary, 2024). There is now a growing list of City of Sanctuary groups across the United Kingdom. Sanctuary cities exist outside of the United Kingdom too and are delivered through different policies, practices and contexts (Bauder, 2017).

Place-Based Marginalisation, Nested Deprivation and Homelessness

Nested deprivation is used to describe pockets of deprivation that exist in otherwise apparently affluent areas (Boswell et al., 2022). Examples of nested deprivation can be seen throughout the United Kingdom, but there has been considerable concern for it in British seaside towns and coastal cities; which now endure some of the highest levels of entrenched deprivation in the country (Asthana and Gibson, 2021, Fiorentino et al., 2023, McDowell and Bonner-Thompson, 2020, Whitty, 2021). Academics have highlighted that many coastal towns have become 'left-behind places' (Fiorentino et al., 2023), leading to the marginalisation of whole communities of people who have become socially excluded (Boswell et al., 2022). The demise of industries that have typically supported such communities such as tourism through globalisation (notably the increasing cheapness through which people can holiday overseas that emerged in the 1970s), and in some areas, the collapse of industrial work such as mining, with few alternative forms of secure, year-round employment, has contributed to the emergence of localised poverty in many coastal and rural communities, leading to people feeling either disconnected from or entrapped by their local economy (Telford, 2021).

A lack of stable employment, and subsequent deprivation within such communities, mean they are associated with particularly poor health outcomes, which is increasingly being discussed by the media, researchers, policymakers and even the Chief Medical Officer (Whitty, 2021). In addition, the availability of poor quality but cheap housing, particularly that designated as Houses in Multiple Occupation (HMO) has been suggested to contribute to inwards migration into these areas from vulnerable groups seeking affordable housing, creating geographies of marginalisation (Bambra, 2022, Ward, 2015) and contributing to increased levels of vulnerably housed and homeless people.

Whilst this is not the case for all coastal communities, and there are some benefits to coastal living, poor healthcare outcomes are often observed, including for largely preventable health issues (Asthana and Gibson, 2021, Norman et al., 2022). The high concentration of cardiovascular disease alongside England's coastline as one example shown in Figure 10.2, visibly highlights a high concentration of poor health in these areas, relative to those that are more central. Often facing high demand; evidence suggests the healthcare services in coastal areas are unable to provide care in line with the agreed service standards for the country (Whitty, 2021).

Case Study: People with an Alcohol Use Disorder, Who Are Vulnerably Housed

Gerry is a Caucasian 54-year-old man. After leaving full-time education at 16, he set up his own small fishing and tourism business in a British Seaside town. In his mid-30s due to various financial challenges and difficulties gaining new work, he closed his business. Gerry was keen to get back on his feet and sought work in gardening. However, the seasonal nature of this work, especially in a British seaside area, meant winters were difficult.

At this time, Gerry had lots of local friends whom he would spend his evenings in the summer, and eventually days in the winter drinking and smoking with. Mounting financial pressures and inability to pay rising rent on time, resulted in him forcibly downsizing his house, and taking up residence in a HMO. Over time, he spent less time at home, or work; but increased his time at the local pub with his friends.

Over the years, work became increasingly hard to get, and Gerry struggled to keep up with the cost of living. Gerry fell further behind on his rent and other bills and was subsequently evicted. He began sleeping on his friend's sofa. At the time,

Gerry had a good relationship with his friends and was not concerned about his vulnerable living situation. He believed he would soon have enough money to secure a place of his own once again, once he was able to find work over the summer. He borrowed money from his friends and continued to drink and smoke heavily.

Over the next five years, Gerry began to get winter chest infections and experienced breathlessness on exertion but wasn't worried as he was not working, and considered it part of the usual winter bugs that circulate in the population. This belief was reinforced by seeing others around him facing similar health issues. However, these issues continued into the summer, and the impact of breathlessness meant Gerry struggled to complete the gardening work he had been offered and often didn't get paid as he was unable to complete the work. Over time, he was offered less and less work, and any work he was offered, took him longer than it used to.

Friends were getting annoyed as Gerry had been sofa surfing between different friends' homes for five years now and had not managed to secure a more permanent living situation. He began to experience psychotic episodes, which sometimes made him challenging to be around. To reduce pressure on his friends, Gerry started to spend nights sleeping rough. At this point, Gerry began injecting heroin. Work continued to become increasingly difficult, which was compounded by a lack of permanent address, meaning his employment-related post had to be handled by the local job centre, which he found embarrassing.

By his early 50s, Gerry had begun sleeping rough most nights, after he began finding it increasingly difficult to access shelter in his friends' homes. He continued to experience psychotic episodes, was still drinking and was using heroin regularly to self-medicate as a result of the challenges he faced in rough sleeping. Gerry's first winter sleeping rough was cold, and lonely, and involved regular acts of violence directed at him. Gerry felt very unwell one night and called in a favour from one of the few friends he had continued contact with. He was found cold and unconscious on the sofa the next morning by his friend, they called 999, and he was pronounced dead at the scene. His cause of death was an acute exacerbation of COPD and exposure. His friend was asked about his last wishes. Gerry had never discussed these.

You may wish to consider the following points:

- In what ways did stigma contribute to Gerry's help-seeking behaviour?
- What were the missed opportunities for intervention that might have prevented Gerry's death?

Clinical Considerations

Meeting the needs of those who are homeless and who have poor mental health and substance use disorders can be challenging (Stablein et al., 2021). For individuals with poor

mental health who are engaged in unhealthy behaviours, such as substance misuse, changing what to many is seen as self-management behaviour relating to their difficult situation, when their living situation continues to be poor, and with limited support is extremely difficult (Carver et al., 2020, Paudyal et al., 2020). A recent review (Woodward et al., 2023) has highlighted that those experiencing deprivation who have multiple long-term conditions face many compounding challenges and barriers to self-management practices including:

- Financial barriers restricting access to basic resources needed to maintain health, such as utilities such as heating, water, transport costs to attend appointments, cost of medications and cost of food, particularly where certain diets are indicated as is often the case in long-term condition self-management.
- Poor health literacy and understanding of their health needs. This also related to financial barriers, which limited opportunities and exposures to opportunities whereby a better understanding about health could be obtained.

Case management is a relevant consideration in people who find themselves in this situation – a recent review has highlighted that case management may support improved mental health, and reduce substance misuse and potential levels of homelessness when compared to normal care, and that this is particularly effective when this care is provided by multidisciplinary teams, with low caseloads, and who are embedded within the local community (Luchenski et al., 2018).

Finally, recognising a lack of housing as one of the social determinants of people's situations; one way of addressing this issue is the Housing First (as opposed to Treatment First) approach, which provides people with housing, and through this, attempts to engage them in supportive healthcare services that meet their needs and help them to change their behaviour over time (Carver et al., 2020, Woodhall-Melnik and Dunn, 2016). The main principle of this approach is that those engaged in harmful behaviours who are homeless may be more able to change their behaviour, once they have access to secure, safe accommodation (O'Campo et al., 2022). Evidence has suggested that such programmes can be useful in enhancing quality of life and recovery (O'Campo et al., 2022, Woodhall-Melnik and Dunn, 2016) and studies have also found that the Housing First Programme can increase people's social integration and social network size (Kirst et al., 2020). Increasingly, research looking into inclusion health is examining findings alongside those with lived experience, including that shown by Luchenski et al. (2018). This can be done through engagement workshops, and other forms of patient and public involvement and engagement (PPIE), which we will explore at the end of this chapter.

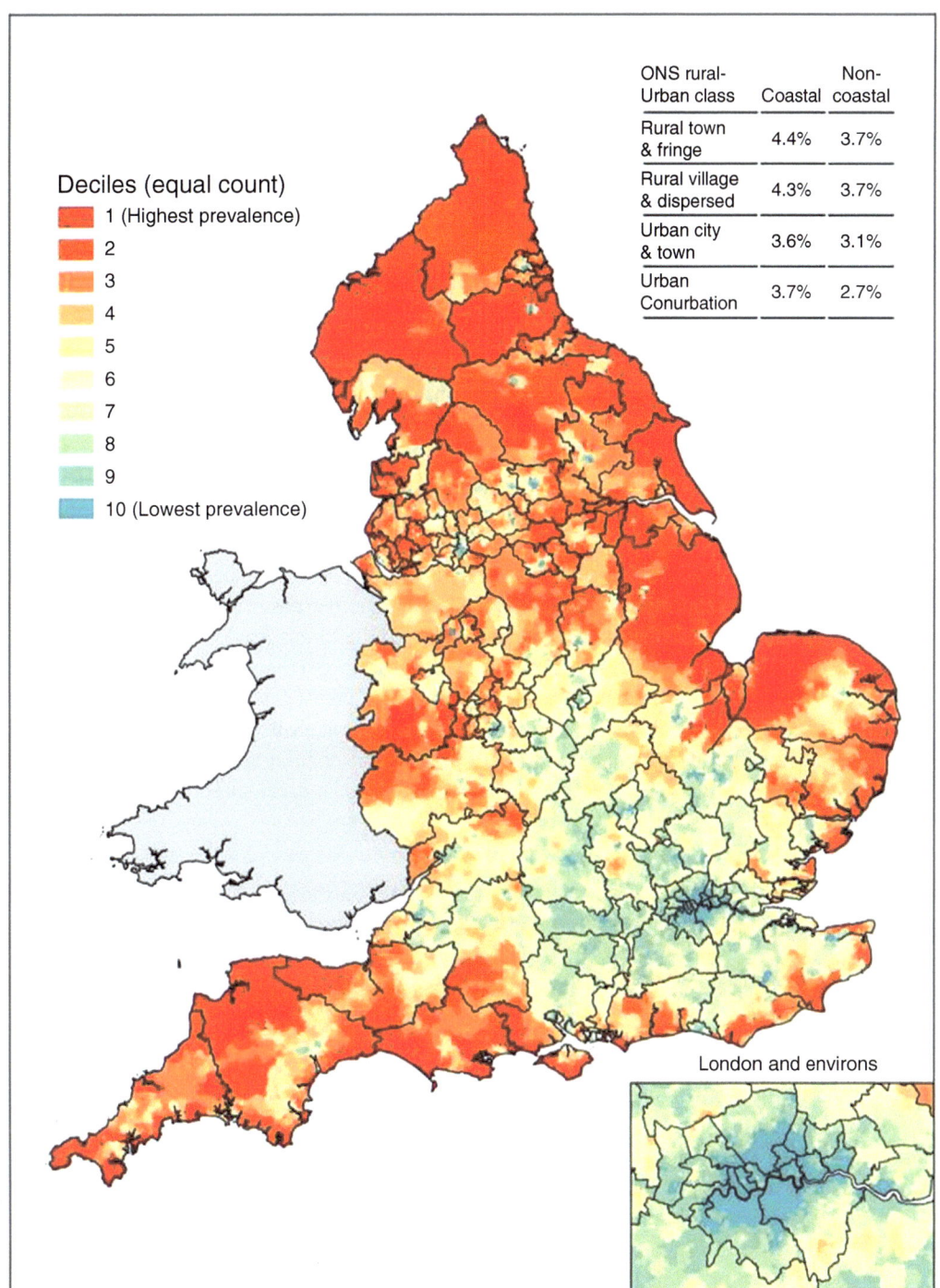

ONS rural-Urban class	Coastal	Non-coastal
Rural town & fringe	4.4%	3.7%
Rural village & dispersed	4.3%	3.7%
Urban city & town	3.6%	3.1%
Urban Conurbation	3.7%	2.7%

Deciles (equal count)
- 1 (Highest prevalence)
- 2
- 3
- 4
- 5
- 6
- 7
- 8
- 9
- 10 (Lowest prevalence)

London and environs

FIGURE 10.2   Crude prevalence of coronary heart health by lower layer super output area (LSOA) in England. **Source:** Asthana and Gibson. (2021)/Averting a public health crisis in England's coastal communities: A call for public health research and policy/Oxford University Press/CC by 4.0.

Racial Inequalities in Cancer Care

Race, as we highlighted earlier, can result in exclusion in some contexts (Cuesta et al., 2024). Whilst not a specific target of inclusion health, racial inequalities and discrimination are commonly experienced in relation to health and access to healthcare (Duveau et al., 2022, Fitzgerald and Hurst 2017,

White et al., 2021) and therefore, our last case study will consider this unequal access.

Globally many cities are now considered to be 'super-diverse', following years of 'diversifying diversity' (Barwick and Beaman, 2019, Vertovec, 2007). In the United Kingdom, as with elsewhere, due to people migrating from an increasing number of places, for a diversity of reasons, the demographic makeup of the country is far more diverse; being composed of people from all over the world who have significant differences in terms of cultures, needs, connections with local communities and socio-economic status.

The varying cultures, values and needs of these increasingly diverse populations, necessitate the need for healthcare professionals, and people in healthcare systems to be able to deliver culturally sensitive, competent, safe and effective care to meet the populations' super-diverse needs across different care settings. Whilst the diversity of the healthcare workforce, including in the United Kingdom, is increasing; most healthcare systems' ethnic and racial compositions do not reflect the same levels of diversity as the populations seeking care. This in turn results in a lack of representation in positions that have the most influence on how care is delivered (Salsberg et al., 2021, Wilbur et al., 2020).

It is now established that there are ethnic and racial inequalities in cancer care, diagnosis and participation in screening programmes (Jones et al., 2014, Martins et al., 2022, Massat et al., 2015, Pinder et al., 2016, Von Wagner et al., 2011). Screening programmes are important in allowing for the early identification and treatment of various cancers; increasing the probability of survival and minimising the possibility of associated morbidity (Bretthauer et al., 2023, Hewitson et al., 2008). Despite this, the uptake of screening varies across ethnic and racial groups, and may relate to differences in stigma, which can result in some groups being diagnosed significantly later, and therefore facing poorer outcomes (Jack et al., 2014, Marlow et al., 2015, Martins et al., 2022, Massat et al., 2015, Richardson-Parry et al., 2023, Von Wagner et al., 2011, Vrinten et al., 2019). The reasons to not take up cancer screening are varied and complex and will differ across individuals (Richardson-Parry et al., 2023). Research has highlighted some factors that influence poor uptake, including poor health literacy and understanding of the importance of screening, cultural beliefs around health and screening, and healthcare services lacking in cultural sensitivity and competence (Dawadi et al., 2022, Kerrison et al., 2023, Ogunsiji et al., 2013). Health literacy is important because when it is lacking, people are less able to acquire, understand and use health information that may benefit the healthcare-related decisions that they make (Sørensen et al., 2012). Research has highlighted significant disparities in relation to health literacy, with worse literacy being seen in disadvantaged groups (MacLeod et al., 2017). This phenomenon is arguably rooted in historic inequalities and unequal power structures. In the context of breast cancer, black women have increased risk (Gathani et al., 2021), but have lower awareness of breast cancer and its risk factors (Forbes et al., 2011, Jones et al., 2015, Rebner and Pai, 2020) and this, combined with confidence in accessing care and barriers to screening uptake (Rebner and Pai, 2020), increases the risk of breast cancer being picked up late, with black women being more likely to be diagnosed with advanced or metastatic breast cancer than white women (Gathani et al., 2021; Hirko et al., 2022, Januszewski et al., 2014).

Case Study: Health Literacy and Participation in Screening Programmes

Asha is a British-born Ghanaian woman. As a second-generation immigrant, she has lived in the city all her life, meeting her husband there, and subsequently having twins with him 15 years ago. The area she lives in has high levels of deprivation and is poorly connected to local services, including healthcare.

She has worked as a support worker in a local care home for young people with complex needs for several years and loves being able to entertain the children she works with, by reading them stories and singing to them. She is generally the life and soul of a party. When she was younger, she used to sing at social events, and she is very good at it, but since having the twins, she has prioritised her time with them, and her involvement with her local church. Her faith is incredibly important to her, and she is well-liked by her local church community.

She has a known family history of cancer, having lost her mother to breast cancer when she was 12, but her subsequent increased risk has never been explained to her. She doesn't perform any breast self-examinations, as she has never been taught how to, and how often she should do so, nor had the importance of this highlighted to her.

Asha was offered breast cancer screening but didn't really know why she had been offered it, or that it is important to detect breast cancer early. With her busy schedule, she accidentally missed the first appointment she was offered due to a clash with her work schedule. She was embarrassed that she had wasted people's time, and as she had no symptoms suggesting that anything was wrong, decided not to rebook, despite receiving a few reminders, which eventually stopped.

During a shower, Asha felt a hard lump in her breast and dimpling. Feeling embarrassed and that the lump was probably unimportant, she did not speak to anyone for some time. Her husband eventually noticed the lump, several weeks later and encouraged her to speak to her GP. She had to wait several weeks for an appointment, at the time she was given an urgent appointment to see a consultant oncologist, who informed her, without looking up, that she had breast cancer that had metastasised. During treatment, her condition worsened, and she began to receive support from the palliative care team.

You may wish to consider the following points:

- What were Asha's experiences of being a black woman accessing health services, and in particular screening services, in the United Kingdom?
- What were the missed opportunities in Asha's care?
- You may wish to consider writing a timeline of where Asha's care could have been improved.

Clinical Considerations

Research has suggested the need for culturally tailored screening programmes to support uptake (Kerrison et al., 2023), including in the context of breast cancer (Marcu et al., 2022). Some of this work has included black women themselves, to understand how best to tailor existing breast cancer programmes to their needs, with women identifying that programmes must highlight the importance of screening to black women specifically. Programmes must tackle false beliefs around incurability, must ensure that interventions are inclusive and engaging, should support black people to talk more about cancer including to their social networks and support people to identify cancer signs on black skin (Agyemang et al., 2023, Marcu et al., 2022). Research has also highlighted the importance of involving target groups in the design and delivery of interventions and using narratives and storytelling to address culturally specific barriers and needs (Ballard et al., 2021, Marcu et al., 2022).

Inclusive Healthcare Design and Research

With most healthcare research seeking to either understand care needs or examine approaches to improve people's health and well-being, one mechanism through which people can have their voices heard, and for services to subsequently better account for their needs is through PPIE activities (Ocloo et al., 2021). There is now a significant emphasis on public involvement in the focus, design, delivery and implementation of healthcare research, through the recognition that public involvement can positively influence the direction of research, as well as how its findings and outputs are used to inform healthcare provision (de Freitas and Martin, 2015, Ocloo et al., 2021), alongside the rising importance of participatory citizenship movements (Ocloo et al., 2021, Timans et al., 2022). All of this is essential in ensuring healthcare provision meets the diverse needs of those people who use them – by in principle, engaging the public as partners, who can influence how care is delivered and understood.

Despite this, academics have highlighted that those participating in activities relating to this are often those whose healthcare needs are already most adequately addressed, such as those from higher status groups – with better access to services that meet their needs (Martin, 2008, Ocloo et al., 2021). To address the inverse care relationship, those seeking to include those carrying the greatest health burden in the design, delivery and exploration of healthcare should consider:

- Reaching out specifically to underserved communities, rather than expecting them to come to them (Baines and Regan de Bere, 2018).
- Provide adequate training to those wanting to contribute, so that they understand their role and feel confident to take part, in a way that recognises and builds on their existing expertise (Baines and Regan de Bere, 2018)
- Make use of bilingual researchers and make use of interpretation services, whilst ensuring that all staff are culturally competent (Dawson et al., 2018, Sheldon et al., 2024).
- Involving community leaders, who may positively influence others to consider taking part (Jameson et al., 2023, Sheldon et al., 2024).
- Consider making use of local community groups, including health groups, who are already embedded within the local community (Jameson et al., 2023, Oldfield et al., 2019).

Involving those most likely to benefit from healthcare services the most has been shown to improve engagement with the recommendations from research in underserved areas. It turns out that being able to see yourself, and people like you, in the design of healthcare services, and the design of how healthcare is understood and improved, can be incredibly powerful for those who have traditionally been incorrectly deemed 'hard to reach', who are now deemed as 'seldom heard', or 'seldom listened to' (Islam et al., 2021).

In short, communities are seldom heard, and represented, when we as healthcare professionals and researchers fail to reach them.

As we have highlighted throughout this book, people's health is shaped by their social and historical contexts. Wherever you are practicing, the starting point to inclusive care is speaking to your patients. You might have to reflect and work on some of your own biases here. Even just taking a few extra minutes to talk to people can help you to better understand their personal history and their social context (Andermann, 2016). Understanding this helps you to better respond to needs – recognising the impact of social context on health and the ability to manage poor health. Evidence suggests that even just taking a few extra minutes can improve care coordination and experiences for those who are at risk of being marginalised (Mercer et al., 2007). All of this helps us provide better care to those needing care the most.

Conclusion

This chapter has introduced, explored and reflected on the impact of social exclusion on individuals and communities. We have highlighted the importance of inclusion in health provision, recognising the importance of poorer health outcomes and experiences of those from marginalised populations. Whilst we have not had the opportunity within the pages of this chapter to fully unpack the issues experienced by those facing marginalisation, we have been able to explore through case studies the impact of forced displacement on health, how nested deprivation, homelessness and multi-morbidity can impact on health and care, and the importance of ensuring preventative programmes are accessible and adequately promoted to all. As research forms such an important part of contemporary healthcare provision, we have also discussed the importance of including those who are socially excluded, alongside evidence-based strategies that promote inclusion.

References

Agyemang, L. S., Wagland, R., Foster, C., McLean, C. & Fenlon, D. 2023. To disclose or not to disclose: an ethnographic exploration of factors contributing to the (non) disclosure of Ghanaian women's breast cancer diagnosis to social networks. *BMC Womens Health*, 23, 366.

Aldridge, R. W., Story, A., Hwang, S. W., Nordentoft, M., Luchenski, S. A., Hartwell, G., Tweed, E. J., Lewer, D., Vittal Katikireddi, S. & Hayward, A. C. 2018. Morbidity and mortality in homeless individuals, prisoners, sex workers, and individuals with substance use disorders in high-income countries: a systematic review and meta-analysis. *Lancet*, 391, 241–250.

Amnesty International. 2024. Refugees, Asylum Seekers, and Migrants [Online]. Available: https://www.amnesty.org/en/what-we-do/refugees-asylum-seekers-and-migrants/#definitions [Accessed].

Andermann, A. 2016. Taking action on the social determinants of health in clinical practice: a framework for health professionals. *CMAJ*, 188, E474–e483.

Asif, Z. & Kienzler, H. 2022. Structural barriers to refugee, asylum seeker and undocumented migrant healthcare access. Perceptions of Doctors of the World caseworkers in the UK. *SSM - Mental Health*, 2, 100088.

Asthana, S. & Gibson, A. 2021. Averting a public health crisis in England's coastal communities: a call for public health research and policy. *Journal of Public Health*, 44, 642–650.

Baines, R. L. & Regan de Bere, S. 2018. Optimizing patient and public involvement (PPI): identifying its "essential" and "desirable" principles using a systematic review and modified Delphi methodology. *Health Expectations*, 21, 327–335.

Ballard, A. M., Davis, A. & Hoffner, C. A. 2021. The impact of health narratives on persuasion in African American women: a systematic review and meta-analysis. *Health Communication*, 36, 560–571.

Bambra, C. 2022. Placing intersectional inequalities in health. *Health & Place*, 75, 102761.

Barwick, C. & Beaman, J. 2019. Living for the neighbourhood: marginalization and belonging for the second-generation in Berlin and Paris. *Comparative Migration Studies*, 7, 1.

Bauder, H. 2017. Sanctuary cities: policies and practices in international perspective. *International Migration*, 55, 174–187.

Bendavid, E., Boerma, T., Akseer, N., Langer, A., Malembaka, E. B., Okiro, E. A., Wise, P. H., Heft-Neal, S., Black, R. E., Bhutta, Z. A., Bhutta, Z., Black, R., Blanchet, K., Boerma, T., Gaffey, M., Langer, A., Spiegel, P., Waldman, R. & Wise, P. 2021. The effects of armed conflict on the health of women and children. *The Lancet*, 397, 522–532.

Benoit, C., McCarthy, B. & Jansson, M. 2015. Stigma, sex work, and substance use: a comparative analysis. *Sociology of Health & Illness*, 37(3), 437–451.

BMA. 2024. Refugee and asylum seeker patient health toolkit. BMA. Available online: https://www.bma.org.uk/advice-and-support/ethics/refugees-overseas-visitors-and-vulnerable-migrants/refugee-and-asylum-seeker-patient-health-toolkit/unique-health-challenges-for-refugees-and-asylum-seekers.

Boswell, J., Denham, J., Furlong, J., Killick, A., Ndugga, P., Rek, B., Ryan, M. & Shipp, J. 2022. Place-based politics and nested deprivation in the U.K.: beyond cities-towns, 'Two Englands' and the 'Left Behind'. *Representation*, 58, 169–190.

Bradby, H., Lindenmeyer, A., Phillimore, J., Padilla, B. & Brand, T. 2020. 'If there were doctors who could understand our problems, I would already be better': dissatisfactory health care and marginalisation in superdiverse neighbourhoods. *Sociology of Health & Illness*, 42, 739–757.

Brandenberger, J., Tylleskär, T., Sontag, K., Peterhans, B. & Ritz, N. 2019. A systematic literature review of reported challenges in healthcare delivery to migrants and refugees in high-income countries- the 3C model. *BMC Public Health*, 19, 1–11.

Bretthauer, M., Wieszczy, P., Løberg, M., et al. 2023. Estimated lifetime gained with cancer screening tests: a meta-analysis of randomized clinical trials. *JAMA Internal Medicine*, 183(11), 1196–1203.

Campbell-Stephens, R. M. 2021. *Educational Leadership and the Global Majority*, 1st Edition, Palgrave Macmillan.

Carver, H., Ring, N., Miler, J. & Parkes, T. 2020. What constitutes effective problematic substance use treatment from the perspective of people who are homeless? a systematic review and meta-ethnography. *Harm Reduction Journal*, 17, 10.

Charlson, F., Van Ommeren, M., Flaxman, A., Cornett, J., Whiteford, H. & Saxena, S. 2019. New WHO prevalence estimates of mental disorders in conflict settings: a systematic review and meta-analysis. *The Lancet*, 394, 240–248.

Cheraghi-Sohi, S., Panagioti, M., Daker-White, G., Giles, S., Riste, L., Kirk, S., Ong, B. N., Poppleton, A., Campbell, S. & Sanders, C. 2020. Patient safety in marginalised groups: a narrative scoping review. *International Journal for Equity in Health*, 19, 26.

City of Sanctuary. 2024. List of City of Sanctuary Groups [Online]. City of Sanctuary Available: https://data.cityofsanctuary.org/groups/list [Accessed].

Crenshaw, K. 1989. Demarginalizing the intersection of race and sex: a black feminist critique of antidiscrimination doctrine, feminist theory and antiracist politics. *University of Chicago Legal Forum*, 1989, 139–167.

Cuadrado, C., Libuy, M. & Moreno-Serra, R. 2023. What is the impact of forced displacement on health? a scoping review. *Health Policy and Planning*, 38(3), 394–408.

Cuesta, J., López-Noval, B. & Niño-Zarazúa, M. 2024. Social exclusion concepts, measurement, and global estimate. *PLoS One*, 19(2).

Cuibus, M. V. & Walsh, P. W. 2025. *Unauthorised migration in the UK*, The Migration Observatory at the University of Oxford. https://migrationobservatory.ox.ac.uk/resources/briefings/unauthorised-migration-in-the-uk/.

Davidson, N., Hammarberg, K., Romero, L. & Fisher, J. 2022. Access to preventative sexual and reproductive health care for women from refugee-like backgrounds: a systematic review. *BMC Public Health*, 22.

Dawadi, A., Lucas, T., Drolet, C. E., Thompson, H. S., Key, K., Dailey, R. & Blessman, J. 2022. Healthcare provider cultural competency and receptivity to colorectal cancer screening among African Americans. *Psychology, Health & Medicine*, 27, 2073–2084.

Dawson, S., Campbell, S. M., Giles, S. J., Morris, R. L. & Cheraghi-Sohi, S. 2018. Black and minority ethnic group involvement in health and social care research: a systematic review. *Health Expectations*, 21, 3–22.

de Freitas, C. & Martin, G. 2015. Inclusive public participation in health: policy, practice and theoretical contributions to promote the involvement of marginalised groups in healthcare. *Social Science & Medicine*, 135, 31–39.

Duveau, C., Demoulin, S., Dauvrin, M., Lepièce, B. & Lorant, V. 2022. Implicit and explicit ethnic biases in multicultural primary care: the case of trainee general practitioners. *BMC Primary Care*, 23(1), 91.

European Parliament. 2015. Refugee status under international law [Online]. European Parliament Available: https://www.europarl.europa.eu/RegData/etudes/ATAG/2015/569051/EPRS_ATA%282015%29569051_EN.pdf [Accessed].

Fitzgerald, C. & Hurst, S. 2017. Implicit bias in healthcare professionals: a systematic review. *BMC Medical Ethics*, 18(1), 1–18.

Filia, K., Menssink, J., Gao, C. X., Rickwood, D., Hamilton, M., Hetrick, S. E., Parker, A. G., Herrman, H., Hickie, I., Sharmin, S., McGorry, P. D. & Cotton, S. M. 2022. Social inclusion, intersectionality, and profiles of vulnerable groups of young people seeking mental health support. *Social Psychiatry and Psychiatric Epidemiology*, 57, 245–254.

Fiorentino, S., Sielker, F. & Tomaney, J. 2023. Coastal towns as 'left-behind places': economy, environment and planning. *Cambridge Journal of Regions, Economy and Society*, 17, rsad045.

Flynn, P. M., Betancourt, H., Emerson, N. D., Nunez, E. I. & Nance, C. M. 2020. Health professional cultural competence reduces the psychological and behavioral impact of negative healthcare encounters. *Cultural Diversity & Ethnic Minority Psychology*, 26, 271–279.

Forbes, L. J. L., Atkins, L., Thurnham, A., Layburn, J., Haste, F. & Ramirez, A. J. 2011. Breast cancer awareness and barriers to symptomatic presentation among women from different ethnic groups in East London. *British Journal of Cancer*, 105, 1474–1479.

Gathani, T., Reeves, G., Broggio, J. & Barnes, I. 2021. Ethnicity and the tumour characteristics of invasive breast cancer in over 116,500 women in England. *British Journal of Cancer*, 125, 611–617.

Goffman, E. 1963. *Stigma: Notes on the Management of a Spoiled Identity*, Prentice Hall.

Grasser, L. R. 2022. Addressing mental health concerns in refugees and displaced populations: Is enough being done? risk management and healthcare. *Policy*, 6(15), 909–922.

Haque, R., Parr, N. & Muhidin, S. 2020. Climate-related displacement, impoverishment and healthcare accessibility in mainland Bangladesh. *Asian Population Studies*, 16, 220–239.

Hart, J. T. 1971. The inverse care law. *Lancet*, 1, 405–412.

Hatzenbuehler, M. L., Phelan, J. C. & Link, B. G. 2013. Stigma as a fundamental cause of population health inequalities. *American Journal of Public Health*, 103, 813–821.

Head, M. G., Brackstone, K., Crane, K., Walker, I. V. & Perelli-Harris, B. 2022. *Understanding health needs of Ukrainian refugees and displaced populations*, University of Southamptin. https://doi.org/10.6084/m9.figshare.20231346.

Hewitson, P., Glasziou, P., Watson, E., Towler, B. & Irwig, L. 2008. Cochrane systematic review of colorectal cancer screening using the fecal occult blood test (hemoccult): an update. *The American Journal of Gastroenterology*, 103, 1541–1549.

Hirko, K. A., Rocque, G., Reasor, E., Taye, A., Daly, A., Cutress, R. I., Copson, E. R., Lee, D. W., Lee, K. H., Im, S. A. & Park, Y. H. 2022. The impact of race and ethnicity in breast cancer- disparities and implications for precision oncology. *BMC Medicine*, 20, 72.

Hodson, N., Ford, E. & Cooper, M. 2019. Adherence to guidelines on documentation required for registration to London GP practice websites: a mixed-methods cross-sectional study. *The British Journal of General Practice*, 69, e731–e739.

Hui, A., Latif, A., Hinsliff-Smith, K. & Chen, T. 2020. Exploring the impacts of organisational structure, policy and practice on the health inequalities of marginalised communities: Illustrative cases from the UK healthcare system. *Health Policy*, 124, 298–302.

Islam, S., Joseph, O., Chaudry, A., Forde, D., Keane, A., Wilson, C., Begum, N., Parsons, S., Grey, T., Holmes, L. & Starling, B. 2021. "We are not hard to reach, but we may find it hard to trust" . . . . Involving and engaging 'seldom listened to' community voices in clinical translational health research: a social innovation approach. *Research Involvement and Engagement*, 7, 46.

Jack, R. H., Møller, H., Robson, T. & Davies, E. A. 2014. Breast cancer screening uptake among women from different ethnic groups in London: a population-based cohort study. *BMJ Open*, 4.

Jameson, C., Haq, Z., Musse, S., Kosar, Z., Watson, G. & Wylde, V. 2023. Inclusive approaches to involvement of community groups in health research: the co-produced CHICO guidance. *Research Involvement and Engagement*, 9, 76.

Januszewski, A., Tanna, N. & Stebbing, J. 2014. Ethnic variation in breast cancer incidence and outcomes—the debate continues. *British Journal of Cancer*, 110, 4–6.

Jawad, M., Hone, T., Vamos, E. P., Roderick, P., Sullivan, R. & Millett, C. 2020. Estimating indirect mortality impacts of armed conflict in civilian populations: panel regression analyses of 193 countries, 1990-2017. *BMC Medicine*, 18, 266.

Jones, C. E., Maben, J., Jack, R. H., Davies, E. A., Forbes, L. J., Lucas, G. & Ream, E. 2014. A systematic review of barriers to early presentation and diagnosis with breast cancer among black women. *BMJ Open*, 4, e004076.

Jones, C. E., Maben, J., Lucas, G., Davies, E. A., Jack, R. H. & Ream, E. 2015. Barriers to early diagnosis of symptomatic breast cancer: a qualitative study of Black African, Black Caribbean and White British women living in the UK. *BMJ Open*, 5, e006944.

Kang, T. S., Head, M. G., Brackstone, K., Buchko, K. & Goodwin, R. 2024. Functional disability, health care access, and mental health in Ukrainians displaced by the 2022 Russian invasion. *Psychiatry Research*, 342.

Kerrison, R. S., Gil, N., Travis, E., Jones, R., Whitaker, K. L., Rees, C., Duffy, S. & von Wagner, C. 2023. Barriers to colonoscopy in UK colorectal cancer screening programmes: qualitative interviews with ethnic minority groups. *Psycho-Oncology*, 32, 779–792.

Kirst, M., Friesdorf, R., Ta, M., Amiri, A., Hwang, S. W., Stergiopoulos, V. & O'Campo, P. 2020. Patterns and effects of social integration on housing stability, mental health and substance use outcomes among participants in a randomized controlled housing first trial. *Social Science & Medicine*, 265, 113481.

Lebano, A., Hamed, S., Bradby, H., Gil-Salmeron, A., Dura-Ferrandis, E., Garces-Ferrer, J., Azzedine, F., Riza, E., Karnaki, P., Zota, D. & Linos, A. 2020. Migrants' and refugees' health status and healthcare in Europe: a scoping literature review. *BMC Public Health*, 20(1039).

Lekas, H.-M., Pahl, K. & Fuller Lewis, C. 2020. Rethinking cultural competence: shifting to cultural humility. *Health Services Insights*, 13, 1178632920970580.

Link, B. G. & Phelan, J. C. 2001. Conceptualizing stigma. *Annual Review of Sociology*, 27, 363–385.

Logie, C. H., Mackenzie, F., Malama, K., Lorimer, N., Lad, A., Zhao, M., Narasimhan, M., Fahme, S., Turan, B., Kagunda, J., Konda, K., Hasham, A. & Perez-Brumer, A. 2024. Sexual and reproductive health among forcibly displaced persons in urban environments in low and middle-income countries: scoping review findings. *Reproductive Health*, 21(51).

Luchenski, S., Maguire, N., Aldridge, R. W., Hayward, A., Story, A., Perri, P., Withers, J., Clint, S., Fitzpatrick, S. & Hewett, N. 2018. What works in inclusion health: overview of effective interventions for marginalised and excluded populations. *The Lancet*, 391, 266–280.

Macleod, S., Musich, S., Gulyas, S., Cheng, Y., Tkatch, R., Cempellin, D., Bhattarai, G. R., Hawkins, K. & Yeh, C. S. 2017. The impact of inadequate health literacy on patient satisfaction, healthcare utilization, and expenditures among older adults. *Geriatric Nursing*, 38, 334–341.

Marcu, A., Marke, L., Armes, J., Whitaker, K. L. & Ream, E. 2022. Adapting a breast cancer early presentation intervention for Black women: a focus group study with women of Black African and Black Caribbean descent in the United Kingdom. *European Journal of Cancer Care*, 31, e13652.

Marlow, L. A., Wardle, J. & Waller, J. 2015. Understanding cervical screening non-attendance among ethnic minority women in England. *British Journal of Cancer*, 113(5), 833–839.

Marmot, M. 2018. Inclusion health: addressing the causes of the causes. *The Lancet*, 391, 186–188.

Martin, G. P. 2008. Representativeness, legitimacy and power in public involvement in health-service management. *Social Science & Medicine*, 67, 1757–1765.

Martins, T., Abel, G., Ukoumunne, O. C., Mounce, L. T. A., Price, S., Lyratzopoulos, G., Chinegwundoh, F. & Hamilton, W. 2022. Ethnic inequalities in routes to diagnosis of cancer: a population-based UK cohort study. *British Journal of Cancer*, 127, 863–871.

Massat, N. J., Douglas, E., Waller, J., Wardle, J. & Duffy, S. W. 2015. Variation in cervical and breast cancer screening coverage in England: a cross-sectional analysis to characterise districts with atypical behaviour. *BMJ Open*, 5, e007735.

Matlin, S. A., Depoux, A., Schütte, S., Flahault, A. & Saso, L. 2018. Migrants' and refugees' health: towards an agenda of solutions. *Public Health Reviews*, 39, 27.

McDowell, L. & Bonner-Thompson, C. 2020. The other side of coastal towns: young men's precarious lives on the margins of England. *Environment and Planning A: Economy and Space*, 52, 916–932.

McVicar, D., Moschion, J. & van Ours, J. 2015. From substance use to homelessness or vice versa? *Social Science & Medicine*, 136–137.

Mercer, S. W., Fitzpatrick, B., Gourlay, G., Vojt, G., McConnachie, A. & Watt, G. C. 2007. More time for complex consultations in a high-deprivation practice is associated with increased patient enablement. *British Journal of General Practice*, 57, 960–966.

Mercer, S. W., Patterson, J., Robson, J. P., Smith, S. M., Walton, E. & Watt, G. 2021. The inverse care law and the potential of primary care in deprived areas. *The Lancet*, 397, 775–776.

Muncan, B., Walters, S. M., Ezell, J. & Ompad, D. C. 2020. "They look at us like junkies": influences of drug use stigma on the healthcare engagement of people who inject drugs in New York City. *Harm Reduction Journal*, 17, 53.

NHS. 2023. A national framework for NHS- action on inclusion health [Online]. NHS. Available: https://www.england.nhs.uk/long-read/a-national-framework-for-nhs-action-on-inclusion-health/.

Norman, P., Exeter, D., Shelton, N., Head, J. & Murray, E. 2022. (Un-) healthy ageing: Geographic inequalities in disability-free life expectancy in England and Wales. *Health & Place*, 76, 102820.

O'Campo, P., Stergiopoulos, V., Davis, O., Lachaud, J., Nisenbaum, R., Dunn, J. R., Ahmed, N. & Tsemberis, S. 2022. Health and social outcomes in the housing first model: testing the theory of change. *EClinicalMedicine*, 47.

O'Donnell, C. A., Burns, N., Mair, F. S., Dowrick, C., Clissmann, C., van den Muijsenbergh, M., van Weel-Baumgarten, E., Lionis, C., Papadakaki, M., Saridaki, A., de Brun, T. & Macfarlane, A. 2016. Reducing the health care burden for marginalised migrants: the potential role for primary care in Europe. *Health Policy*, 120, 495–508.

O'Donnell, P., Moran, L., Geelen, S., O'Donovan, D., van den Muijsenbergh, M. & Elmusharaf, K. 2021. "There is people like us and there is people like them, and we are not like them." Understating social exclusion – a qualitative study. *PLoS One*, 16, e0253575.

Ocloo, J., Garfield, S., Franklin, B. D. & Dawson, S. 2021. Exploring the theory, barriers and enablers for patient and public involvement across health, social care and patient safety: a systematic review of reviews. *Health Research Policy and Systems*, 19, 8.

Office for Health Improvement and Disparities 2022. SPOTLIGHT: Improving Inclusion Health Outcomes. Available online at: https://analytics.phe.gov.uk/apps/spotlight/.

Ogunsiji, O., Wilkes, L., Peters, K. & Jackson, D. 2013. Knowledge, attitudes and usage of cancer screening among West African migrant women. *Journal of Clinical Nursing*, 22, 1026–1033.

Oldfield, B. J., Harrison, M. A., Genao, I., Greene, A. T., Pappas, M. E., Glover, J. G. & Rosenthal, M. S. 2019. Patient, family, and community advisory councils in health care and research: a systematic review. *Journal of General Internal Medicine*, 34, 1292–1303.

Paudyal, V., Maclure, K., Forbes-McKay, K., McKenzie, M., Macleod, J., Smith, A. & Stewart, D. 2020. 'If I die, I die, I don't care about my health': Perspectives on self-care of people experiencing homelessness. *Health & Social Care in the Community*, 28, 160–172.

Pinder, R. J., Ferguson, J. & Møller, H. 2016. Minority ethnicity patient satisfaction and experience: results of the national cancer patient experience survey in England. *BMJ Open*, 6, e011938.

Phelan, J. C., Link, B. G. & Dovidio, J. F. 2008. Stigma and prejudice: one animal or two? *Social Science & Medicine*, 67, 358–367.

Platts-Fowler, D. & Robinson, D. 2015. A Place for integration: refugee experiences in two English cities. *Population, Space and Place*, 21, 476–491.

Rebner, M. & Pai, V. R. 2020. Breast cancer screening recommendations: African American women are at a disadvantage. *Journal of Breast Imaging*, 2, 416–421.

Richardson-Parry, A., Baas, C., Donde, S., Ferraiolo, B., Karmo, M., Maravic, Z., Munter, L., Ricci-Cabello, I., Silva, M., Tinianov, S., Valderas, J. M., Woodruff, S. & van Vugt, J. 2023. Interventions to reduce cancer screening inequities: the perspective and role of patients, advocacy groups, and empowerment organizations. *International Journal for Equity in Health*, 22, 19.

Ruiz, A. M., Luebke, J., Klein, K., Moore, K., Gonzalez, M., Dressel, A. & Mkandawire-Valhmu, L. 2021. An integrative literature review and critical reflection of intersectionality theory. *Nursing Inquiry*, 28, e12414.

Salsberg, E., Richwine, C., Westergaard, S., Martinez, M. P., Oyeyemi, T., Vichare, A. & Chen, C. P. 2021. Estimation and comparison of current and future racial/ethnic representation in the US health care workforce. *JAMA Network Open*, 4, e213789–e213789.

Saunders, S. L., Sutcliffe, K. L., McOrist, N. S. & Levett, K. M. 2022. The associations between women who are immigrants, refugees or asylum seekers, access to universal healthcare and the timely uptake of antenatal care: a systematic review. *ANZJOG*, 63(2), 134–145.

Scott, R., Forde, E. & Wedderburn, C. 2022. Refugee, migrant and asylum seekers' experience of accessing and receiving primary healthcare in a UK city of sanctuary. *Journal of Immigrant and Minority Health*, 24, 304–307.

Sheldon, E., Ezaydi, N., Ditmore, M., Fuseini, O., Ainley, R., Robinson, K., Hind, D. & Lobo, A. J. 2024. Patient and public involvement in the development of health services: engagement of underserved populations in a quality improvement programme for inflammatory bowel disease using a community-based participatory approach. *Health Expectations*, 27, e14004.

Shulman, C., Hudson, B. F., Low, J., Hewett, N., Daley, J., Kennedy, P., Davis, S., Brophy, N., Howard, D., Vivat, B. & Stone, P. 2018. End-of-life care for homeless people: a qualitative analysis exploring the challenges to access and provision of palliative care. *Palliative Medicine*, 32, 36–45.

Siddiqui, F. R. 2014. Annotated bibliography on participatory consultations to help aid the inclusion of marginalized perspectives in setting policy agendas. *International Journal for Equity in Health*, 13, 124.

Sørensen, K., van den Broucke, S., Fullam, J., Doyle, G., Pelikan, J., Slonska, Z., Brand, H. & Consortium Health Literacy project, E 2012. Health literacy and public health: a systematic review and integration of definitions and models. *BMC Public Health*, 12, 80.

Stablein, G. W., Hill, B. S., Keshavarz, S. & Llorente, M. D. 2021. Homelessness and substance use disorders. *In:* Ritchie, E. C. & Llorente, M. D. (eds.) *Clinical Management of the Homeless Patient: Social, Psychiatric, and Medical Issues*, Cham: Springer International Publishing, 179–194.

Telford, L. 2021. 'There is nothing there': Deindustrialization and loss in a coastal town. *Competition and Change*, 26, 197–214.

Timans, R., de Jong, J., Brabers, A., Horsselenberg, M. & Damen, L. 2022. Citizen participation in healthcare: a field perspective. *European Journal of Public Health*, 32, ckac131–ckac545.

Tweed, E. J., Popham, F., Thomson, H. & Katikireddi, S. V. 2022. Including 'inclusion health'? A discourse analysis of health inequalities policy reviews. *Critical Public Health*, 32, 700–712.

UK Government 2023. Guidance. NHS entitlements: migrant health guide. Available online at: https://www.gov.uk/guidance/nhs-entitlements-migrant-health-guide.

UNHCR. 2020. Global trends: forced displacement in 2020 [Online]. UNHCR: The UN Refugee Agency. Available: https://www.unhcr.org/statistics/unhcrstats/60b638e37/global-trends-forced-displacement-2020.html [Accessed].

UNHCR. 2023b. Focus area strategic plan for climate action [Online]. UNHRC: The UN Refugee Agency. Available: https://reporting.unhcr.org/climate-action-focus-area-strategic-plan-20242030?_gl=1*yd0wt9*_rup_ga*MzI0ODg2NDg4LjE3MDU0MTA5MzM.*_rup_ga_EVDQTJ4LMY*MTcwNTQxMDkzMy4xLjEuMTcwNTQxMjM2Ny4wLjAuMA..*_ga*MzI0ODg2NDg4LjE3MDU0MTA5MzM.*_ga_FXYR2Y8W7G*MTcwNTQxMDkzMy4xLjEuMTcwNTQxMjM2Ny4wLjAuMA..#_ga=2.210673045.1438515956.1705410933-324886488.1705410933 [Accessed 2024].

UNHCR. 2023a. Global Trends: forced Displacement in 2022 [Online]. UNHRC: The UN Refugee Agency. Available: https://www.unhcr.org/global-trends-report-2022 [Accessed].

Van Rosse, F., de Bruijne, M., Suurmond, J., Essink-Bot, M.-L. & Wagner, C. 2016. Language barriers and patient safety risks in hospital care. a mixed methods study. *International Journal of Nursing Studies*, 54, 45–53.

Vanderpyl, L., Charania, N., Treharne, G. J. & Naasan, Z. A. 2024. The potential of a rights-base approach to refugee-focused mental health policy in Aotearoa New Zealand. *Kōtuitui: New Zealand Journal of Social Sciences Online*, 1–25.

Vertovec, S. 2007. Super-diversity and its implications. *Ethnic and Racial Studies*, 30, 1024–1054.

Vrinten, C., Gallagher, A., Waller, J. & Marlow, L. A. V. 2019. Cancer stigma and cancer screening attendance: a population based survey in England. *BMC Cancer*, 19(1), 1–10.

Von Wagner, C., Baio, G., Raine, R., Snowball, J., Morris, S., Atkin, W., Obichere, A., Handley, G., Logan, R. F. & Rainbow, S. 2011. Inequalities in participation in an organized national colorectal cancer screening programme: results from the first 2.6 million invitations in England. *International Journal of Epidemiology*, 40, 712–718.

Ward, K. J. 2015. Geographies of exclusion: seaside towns and houses in multiple occupancy. *Journal of Rural Studies*, 37, 96–107.

Watt, G. 2018. The inverse care law revisited: a continuing blot on the record of the National Health Service. *The British Journal of General Practice*, 68, 562–563.

Webber, F. 2019. On the creation of the UK's 'hostile environment'. *Race & Class*, 60, 76–87.

Whitty, C. 2021. Chief Medical Officer's Annual Report 2021: Health in Coastal Communities

White, A., Thornton, R. L. J. & Greene, J. A. 2021. Remembering past lessons about structural racism - recentering black theorists of health and society. *The New England Journal of Medicine*, 385, 850–855.

Wilbur, K., Snyder, C., Essary, A. C., Reddy, S., Will, K. K. & Mary, S. 2020. Developing workforce diversity in the health professions: a social justice perspective. *Health Professions Education*, 6, 222–229.

Woodhall-Melnik, J. R. & Dunn, J. R. 2016. A systematic review of outcomes associated with participation in housing first programs. *Housing Studies*, 31, 287–304.

Woodward, A., Davies, N., Walters, K., Nimmons, D., Stevenson, F., Protheroe, J., Chew-Graham, C. A. & Armstrong, M. 2023. Self-management of multiple long-term conditions: a systematic review of the barriers and facilitators amongst people experiencing socio-economic deprivation. *PLoS One*, 18, e0282036.

Woodward, A., Howard, N. & Wolffers, I. 2014. Health and access to care for undocumented migrants living in the European Union: a scoping review. *Health Policy and Planning*, 29, 818–830.

Zimmerman, C., Kiss, L. & Hossain, M. 2011. Migration and health: a framework for 21st century policy-making. *PLoS Medicine*, 8.

CHAPTER 11

Disability, Society and Health

Chris Allen[1], Simon Hall[1], Erica Goddard[2], and Neil Summers[2]

[1] *School of Health Sciences, University of Southampton, Southampton, UK*
[2] *School of Health, Wellbeing & Social Care, The Open University, Milton Keynes, UK*

Introduction

Our lives are 'embodied', with bodies and minds being central to everything we do, and every aspect of daily living. For many, bodies and minds are taken for granted until something changes that draws attention to limitations and societies lack of accommodation of these. However, for those born with impairments, or who have become impaired through the course of their lives, significant barriers and disadvantages are experienced that extend beyond the actual impairment. The focus of this chapter is to consider the human body and mind in relation to impairment and disability through the life course, whilst highlighting the complex societal exclusionary practices those living with a disability experience.

This chapter serves as an overview of some of the key considerations of social science around disability and differential experiences for those with physical, mental, cognitive and sensory impairments. The experiences of those with disabilities relate to many of the concepts explored elsewhere in this book, including how health is seen and understood, inequalities, stigma, stereotypes and marginalisation. Because of this, we recommend reading this chapter alongside Chapters 3, 8–10 specifically.

LEARNING OUTCOMES

By the end of this chapter, you will be able to:

- Understand the strengths and limitations of the different models of disability, including the highly influential medical and social models of disability.
- Identify the history and context of important legislation relating to those living with physical, mental, cognitive and sensory impairments and their rights.
- Recognise the various forms of social disadvantage those that living with physical, mental, cognitive and sensory impairments face, across the life course.

Embodiment

> ### Key Terms and Definitions
>
> **Impairment:** Something someone lives with, that might limit them in some way.
>
> **Disability:** In the context of the law, this generally refers to having an impairment that has a substantial and long-term impact on a person's ability to perform everyday activities.
>
> **Medical model of disability:** Suggests that people are disabled by their impairments and that these impairments where possible should be 'fixed'.
>
> **Social model of disability:** Suggests that it is society that disables people, through poorly accommodating people's differences.
>
> **Disablism/ableism:** Prejudicial or biased attitudes towards those with a disability or viewing people without a disability more positively.

'Embodiment' simply refers to us living through our bodies. Everyday activities and needs such as communicating, building and maintaining relationships with others, sex, taking part in cherished activities, playing sports, exercising, employment and education, and other aspects of daily living, are all fulfilled through our bodies and our minds, which we can become particularly aware of, when they limit or negatively impact on us in some way. Exactly how these everyday activities are performed and experienced varies, due to intrinsic factors (such as having a reduced range of movement in a limb or experiencing fatigue) and extrinsic factors (such as public spaces being inaccessible or people negatively evaluating those living with an impairment). This 'embodied experience', is unique to each us, and how we experience the

Social Sciences for Healthcare Professionals, First Edition. Edited by Chris Allen.
© 2026 John Wiley & Sons Ltd. Published 2026 by John Wiley & Sons Ltd.

TABLE 11.1	How our bodies and minds impact social life, and the life course.
Identity	Our bodies can represent who we are. This can include how well we look after our body and our mind, what exercise we do, what we eat and drink, etc.
Stigma	When we have a real or perceived difference, this can affect the way others respond to us, and the way we see ourselves.
Body politics	Our bodies can represent a form of 'status', and in some cases, a 'master status'. Because of this, and regardless of capability, someone with perceived or actual differences that are undesirable in society, might be afforded very different opportunities and life chances, than someone without.
Consumption	Societies generally desire bodies that look healthy. People's consumption patterns are influenced by trying to acquire a desired body type (e.g., weight loss pills, Botox, hair transplants, etc.). This is in large part, fuelled by commercialisation and the strive for 'perfect bodies'.

social world (Krieger, 2005, Leder, 1990, Nettleton and Watson, 1998, Scully, 2006); and relates to how we look, what we can do and how we behave. All of which impacts how we see ourselves, and how others see and respond to us. When what we can do is in some ways limited in comparison to what others are able to do, we can feel embarrassed and ashamed and others can also treat us more negatively. Both responses are products of our social world – what is seen as 'normal'. Someone living with an impairment, whatever it may be, may have radically different needs in relation to access to and engagement with such activities – and as a result, may be disadvantaged in several important domains of social and economic life, in part due to intrinsic factors, but also due to how society responds or poorly accommodates differences both in its design, as well as through the systematic differences in privilege, power and status afforded to different groups (Brown et al., 2023, Thomson, 1997).

Whilst recognising that society often does respond poorly to those who are seen as deviating from a perceived 'norm', impairments do not need to be seen as negative, and many people are proud of their disabled identity (Smith and Sparkes, 2022). Rather than something to be 'fixed', their 'differences' are simply part of them. Indeed, much of what may be considered an impairment, should not limit participation in social and economic life. Yet, as we will explore later in this chapter, how accommodating or not society is towards those with impairments, is embedded in society's culture, norms and values and what is and what is not seen as 'normal' (Goodley, 2014). As we have alluded to in an earlier chapter, when discussing stigma and stereotypes, the 'othering' of people with disabilities and the extent to which they are 'psycho-emotionally' disabled, will vary from culture to culture. The visible and invisible differences can result in stigma (both felt and enacted) that can result in discriminatory behaviours and practices, and that result in people undergoing significant impression management[1], which may reduce engagement with many aspects of social and economic life, as well as leading to either avoidance or

poorer experiences of healthcare services (Gréaux et al., 2023). Whilst those living with impairments often experience this, some experience it more, for example, those living with severe mental illness and those living with a learning disability.

There are myriad ways in which our bodies and our minds shape our lives. How we see ourselves, how others see us, how much of a voice we have, what resources we can accrue and even our consumption. Some of these are summarised in Table 11.1.

What Is Disability?

Whilst you may have some intuitive sense of what a disability is, it is difficult to precisely define what is and what is not a disability (Bickenback, 2020, Mitra, 2006). As we saw in the context of medicalisation in Chapter 3, even what is, and what is not considered an 'impairment' is subject to change over time, and in different social contexts. Generally, definitions of disability point towards impairments that make it more difficult for someone to do normal daily activities. In fact, this definition is commonly used to define disability in law, for example in the United Kingdom, the 2010 Equality Act defines disability as any physical or mental impairment that has a substantial[2] and long-term[3] impact on a person's ability to do normal daily activities.

However, disability is complex, and no uniform definition exists (Bickenback, 2020, Leonardi et al., 2006). Individual definitions of disability tend to reflect their intended use. For example, legal definitions of disability need to be inclusive, medical definitions point towards an underlying aetiology, and definitions used to determine eligibility, such as in the UK Personal Independence Payments or 'PIP', tend to be more restricted and centre on the performance of certain tasks

---

[1] A great deal of energy can be exerted by those with impairments to finally balance having their needs met, with concealing differences for fear of how others may respond to them.

[2] 'Substantial' under this definition generally suggests that the difficulties in doing daily activities are not trivial – for example, it takes someone significantly more time to make a meal or to get dressed.

[3] Often seen as being 12 months or more, meaning that those with acute illness that fully resolves would likely not be seen as having a disability, though they may still experience physical and cognitive impairment.

(Bickenback, 2020). As with changes to the classification of health and disease, changes in definitions and classifications of disability can result in people's disability status changing overnight.

Attitudes Towards Disability

In a UK context, changing attitudes towards those with physical impairments increased following the Second World War, in which there were an increasing number of people with combat-related impairments (Barnes, 2020). Shifting attitudes have been supported by the work of disability activists, alongside demographic changes that make it more likely that an increasingly large proportion of the population will see (in others) and experience (in themselves) impairments (Barnes, 2020).

The United Kingdom, as with elsewhere, has an aging population (covered more in Chapter 7), which has seen a continuously increasing number of people living with various impairments that impact on their physical and mental abilities (WHO, 2011). To varying extents, we are all on this potential trajectory, with our risk of experiencing impairment increasing as we age. Currently around 1/6 of the world's population (roughly 1.3 billion people) are living with some form of disability (WHO, 2023). In the United Kingdom, around 24% of the population has a disability, with a greater proportion being older adults (Kirk-Wade, 2023). Despite this, it is common for people to underestimate the prevalence of disability in their society, or to believe they do not know anyone with a disability, when in fact, they likely do (Dixon et al., 2018). Underestimation may occur due to narrow societal views of what constitutes a disability (e.g. a wheelchair symbol depicting disabled parking when many people with a disability do not need a wheelchair), hidden disabilities (including chronic pain, chronic fatigue, etc.) and age-related decline simply being seen as a part of the 'normal' aging process rather than constituting an impairment (Dixon et al., 2018).

How Is Disability Understood?

There are several ways we can use social and biological sciences to understand disability. These understandings can in turn give us indications as to what support may be appropriate. As a broad starting point, we can examine disability through a biomedical lens. This helps us to make sense of people's signs (what we can see) and symptoms (what they experience) and try to resolve these, where this is possible and appropriate (through, e.g. medication, surgery or other therapeutic interventions), or where this is not possible or appropriate, addressing through the same, any particularly unpleasant symptoms that may result from such impairments, such as where they cause pain, discomfort or

fatigue, or where they result in embarrassment, such as incontinence or difficulties having sex (Dueñas et al., 2016, Gotaas et al., 2021, Riemsma et al., 2017, Scott et al., 2021). Psychology can help us make sense of and put in place support where these biological differences, their resultant impairments, and the unpleasant signs and symptoms they produce, impact on how people see themselves, and how they feel (Dunn and Burcaw, 2013, Goodley, 2020). Finally, sociology can help us understand how society sees and accommodates those with different impairments, and this can help us understand differential power, inequalities and how those with a disability can be better accommodated in a society's configuration and design, reducing the disadvantages and unfair treatment those with impairments often face (Barry and Yuill, 2022). Disability studies are multidisciplinary and includes contributions from all of these, as well as other academic fields, though its dominant model, the social model of disability, poorly aligns with medicine and psychologies focus on individuals and their behaviour (Barnes, 2020, Goodley, 2020). In the context of healthcare professionals, viewing disability through the biomedical lens has traditionally been common, but other important disability models exist, some of which have become highly influential in changing how disability is seen and understood, including in international legislation and classification of functioning and disability (WHO, 2007).

Essentially, there are two main ways in which disability can be conceptualised and therefore understood. These challenge us to think about what 'disability' and 'impairment' is.

In answering the following question, you are encouraged to think about which reflects your approach towards those with an impairment.

So, is a disability:

1. A physical difference or impairment that results in one's abilities being limited in some way.

   Or is it:

2. The barriers and attitudes towards people with a physical difference or impairment that prevents them from doing the things that those without these differences can do.

The first conceptualisation focusses on the limitations of individuals with a disability (this is the medical model – something is 'wrong' with the body, and this must be 'fixed'). The second conceptualisation instead values people's diverse needs. Its focus is primarily on how society responds to and includes those with impairments. This is the social model of disability (Barnes, 2020, Goering, 2015, Oliver, 2013, Shakespeare, 2017). These distinctions are relevant, as they ultimately influence our responses to the needs of those living with an impairment. How we conceptualise disability relates to how those with an impairment are seen, including their capabilities and whether it is their perceived deficits or strengths that we choose to focus on. It also influences how much we demand that societies work to remove barriers to social and economic participation for those with physical, mental, cognitive or sensory impairments.

The Medical Model

Let's start by focussing on the medical model, which tradition-ally has been the main lens through which healthcare profes-sionals and healthcare systems have viewed disability (Hogan, 2019), and until relatively recent developments that were largely led by disability activists and academics, was *the* dominant way disability was seen and understood. By inter-preting disability as a medical condition, we (inadvertently perhaps) imply that there is something 'wrong' with someone (Oliver, 2013). Disability through this lens is seen as an individ-ual personal tragedy. This leads to people being seen as in some way deficient, and with perceived deficits that medicine and the professions allied to it must correct through treatment, therapy or other types of intervention, or which may require the person to either:

1. Accept and adapt to their limitations

or

2. be reliant on others.

This can result in the stereotyping (see Chapter 9) of those with a disability, leading to them becoming objects of unwanted pity and/or charity and overhelping, being feared, or being actively avoided; sometimes through people's fear or concern of saying or doing the wrong thing (Barnes, 2020, Fiske, 2012, Hughes, 2020, Nario-Redmond, 2010, Reeve, 2020). The medical deficit model fits with earlier functionalist (see Chapter 2) understandings about health and illness, notably that of Talcott Parsons and the 'sick role' highlighting sickness and disability as a form of 'social deviance' that involves certain rights and obligations (Parsons, 1951, Perry, 2011, Varul, 2010). Being disabled marks you as 'deviant' and if you have a recognised impairment, you should submit to medical care and try to get better (Parsons, 1951, Varul, 2010). Whilst medical diagnosis can be validating (particularly in giving a name to something, and helping people make sense of what they are experiencing), for many there is no clear identifiable cause that can or indeed should be addressed, and labels are often not chosen (Moss and Teghtsoonian, 2008). With many forms of impairment not being curable, classification and labelling systems may only serve to highlight people's differences, and the impact of this is that disability becomes an ascribed social status – in some cases a 'master status' (Barnartt, 2013), that highlights that something is 'wrong' with someone, as opposed to something being 'wrong' with society in terms of how it responds to peoples differences. This, in turn, can influence how people are seen, and where they are situated within the social hierarchies that emerge through social stratification. This is significant, because the impact an impairment may have on someone's everyday life, is often linked to their access to material and social resources, and often not because of the impairment but because of society (Eide and Ingstad, 2011, Horner-Johnson, 2021, Reeve, 2020).

The Social Model of Disability

Contrasting this is the social model of disability. In the 1970s, out of concern for the disadvantage experienced by those with a physical impairment, through the efforts of significant disability activists, the Union of the Physically Impaired Against Segregation (UPIAS) was created, and its members argued that disability represented a form of 'social oppression', not dissimilar to that experienced by other marginalised groups, such as those minoritised based on gender, sexual orientation and race (Barnes, 2020). Michael Oliver, a key academic and disabled activist, building on the earlier work of the UPIAS (1976), formulated the Social Model of Disability to promote UPIAS's definition of disability to care professionals, specifically prospective social workers (Oliver, 1981, Oliver 1990, Tregaskis, 2002). Oliver, in a now much-cited and highly influential text, highlighted that a disability is a disadvantage or restriction of activity caused by contemporary social organisation, that fails to account for the needs of those with physical impairments and due to this, actually excludes them from participating in important aspects of social life (Oliver, 1990).

> ### Stop and Think: Are Impairment and Disability Distinct?
>
> Take a moment to consider the social model of disability.
>
> - What benefits do you think such a model might bring?
> - Can you think of any limitations to the social model of disability?
> - Think about someone you have provided care to, who is recognised as having either a physical, men-tal, cognitive or sensory impairment. If you could change the social world around them, to remove barriers to their participation in all aspects of social and economic life, would they still be disadvantaged by the impairments that they have?
> - Would your answer here change, if the person you are thinking about has a relatively mild impairment, or has an impairment that gives them more signifi-cant difficulties?

A key question to ask here is whether the person would still be disadvantaged if all social and material barriers were removed. Many highlight that the social model has limitations, especially in its application to those with very severe impairments (Barnes, 2020). Even if it was possible to remove such barriers, those with more severe physical, mental, cognitive or sensory impairments may still find aspects of daily living challenging and may require at least some support from others to do the things that they want to be able to do and be who they want to be (Prah Ruger and Mitra, 2015). In this sense, the nature of marginalisation of those with a disability is different from that experienced by other marginalised groups, such as those who are marginalised based on their biological sex, gender, sexual orientation, race, ethnicity and those who have migrated, because the disadvantages that are experienced in these cases are entirely the product of societies, whereas in the context of disability, whilst contested by the social model of disability, at least some of the disadvantage experienced is due to intrinsic factors (i.e. peoples impairment[s]).

Let's take the example of a relatively young, working-age (let's say 51) stroke survivor. The long-term effects of their stroke have left them hemiplegic (meaning they are unable to move one side of their body), expressively dysphasic (meaning they are unable to form words and coherent sentences) and dysphagic (meaning they have some difficulty swallowing food and water). If all material and social barriers are removed from society (i.e. by addressing the extrinsic issues), it is difficult to see how this person could enjoy the same freedoms, and capabilities, as those who have not had a severe neurological event. People's mobility, their pain and chronic fatigue, may limit opportunities to participate in social and economic life, even where society seeks to accommodate differences.

Another important point is that disability is not binary (disabled/not disabled). There is considerable diversity in relation to impairment 'effects', and the extent to which those with impairments need support and/or healthcare interventions. For example, the needs of someone with quadriplegia will be very different to the needs of someone experiencing sensory loss. Impairments such as sensory loss are also not binary (e.g. deaf/not deaf, blind/not blind – there is considerable variety within impairments). Those with impairments might be otherwise healthy, their condition being stable and requiring no more medical intervention than those of a similar age; but for some, their condition may fluctuate significantly and may require timely access to care or medical intervention to prevent their condition or their symptoms from getting worse. In summary, experiences of disadvantage will vary by impairment and by people and will be influenced by other intersecting forms of disadvantage (Kavanagh et al., 2015, Wickenden, 2023).

Despite its limitations, the social model has been highly influential in the positive repositioning of disability in society; rather than seeing disability as an individual issue, it highlights the oppression and barriers that those with a disability face (Barnes, 2020). Barriers to participation, that those with 'normative' bodies do not experience, and which those with 'nonstandard' bodies and minds, alongside their allies, have fought for, over many years, by highlighting that people's differences should not result in their exclusion from economic and social life (Barnes, 2020, Oliver, 2013).

Stop and Think: Does Society Poorly Accommodate People's Differences?

Take a moment to consider the alterable aspects that make society inaccessible for those with physical, mental, cognitive and sensory impairments.

You might have considered:

- Material features of buildings that do not account for physical differences, such as steps, instead of ramps, and a lack of elevators to access different levels.
- Toilets and bathrooms that are inaccessible, or difficult to use.
- The use of stiles, limiting access to the countryside and nature, for some people with disabilities.
- People parking on curbs, limiting people's access to safe pavements and sidewalks.
- Poorly designed websites, or other information sources, that do not account for people's cognitive or sensory differences.
- Information being provided using inaccessible, and complex language, that is full of jargon.
- Noisy and busy social and work environments.
- Staff in banks and shops not providing, or equipping staff with the skills to use alternative communication strategies such as sign language and Makaton.

Did you think of any others?

Largely through the social model, there have been significant changing attitudes towards those with various forms of impairment. Using the social model, societies can think of disability in different, more inclusive ways across several domains for example in access to employment, education, healthcare access, transport and participation in many other aspects of social and economic life (Barnes, 2020, Oliver, 2013). Initially used in the context of physical impairments, the social model of disability has since been used to consider all forms of impairment and society's response to them which we will expand upon later in this chapter. It has gone on to form the basis of policy from international institutions such as the World Health Organisation (WHO), the United Nations (UN) and the World Bank (Watson and Vehmas, 2022).

The social model of disability is particularly visible within attempts to address structural disablism, such as a range of national, and international laws and commitments to those living with a disability, and in particular, throughout the United Nations Convention of the Rights of Persons with Disabilities (UN, 2007), which represented a paradigm shift in how societies have responded to disability. A summary of the convention is provided below.

United Nations Convention on the Rights of Persons with Disabilities (CRPD) (UN, 2007)

There is a long history of campaigning for disability rights that preceded the CRPD (See Series, (2020) for a useful overview). The post-World War 2 Universal Declaration of Human Rights was intended to be 'universal' – a protection for *all* people, yet academics and activists highlighted its shortcomings in relation to the rights of those with disabilities, and concerns that the rights of people with disabilities were falling behind the rights and protections of other marginalised groups.

Take this oft-quoted line from Article 2 of the declaration, for example:

'Everyone is entitled to all the rights and freedoms set forth in this Declaration, without distinction of any kind, such as race, colour, sex, language, religion, political or other opinion, national or social origin, property, birth, or other status'.

Whilst possibly captured in 'other status', disability is noticeably missing.

The United Nations Convention on the Rights of Persons with Disabilities (CRPD) represents the first treaty to be developed by those with a disability, for those with a disability (Kanter, 2015). Whilst not establishing any new rights per se, and whilst its exact legal status varies from society to society, it is widely recognised that the CRPD represented a fundamentally new way of seeing disability, including the rights and inclusion of those living with a disability ('nothing about us without us'), and how we should as a society respond, including working on addressing stereotypes and recognising the many and varied contributions to society that those with disabilities make (Series, 2020).

The CRPD highlights disability as a broad and 'evolving concept', and within its articles, the social model of disability is clearly visible, as well as emphasising the interactions of intrinsic (the individual) and extrinsic (i.e. the environment), seen in the ICF (see Chapter 3).

Disability and Discrimination

Despite shifting attitudes towards those with impairments, it is not uncommon for people to still experience unfair and discriminatory treatment based on their real or perceived differences. In a recent UK-based survey, 32% of disabled respondents highlighted significant negative and prejudicial attitudes towards their disability, in contrast to just 22% of non-disabled respondents believing that such attitudes are highly prevalent (Dixon et al., 2018). The 'disability perception gap' suggests that those with a disability are often seen as significantly less capable than they are, which has knock-on implications for how people respond to them in everyday life and the opportunities that disabled people can access (Dixon et al., 2018). In these cases, it is not the impairments that disable people, it is society's unhelpful and discriminatory attitudes and responses towards them that cause their disadvantage. In addition, dominant organisational ideals, workplace culture, job design and

person specifications, and labour market changes, tend to be centred around the needs of a 'typical' worker who has no impairments (Foster and Wass, 2013). In part because of this, those with a disability enjoy lower levels of well-paid secure employment (Hästbacka et al., 2016, Powell, 2024, Qiu et al., 2023).

The more limited access to well-paid secure employment, and before that, educational attainment through barriers too and disrupted schooling, can often, amongst other challenges, result in those with an impairment being more likely to live in poverty than those without (Tinson et al., 2016, Palmer, 2011). People with impairments may also have more limited opportunities to participate in other aspects of society too and may find it more difficult to form social bonds beyond close ties and are far more likely to be socially isolated, experience loneliness more often (explored more in Chapter 16) and have lower perceived social support than those who do not (Emerson et al., 2021).

Disability can itself be considered a socio-determinant of health, alongside other personal constitutional factors such as age, gender, race and ethnicity and their intersections. As we explored in Chapter 8, there as several determinants that may relate to the poorer health outcomes experienced by those with a disability, meaning that those with an impairment are disadvantaged in ways that make them more likely to need healthcare (Gréaux et al., 2023). However, for those with a disability, access to healthcare is often not straightforward, and people often experience significant challenges and barriers to accessing healthcare, alongside bias, discriminatory treatment and poorer healthcare outcomes when they do manage to access it (Gréaux et al., 2023, McClintock et al., 2018, Sakellariou and Rotarou, 2017).

In the rest of this chapter, we will consider disabilities in the context of children, young people and adults with learning difficulties. We will also briefly consider disability in the context of mental ill health. We will consider access in relation to key determinants of health, such as education and employment, as well as access to healthcare.

Children and Young People with Disabilities

The sociologist Michel Foucault (1926–1984) pointed out that we are judged against a perceived 'norm' throughout our lives and that 'judges of normality are present everywhere' – be it the 'teacher-judge', 'doctor-judge', 'social-worker' judge, etc. (Foucault, 1995). This 'judge' is a person who (normally) the state gives power to make decisions about what is, or what is not 'normal' ways of being and behaving. Such judgements are a defining feature of children's and young people's lives in western and industrialised nations. Throughout childhood, and even before a child is born, children are 'measured' and pitched against their peers. This can include developmental assessments of their size, weight, height, physical health, communication, agility, cognition and play (amongst other things) (CDC, 2024, UK Government, 2014b). This benchmarking largely occurs in education and these measures rely on an average or 'norm' being identified, which, as with other life course stages, rather than recognising the diversity that occurs across people, can instead result in people being positively, or negatively classified relative to their peers. When applied such descriptions, which are themselves socially constructed, become laden with all sorts of meanings, that can potentially stigmatise those falling outside of the normative measures of attainment (Uba and Nwoga, 2016). Those deemed as 'falling behind' or 'underachieving', may in turn experience discrimination, poor educational investment and resultant poorer long-term outcomes (Algraigray and Boyle, 2017, Hodkinson, 2020).

Because education and educational attainment is such a central aspect of the lives of children and young people with disabilities, and because it is such an important determinant of health, with life course implications (Zajacova and Lawrence, 2018), it forms the basis of our discussion of childhood disability. In the United Kingdom, as with elsewhere, education is based on a classification system which measures age-related levels of attainment in a range of criteria. There is diversity in children's attainment against these, but students falling below a certain expected 'threshold' for their age, are 'labelled' as having a Special Educational Need or Disability (SEND) (Uba and Nwoga, 2016, UK Government, 2014b). SEND as a term has come to represent a diverse group of children and young people, with different levels of physical, psychological, cognitive and sensory impairment, and different levels of needs relating to these (UK Government, 2014a, UK Government, 2014b).

Approximately 11% of all children in the United Kingdom have some form of disability, and this figure has almost doubled over the last decade (Kirk-Wade, 2023). The reasons for this increase in a United Kingdom context are complex (Taberner, 2023), but include greater recognition, increasing medicalisation and the widening of criteria for some conditions, leading to higher rates of diagnosis (Russell et al., 2022, Taberner, 2023, Underwood, 2008), alongside the inclusion of social and behavioural difficulties in childhood disability statistics (Kirk-Wade, 2023). The impact of these differences on everyday life varies from child to child. Whilst children can have physical, sensory, learning and mental health disabilities, many have a combination of these, alongside other forms of intersecting disadvantage (covered in Chapter 8) (Emerson and Hatton, 2007). Such differences, as with other life course stages (see Chapter 15), mean that when we talk about children with disabilities, we are not describing one large homogenous group of similarly impaired children, but are in fact talking about children with a variety of different types of impairments, that impact on their lives in many different ways, and who therefore have very different capabilities and needs.

Children and young people with disabilities have previously been segregated into specialist education institutions, but significant progress has been made and now most live with their families and attend mainstream school environments

(Hodkinson, 2020). In the United Kingdom, the 2014 Child and Family Act, and its accompanying SEND Code of Practice (2014) aimed to make education more inclusive for those with impairments by focussing on broad categories of 'need' (such as communication and interaction, cognition and learning, social, emotional and mental health, sensory and physical).

Such measurements and in some cases diagnostic classifications make labels inevitable and even a requirement, particularly where it becomes relevant to what support children and young people receive (Algraigray and Boyle, 2017, Brady et al., 2023). Families and professionals have spoken of the positive outcomes for children with the label of SEND (Sales and Vincent, 2018), but whilst classifications can be useful in helping children access support and understanding their differences, they can also be unhelpful because they can impact on how they are perceived by others, and in turn how they perceive themselves (Brady et al., 2023). For example, the way in which school classes are organised in relation to academic attainment (bottom, middle and top sets), and teacher's own preconceived understandings which are influenced by wider society's bias towards those with a disability, can lead to assumptions about disabled children and what they (and their bodies) are likely to be able to achieve (Bodfield and Culshaw, 2023, Goodley and Runswick Cole, 2015, Holt, 2004). The way that children learn and are assessed may disadvantage some children who have bodies that are unable to perform in the expected way, at the expected time, using expected methods; for instance, children who learn more slowly or struggle with handwriting, or who are easily distracted.

SEND policies have been criticised for creating a dependence on formal diagnosis, through aligning to a deficit or medical model of disability, that typically centres on problems and difficulties with individual children, rather than focussing on their strengths, or with wider social systems and how they disable those with differences, as well as reproducing social, economic and political inequalities (Bodfield and Culshaw, 2023, Hunter et al., 2020, Keville et al., 2024). The concepts of 'inclusion' and 'need', which are central to special education, suggest the child is somehow 'lacking', deficient in some way, non-normative, and potentially even marginalised when placed outside of the more socially desired mainstream schooling option (Hodkinson, 2020). Concern also exists around the racialisation of special educational needs. In one recent study, children with other intersecting disadvantages, such as black Caribbean or Pakistani children were more likely to be identified as meeting categories of educational need than white, Indian or Chinese pupils (Strand and Lindorff, 2018).

Discrimination can surface in other ways too. Children with more complex disabilities, such as children with learning disabilities and autism, often have multiple needs that are addressed through a centrally co-ordinated 'education health care plan' (EHCP) (Keville et al., 2024). These person-centred plans should be based on the wishes and aspirations of the child, but research has suggested that children are often not given the opportunity to contribute to their plan due to the perception that they cannot communicate their needs or do not understand the process

(Sharma, 2021). Similarly, children with severe learning disabilities are often excluded from decision-making altogether, due to misconceptions that they are unable to contribute in a meaningful way (Sapiets, 2021). The different ways children and young people communicate mean that augmentative communication strategies (such as Talking Mats, picture symbols, Makaton and sign language) should be adopted to ensure that what children may feel, like or want – is adequately captured and understood (Sapiets, 2021).

Alongside changes to education provision, the importance of care for children with a disability has gained increasing recognition and focus across health and social care services. However, research suggests that long-term education and health-related outcomes for children with a disability continue to be comparatively poor, and they are more likely to experience social exclusion and fewer opportunities to gain meaningful employment in adulthood (Department for Education, 2023, Ofsted, 2021). One of the key aims of the SEND Code of Practice 2014 was to enhance opportunities for employment for disabled young people transitioning to adulthood. The relative merits and assumptions behind this aim have been discussed (Hunter et al., 2020), but it is widely recognised that higher education (Tinson et al., 2016), as well as employment remains out of reach to a great many people with physical, mental or cognitive impairments (Department for Education, 2023, Ofsted, 2021). Evidence suggests individuals 'labelled' as having SEND at school are less likely to be in employment compared to peers with a similar level of attainment and are likely to be in lower-income jobs (Anderson, 2023).

Other social inequalities that children and young people with disabilities experience are well recognised (Emerson and Hatton, 2007). They are more likely to live in poverty, be in a single-parent household, or be placed in long-term care, but the extent of this is linked to socio-economic status, with those from higher socio-economic status groups being less likely to experience such hardships (Bixby, 2023). In Chapter 15, we introduce you to the concept of 'linked' lives and this is particularly visible in considering the material advantages and disadvantages seen in this stage of the life course. Parents and carers, but particularly those parents and carers with the least resources, are more likely to experience mental health problems, though this likely relates to the nature of the impairment, as well as other factors, such as the age of the parents/carer (Bixby, 2023, Holland et al., 2018). In addition, caring responsibilities, as with caring in other life course stages, may make it harder for parents to secure and maintain paid work, further exacerbating the family's overall material disadvantage (Bixby, 2023, Nicoriciu and Elliot, 2023).

Learning Disability

As with other disabilities discussed in this chapter, we all have different intrinsic capabilities, and because of this, our needs are varied and diverse. There is significant lay, academic and professional debate about what constitutes a learning disability. As with impairments more broadly, what is, and what is not an 'impairment' is socially constructed, and subject to change over time. For example, at what point precisely does someone's learning difference constitute a disability as opposed to simply being a part of natural variation in human cognition and intellectual ability? As with other disabilities discussed in this chapter, for some on this continuum, their intellectual abilities can intrinsically make some aspects of participation more challenging, but society itself, and the way others respond, can and often does interact with the challenges their intrinsic capabilities present them with. For example, arguments exist that learning disability is a social phenomenon, a product of our education systems that generally seek to assess, test and classify children (who become adults) against a 'norm' for intellectual ability. Such an understanding of learning disability can impact those given such a label, who must then demonstrate that they are competent before accessing the same freedoms that others enjoy automatically (Stalker, 2022). Those falling into this category might not be listened to, or respected, and may be subject to other people's unwanted pity, overhelping, judgements and decisions about how they live and what they should be able to do (Stalker, 2022). Historically, those whose intellectual differences have resulted in their labelling, have been oppressed and devalued by society, often facing marginalisation and discrimination that leads to their exclusion, denial of equal rights and opportunities, and even abuse (Trent, 2017). Despite experiencing many of the same oppressive forces as those with physical disabilities, those with a learning disability were excluded from the original formulation put forward by the Union of the Physically Impaired Against Segregation (1976), which largely highlighted the body as the source of impairments; and it has been argued that they have also been excluded from many of the debates around disability that have occurred since (Stalker, 2022).

As a historically segregated group, in countries such as the United Kingdom, where there has been an increased focus on inclusion, whilst some improvement has been seen, those with a learning disability still commonly encounter negative and prejudicial attitudes and behaviours (Scior and Werner, 2016, Wilson and Scior, 2014). For example, within a social care context, abuse continues to be a significant concern, highlighting the ongoing struggle for the rights and protection of individuals with learning disabilities in even more affluent societies, with well-documented cases such as that of Winterbourne View Hospital, and more recently Whorlton View (Richards, 2020, Willis, 2020). Those with a learning disability are less likely to be employed, highlighting the systematic inequalities faced by this group (McTier et al., 2016, Moore et al., 2020, Woman and Equalities Committee, 2024). In addition, Implicit-Association Tests (IAT), which look to see if people have an implicit bias towards specific groups, highlight that people often implicitly see those with a learning disability more negatively than those without (Wilson and Scior, 2014), and research has highlighted implicit bias such as this, alongside discriminatory and prejudicial attitudes are sometimes held by those delivering care (Ali et al., 2013, Pelleboer-Gunnink et al., 2017).

Inclusive Healthcare Provision for Those with a Learning Disability

Accessing healthcare is a fundamental right for all individuals (Ali et al., 2013, UN, 2007), yet people with learning disabilities often encounter significant barriers, abuse, mistreatment and inadequate or discriminatory practices (Desroches et al., 2022, Krahn et al., 2015, Lee et al., 2024, Pelleboer-Gunnink et al., 2017). In this section, we will unpack and examine some of the challenges faced by individuals with learning disabilities in accessing healthcare in the United Kingdom and elsewhere, exploring known factors such as communication barriers, discriminatory attitudes, inadequate training amongst healthcare professionals and known systemic barriers that limit the ability for those with a learning disability to shape their care and healthcare provision for people with their needs (Ali et al., 2013, Desroches et al., 2022, Krahn et al., 2015, Pelleboer-Gunnink et al., 2017).

Individuals with learning disabilities continue to experience communication difficulties with healthcare professionals when accessing care (McCormick et al., 2021). For some, non-verbal and alternative communication strategies may be needed that are responsive and adaptable to people's diverse needs and preferences (Lee et al., 2024, McCormick et al., 2021). A lack of effective and inclusive communication can lead to misunderstandings, dismissed symptoms, misdiagnoses, a lack of or inadequate treatment and involvement, that can compromise outcomes and the quality of care received by those with learning disabilities (McCormick et al., 2021). In addition, people with learning disabilities may struggle to articulate their health concerns or understand medical information, hindering effective communication with healthcare professionals (Adam et al., 2020, Hallyburton, 2022, McCormick et al., 2021). Without adequate support, those with a learning disability are often sidelined in decision-making, including in relation to end-of-life care (Adam et al., 2020, Tuffrey-Wijne et al., 2020, Wagemans et al., 2010). Training in learning disability awareness and communication skills is often emphasised as being important in ensuring equitable access to high-quality care (Costello et al., 2007, Rotenberg et al., 2022, Trollor et al., 2016, Trollor et al., 2018), and is now a statutory requirement in some countries (NHS England, 2024). To improve healthcare services for people with learning disabilities, students and the healthcare workforce need opportunities to have contact, engage and learn from the needs and perspectives of individuals with disabilities, as well as training in person-centred care and adaptive communication strategies, to better support those with the sensory and cognitive impairments that are particularly common in those with a learning disability (Rotenberg et al., 2022).

There are also structural factors that lead to poor care provision for those with a learning disability. Structural inequalities in healthcare funding and resource allocation have disproportionately affected individuals with learning disabilities, further limiting access to essential healthcare services (Tuffrey-Wijne et al., 2020). Research has highlighted issues such as long waiting times for appointments, complex referral processes and limited access to specialist services tailored to the needs of individuals with learning disabilities (Doherty et al., 2020, Krahn and Fox, 2014, Tuffrey-Wijne et al., 2020). Other systematic issues that arise from bias and discrimination, alongside a lack of training, include misdiagnosis, or a lack of diagnosis altogether, and this can occur due to diagnostic overshadowing where symptoms are incorrectly attributed to an impairment, rather than exploring the presenting complaints underlying aetiology (Hallyburton, 2022, Lee et al., 2024). This can lead to inequities in which health issues may go undiagnosed and subsequently untreated, with potentially catastrophic and now well-documented impacts. Such inequities contribute to the premature death of people with learning disabilities, which is often referred to as 'death by indifference' (Ryan, 2017).

Addressing the challenges we have explored in this section, requires a multifaceted approach encompassing policy reforms, increased awareness and training for healthcare professionals, involvement in planning healthcare provision and improved coordination and integration of healthcare services (Lakhani et al., 2018). To ensure needs are adequately incorporated into healthcare provision, when we consider planning, designing or commissioning of new services, those with a disability should be included from inception (de Haas et al., 2022). The slogan 'nothing about us, without us', which emerged through disability activism (Charlton, 1998), is now commonly deployed in professional and policy contexts when considering the involvement of those receiving health and social care in decisions about what provision should look like. Recognising that those with a disability have unique and important insights into the care that they receive, and what they need from healthcare, it is vitally important that those with a disability are engaged with, regardless of their age or communication difficulties, as opposed to simply soliciting the views of relatives and carers.

Biographical Disruption

Disability is not necessarily something that people are born with, and it is common for people to suddenly, or gradually lose some of their physical and or mental functional abilities (WHO, 2011). However, such changes can also be incredibly sudden, and unexpected, and this can bring about changes in the way people perceive themselves, and their own personal biography – that is, who they perceive themselves to be, and what they believe their future will be like. Michael Bury's (1982) now seminal concept of biographical disruption, which was first used in the study of rheumatoid arthritis, highlights illness as a shock to someone's everyday life, leading them to re-evaluate personal narratives and the taken for granted aspects of their bodily functions (Bury, 1982). As part of this re-evaluation, people necessarily consider how changes might impact on their future life trajectories and opportunities (Bury, 1982). An important theory in medical sociology in particular (Engman, 2019, Larsson and Grassman, 2012); biographical disruption is generalisable to several chronic conditions, including those associated with physical impairment (Asbring, 2001, Faircloth et al., 2004, Locock et al., 2009, Wolfenden and Grace, 2012). It has also been used in the study of mental illness (Apesoa-Varano et al., 2015, Larsson and Grassman, 2012, Perry and Pescosolido, 2012). Academics have highlighted that those with a chronic illness, or disability, rather than re-evaluating expectations for their life and their future, instead incorporate their illness into their existing identity, reflecting instead a process of normalisation (Sanderson et al., 2011) with others highlighting that people can move back and forth between these two states, in a process referred to as 'biographical oscillation' (Bell et al., 2016).

Mental Distress

Survivor-led work, such as the recovery movement that we introduced in Chapter 4, is useful in terms of reorientating focus towards supporting people to live well, despite experiencing mental distress. Such a discourse represents a significant shift in how mental distress is viewed. People can recover, and now, rather than there being fixed requirements for a return to 'normalcy' prior to social and economic integration and inclusion, participation in important domains of social life is seen as important to gain the capabilities needed to manage and recover from mental distress (Davidson et al., 2009). In the context of mental health, the capabilities approach, which we discussed in Chapter 3, provides another useful framework for reorientating our approach to mental ill health and prompting us to think about whether people are equipped to lead a life that they value (White et al., 2016).

In defining severe mental ill health as a disability, new legislation, such as the passing of the Americans with Disabilities Act (ADA)[4], in principle ensured similar protections and rights for those with severe mental ill health as other types of disability (Davidson, 2016). Such legislation emphasised that those experiencing mental ill health should have equal opportunities to participate in society through access to education and employment, as well as healthcare and society's institutions more generally putting in place 'reasonable adjustments'; and that rather than being contingent on recovery, these should be recognised as supporting recovery (Davidson, 2016). However, significant challenges to

participation in economic and social life remain. Where mental health impacts on individuals, as well as on how others perceive and respond to them, it can have a varied and significant impact on people's daily activities, as well as their participation in social, economic and educational opportunities (Cullen et al., 2017, Perry, 2011). The relationship between mental ill health and socioeconomic outcomes is complex and bi-directional. For example, where material disadvantage exists, so too does the risk of physical health issues and multi-morbidity (Marmot, 2010, Marmot et al., 2020, Reilly et al., 2015). In turn, having one or more chronic conditions greatly increases the risk of having co-morbid mental health issues (Pizzol et al., 2023); and those with severe mental illness, also have an increased risk of physical health conditions compared to the general population (Launders et al., 2022). However, they are also more likely to have symptoms of physical ill health overlooked or attributed to their mental health issues (Hallyburton, 2022).

Of the different types of disability discussed in this chapter, those with severe mental ill health, as well as those with a learning disability, are more likely to experience prejudicial attitudes and discrimination, than those with other forms of disability (Henderson et al., 2014, Scior and Werner, 2015). They are less likely to be employed than the general population, which further exacerbates material disadvantage (Stevenson and Farmer, 2017) and the risk of homelessness is high, especially in more severe presentations such as psychosis (Gutwinski et al., 2021, Powell and Maguire, 2018). Other factors exacerbating disadvantage include poorer living and working conditions when in employment, reduced status and lower levels of autonomy – each of which may negatively impact on mental health (Kirkbride et al., 2024, Ridley et al., 2020). Because of the relationship of poverty to poor health outcomes, participation in society and particularly education, training and employment has been recognised as a key intervention for recovery, and the movement of mental healthcare beyond hospitals, and the use of Individual Placement Support has become increasingly common (Barnett et al., 2022).

As we highlighted in Chapter 9, those with complex mental ill health can face significant felt, self and enacted stigma, which can marginalise and work to limit their participation in education, and employment, as well as reducing their access to healthcare (Trevillion et al., 2022). In Chapter 9, some stigma-reducing interventions were discussed and these were broadly broken down into education and contact interventions. One further intervention that has been deployed to support recovery and greater community inclusion of those with poor mental health in the population more generally, is the use of 'Mental Health First Aid' (Morgan et al., 2018). Davidson (2016) highlights that interventions that ensure people with severe mental ill health are adequality supported in their societies and by its various institutions are largely social and relational and may support participation in the same way as does the provision of ramps and wheelchair access for those with physical

---

[4] Which preceded equivalent acts in international law, and in the United Kingdom, the Equalities Act (2010) and the Disability Discrimination Act (1995).

disabilities. 'Mental Health First Aid' is a standardised, educational programme that is designed to increase participants' mental health literacy, including their knowledge, attitudes and behaviours relating to mental ill-health, which in turn is hoped will create more inclusive environments, that empower the public to approach, support and refer individuals who are in distress to supportive services (Hadlaczky et al., 2014, Morgan et al., 2018).

Clinical Considerations

- Those living with physical, mental, cognitive and sensory impairments face disadvantages beyond their intrinsic limitations.
- These disadvantages relate to accessibility and treatment in society more generally (education, employment, etc.), as well as in healthcare settings in particular.
- The social model of disability has been useful in creating more accessible environments, but in the context of healthcare, there is still a long way to go.
- Disability is not binary. The needs of those living with an impairment vary from person to person, and from impairment to impairment. It is important to understand these differences when providing care.
- It is essential to include those living with physical, mental, cognitive and sensory impairments in decisions about their care and be able to adapt to their preferences and communication needs.
- Training can be affective in improving the experiences and outcomes of those accessing healthcare.
- Healthcare professionals have a key role in shaping society's attitudes and values around disability and can be powerful advocates for change.

Conclusion

In this chapter, we have highlighted that there is no single embodied experience. All of our bodies are unstable, and potentially vulnerable to changes that result in impairments across our life course. Whilst the concept of disability tends to be viewed as binary – disabled/nondisabled, it is more useful to consider disability through a lens of a continuum of needs that recognises human diversity and difference and ensures that the way in which society is set up and configured does not create undue disadvantage. Globally, including in western and developed societies, those labelled as having a disability, continue to be disadvantaged by their impairments (intrinsic factors), but also by the societies prevailing prejudicial attitudes towards those living with a disability, as well as the lack of accommodations to those living with physical, mental, cognitive and sensory impairments (extrinsic factors). The social model of disability and following this the UN CRPD have resulted in a paradigm shift in the way disability is seen in many societies, which is improving the lives and prospects for many of those living with a range of disabilities. How exactly disabilities are defined, remains contentious but through recognising the impact of adjustable extrinsic factors, such as building accessibility and employment rights, those that may be defined as disabled, have increasing opportunities for greater participation in many aspects of social and economic life. Despite this, significant disadvantages are still experienced that are amendable to change, especially for those with other forms of intersecting disadvantage. In this regard, the ambitions of the CRPD will not be achieved, until all of societies members enjoy equal rights with others in their society, regardless of any impairments they may have. We are all a part of the society in which we live and work, and as citizens and healthcare professionals, we have a role and are key allies in shaping the prevailing attitudes and values towards impairment.

References

Adam, E., Sleeman, K. E., Brearley, S., Hunt, K. & Tuffrey-Wijne, I. 2020. The palliative care needs of adults with intellectual disabilities and their access to palliative care services: a systematic review. *Palliative Medicine*, 34, 1006–1018.

Algraigray, H. & Boyle, C. 2017. *The SEN label and its effect on special education*, British Psychological Society.

Ali, A., Scior, K., Ratti, V., Strydom, A., King, M. & Hassiotis, A. 2013. Discrimination and other barriers to accessing health care: perspectives of patients with mild and moderate iIntellectual disability and their carers. *PLoS One*, 8, e70855.

Anderson, O. 2023. Post-16 education and labour market activities, pathways and outcomes (LEO). *International Journal of Population Data Science*.

Apesoa-Varano, E. C., Barker, J. C. & Hinton, L. 2015. Shards of sorrow: older men's accounts of their depression experience. *Social Science & Medicine*, 124, 1–8.

Asbring, P. 2001. Chronic illness–a disruption in life: identity-transformation among women with chronic fatigue syndrome and fibromyalgia. *Journal of Advanced Nursing*, 34, 312–319.

Barnartt, S. N. 2013. *Introduction: Disability and Intersecting Statuses*, Emerald Group Publishing Limited.

Barnes, C. 2020. Understanding the Social Model of Disability: Past, Present, Future. *In:* Watson, N. & Vehmas, S. (eds.) *Routledge Handbook of Disability Studies*, Routledge.

Barnett, P., Steare, T., Dedat, Z., Pilling, S., Mccrone, P., Knapp, M., Cooke, E., Lamirel, D., Dawson, S., Goldblatt, P., Hatch, S., Henderson, C., Jenkins, R. K. T., Machin, K., Simpson, A., Shah, P., Stevens, M., Webber, M., Johnson, S. & Lloyd-Evans, B. 2022. Interventions to improve social circumstances of people with mental health conditions: a rapid evidence synthesis. *BMC Psychiatry*, 22, 302.

Barry, A. & Yuill, C. 2022. *Understanding the Sociology of Health: An Introduction*, Sage.

Bell, S. L., Tyrrell, J. & Phoenix, C. 2016. Ménière's disease and biographical disruption: where family transitions collide. *Social Science & Medicine*, 166, 177–185.

Bickenback, J. 2020. The ICF and its relationship to disability studies. *In:* Watson, N. & Vehmas, S. (eds.) *Routledge Handbook of Distality Studies*, Routledge.

Bixby, L. E. 2023. Disability Is Not a Burden: The Relationship between Early Childhood Disability and Maternal Health Depends on Family Socioeconomic Status. *Journal of Health and Social Behavior*, 64, 354–369.

Bodfield, K. S. & Culshaw, A. 2023. The place for diagnosis in the UK education system? *Emotional and Behavioural Difficulties*, 28, 316–328.

Brady, G., Franklin, A. & Collective, R. S. 2023. 'I am more than just my label': rights, fights, validation and negotiation. Exploring theoretical debates on childhood disability with disabled young people. *Sociology of Health & Illness*, 45, 1376–1392.

Brown, R. L., Maroto, M. & Pettinicchio, D. 2023. *The Oxford handbook of the sociology of disability*, Oxford University Press.

Bury, M. 1982. Chronic illness as biographical disruption. *Sociology of Health & Illness*, 4, 167–182.

CDC. 2024. CDC's Developmental Milestones [Online]. CDC Available: https://www.cdc.gov/ncbddd/actearly/milestones/index.html [Accessed].

Charlton, C. 1998. *Nothing about us without us: Disability oppression and empowerment*, University of California Press.

Costello, H., Bouras, N. & Davis, H. 2007. The role of training in improving community care staff awareness of mental health problems in people with intellectual disabilities. *Journal of Applied Research in Intellectual Disabilities*, 20, 228–235.

Cullen, B. A., Mojtabai, R., Bordbar, E., Everett, A., Nugent, K. L. & Eaton, W. W. 2017. Social network, recovery attitudes and internal stigma among those with serious mental illness. *International Journal of Social Psychiatry*, 63, 448–458.

Davidson, L. 2016. The recovery movement: implications for mental health care and enabling people to participate fully in life. *Health Affairs*, 35, 1091–1097.

Davidson, L., Ridgway, P., Wieland, M. & O'connell, M. 2009. A capabilities approach to mental health transformation: a conceptual framework for the recovery era. *Canadian Journal of Community Mental Health*, 28, 35–46.

De Haas, C., Grace, J., Hope, J. & Nind, M. 2022. Doing research inclusively: Understanding what it means to do research with and alongside people with profound intellectual disabilities. *Social Sciences*, 11, 159.

Desroches, M. L., Howie, V. A., Wilson, N. J. & Lewis, P. 2022. Nurses' attitudes and emotions toward caring for adults with intellectual disability: an international replication study. *Journal of Nursing Scholarship*, 54, 117–124.

Dixon, S., Smith, C. & Touchet, A. 2018. The Disability Perception Gap. SCOPE. Available online at: https://assets-eu-01.kc-usercontent.com/73ea709e-f9f8-0168-3842-ebd7ad1e23ac/acb8a67e-86c7-47a8-b809-0d099acd6ac6/disability-perception-gap-report.pdf.

Department for Education. 2023. SEND and alternative provision improvement plan. Available online at: https://www.gov.uk/government/publications/send-and-alternative-provision-improvement-plan.

Doherty, A. J., Atherton, H., Boland, P., Hastings, R., Hives, L., Hood, K., James-Jenkinson, L., Leavey, R., Randell, E. & Reed, J. 2020. Barriers and facilitators to primary health care for people with intellectual disabilities and/or autism: an integrative review. *BJGP open*, 4.

Dueñas, M., Ojeda, B., Salazar, A., Mico, J. A. & Failde, I. 2016. A review of chronic pain impact on patients, their social environment and the health care system. *Journal of Pain Research*, 457–467.

Dunn, D. S. & Burcaw, S. 2013. Disability identity: exploring narrative accounts of disability. *Rehabilitation Psychology*, 58, 148.

Eide, A. H. & Ingstad, B. 2011. *Disability and Poverty: A global challenge*, Bristol University Press.

Emerson, E., Fortune, N., Llewellyn, G. & Stancliffe, R. 2021. Loneliness, social support, social isolation and wellbeing among working age adults with and without disability: cross-sectional study. *Disability and Health Journal*, 14, 100965.

Emerson, E. & Hatton, C. 2007. Mental health of children and adolescents with intellectual disabilities in Britain. *The British Journal of Psychiatry*, 191, 493–499.

Engman, A. 2019. Embodiment and the foundation of biographical disruption. *Social Science & Medicine*, 225, 120–127.

Faircloth, C. A., Boylstein, C., Rittman, M., Young, M. E. & Gubrium, J. 2004. Sudden illness and biographical flow in narratives of stroke recovery. *Sociology of Health & Illness*, 26, 242–261.

Fiske, S. T. 2012. Warmth and competence: stereotype content issues for clinicians and researchers. *Canadian Psychology/Psychologie Canadienne*, 53, 14.

Foster, D. & Wass, V. 2013. Disability in the Labour Market: an Exploration of Concepts of the Ideal Worker and Organisational Fit that Disadvantage Employees with Impairments. *Sociology*, 47, 705–721.

Foucault, M. 1995. *Discipline and Punish: The Birth of the Prison*, Vintage.

Goering, S. 2015. Rethinking disability: the social model of disability and chronic disease. *Current Reviews in Musculoskeletal Medicine*, 8, 134–138.

Goodley, D. 2014. *Dis/ability Studies*, London: Routledge.

Goodley, D. 2020. The Psychology of Disability Studies. *In:* Watson, N. & Vehmas, S. (eds.) *Routledge Handbook of Disability Studies*, Routledge.

Goodley, D. & Runswick Cole, K. 2015. Critical psychologies of disability: boundaries, borders and bodies in the lives of disabled children. *Emotional and Behavioural Difficulties*, 20, 51–63.

Gotaas, M. E., Stiles, T. C., Bjørngaard, J. H., Borchgrevink, P. C. & Fors, E. A. 2021. Cognitive behavioral therapy improves physical function and fatigue in mild and moderate chronic fatigue syndrome: a consecutive randomized controlled trial of standard and short interventions. *Frontiers in Psychiatry*, 12, 580924.

Gréaux, M., Moro, M. F., Kamenov, K., Russell, A. M., Barrett, D. & Cieza, A. 2023. Health equity for persons with disabilities: a global scoping review on barriers and interventions in healthcare services. *International Journal for Equity in Health*, 22, 236.

Gutwinski, S., Schreiter, S., Deutscher, K. & Fazel, S. 2021. The prevalence of mental disorders among homeless people in high-income countries: an updated systematic review and meta-regression analysis. *PLoS Medicine*, 18, e1003750.

Hadlaczky, G., Hökby, S., Mkrtchian, A., Carli, V. & Wasserman, D. 2014. Mental Health First Aid is an effective public health intervention for improving knowledge, attitudes, and behaviour: a meta-analysis. *International Review of Psychiatry*, 26, 467–475.

Hallyburton, A. 2022. Diagnostic overshadowing: an evolutionary concept analysis on the misattribution of physical symptoms to pre-existing psychological illnesses. *International Journal of Mental Health Nursing*, 31, 1360–1372.

Hästbacka, E., Nygård, M. & Nyqvist, F. 2016. Barriers and facilitators to societal participation of people with disabilities: a scoping review of studies concerning European countries. *Alter*, 10, 201–220.

Henderson, C., Noblett, J., Parke, H., Clement, S., Caffrey, A., Gale-Grant, O., Schulze, B., Druss, B. & Thornicroft, G. 2014. Mental health-related stigma in health care and mental health-care settings. *The Lancet Psychiatry*, 1, 467–482.

Hodkinson, A. 2020. Special educational needs and inclusion, moving forward but standing still? A critical reframing of some key issues. *British Journal of Special Education*, 47, 308–328.

Hogan, A. J. 2019. Moving away from the "medical model": the development and revision of the World Health Organization's Classification of Disability. *Bulletin of the History of Medicine*, 93, 241–269.

Holland, J., Pell, G. & KIDS 2018. Children with SEND and the emotional impact on parents. *British Journal of Special Education*, 45, 392–411.

Holt, L. 2004. Children with mind–body differences: performing disability in primary school classrooms. *Children's Geographies*, 2, 219–236.

Horner-Johnson, W. 2021. Disability, intersectionality, and inequity: life at the margins. *In:* Lollar, D. J., Horner-Johnson, W. & Froehlich-Grobe, K. (eds.) *Public Health Perspectives on Disability: Science, Social Justice, Ethics, and Beyond*, New York, NY: Springer US.

Hughes, B. 2020. Invalidating emotions in the non-disabled imaginary. *In:* Watson, D. & Vehmas, S. (eds.) *Routledge Handbook of Disability Studies*, Routledge.

Hunter, J., Runswick-Cole, K., Goodley, D. & Lawthom, R. 2020. Plans that work: improving employment outcomes for young people with learning disabilities. *British Journal of Special Education*, 47, 134–151.

Kanter, A. 2015. *The Development of Disability Right Under International Law: From Charity to Human Rights*, Routledge.

Kavanagh, A. M., Krnjacki, L., Aitken, Z., Lamontagne, A. D., Beer, A., Baker, E. & Bentley, R. 2015. Intersections between disability, type of impairment, gender and socio-economic disadvantage in a nationally representative sample of 33,101 working-aged Australians. *Disability and Health Journal*, 8, 191–199.

Keville, S., Mills, M. & Ludlow, A. K. 2024. Exploring mothers' experiences of accessing an Education Health and Care Plan (EHCP) for an autistic child attending mainstream school in the United Kingdom. *International Journal of Developmental Disabilities*, 1–12.

Kirk-Wade, E. 2023. *UK disability statistics: Prevalence and life experiences Research Briefing*, House of Commons Library House of Commons.

Kirkbride, J. B., Anglin, D. M., Colman, I., Dykxhoorn, J., Jones, P. B., Patalay, P., Pitman, A., Soneson, E., Steare, T., Wright, T. & Griffiths, S. L. 2024. The social determinants of mental health and disorder: evidence, prevention and recommendations. *World Psychiatry*, 23, 58–90.

Krahn, G. L. & Fox, M. H. 2014. Health disparities of adults with intellectual disabilities: what do we know? What do we do? *Journal of Applied Research in Intellectual Disabilities*, 27, 431–446.

Krahn, G. L., Walker, D. K. & Correa-De-Araujo, R. 2015. Persons With Disabilities as an Unrecognized Health Disparity Population. *American Journal of Public Health*, 105, S198–S206.

Krieger, N. 2005. Embodiment: a conceptual glossary for epidemiology. *Journal of Epidemiology & Community Health*, 59, 350–355.

Lakhani, A., Mcdonald, D. & Zeeman, H. 2018. Perspectives of self-direction: a systematic review of key areas contributing to service users' engagement and choice-making in self-directed disability services and supports. *Health & Social Care in the Community*, 26, 295–313.

Larsson, A. T. & Grassman, E. J. 2012. Bodily changes among people living with physical impairments and chronic illnesses: biographical disruption or normal illness? *Sociology of Health & Illness*, 34, 1156–1169.

Launders, N., Dotsikas, K., Marston, L., Price, G., Osborn, D. P. J. & Hayes, J. F. 2022. The impact of comorbid severe mental illness and common chronic physical health conditions on hospitalisation: a systematic review and meta-analysis. *PLoS One*, 17, e0272498.

Leder, D. 1990. *The Absent Body*, The University of Chicago Press.

Lee, A. C., Herrieven, E. & Harrower, N. A. 2024. Health inequalities for people with learning disabilities: why it matters and what emergency physicians need to know. *British Journal of Hospital Medicine*, 85, 1–7.

Leonardi, M., Bickenbach, J., Ustun, T. B., Kostanjsek, N. & Chatterji, S. 2006. The definition of disability: what is in a name? *The Lancet*, 368, 1219–1221.

Locock, L., Ziebland, S. & Dumelow, C. 2009. Biographical disruption, abruption and repair in the context of motor neurone disease. *Sociology of Health & Illness*, 31, 1043–1058.

Marmot, M., Allen, J., Boyce, T., Goldblatt, P. & Morrison, J. 2020. Health Equity in England: The Marmot Review 10 Years On [Online]. The Health Foundation Available: https://www.health.org.uk/publications/reports/the-marmot-review-10-years-on [Accessed].

Marmot, M. G. 2010. Fair society, healthy lives: the Marmot Review: strategic review of health inequalities in England post- 2010.

Mcclintock, H. F., Kurichi, J. E., Barg, F. K., Krueger, A., Colletti, P. M., Wearing, K. A. & Bogner, H. R. 2018. Health care access and quality for persons with disability: patient and provider recommendations. *Disability and Health Journal*, 11, 382–389.

Mccormick, F., Marsh, L., Taggart, L. & Brown, M. 2021. Experiences of adults with intellectual disabilities accessing acute hospital services: a systematic review of the international evidence. *Health & Social Care in the Community*, 29, 1222–1232.

Mctier, A., Macdougall, L., Mcgregor, A., Hirst, A. & Rinne, S. 2016. Mapping the Employability Landscape for People with Learning Disabilities in Scotland. Scottish Commission for Learning Disability. Available online: https://www.scld.org.uk/wp-content/uploads/2016/08/SCLD-Report-Web.pdf.

Mitra, S. 2006. The Capability Approach and Disability. *Journal of Disability Policy Studies*, 16, 236–247.

Moore, K., Mcdonald, P. & Bartlett, J. 2020. Emerging trends affecting future employment opportunities for people with intellectual disability: the case of a large retail organisation. *In: New lenses on intellectual disabilities*, Routledge.

Morgan, A. J., Ross, A. & Reavley, N. J. 2018. Systematic review and meta-analysis of Mental Health First Aid training: effects on knowledge, stigma, and helping behaviour. *PLoS One*, 13, e0197102.

Moss, P. & Teghtsoonian, K. 2008. *Contesting illness: process and practices*, University of Toronto Press.

Nario-Redmond, M. R. 2010. Cultural stereotypes of disabled and non-disabled men and women: consensus for global category representations and diagnostic domains. *British Journal of Social Psychology*, 49, 471–488.

Nettleton, S. & Watson, J. 1998. *The body in everyday life*, Routledge.

NHS England. 2024. The Oliver McGowan Mandatory Training on Learning Disability and Autism [Online]. NHS England Available: https://www.hee.nhs.uk/our-work/learning-disability/current-projects/oliver-mcgowan-mandatory-training-learning-disability-autism [Accessed].

Nicoriciu, A. M. & Elliot, M. 2023. Families of children with disabilities: income poverty, material deprivation, and unpaid care in the UK. *Humanities and Social Sciences Communications*, 10, 519.

Ofsted. 2021. SEND: Old issues, new issues, next steps [Online]. Ofsted. [Accessed].

Oliver, M. 1981. A new model of the social work role in relation to disability. *In:* Campling, J. (ed.) *The handicapped person: a new perspective for social workers*, London: RADAR.

Oliver, M. 1990. Critical texts in social work and the welfare state the politics of disablement. Recuperado de. https://disability-studies. leeds.ac.uk/library/.

Oliver, M. 2013. The social model of disability: thirty years on. *Disability & Society*, 28, 1024–1026.

Palmer, M. 2011. Disability and poverty: a conceptual review. *Journal of Disability Policy Studies*, 21, 210–218.

Parsons, T. 1951. *The Social System*, England: Routledge.

Pelleboer-Gunnink, H. A., Van Oorsouw, W., Van Weeghel, J. & Embregts, P. 2017. Mainstream health professionals' stigmatising attitudes towards people with intellectual disabilities: a systematic review. *Journal of Intellectual Disability Research*, 61, 411–434.

Perry, B. L. 2011. The labeling paradox: stigma, the sick role, and social networks in mental illness. *Journal of Health and Social Behavior*, 52, 460–477.

Perry, B. L. & Pescosolido, B. A. 2012. Social network dynamics and biographical disruption: the case of "first-timers" with mental illness. *American Journal of Sociology*, 118, 134–175.

Pizzol, D., Trott, M., Butler, L., Barnett, Y., Ford, T., Neufeld, S. A. S., Ragnhildstveit, A., Parris, C. N., Underwood, B. R., López Sánchez, G. F., Fossey, M., Brayne, C., Fernandez-Egea, E., Fond, G., Boyer, L., Shin, J. I., Pardhan, S. & Smith, L. 2023. Relationship between severe mental illness and physical multimorbidity: a meta-analysis and call for action. *BMJ Mental Health*, 26, e300870.

Powell, A. 2024. *Disabled people in employment: Research Briefing*, House of Commons Library.

Powell, K. & Maguire, N. 2018. Paranoia and maladaptive behaviours in homelessness: the mediating role of emotion regulation. *Psychology and Psychotherapy: Theory, Research and Practice*, 91, 363–379.

Prah Ruger, J. & Mitra, S. 2015. *Health, disability and the capability approach: An introduction*, Taylor & Francis.

Qiu, N., Jiang, Y., Sun, Z. & Du, M. 2023. The impact of disability-related deprivation on employment opportunity at the neighborhood level: does family socioeconomic status matter? *Frontiers in Public Health*, 11, 1232829.

Reeve, D. 2020. Psycho-Emotional Disablism: The missing links? In: Watson, N. & Vehmas, S. (eds.) *Routledge Handbook of Disability Studies*, Routledge.

Reilly, S., Olier, I., Planner, C., Doran, T., Reeves, D., Ashcroft, D. M., Gask, L. & Kontopantelis, E. 2015. Inequalities in physical comorbidity: a longitudinal comparative cohort study of people with severe mental illness in the UK. *BMJ Open*, 5, e009010.

Richards, M. 2020. Whorlton Hall, Winterbourne… person-centred care is long dead for people with learning disabilities and autism. *Disability & Society*, 35, 500–505.

Ridley, M., Rao, G., Schilbach, F. & Patel, V. 2020. Poverty, depression, and anxiety: causal evidence and mechanisms. *Science*, 370.

Riemsma, R., Hagen, S., Kirschner-Hermanns, R., Norton, C., Wijk, H., Andersson, K.-E., Chapple, C., Spinks, J., Wagg, A., Hutt, E., Misso, K., Deshpande, S., Kleijnen, J. & Milsom, I. 2017. Can incontinence be cured? A systematic review of cure rates. *BMC Medicine*, 15, 63.

Rotenberg, S., Rodríguez Gatta, D., Wahedi, A., Loo, R., Mcfadden, E. & Ryan, S. 2022. Disability training for health workers: a global evidence synthesis. *Disability and Health Journal*, 15, 101260.

Russell, G., Stapley, S., Newlove-Delgado, T., Salmon, A., White, R., Warren, F., Pearson, A. & Ford, T. 2022. Time trends in autism diagnosis over 20 years: a UK population-based cohort study. *Journal of Child Psychology and Psychiatry*, 63, 674–682.

Ryan, S. 2017. *Justice for laughing boy: Connor Sparrowhawk-A death by indifference*, Jessica Kingsley Publishers.

Sakellariou, D. & Rotarou, E. S. 2017. Access to healthcare for men and women with disabilities in the UK: secondary analysis of cross-sectional data. *BMJ Open*, 7, e016614.

Sales, N. & Vincent, K. 2018. Strengths and limitations of the Education, Health and Care plan process from a range of professional and family perspectives. *British Journal of Special Education*, 45, 61–80.

Sanderson, T., Calnan, M., Morris, M., Richards, P. & Hewlett, S. 2011. Shifting normalities: interactions of changing conceptions of a normal life and the normalisation of symptoms in rheumatoid arthritis. *Sociology of Health & Illness*, 33, 618–633.

Sapiets, S. 2021. Valuing the views of children with a learning disability. Engaging with children and young people with severe or profound and multiple learning disabilities. The Challenging Behaviour Foundation/MENCAP. Available online at: https://www. challengingbehaviour.org.uk/wp-content/uploads/ 2021/03/Valuing-the-views-of-children-with-a-learning-disability. pdf.

Scior, K. & Werner, S. 2015. *Changing attitudes to learning disability: A review of the literature*. Mencap.

Scior, K. & Werner, S. 2016. *Intellectual Disability and Stigma: Stepping out from the Margines*, Springer Link.

Scott, K. M., Hastings, J. A. & Temme, K. E. 2021. 22 - Sexual Dysfunction And Disability. *In:* Cifu, D. X. (ed.) *Braddom's Physical Medicine and Rehabilitation (Sixth Edition)*, Philadelphia: Elsevier.

Scully, J. L. 2006. Disabled Embodiment And An Ethic Of Care. *In:* Rehmann-Sutter, C., Düwell, M. & Mieth, D. (eds.) *Bioethics in Cultural Contexts: Reflections on Methods and Finitude*, Dordrecht: Springer Netherlands.

Series, L. 2020. Disability and Human Rights. *In:* Watson, N. & Vehmas, S. (eds.) *Routledge Handbook of Disability Studies*, Routledge.

Shakespeare, T. 2017. *Disability: The Basics* Routledge.

Sharma, P. 2021. Barriers faced when eliciting the voice of children and young people with special educational needs and disabilities for their Education, Health and Care Plans and Annual Reviews. *British Journal of Special Education*, 48, 455–476.

Smith, B. & Sparkes, A. 2022. Disability, Sport, and Physical Activity. *In:* Watson, N. & Vehmas, S. (eds.) *Routledge Handbook of Disability Studies*, Routledge.

Stalker, K. 2022. Theorising the position of people with learning difficulties within disability studies. *In:* Watson, N. & Vehmas, S. (eds.) *Routledge Handbook of Disabilities Studies*, Routledge.

Stevenson, D. & Farmer, P. 2017. Thriving at Work: a review of mental health and employers. *Department for Work and Pensions.* https://assets. publishing.service.gov.uk/media/5a82180e40f0b6230269acdb/thriving-at-work-stevenson-farmer-review.pdf.

Strand, S. & Lindorff, A. 2018. Ethnic disproportionality in the identification of Special Educational Needs (SEN) in England: eExtent, causes and consequences. *Economic and Social Research Council.* Available online: https://www.education.ox.ac.uk/wp-content/ uploads/2018/08/Executive-Summary_2018-12-20.pdf.

Taberner, J. E. 2023. There are too many kids with special educational needs. *Frontiers in Education*, 8. Frontiers Media SA, 1125091.

Thomson, G. 1997. *Extraordinaty bodies: Figuring physical disability in America culture and literature*, New York: Columbia University Press.

Tinson, A., Aldridge, H., Born, T. B. & Hughes, C. 2016. *Disability and poverty. Why disability must be at the centre of poverty reduction*, York: New Policy Institute.

Tregaskis, C. 2002. Social Model Theory: the story so far. *Disability & Society*, 17, 457–470.

Trent, J. 2017. *Inventing the feeble mind: A history of intellectual disability in the United States*, Oxford University Press.

Trevillion, K., Stuart, R., Ocloo, J., Broeckelmann, E., Jeffreys, S., Jeynes, T., Allen, D., Russell, J., Billings, J., Crawford, M. J., Dale, O., Haigh, R., Moran, P., Mcnicholas, S., Nicholls, V., Foye, U., Simpson, A., Lloyd-Evans, B., Johnson, S. & Oram, S. 2022. Service user perspectives of community mental health services for people with complex emotional needs: a co-produced qualitative interview study. *BMC Psychiatry*, 22, 55.

Trollor, J. N., Eagleson, C., Turner, B., Tracy, J., Torr, J. J., Durvasula, S., Iacono, T., Cvejic, R. C. & Lennox, N. 2018. Intellectual disability content within tertiary medical curriculum: how is it taught and by whom? *BMC Medical Education*, 18, 182.

Trollor, J. N., Ruffell, B., Tracy, J., Torr, J. J., Durvasula, S., Iacono, T., Eagleson, C. & Lennox, N. 2016. Intellectual disability health content within medical curriculum: an audit of what our future doctors are taught. *BMC Medical Education*, 16, 105.

Tuffrey-Wijne, I., Finlayson, J., Bernal, J., Taggart, L., Lam, C. K. K. & Todd, S. 2020. Communicating about death and dying with adults with intellectual disabilities who are terminally ill or bereaved: a UK-wide survey of intellectual disability support staff. *Journal of Applied Research in Intellectual Disabilities*, 33, 927–938.

Uba, C. D. & Nwoga, K. A. 2016. Understanding stigma from a sociocultural context: mothers' experience of stigma directed towards children with special educational needs. *International Journal of Inclusive Education*, 20, 975–994.

UK Government 2014a. *Children and Families Act 2014*, Available online: UK Government. at: https://www.legislation.gov.uk/ukpga/2014/6/contents.

UK Government 2014b. *SEND code of practice: 0 to 25*, Available online: UK Government. at: https://www.gov.uk/government/publications/send-code-of-practice-0-to-25.

UN 2007. Convention on the Rights of Persons with Disabilities.

Underwood, K. 2008. *The Construction of Disability in our Schools: Teacher and Parent perspectives on the experience of labelled students*, Sense Publishers.

UPIAS 1976. *Fundamental Principles of Disability*, London: Union of the Physically Impaired Against Segregation.

Varul, M. Z. 2010. Talcott Parsons, the Sick Role and Chronic Illness. *Body & Society*, 16, 72–94.

Wagemans, A., Van Schrojenstein Lantman-De-Valk, H., Tuffrey-Wijne, I., Widdershoven, G. & Curfs, L. 2010. End-of-life decisions: an important theme in the care for people with intellectual disabilities. *Journal of Intellectual Disability Research*, 54, 516–524.

Watson, N. & Vehmas, S. 2022. *Routledge Handbook of Disabilities Studies*, Routledge.

White, R. G., Imperiale, M. G. & Perera, E. 2016. The Capabilities Approach: fostering contexts for enhancing mental health and wellbeing across the globe. *Globalization and Health*, 12, 16.

WHO 2011. World Report on Disability 2011.

WHO. 2023. Disability [Online]. World Health Organization. Available: https://www.who.int/news-room/fact-sheets/detail/disability-and-health [Accessed].

WHO. 2007. International Classification of Functioning, Disability and Health (ICF). Available online at: https://www.who.int/standards/classifications/international-classification-of-functioning-disability-and-health.

Wickenden, M. 2023. Disability and other identities?-how do they intersect? *Frontiers in Rehabilitation Sciences*, 4, 1200386.

Willis, D. 2020. Whorlton Hall, Winterbourne View and Ely Hospital: learning from failures of care. *Learning Disability Practice*, 23.

Wilson, M. C. & Scior, K. 2014. Attitudes towards individuals with disabilities as measured by the implicit association test: a literature review. *Research in Developmental Disabilities*, 35, 294–321.

Wolfenden, B. & Grace, M. 2012. Identity continuity in the face of biographical disruption: 'It's the same me'. *Brain Impairment*, 13, 203–211.

Woman And Equalities Committee 2024. Inequalities in healthcare and employment for people with a learning disability and autistic people. House of Commons. Available online at: https://committees.parliament.uk/publications/44825/documents/222674/default/.

Zajacova, A. & Lawrence, E. M. 2018. The relationship between education and health: reducing disparities through a contextual approach. *Annual Review of Public Health*, 39, 273–289.

PART 3

Understanding Health Behaviors, Health Behavior Change, and Public Health

CHAPTER 12

Understanding Unhealthy Behaviour

Chris Allen, Sam Woodnutt, and Gilly Mancz
School of Health Sciences, University of Southampton, Southampton, UK

Introduction

Our health behaviours (healthy and harmful) are known to contribute to our health outcomes. In Chapter 8, various factors such as social, cultural, psychological and economic were shown to contribute to an individual's likeliness, or disposition to follow certain health-enhancing as well as certain health-damaging behaviours. However, as we explore in this chapter, no single isolated factor explains why people engage in different behaviours. In the next two chapters, we will use theory to explain *why* people engage in unhealthy behaviours in the first place and then seek to understand *how* health behaviour change can be promoted through a range of evidence-based approaches. Then, in Chapter 14, we open up the moral and ethical debates that exist around whether governments should take action to promote behaviour change, or whether we should as a society, simply let people make their own choices. Because of this, these three chapters are best read together, especially the first two.

This first chapter is all about the *why*. Why, as individuals and as a society, do so many of us continue to do things such as over-consume unhealthy food, even when we know this might be harmful, and even when we are trying to cut back? The following two chapters are all about the *how*. How can healthcare professionals, and society more generally, change people's unhealthy behaviours? Understanding the *why* (this chapter), helps us better understand *how* best to support people to change their behaviours, within the social context in which they are practised, using evidence-based behaviour change strategies. Many of the theories and models that explain the *why*, also underpin consideration of the *how*, which are discussed in the following two chapters.

LEARNING OUTCOMES

By the end of this chapter, you will be able to:

- Identify the various influences and explanations for why people engage in behaviours that they know are unhealthy for them.
- Understand the various health behaviour theories that have been used to explain why people continue to engage in behaviours that are unhealthy.

What Are Unhealthy Behaviours?

> **Key Terms and Definitions**
>
> **Agency:** The capacity of an individual to be able to exercise control over their decisions and what they do.
>
> **Habitus:** How people see and respond to their social world in terms of their habits, behaviours and how they act.
>
> **Self-efficacy:** Generally relates to an individual's belief that they have the capability to do something.

Global burden of disease research consistently highlights the harmful impact of behaviours such as diet, inactivity, alcohol consumption and smoking on health (Afshin et al., 2019, Degenhardt et al., 2018, Katzmarzyk et al., 2022, Khan Minhas

---

Social Sciences for Healthcare Professionals, First Edition. Edited by Chris Allen.
© 2026 John Wiley & Sons Ltd. Published 2026 by John Wiley & Sons Ltd.

et al., 2024, Shield et al., 2020). Health behaviours such as these are known contributors to the genesis of many chronic conditions and are related to premature mortality and morbidity (Afshin et al., 2019, Åkesson et al., 2014, Ford et al., 2009, Kerr and Booth, 2022, Khan Minhas et al., 2024, Kvaavik et al., 2010, Matheson et al., 2012). The link between many of these behaviours and poorer morbidity and mortality is not in any way new. In fact, the links between poor diet, smoking and physical inactivity and increasing morbidity have been established through epidemiological research since at least the 1950s, in seminal studies such as the Framingham Heart studies (Andersson et al., 2019, Dawber et al., 1951), and several well-known studies of smoking outcomes including in doctors[1] (Doll and Hill, 1954, Doll et al., 2004). Now, it is widely recognised as an urgent situation that needs to be addressed, with the increasing strain that such behaviours and their resultant health impacts place on global healthcare systems, and the attendant financial and social impacts of this to individuals and to society (Hajat and Stein, 2018, Kazibwe et al., 2021, Murphy et al., 2019, Murphy et al., 2020). The causes of unhealthy behaviours, as we go on to discuss, are many and varied. Lifestyle and behaviour factors certainly do tend to be patterned by culture and socio-economic status, with those from disadvantaged groups being more likely to engage in harmful health behaviours for a variety of reasons, including as we will explore, factors outside of the control of individuals (Bartley, 2017, Katainen and Gronow, 2024, Weyers et al., 2010). However, there are other causes relating to individuals, and populations, that are also important to understand, often in the context of specific behaviours.

Diet

Our dietary needs differ across the life course, and in response to different health states (e.g. being pregnant), and different health conditions (for example, having diabetes) (Ley et al., 2014, Raghavan et al., 2019). Over many years, studies continue to consistently demonstrate the relationship between the quantity and quality of our diets and our health (Katz et al., 2018). The relationship between extremes of weight (i.e. either being very overweight or very underweight) and health is well understood (Bhaskaran et al., 2018, Flegal et al., 2013). Types and volumes of food consumption are often cited as problematic, with associated increased incidence and prevalence of overweight and obesity now an established health issue worldwide (Dai et al., 2020, Ng et al., 2014). The causes of obesity are complex but can be reduced to being caused by the energy (i.e. calories) someone consumes consistently outreaching what they use (Townshend and Lake, 2017). With healthier foods tending to be more expensive, food choice is often guided by what people can afford (Darmon and Drewnowski, 2015). There is also a likely evolutionary basis

for energy-dense food consumption (Ahlstrom et al., 2017). For example, for hunter-gatherers coming across a sizeable portion of energy-dense food was rare and they would have had few opportunities to store it for later consumption. Nor would they be able to predict when they might have access again, hence a large amount of food may be consumed all at once – but then often not again for a whilst. In modern times, energy-dense food is abundantly available in much of the world. But dietary influences often also relate to culture, and social influences, especially those around obesity (Katainen and Gronow, 2024). However, the many and varied determinants that underpin this, as with other health behaviours are complex, extend far beyond an individual's own choices and include a full range of broader determinants, often coined as the 'obesogenic environment' as shown in Figure 12.1 (Allender et al., 2015, Townshend and Lake, 2017).

The obesogenic environment serves as a useful reminder of the underlying complexity and influences of health behaviours (Allender et al., 2015). Establishing a true causal pathway for obesity is challenging, with so many factors contributing towards it across all levels of a society (Townshend and Lake, 2017), alongside established social network influences (Christakis and Fowler, 2007, Serrano Fuentes et al., 2019, 2022).

Activity Levels

As with other behaviours discussed here, our preferences and behaviours around physical activity are often determined by culture, and our social and community networks (Mötteli and Dohle, 2020). Research has highlighted that those who are physically inactive, are likely to be situated within social networks where such inactivity is also relatively normal (Mötteli and Dohle, 2020). As with diet, studies consistently demonstrate that physical inactivity is one of the leading risk factors for premature mortality and morbidity, such as type 2 diabetes, stroke, cardiovascular disease, mental ill health and many forms of cancer (Dai et al., 2020, Katzmarzyk et al., 2022). The World Health Organizations' recommendations for levels of physical activity vary across the life course, and there are different recommendations for different health states and conditions (WHO, 2024). However, it is generally recognised that people's lived environments as well as their access to social and material resources, can facilitate and constrain participation in physical activity (Müller et al., 2024).

Alcohol Consumption

As with other health behaviours, alcohol consumption is influenced by social and community networks (Rosenquist et al., 2010). Alcohol consumption, be it irregular, but heavy drinking (such as 'binge drinking'), or more frequent and consistent consumption can have a deleterious impact on health and well-being in different ways (Griswold et al., 2018, Roche

---

[1] These doctors were purposefully sampled due to the ease with which they could be recruited and followed up by researchers (Doll and Hill, 1954; Doll et al., 2004).

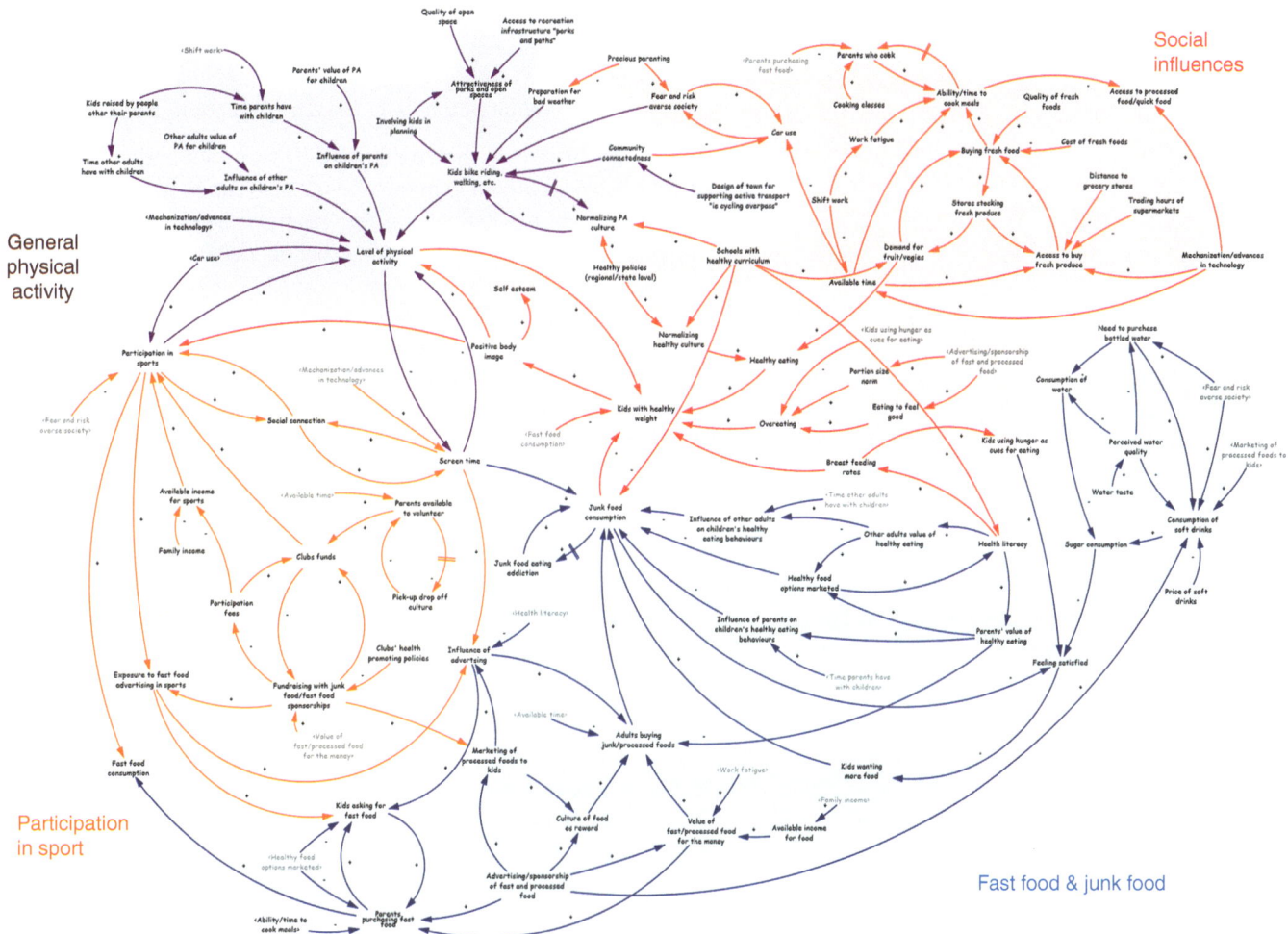

FIGURE 12.1   Causal loop diagram of causes of childhood obesity in the community. **Source:** Allender et al. (2015) / PLOS / CC BY 4.0.

et al., 2015). For example, binge drinking harms relate to intoxication and the accidents and injuries that might follow, both to the person consuming alcohol and to others (Sontate et al., 2021, Waller, 2020). In contrast, more frequent consumption can cause chronic illness, such as through damaging livers, and vascular and neurological systems (Biddinger et al., 2022, Cheungpasitporn et al., 2015, Kamal et al., 2020, Singal and Mathurin, 2021, Subramaniyan et al., 2021).

We know that the harms of drinking disproportionately fall on those experiencing some form of socio-economic disadvantage, with higher levels of alcohol-related harm being experienced in lower SES groups, even when patterns of consumption are broadly similar (Boyd et al., 2021, Katikireddi et al., 2017). Harmful alcohol consumption can also negatively impact on individuals' socio-economic status, through its effects (both physical and mental) and harmful impact on social relationships (those with alcohol use disorders typically have smaller social networks), employment and other domains of social life (Jørgensen et al., 2019, Mowbray et al., 2014). Those engaging in harmful alcohol consumption face stigma (see Chapter 9), that can serve to reduce their access to care and support services as well as limit access to broader socio-economic opportunities (Kumar et al., 2022).

Smoking

As with the other health behaviours we have discussed, smoking is associated with significant early mortality and morbidity (He et al., 2022, GBD Tobacco Collaborators, 2017). In fact, as recent policy papers have indicated, cigarettes are unique in being the one legal consumable that when used exactly as instructed, will kill most of its users, and unlike other behaviours discussed in this chapter, even infrequent use is harmful (Khan, 2022). The average smoker's life expectancy is around 10 years lower, and they are more likely to need ongoing care and support earlier in their lives than non-smokers (Doll et al., 2004, Khan, 2022, Pirie et al., 2013, Royal College of Physicians, 2018). As with other health behaviours, SES can act as a buffer to some degree, for example, evidence has suggested that the harms of smoking are disproportionately experienced by those with socio-economic status, but these differences in harms are not as significant as the gaps between smokers and non-smokers (Gruer et al., 2009). Despite it being widely accepted that smoking is harmful, a large number of people still smoke (Khan, 2022, Royal College of Physicians, 2018)

Many of those who smoke state that were they to be given the choice again, they would never have started. This underpins the highly addictive nature of tobacco smoking. In fact, evidence suggests that most smokers require more than 30 attempts to quit (Chaiton et al., 2016). These attempts are more likely if attempted with others (Christakis and Fowler, 2008; Nagawa et al., 2020), and as with the other behaviours considered here, social and community networks are highly influential in shaping smoking behaviours in the first place (Christakis and Fowler, 2008).

Why Do We Engage in Unhealthy Behaviour?

Our discussion has already given some strong teasers of the complex interconnected influences of health behaviours. Indeed, there are various factors (social, economic, psychological, cultural) that contribute to an individual's likeliness to follow certain healthy, or unhealthy behaviours (Allender et al., 2015, Bartley, 2017, Christakis and Fowler, 2013, Katainen and Gronow, 2024, McCartney et al., 2019, 2021, Wami et al., 2020, Williams, 2019). We also highlighted some of these in Chapter 8 when we considered the socio-determinants of health. People and society, as we have explored, are incredibly complex. People do not always behave in ways that seem rational, and behaviour is not always fully predictable; behaviours such as smoking and drinking that are now widely understood to cause harm are still widely practised.

Structure and Agency

It is sometimes useful to think about health behaviours in terms of social structures and individual agency. In considering health behaviours, understanding the extent to which someone perceives their behaviour as being harmful (both now and in the future), and how this relates to their decision-making is, of course, important to understand. There is a long history of seeing health behaviour through this lens – essentially seeing health behaviours as the product of conscious decision-making, in which personal barriers are considered, and potential consequences evaluated.

Stop and Think: Would People Be Surprised?

Let's consider that as part of a university module on health promotion, you have been asked to attend a town centre with information leaflets about smoking risks, and you have been encouraged to chat with people about these risks. As part of this activity, you have been asked to record if people were aware of the risks of smoking, and the potential impact it could have on their health. You were also asked to find out if people experienced any potential barriers.

- Are you likely to find **anyone** that was unaware of the risks?
- What potential barriers might people articulate?

Obviously, the extent to which the public understand the risks attached to their behaviours varies across different types of behaviour. For example, people may be less certain of the impact of other behaviours, such as vaping (Pepper et al., 2019), and misbeliefs do exist, for example, around the harms of vaccination (Bussink-Voorend et al., 2022). However, for many of the behaviours that are most harmful to our health (poor diet, inactivity, drinking, smoking, etc.), the health messaging is already very much out there. Therefore, when considering the root causes of unhealthy behaviours, it is worth underlining that these are far more *complex* than simply not having access to information on health impacts.

In addition, we might also want to consider how much control people have over their behaviour, and how much they enjoy it (sometimes referred to as positive affect). For example, to what extent can people control their impulses and their subsequent behaviour, and how much do individual personal characteristics account for and explain this? A lot of this we can directly observe (such as whether someone engages with a behaviour), alongside associative behavioural tendencies (much like Pavlov's dog, discussed in Chapter 4) whereby certain behaviours can be observed after certain exposures (Leung et al., 2014, Watson et al., 2016). However, many of the underpinning cognitive processes are harder to see (for example motivation and positive affect) but are still important in explaining why people do what they do. All of these individual-level considerations are clearly important in understanding an individual's agency; how much are they able to personally influence their own behaviour. However, we cannot look at these individual factors in isolation. People certainly have a choice about the behaviours they follow, but these choices are always (unless people are put into a controlled lab) influenced and constrained by their environment (the structure), as well as their own individual characteristics and their impact on control and decision making (their agency).

Health behaviours are generally practised within the constraints of social structures (Bartley, 2017, Katainen and Gronow, 2024). For example, as we have highlighted in this chapter, and explored in Chapter 8, there is a social pattern to health behaviours with those in higher socio-economic status groups tending to be more likely to follow health-enhancing behaviours, and less likely to engage in unhealthy ones (Pampel et al., 2010). The reverse is also true – lower socio-economic status groups are more likely to engage in unhealthy behaviours and less likely to engage in health-enhancing ones (Bartley, 2017, Katainen and Gronow, 2024). People's social context – their families and personal networks of support, their socio-economic status and access to resources, their culture and their geography are also all highly relevant (Glanz et al., 2024, McCartney et al., 2019, 2021, Wami et al., 2020). Whilst we cannot overlook that social structures play a key role in health behaviours, other factors such as the knowledge an individual has about the behaviour and its impact, their attitudes, how well they manage stress and how motivated they are all have relevance in shaping behaviours (Glanz et al., 2024). In the following sections, we will review the ways health behaviour is currently explained and understood–both in the context of individuals, as well as in groups.

Social Structure

Habitus and People's Cultural and Social Environments

As we explored in Chapter 8, recent work has attempted to show the underlying processes and mechanisms that account for why those in lower socio-economic status groups, are more likely to engage in unhealthy behaviours across the life course (McCartney et al., 2019, Wami et al., 2020). This work has provided some useful visualisations of these underlying social processes and mechanisms, and these are shown in Figure 12.2.

Our early childhood, including the opportunities that we have available to us, our class and the cultures we are exposed to, influences who we are, and how we behave (McCartney et al., 2019, Wami et al., 2020). Culture and class are highly significant, playing a role in even the clothes we wear, the music we enjoy and the identity markers or symbols we have (Bourdieu, 2018). These factors also influence our health behaviours and once established, can be particularly challenging to change throughout the life course, and often result in significant inequalities in health being experienced (Bartley, 2017). But this all occurs within a broader social system that shapes the relative power and influence of people from different social classes (McCartney et al., 2019, Wami et al., 2020). This allows individuals and groups to be discriminated or marginalised, which can also shape health behaviours, and constrain people's efforts to follow healthier lifestyles (McCartney et al., 2019, Wami et al., 2020), especially where tactics of 'social closure' and 'opportunity hoarding' (discussed in Chapter 6) are deployed by dominant classes, to the detriment of those in lower socioeconomic status groups, who end up having more restricted access to such opportunities and more restricted access to well-paid and meaningful labour market opportunities (Weber, 1978). As well as this, market conditions also powerfully shape people's health behaviours, and sometimes companies promoting harmful behaviours, particularly aggressively target lower-status groups. It is the behaviours of these companies, who we now turn our attention too, as they can have a significant role in influencing the health behaviours of a society.

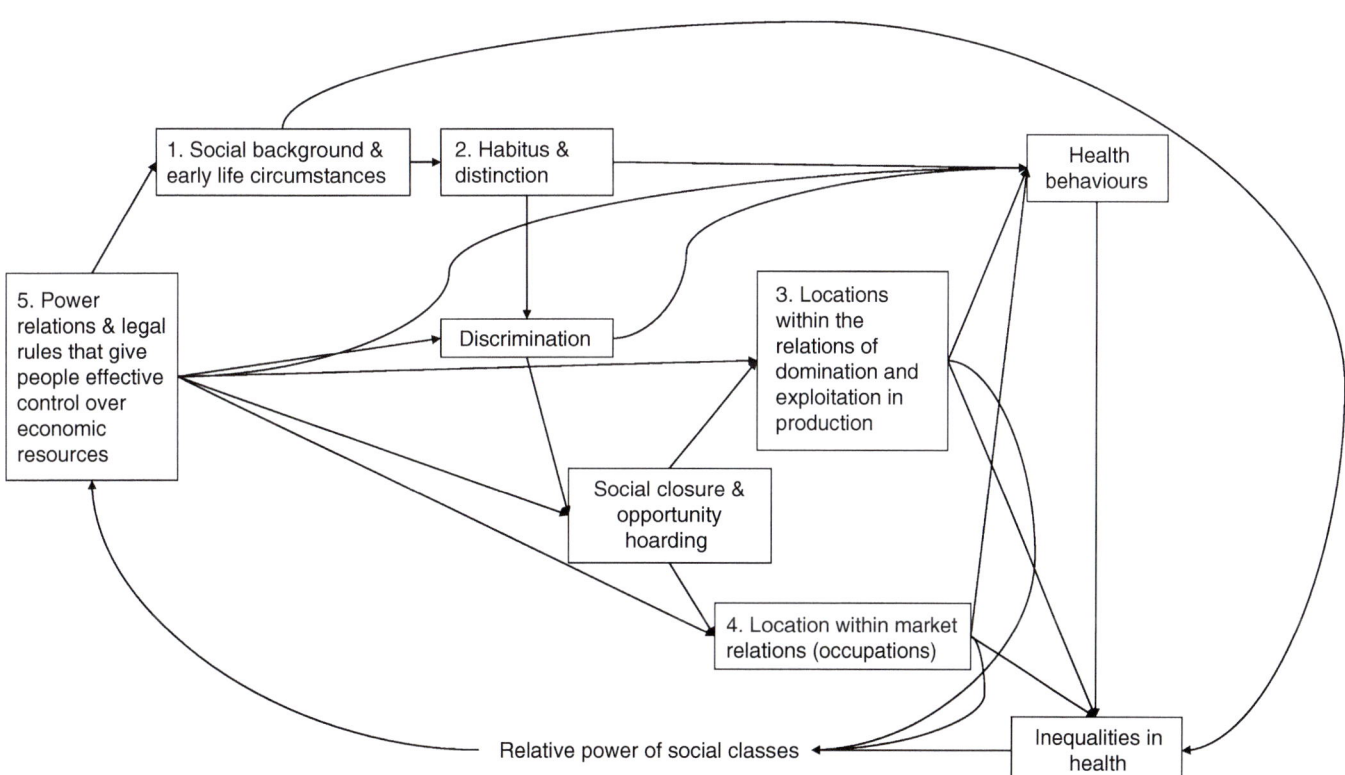

FIGURE 12.2 How class relations explain inequalities in health outcomes. **Source:** Wami et al. (2020) / Springer Nature / CC BY 4.0.

The Commercial Determinants of Health

As we explored in Chapter 8, we know that the conditions in which we are born, where we grow up, where we live, work and age, have a significant impact on our health and our well-being (Bartley, 2017, Marmot, 2010, Marmot et al., 2008, 2020). As too does the consumption of unhealthy commodities such as foods that are high in fat, sugar or salt, tobacco, and alcohol, which as we have highlighted are inequitably consumed. Commercialisation, and the commercial determinants of health, shape our behaviours (both positively and negatively) and our environments across the life course (Gilmore et al., 2023, Kickbusch et al., 2016, WHO, 2023). Whilst no uniform definition exists, definitions of the commercial determinants of health generally point towards the mismatch between companies striving to maximise profits (of which many in a society do rely on – e.g., for employment, income, investments, etc.), with a societies need to improve population health and well-being (Gilmore et al., 2023, Kickbusch et al., 2016). The role industry has on health behaviours, has even led to claims of 'industrial epidemics', or 'profit-driven diseases' (Gilmore et al., 2023). Of course, it should not be forgotten that businesses often play a vitally important role in the promotion of health too, and many of the advances in healthcare that societies now enjoy (some of which are expanded upon in Chapter 20) are through the work and innovation that takes part within sometimes highly profitable companies (including, e.g. the COVID-19 vaccination, albeit potentially exacerbating inequality) (Freeman et al., 2023). However, Kickbusch et al. (2016) highlight that wealth creation is often prioritised over health creation, and this is particularly the case with unhealthy commodities, such as the production and sale of tobacco. In particular, the commercial determinants of health reflect organisations' influence on population health through their influence on behaviours (availability, cost, marketing, desirability, etc.), and the social environments in which people live, and ultimately shape health outcomes through:

- **Marketing:** Companies are known to use aggressive marketing strategies, including towards children to promote their products, which enhances both their desirability and their acceptability in the populations they target (Cairns et al., 2013, Freudenberg and Galea, 2008, Ireland et al., 2019, Knai et al., 2018, Savell et al., 2015). Marketing has the capacity to change our social norms, normalising the consumption of harmful products (Petticrew et al., 2020).
- **Lobbying governments and policymakers:** To object, undermine, influence and sometimes delay government attempts to address health behaviours using many of the strategies expanded upon in Chapter 14, such as decisions taken to curb consumption, through taxes, minimum pricing, regulations and legislation around who can buy the product, how the product can be marketed and how the product must be packaged (Kickbusch et al., 2016).

- **Globalisation and supply chains:** This has been both good and bad. In terms of positives, this has increased the supply of products, which includes the range of options that are available to people (some of which are healthy). However, it has also increased the supply of unhealthy products to consumers (e.g. McDonalds, etc. popping up in countries that in a now bygone era, did not have much exposure to fast food). High supply can also lead to competition, and the driving down of prices and discounting of unhealthy products, making them more *affordable* (Kickbusch et al., 2016). Sometimes product availability can also be tied to certain groups. For example, the density and therefore exposure of outlets selling tobacco and alcohol is often higher in lower socio-economic status areas – a deliberate targeting of vulnerability, through seeking to profit from increased demand (for several reasons) in these areas (Caryl et al., 2020, Shortt et al., 2015). One study that used GPS data to track exposure, found that children in more deprived areas had up to 7 times more tobacco exposure than those living in less deprived areas (Caryl et al., 2020).
- **Corporate social responsibility:** Many companies have made explicit that they practice within a corporate social responsibility framework (Petticrew et al., 2020). However, critics have argued that these tactics are often deployed as a smokescreen strategy for buffing against a company's poor public image (Dorfman et al., 2012, Petticrew et al., 2020). Companies often want to paint themselves as part of the solution, rather than the locus of the issue (Petticrew et al., 2020). For example, for those producing very harmful substances, such as tobacco, the most socially responsible thing for that company to do, would surely be to cease its production of tobacco.

Personal and Individual Level Factors

Addiction and Habits

Early understanding of health behaviours, and in particular theories such as the health beliefs model (discussed later in this chapter), tended to suggest that the decision of whether to engage in a certain health behaviour or not, involved deliberative and conscious decision-making, taking into account what is involved, what potential barriers might be faced and what the potential consequences to behaviours may be (Glanz et al., 2024, Glanz and Bishop, 2010). Essentially intentional actions are driven by conscious decisions about the behaviour (i.e. things we have had the opportunity to think about and don't just do habitually, or impulsively). However, a lot of our health behaviours are governed by unconscious cognitive processes and actions (Gardner et al., 2022). We often do things in response to our situation and our environments automatically – without really thinking about what it is we are actually doing (Orbell and Verplanken, 2010). We touched on some of this in Chapter 4 in relation to behaviourism. Classical conditioning and behaviourism suggest that we can develop associations between actions or behaviours and emotions. Some of the habits we form are 'healthy' or 'functional' and some are 'unhealthy' or 'dysfunctional'. However, for many habits, consumption is unhealthy regardless of the relationship we form with it – for example, smoking, illicit substance misuse or alcohol excess. With an addiction, the relationship rather than the behaviour can be more important. For example, an addiction to exercise could lead to detrimental health effects as much as an addiction to an unhealthy substance (Berczik et al., 2012).

In the following sections, we will explore addiction. Within the confines of this chapter, we do not have the scope to discuss all that is known about addiction (this subject fills entire textbooks). We will have the opportunity to consider how it relates to behaviour though. Many of the same principles that apply to addiction to substances such as alcohol or illicit drugs, also apply to other non-chemical addictions (e.g. gambling). However, the inner psychological mechanisms are often easier to see, when they do not involve intoxicating substances, which bring with them their own physiological and psychological impacts (Wackernah et al., 2014, Wikler, 2013).

But first, what is addiction? Addiction is complex, and there have been several proposed definitions for it (West and Brown, 2013). Literature on addiction generally points towards two aspects of addiction. These are: *dependence* and *compulsion* (West and Brown, 2013). First, dependence refers to a feeling or urge to seek relief from internal discomfort through enacting a given behaviour (such as taking a drug). Compulsion, on the other hand, refers to an inability to control the urges, and continuation of the behaviour despite known negative consequences (e.g. drug-taking with known legal/health consequences, or harmful alcohol consumption, etc.) (Koob and Volkow, 2010).

For some addictions, there are more obvious neurochemical processes that reinforce and make repeated behaviour more likely. For example, alcohol use can bring about drug-related effects on the brain and the formation of an addiction (Miller, 2013, Verheul and van den Brink, 2000). Alcohol is a psychoactive substance that acts on neurotransmitters (the chemicals that nerves use to carry signals) in the brain, specifically gamma-aminobutyric acid (GABA) and glutamate (Vengeliene et al., 2008). Alcohol use essentially disrupts the brain's use of these neurotransmitters, and as such is associated with feeling calm and happy (alongside other disruptions such as impaired balance, speech and judgement depending on the dose). However, prolonged use can change the way the body stores and releases these neurochemicals, resulting in dependency (Davis and Wu, 2001, Miller, 2013). When people are alcohol dependent, they cannot just stop drinking even if they want to as this could result in harm (Hillbom et al., 2003). Those who are dependent on alcohol, generally require healthcare professional support and often require medication (that acts on the brain), to support them in reducing consumption slowly, rather than abruptly (Kumar et al., 2009).

> ### Stop and Think: Who Is More Predisposed to Alcohol Excess
>
> Now that you know that alcohol has a potentially calming and uplifting effect on the brain, who do you think may be more vulnerable to using alcohol excessively, and even developing an addiction to it and why?
>
> You might have considered the following:
>
> - People with anxiety
> - People with stressful or chaotic jobs/lives
> - People who have experienced trauma
> - People without other ways of managing their emotions or stress

Addiction can also occur through reward-seeking behaviours. This is generally the case where behaviours do not involve external chemicals (such as alcohol or drugs) influencing the brain, and these are generally related more to emotional states, with the body releasing its own internal chemicals in response to these (Keren et al., 2018). For example: exercise addiction. Although exercise (in moderation) has an overall positive effect on health, excessive exercise likely has adverse physiological and psychological effects (Weinstein and Weinstein, 2014). Exercise at certain intensities is associated with the release of endorphins (which are associated with feelings of euphoria and happiness, i.e. positive affect, see below), which have shown to have benefits on a range of health conditions (Tripathi et al., 2023). However, someone who develops a dependency on exercise, and then feels a compulsion to seek relief, reward or happiness through exercise (despite there being negative health outcomes associated with the intensity or amount of exercise they are doing) is at risk of developing an addiction to exercise. The neurochemical processes underlying other behavioural addictions such as gambling (Conversano et al., 2012) and sex (Chatzittofis et al., 2022) are thought to be similar. The development of an addiction is currently considered to be a complex interplay between what is being consumed or what behaviours are being enacted, someone's individual characteristics including their traits, and a person's environment (MacKillop and Ray, 2017), which we discuss later.

Hedonism and Affective Responses

Anyone who has tussled with changing a behaviour will likely relate to the good and bad feelings that go with these. Chips or French fries are after all, for most people, quite tasty. Obviously, other cognitive processes underpin our decision to eat chips (otherwise eating chips is all we would do), but one of the most powerful amongst these is arguably the pleasure people get from their consumption. Our previous enjoyment of eating unhealthy foods makes us more likely to eat them again (Glanz et al., 2024, Williams, 2019). At least some of this positive affect may come from the environments such consumption occurs in (such as a meal with friends or drinks at a pub). Likewise, a lot of what we need to do to be healthier, for many people isn't particularly enjoyable, for example, cycling in busy and dangerous traffic. Clearly at least a part of this lack of enjoyment is related to the environment in which people are often forced to exercise in, making what could otherwise be enjoyable, unpleasant. However, previous lack of enjoyment, also makes us less likely to do that activity again (Glanz et al., 2024, Williams, 2019).

We can think of these affective responses as rewards and reinforcement, and these, at least in part, do guide our behaviours (Glanz et al., 2024, Williams, 2019). Indeed, our affective responses are important aspects of reinforcement theories of addiction and other potentially harmful types of consumption and can be considered as affective determinants of health behaviours (Williams and Evans, 2014). Though clearly there is more going on here than just us liking some things and not liking others. Whilst interest in affective states and behaviour is not new (e.g. it underpins the work of early philosophers and economists such as Jeremy Bentham), academic research now seeks to understand how positive and negative affect can influence our self-regulation and impulses, decision-making and subsequent health behaviours (Glanz et al., 2024, Williams, 2019). It is also widely recognised that in relation to what we consume, we discount the future heavily. This means that we generally prefer smaller short-term rewards (such as the short-term joy of eating chips), over longer-term, larger rewards (such as being a healthy weight) (Kakoschke et al., 2023). This same relationship exists for uncomfortable activities, that might benefit us in the future (like going for a run in the wind and rain) (Kakoschke et al., 2023). There is likely an evolutionary basis to why we discount the future so heavily (Ahlstrom et al., 2017; Kakoschke et al., 2023).

Personality and Behaviour

Whilst being cautious not to overlook the broader social determinants that have so much impact on the behaviours people adopt, it is relevant to highlight the work of social scientists, particularly health psychologists, who have attempted to understand the impact of people's personalities, including the commonly discussed 'big 5' personality traits (notably extraversion, conscientiousness, openness to experience, agreeableness and neuroticism) on health-enhancing and health-harming behaviours, to understand who might be more predisposed to certain harmful behaviours or conversely health-enhancing behaviours (Hampson et al., 2007, Joyner et al., 2018, Joyner and Loprinzi, 2018, Kim, 2016, Turiano et al., 2018, Umberson et al., 2010). In particular, the health behaviour model of personality provides one framework for understanding health behaviours in the context of personality (Smith, 2006). Widely used, the 'big 5' personality traits pop up in all sorts of studies examining people's behaviours in a range of different social contexts, for example, within this book they are also briefly covered in the context of leadership and teamwork. You will already be familiar with many of these, as they form the basis of everyday conversations about people and what they are like. For example, many of you will quickly know what extraversion is, and will already have some idea about what extraverted (or conversely introverted) people are like and how they behave. Essentially, the 'big 5' traits are as follows:

- **Conscientiousness:** Generally, refers to how disciplined, goal-orientated, responsible and reliable a person is, and can include their ability to control their impulses (Gartland et al., 2021, Turiano et al., 2018).
- **Neuroticism:** Generally, those with high neuroticism are seen as being less emotionally stable, more anxious and less able to control and manage their emotions, as well as being more likely to be negatively impacted by stress (Turiano et al., 2018).
- **Agreeableness:** Is essentially how prosocial someone is – how cooperative and empathetic they are towards others (Turiano et al., 2018).
- **Extraversion:** Those with high extraversion are often described as being outgoing, highly sociable and energetic. In contrast, introverts tend to be quieter and more inhibited in their behaviours, especially in groups (Turiano et al., 2018).
- **Openness to experience:** How open to new experiences people are. Those with low levels of openness to experience may have a narrower range of interests and may be less likely to seek out new activities (Turiano et al., 2018).

Unsurprisingly, especially in the context of impulse control, those who have high levels of conscientiousness have been argued to be more likely to follow health-enhancing behaviours (Bogg and Roberts, 2004, Gartland et al., 2021, O'Connor, 2020). In addition, those with high neuroticism are also more likely to follow health-harming behaviour, especially through the adoption of maladaptive coping strategies (Rochefort et al., 2019), but conversely, may also be more health vigilant, especially when combined with conscientiousness (Graham et al., 2020).

Theoretical Models of Health Behaviour

Stop and Think: Unhealthy Behaviour and Theory in Action

Case Study 1 – Jamal

Jamal is a 30-year-old truck driver. Once in great shape, since injuring his back several years ago, his levels of activity have decreased significantly. His job involves very long hours, and he is away from home often, generally working a range of very unsociable shifts. Often restricted in terms of the food that he can access when on the road, he generally eats food from the various fast food vendors who serve the nation's network of roads. Often at these vendors, he is able to eat with other long-haul drivers, a few of whom have become regular contacts, especially those who are a similar age. He enjoys the burger and fries that they serve and likes eating this in the company of his new friends, in between long periods of relative isolation whilst behind the wheel.

Case Study 2 – Rita

Rita is 58 years old and has smoked for most of her adult life. She has recently been diagnosed with COPD and has been strongly encouraged to quit smoking. She currently finds most physical activity tough. She has attended a pulmonary rehabilitation class following her diagnosis and this has helped her manage her breathlessness, especially on exertion. She is keen to do some more exercise and has co-opted some of the other pulmonary rehabilitation attendees to go with her on a Tuesday morning. However, she isn't sure if she needs to give up smoking. She enjoys it, has already been diagnosed with COPD anyway, and now that she knows how to manage her breathlessness better, she is not sure why she even needs to give it up.

Having read the two case studies, as you step through the following theories, combined with the discussion thus far, consider how the relevant theories might be used to explain why Jamal and Rita might find it so hard to change their established behaviours.

As we explored in Chapter 2, a theory is simply a set of interrelated concepts that seek to make sense of an event or to make predictions about how events or situations might unfold in the future. In the context of health behaviour theory, there are several explanatory models that have relevance to our understanding of *why* people engage in certain behaviours that might be detrimental to their health and well-being; often even when they recognise that this behaviour may be harmful to themselves, and even others around them (Glanz et al., 2024, Glanz and Bishop, 2010).

As with other theories, health behaviour theories often have relatively similar general ideas; albeit using different terminologies and having different focuses (Glanz et al., 2024, Glanz and Bishop, 2010, Williams, 2019). As we showed in Chapter 2, good theories can give us hints about what to look at and can be tested in a variety of contexts. Many of these theories have formed the basis of the interventions that are discussed in the following chapters.

We do not have scope to explore every theory that is relevant to unhealthy behaviour within this chapter, but we will summarise some of the most influential ones – including the

Health Belief Model (Rosenstock, 1966, 1974a), and the Social Cognitive Theory (Bandura and Cervone, 2023). These are all examples of explanatory theories as they help us to understand why people do what they do. Most explanatory models and theories of health behaviour include a focus on cognition (beliefs, motivations, etc.) (Williams, 2019).

Many health behaviour models include consideration of expectancies and their values when explaining behaviour. For example, people may be more likely to eat more fruit and vegetables, if they believe it will reduce their risk of morbidity and mortality (Glanz et al., 2024, Williams, 2019). We might think of this as an 'outcome expectancy'. I follow *this* behaviour, and this is the outcome I *expect*. 'Outcome values' are also important. How much are the expected outcomes valued? The more value derived from such expectancies, the more likely someone is to follow a healthy behaviour (Glanz et al., 2024, Williams, 2019). Generally, people are more likely to change their behaviour *if* they believe their behaviour will result in a positive outcome AND *if* they value that expected outcome. For example, 'eating less doughnuts and chips (substitute for any energy-dense food of your choice), will help me lose weight, and I value being a healthy weight'. 'By smoking less, I will get less out of breath when I go swimming, and I value being able to go swimming without feeling short of breath'. Not believing that eating less doughnuts and chips will help weight loss, or that smoking cessation will improve breathlessness, or not valuing weight loss, or more comfortable swimming, will likely result in no change in behaviour. However, this does not fully explain health behaviour, because most recognise that if they follow a better diet/engage with smoking cessation, they will be able to be healthier, and most people value their health – yet doughnuts and chips are still consumed and smoking remains popular, as do many other unhealthy behaviours. There is therefore a need to move beyond a simple expectancy value formulation, and theories and models generally also emphasise the importance of people's behavioural *motivations*, *intentions* and *goals*. They also often emphasis a social component, which is often tied to social values and beliefs, as well as a social efficacy component (essentially the belief that a change is possible) (Bandura and Cervone, 2023, Glanz et al., 2024, Glanz and Bishop, 2010, Williams, 2019). Rather than just expecting that a behaviour will elicit a positive outcome, and valuing this outcome, changing behaviour involves the motivation, intention and deliberative goal setting to make a change *actually* happen (Glanz et al., 2024, Williams, 2019). And importantly, it really helps if the intended behaviour does not involve resisting social norms (such as if all your friends smoke), and if people have access to people in their social networks who will be supportive of a change and may wish to change their behaviour too (Christakis and Fowler, 2013). People are far more likely to change their behaviour when they do this alongside others (Christakis and Fowler, 2013, Umberson et al., 2010) and social influences can influence someone's beliefs about whether a change is *actually* possible (i.e. their levels of self-efficacy).

Health Belief Model

The health beliefs model emerged in the 1950s and was initially developed to help understand why people pursue behaviours that they know or are told are harmful (Rosenstock, 1966). The model arose through concerns at the time that people were not readily taking up disease prevention or detection programmes (most notably at the time, for Tuberculosis), despite such programmes being highlighted as beneficial and despite them typically incurring no, or only a very nominal cost (Rosenstock, 1974b).

The health beliefs model can also help us to make sense of situations such as those shown in the Volvo case study provided. Why do people continue to engage in unhealthy behaviours when they know the risks involved (dying in a car crash), and what they are being advised to change might seem relatively insignificant (putting on a seat belt)? The model attempts to capture the cognitive processes that make a given behaviour more or less attractive (Glanz et al., 2024, Glanz and Bishop, 2010). Its key considerations can be broken down into the *threat* of the illness or disease as understood through the individual's perceived likelihood of experiencing a health issue, and the perceived severity and consequences of experiencing the health issue – as well as the perceived benefits and barriers to changing established behaviours in response to such concerns (Abraham and Sheeran, 2015, Glanz et al., 2024, Glanz and Bishop, 2010, Williams, 2019). The model can also help us to think about what might need to change to make a desired health behaviour more attractive. One significant limitation of the model is it does not account for behaviours that are habitual, or even addictive, as it principally thinks about behaviours as being conscious and deliberative.

Case Study: Volvo, the Three-Point Safety Belt and Diffusion of Innovations Theory

The three-point safety belt has a relatively interesting history, especially in the context of behaviour – and questions around why people do not do things that they know could save their life that require very little effort and very little discomfort. The three-point safety belt was initially designed by engineer Nils Bohlin in the 1950s (Bell, 2021). As far as public health innovations go, few have saved as many lives as the three-point safety belt. Volvo, the owners of the technology having invested significantly in it, rather than seeking to make a profit from it (i.e. exercising corporate social responsibility) opted instead to make their technology available to other car manufacturers for free (Bell, 2021). Great news then, a new technology, that could significantly improve people's chances of survival in a crash, increasingly available, and being more comfortable than previous seat belts, were arguably more likely to be worn (Bell, 2021).

But did people use them? No. At least not initially. Sometimes people just do not act rationally.

Changing practices around seatbelt use followed sustained public health campaigns and legislative actions to mandate their use. Even now, cars are built with technologies that force use, through playing irritating noises, etc., until the occupant eventually concedes (by putting on their seatbelt). Ultimately, people find it hard to adopt new ways of behaving, even when the benefits are clear, and what is being asked from them is very minimal.

How to Make Sense of This to Support Uptake

There are a few theories for behaviour that can help us understand people's behaviours in cases such as this. The most widely known are the Health Belief Model, as well as Rogers' seminal Diffusion of Innovations theory (Rogers et al., 2014). We expand on the latter in Chapter 20 in the context of innovations. The speed at which an innovation is adopted by a society relates to many things, including relative advantage (is it seen as better than what already exists), compatibility (is it compatible with people's needs, values and expectations) and observability (can the benefits be seen) (Rogers and Shoemaker, 1971, Rogers et al., 2014).

Social Cognitive Theory

Social cognitive theory has been used across the social health sciences, and in a range of clinical and educational contexts (Luszczynska and Schwarzer, 2020). The theory was developed from social learning theory, which suggests that individuals want to be active and engaged in controlling what happens to them, that reciprocal interactions between behaviours and their influencing and controlling conditions underpin human behaviour; essentially behaviours are influenced and learned through observing others (Bandura, 1971). In addition, the theory identifies two key concepts that directly and indirectly influence behaviours, these are: self-efficacy and outcomes expectations. We will explore this theory in greater depth in the following chapter, as it forms the basis of some commonly used health behaviour interventions.

The Social Ecological Model

Taking a broader focus, but still consistent with social cognitive concepts, are Social Ecological models of behaviour, that arose through various studies of behaviours in urban environments.

These studies generally sought to explain the dynamic interplay of various personal and environmental factors on behaviours and human development, highlighting the relevance of creating environments that are promote healthier behaviours and lifestyles (Glanz et al., 2024, Williams, 2019). The Socioecological framework takes a broader perspective on health behaviours, highlighting that whilst cognitive and social factors are important, health behaviours are in fact practised within a far more complex and multi-layered open system. Essentially, socioecological theories highlight that it is not enough to believe a change will lead to positive outcomes, value these positive outcomes, have the motivation and intention to follow through on the proposed change, believe you can do it, and have support, if the overarching social environment is not supportive of the change. For example, believing that swimming will bring about improved health, valuing this outcome, and having the belief and social support to do this, will still not be possible if there are no accessible and affordable swimming facilities or open water, where people can safely swim, as well as the broader social, political and economic influences that increase the likelihood of publicly available, affordable and accessible swimming facilities being made available to those who want to and can swim. Likewise, cutting back on the doughnuts and chips requires access to healthy, accessible, affordable and desirable alternative food options, which reflects the social environments that people live and work in, alongside the commercial determinants of health that we discussed earlier.

Urie Brofenbreener's (1917–2005) seminal 'ecological systems theory'; or 'ecological framework for human development' suggests a **systems approach** is useful for understanding human behaviours and development (Bronfenbrenner, 2000, Glanz et al., 2024, Williams, 2019). Whilst we have highlighted individual factors that have been examined, particularly in the field of psychology, we have emphasised throughout this book, and this chapter, the importance of social structure and social context in shaping what people do and how they behave. Bronfenbrenner's work was underpinned by the concern that it is not appropriate to study how people (in the original context children) behave, exclusively in a lab, where behaviour is manipulated and studied, causing them to potentially do some 'strange things, in response to strange situations'. These behaviours often poorly reflect real-life behaviour, and how it develops within everyday settings and contexts, where more varied and diverse influences exist and cannot be easily controlled or manipulated (Glanz et al., 2024, Williams, 2019). In early work, Bronfenbrenner highlighted that individual factors (such as biological and genetic factors) cannot alone explain behaviour and human development, highlighting the importance of examining broader (interpersonal, cultural, organisational, environmental, political, economic, etc.) social influences in understanding what we do and how we behave (Bronfenbrenner, 2000, Williams, 2019).

Our behaviours are determined by not just our own biology, and personal characteristics, but also our social networks (expanded upon in Chapter 15), as well as the broader social environment in which we live and work, and the impact of the political environment (discussed in Chapters 5 and 14) and the commercial determinants of health (discussed earlier in this chapter). Behaviours are both shaped by and ultimately shape the social environment. When harmful commodities are more available in areas facing higher levels of deprivation, they are more likely to be consumed, and their consumption in turn, increases their supply to meet a perceived local demand, as one example. Likewise, our own health behaviours, as we explore in a later chapter, influence the behaviours of others. In addition, where lots of people are following behaviours that are harmful to themselves and broader society, governments might be prompted to take action to restrict, or disincentivise consumption, using some of the strategies we will explore in Chapter 14. Essentially, social-ecological modules (of which there are several) highlight a whole cocktail of a person's various personal and social influences and exposures, in which everything is connected, and which generally occur across several interrelated systems that all shape and influence one another; not too dissimilar to the obesogenic environments, that we used to highlight how many things within a society contribute to obesity at the start of this chapter.

Whilst the Socioecological Framework is useful in highlighting the myriads of biological, psychological, social, cultural economic and political impacts on people's behaviour, it is not possible to use it to determine exactly how all these factors interact and hang together (which is most relevant, etc.) to shape what people do. It does however allow us to consider things from an 'upstream' perspective (discussed in Chapter 14). Through this, we can consider not only what individuals do, but also how societies shape what they do. Of course, though, this does move us away from important personal factors that may also relate to behaviour, such as positive affect (enjoying a behaviour), motivation and belief to change.

Clinical Considerations

- Those in lower socio-economic status groups are more likely to engage in unhealthy behaviours, but these behaviours are often engaged with, in challenging social contexts.
- People's health behaviours are determined by many things, many of which lie outside of an individual's personal control.
- For an individual to change their behaviour, they must:
  - Have *expectations* about the outcomes associated with their changing behaviour;
  - *Value* these outcomes;
  - Have positive *support* and strategies to avoid unwanted negative *social influence*;
  - *Believe* that it is possible to change their behaviour;
  - As well as having access to the resources, and an environment that enables the change.

Conclusion

In this chapter, we have explored why people engage in behaviours that they know are unhealthy (such as smoking, drinking harmful levels of alcohol, diet and inactivity) and that are known to contribute to the global burden of disease and early mortality. We have looked at this in the context of people's agency and the choices that they make, as well as the impact the social environment has on behaviour, including some consideration of the commercial determinants of health. Several theories have been introduced, including the Health Beliefs Model and Social Cognitive Theory, which have been used to help explain people's behaviours. In the next chapter, we build on this, to explore some evidence-based interventions for how behaviour change can be supported in those wanting to change their behaviours.

References

Abraham, A. & Sheeran, P. 2015. The health belief model. *In:* Conner, M. & Norman, P. (eds.) *Predicting and Changing Health Behaviour*, Open University Press.

Afshin, A., Sur, P. J., Fay, K. A., Cornaby, L., Ferrara, G., Salama, J. S., Mullany, E. C., Abate, K. H., Abbafati, C., Abebe, Z., Afarideh, M., Aggarwal, A., Agrawal, S., Akinyemiju, T., Alahdab, F., Bacha, U., Bachman, V. F., Badali, H., Badawi, A., Bensenor, I. M., Bernabe, E., Biadgilign, S. K. K., Biryukov, S. H., Cahill, L. E., Carrero, J. J., Cercy, K. M., Dandona, L., Dandona, R., Dang, A. K., Degefa, M. G., El Sayed Zaki, M., Esteghamati, A., Esteghamati, S., Fanzo, J., Farinha, C. S. E. S., Farvid, M. S., Farzadfar, F., Feigin, V. L., Fernandes, J. C., Flor, L. S., Foigt, N. A., Forouzanfar, M. H., Ganji, M., Geleijnse, J. M., Gillum, R. F., Goulart, A. C., Grosso, G., Guessous, I., Hamidi, S., Hankey, G. J., Harikrishnan, S., Hassen, H. Y., Hay, S. I., Hoang, C. L., Horino, M., Ikeda, N., Islami, F., Jackson, M. D., James, S. L., Johansson, L., Jonas, J. B., Kasaeian, A., Khader, Y. S., Khalil, I. A., Khang, Y.-H., Kimokoti, R. W., Kokubo, Y., Kumar, G. A., Lallukka, T., Lopez, A. D., Lorkowski, S., Lotufo, P. A., Lozano, R., Malekzadeh, R., März, W., Meier, T., Melaku, Y. A., Mendoza, W., Mensink, G. B. M., Micha, R., Miller, T. R., Mirarefin, M., Mohan, V., Mokdad, A. H., Mozaffarian, D., Nagel, G., Naghavi, M., Nguyen, C. T., Nixon, M. R., Ong, K. L., Pereira, D. M., Poustchi, H., Qorbani, M., Rai, R. K., Razo-García, C., Rehm, C. D., Rivera, J. A., Rodríguez-Ramírez, S., Roshandel, G., Roth, G. A., et al. 2019. Health effects of dietary risks in 195 countries, 1990–2017: a systematic analysis for the Global Burden of Disease Study 2017. *The Lancet*, 393, 1958–1972.

Ahlstrom, B., Dinh, T., Haselton, M. G. & Tomiyama, A. J. 2017. Understanding eating interventions through an evolutionary lens. *Health Psychology Review*, 11, 72–88.

Åkesson, A., Larsson, S. C., Discacciati, A. & Wolk, A. 2014. Low-risk diet and lifestyle habits in the primary prevention of myocardial infarction in men: a population-based prospective cohort study. *Journal of the American College of Cardiology*, 64, 1299–1306.

Allender, S., Owen, B., Kuhlberg, J., Lowe, J., Nagorcka-Smith, P., Whelan, J. & Bell, C. 2015. A Community Based Systems Diagram of Obesity Causes. *PLoS One*, 10, e0129683.

Andersson, C., Johnson, A. D., Benjamin, E. J., Levy, D. & Vasan, R. S. 2019. 70-year legacy of the Framingham Heart Study. *Nature Reviews Cardiology*, 16, 687–698.

Bandura, A. 1971. Social Learning Theory. [Online]. https://www.asecib.ase.ro/mps/Bandura_SocialLearningTheory [Accessed].

Bandura, A. & Cervone, D. 2023. *Social Cognitive Theory: An Agentic Perspective on Human Nature*, John Wiley and Sons.

Bartley, M. 2017. *Health Inequality: An introduction to concepts theories and methods*, Cambridge Polity.

Bell, D. 2021. Volvo's gift to the world, modern seat belts have saved millions of lives. [Online]. Forbes. Available: https://www.forbes.com/sites/douglasbell/2019/08/13/60-years-of-seatbelts-volvos-great-gift-to-the-world/ [Accessed].

Berczik, K., Szabó, A., Griffiths, M. D., Kurimay, T., Kun, B., Urbán, R. & Demetrovics, Z. 2012. Exercise addiction: symptoms, diagnosis, epidemiology, and etiology. *Substance Use & Misuse*, 47, 403–417.

Bhaskaran, K., Dos-Santos-Silva, I., Leon, D. A., Douglas, I. J. & Smeeth, L. 2018. Association of BMI with overall and cause-specific mortality: a population-based cohort study 3.6 million adults in the UK. *The Lancet Diabetes & Endocrinology*, 6, 944–953.

Biddinger, K. J., Emdin, C. A., Haas, M. E., Wang, M., Hindy, G., Ellinor, P. T., Kathiresan, S., Khera, A. V. & Aragam, K. G. 2022. Association of habitual alcohol intake with risk of cardiovascular disease. *JAMA Network Open*, 5, e223849–e223849.

Bogg, T. & Roberts, B. W. 2004. Conscientiousness and health-related behaviors: a meta-analysis of the leading behavioral contributors to mortality. *Psychological Bulletin*, 130, 887.

Bourdieu, P. 2018. The forms of capital. *In: The sociology of economic life*, Routledge.

Boyd, J., Bambra, C., Purshouse, R. C. & Holmes, J. 2021. Beyond behaviour: how health inequality theory can enhance our understanding of the 'Alcohol-Harm Paradox'. *International Journal of Environmental Research and Public Health*, 18.

Bronfenbrenner, U. 2000. *Ecological systems theory*, American Psychological Association.

Bussink-Voorend, D., Hautvast, J. L. A., Vandeberg, L., Visser, O. & Hulscher, M. E. J. L. 2022. A systematic literature review to clarify the concept of vaccine hesitancy. *Nature Human Behaviour*, 6, 1634–1648.

Cairns, G., Angus, K., Hastings, G. & Caraher, M. 2013. Systematic reviews of the evidence on the nature, extent and effects of food marketing to children. A retrospective summary. *Appetite*, 62, 209–215.

Caryl, F., Shortt, N. K., Pearce, J., Reid, G. & Mitchell, R. 2020. Socioeconomic inequalities in children's exposure to tobacco retailing based on individual-level GPS data in Scotland. *Tobacco Control*, 29, 367.

Chaiton, M., Diemert, L., Cohen, J. E., Bondy, S. J., Selby, P., Philipneri, A. & Schwartz, R. 2016. Estimating the number of quit attempts it takes to quit smoking successfully in a longitudinal cohort of smokers. *BMJ Open*, 6, e011045.

Chatzittofis, A., Boström, A. D. E., Savard, J., Öberg, K. G., Arver, S. & Jokinen, J. 2022. Neurochemical and Hormonal Contributors to Compulsive Sexual Behavior Disorder. *Current Addiction Reports*, 9, 23–31.

Cheungpasitporn, W., Thongprayoon, C., Kittanamongkolchai, W., Brabec, B. A., O'corragain, O. A., Edmonds, P. J. & Erickson, S. B.

2015. High alcohol consumption and the risk of renal damage: a systematic review and meta-analysis. *QJM*, 108, 539–548.

Christakis, N. A. & Fowler, J. H. 2007. The spread of obesity in a large social network over 32 years. *New England Journal of Medicine*, 357, 370–379.

Christakis, N. A. & Fowler, J. H. 2008. The collective dynamics of smoking in a large social network. *New England Journal of Medicine*, 358, 2249–2258.

Christakis, N. A. & Fowler, J. H. 2013. Social contagion theory: examining dynamic social networks and human behavior. *Statistics in Medicine*, 32, 556–577.

Conversano, C., Marazziti, D., Carmassi, C., Baldini, S., Barnabei, G. & Dell'osso, L. 2012. Pathological gambling: a systematic review of biochemical, neuroimaging, and neuropsychological findings. *Harvard Review of Psychiatry*, 20, 130–148.

Dai, H., Alsalhe, T. A., Chalghaf, N., Riccò, M., Bragazzi, N. L. & Wu, J. 2020. The global burden of disease attributable to high body mass index in 195 countries and territories, 1990-2017: an analysis of the Global Burden of Disease Study. *PLoS Medicine*, 17, e1003198.

Darmon, N. & Drewnowski, A. 2015. Contribution of food prices and diet cost to socioeconomic disparities in diet quality and health: a systematic review and analysis. *Nutrition Reviews*, 73, 643–660.

Davis, K. M. & Wu, J.-Y. 2001. Role of glutamatergic and GABAergic systems in alcoholism. *Journal of Biomedical Science*, 8, 7–19.

Dawber, T. R., Meadors, G. F. & Moore, F. E., Jr. 1951. Epidemiological approaches to heart disease: the Framingham Study. *American Journal of Public Health and the Nations Health*, 41, 279–286.

Degenhardt, L., Charlson, F., Ferrari, A., Santomauro, D., Erskine, H., Mantilla-Herrara, A., Whiteford, H., Leung, J., Naghavi, M. & Griswold, M. 2018. The global burden of disease attributable to alcohol and drug use in 195 countries and territories, 1990–2016: a systematic analysis for the Global Burden of Disease Study 2016. *The Lancet Psychiatry*, 5, 987–1012.

Doll, R. & Hill, A. B. 1954. The Mortality of Doctors in Relation to Their Smoking Habits. *British Medical Journal*, 1, 1451.

Doll, R., Peto, R., Boreham, J. & Sutherland, I. 2004. Mortality in relation to smoking: 50 years' observations on male British doctors. *BMJ*, 328, 1519.

Dorfman, L., Cheyne, A., Friedman, L. C., Wadud, A. & Gottlieb, M. 2012. Soda and tobacco industry corporate social responsibility campaigns: how do they compare? *PLoS Medicine*, 9, e1001241.

Flegal, K. M., Kit, B. K., Orpana, H. & Graubard, B. I. 2013. Association of all-cause mortality with overweight and obesity using standard body mass index categories: a systematic review and meta-analysis. *JAMA*, 309, 71–82.

Ford, E. S., Bergmann, M. M., Kröger, J., Schienkiewitz, A., Weikert, C. & Boeing, H. 2009. Healthy living is the best revenge: findings from the European Prospective Investigation Into Cancer and Nutrition-Potsdam study. *Archives of Internal Medicine*, 169, 1355–1362.

Freeman, T., Baum, F., Musolino, C., Flavel, J., Mckee, M., Chi, C., Giugliani, C., Falcão, M. Z., De Ceukelaire, W. & Howden-Chapman, P. 2023. Illustrating the impact of commercial determinants of health on the global COVID-19 pandemic: Thematic analysis of 16 country case studies. *Health Policy*, 134, 104860.

Freudenberg, N. & Galea, S. 2008. The impact of corporate practices on health: implications for health policy. *Journal of Public Health Policy*, 29, 86–104.

Gardner, B., Rebar, A. L. & Lally, P. 2022. How does habit form? Guidelines for tracking real-world habit formation. *Cogent Psychology*, 9, 2041277.

Gartland, N., Wilson, A., Lawton, R. & O'connor, D. B. 2021. Conscientiousness and engagement with national health behaviour guidelines. *Psychology, Health & Medicine*, 26, 421–432.

GBD Tobacco Collaborators 2017. Smoking prevalence and attributable disease burden in 195 countries and territories, 1990-2015: a systematic analysis from the Global Burden of Disease Study 2015. *Lancet*, 389, 1885–1906.

Gilmore, A. B., Fabbri, A., Baum, F., Bertscher, A., Bondy, K., Chang, H.-J., Demaio, S., Erzse, A., Freudenberg, N., Friel, S., Hofman, K. J., Johns, P., Abdool Karim, S., Lacy-Nichols, J., De Carvalho, C. M. P., Marten, R., Mckee, M., Petticrew, M., Robertson, L., Tangcharoensathien, V. & Thow, A. M. 2023. Defining and conceptualising the commercial determinants of health. *The Lancet*, 401, 1194–1213.

Glanz, K. & Bishop, D. B. 2010. The role of behavioral science theory in development and implementation of public health interventions. *Annual Review of Public Health*, 31, 399–418.

Glanz, K., Rimer, B. & Viswanath, K. 2024. *Health Behaviour: Theory, Research and Practice*, Wiley.

Graham, E. K., Weston, S. J., Turiano, N. A., Aschwanden, D., Booth, T., Harrison, F., James, B. D., Lewis, N. A., Makkar, S. R., Mueller, S., Wisniewski, K. M., Yoneda, T., Zhaoyang, R., Spiro, A., Willis, S., Schaie, K. W., Sliwinski, M., Lipton, R. A., Katz, M. J., Deary, I. J., Zelinski, E. M., Bennett, D. A., Sachdev, P. S., Brodaty, H., Trollor, J. N., Ames, D., Wright, M. J., Gerstorf, D., Allemand, M., Drewelies, J., Wagner, G. G., Muniz-Terrera, G., Piccinin, A. M., Hofer, S. M. & Mroczek, D. K. 2020. Is healthy neuroticism associated with health behaviors? A coordinated integrative data analysis. *Collabra: Psychology*, 6, 32.

Griswold, M. G., Fullman, N., Hawley, C., Arian, N., Zimsen, S. R. M., Tymeson, H. D., Venkateswaran, V., Tapp, A. D., Forouzanfar, M. H., Salama, J. S., Abate, K. H., Abate, D., Abay, S. M., Abbafati, C., Abdulkader, R. S., Abebe, Z., Aboyans, V., Abrar, M. M., Acharya, P., Adetokunboh, O. O., Adhikari, T. B., Adsuar, J. C., Afarideh, M., Agardh, E. E., Agarwal, G., Aghayan, S. A., Agrawal, S., Ahmed, M. B., Akibu, M., Akinyemiju, T., Akseer, N., Asfoor, D. H. A., Al-Aly, Z., Alahdab, F., Alam, K., Albujeer, A., Alene, K. A., Ali, R., Ali, S. D., Alijanzadeh, M., Aljunid, S. M., Alkerwi, A. A., Allebeck, P., Alvis-Guzman, N., Amare, A. T., Aminde, L. N., Ammar, W., Amoako, Y. A., Amul, G. G. H., Andrei, C. L., Angus, C., Ansha, M. G., Antonio, C. A. T., Aremu, O., Ärnlöv, J., Artaman, A., Aryal, K. K., Assadi, R., Ausloos, M., Avila-Burgos, L., Avokpaho, E. F., Awasthi, A., Ayele, H. T., Ayer, R., Ayuk, T. B., Azzopardi, P. S., Badali, H., Badawi, A., Banach, M., Barker-Collo, S. L., Barrero, L. H., Basaleem, H., Baye, E., Bazargan-Hejazi, S., Bedi, N., Béjot, Y., Belachew, A. B., Belay, S. A., Bennett, D. A., Bensenor, I. M., Bernabe, E., Bernstein, R. S., Beyene, A. S., Beyranvand, T., Bhaumik, S., Bhutta, Z. A., Biadgo, B., Bijani, A., Bililign, N., Birlik, S. M., Birungi, C., Bizuneh, H., Bjerregaard, P., Bjørge, T., Borges, G., Bosetti, C., Boufous, S., Bragazzi, N. L., Brenner, H., Butt, Z. A., et al. 2018. Alcohol use and burden for 195 countries and territories, 1990–2016: a systematic analysis for the Global Burden of Disease Study 2016. *The Lancet*, 392, 1015–1035.

Gruer, L., Hart, C. L., Gordon, D. S. & Watt, G. C. 2009. Effect of tobacco smoking on survival of men and women by social position: a 28 year cohort study. *BMJ*, 338, b480.

Hajat, C. & Stein, E. 2018. The global burden of multiple chronic conditions: a narrative review. *Preventive Medicine Reports*, 12, 284–293.

Hampson, S. E., Goldberg, L. R., Vogt, T. M. & Dubanoski, J. P. 2007. Mechanisms by which childhood personality traits influence adult health status: educational attainment and healthy behaviors. *Health Psychology*, 26, 121.

He, H., Pan, Z., Wu, J., Hu, C., Bai, L. & Lyu, J. 2022. Health effects of tobacco at the global, regional, and national levels: results from the 2019 global burden of disease study. *Nicotine & Tobacco Research*, 24, 864–870.

Hillbom, M., Pieninkeroinen, I. & Leone, M. 2003. Seizures in alcohol-dependent patients: epidemiology, pathophysiology and management. *CNS Drugs*, 17, 1013–1030.

Ireland, R., Bunn, C., Reith, G., Philpott, M., Capewell, S., Boyland, E. & Chambers, S. 2019. Commercial determinants of health: advertising of alcohol and unhealthy foods during sporting events. *Bulletin of the World Health Organization*, 97, 290–295.

Jørgensen, M. B., Pedersen, J., Thygesen, L. C., Lau, C. J., Christensen, A. I., Becker, U. & Tolstrup, J. S. 2019. Alcohol consumption and labour market participation: a prospective cohort study of transitions between work, unemployment, sickness absence, and social benefits. *European Journal of Epidemiology*, 34, 397–407.

Joyner, C. & Loprinzi, P. D. 2018. Longitudinal effects of personality on physical activity among college students: examining executive function as a potential moderator. *Psychological Reports*, 121, 344–355.

Joyner, C., Rhodes, R. E. & Loprinzi, P. D. 2018. The prospective association between the five factor personality model with health behaviors and health behavior clusters. *Europe's Journal of Psychology*, 14, 880–896.

Kakoschke, N., Cox, D., Ryan, J., Gwilt, I., Davis, A., Jansons, P., De Courten, B. & Brinkworth, G. 2023. Disrupting future discounting: a commentary on an underutilised psychological approach for improving adherence to diet and physical activity interventions. *Public Health Nutrition.*, 26(5).

Kamal, H., Tan, G. C., Ibrahim, S. F., Shaikh, M. F., Mohamed, I. N., Mohamed, R. M. P., Hamid, A. A., Ugusman, A. & Kumar, J. 2020. Alcohol use disorder, neurodegeneration, Alzheimer's and Parkinson's disease: interplay between oxidative stress, neuroimmune response and excitotoxicity. *Frontiers in Cellular Neuroscience*, 14, 282.

Katainen, A. & Gronow, A. 2024. Habits and the socioeconomic patterning of health-related behaviour: a pragmatist perspective. *Social Theory & Health*, 22, 36–52.

Katikireddi, S. V., Whitley, E., Lewsey, J., Gray, L. & Leyland, A. H. 2017. Socioeconomic status as an effect modifier of alcohol consumption and harm: analysis of linked cohort data. *The Lancet Public Health*, 2, e267–e276.

Katz, D. L., Frates, E. P., Bonnet, J. P., Gupta, S. K., Vartiainen, E. & Carmona, R. H. 2018. Lifestyle as medicine: the case for a true health initiative. *American Journal of Health Promotion*, 32, 1452–1458.

Katzmarzyk, P. T., Friedenreich, C., Shiroma, E. J. & Lee, I.-M. 2022. Physical inactivity and non-communicable disease burden in low-income, middle-income and high-income countries. *British Journal of Sports Medicine*, 56, 101–106.

Kazibwe, J., Tran, P. B. & Annerstedt, K. S. 2021. The household financial burden of non-communicable diseases in low-and middle-income countries: a systematic review. *Health research policy and systems*, 19, 96.

Keren, H., O'callaghan, G., Vidal-Ribas, P., Buzzell, G. A., Brotman, M. A., Leibenluft, E., Pan, P. M., Meffert, L., Kaiser, A., Wolke, S., Pine, D. S. & Stringaris, A. 2018. Reward processing in depression: a conceptual and meta-analytic review across fMRI and EEG studies. *The American Journal of Psychiatry*, 175, 1111–1120.

Kerr, N. R. & Booth, F. W. 2022. Contributions of physical inactivity and sedentary behavior to metabolic and endocrine diseases. *Trends in Endocrinology & Metabolism*, 33, 817–827.

Khan, J. 2022. The Khan revieThe Khan Review: Making Smoking Obsolete: Making smoking obsolete. Gov.UK: UK Government.

Khan Minhas, A. M., Sedhom, R., Jean, E. D., Shapiro, M. D., Panza, J. A., Alam, M., Virani, S. S., Ballantyne, C. M. & Abramov, D. 2024. Global burden of cardiovascular disease attributable to smoking, 1990–2019: an analysis of the 2019 Global Burden of Disease Study. *European Journal of Preventive Cardiology*, 31, 1123–1131.

Kickbusch, I., Allen, L. & Franz, C. 2016. The commercial determinants of health. *The Lancet Global Health*, 4, e895–e896.

Kim, J. 2016. Personality traits and body weight: evidence using sibling comparisons. *Social Science & Medicine*, 163, 54–62.

Knai, C., Petticrew, M., Mays, N., Capewell, S., Cassidy, R., Cummins, S., Eastmure, E., Fafard, P., Hawkins, B. & Jensen, J. D. 2018. Systems thinking as a framework for analyzing commercial determinants of health. *The Milbank Quarterly*, 96, 472–498.

Koob, G. F. & Volkow, N. D. 2010. Neurocircuitry of addiction. *Neuropsychopharmacology*, 35, 217–238.

Kumar, C. N., Andrade, C. & Murthy, P. 2009. A randomized, double-blind comparison of lorazepam and chlordiazepoxide in patients with uncomplicated alcohol withdrawal. *Journal of Studies on Alcohol and Drugs*, 70, 467–474.

Kumar, S., Schess, J., Velleman, R. & Nadkarni, A. 2022. Stigma towards dependent drinking and its role on caregiving burden: a qualitative study from Goa, India. *Drug and Alcohol Review*, 41, 778–786.

Kvaavik, E., Batty, G. D., Ursin, G., Huxley, R. & Gale, C. R. 2010. Influence of individual and combined health behaviors on total and cause-specific mortality in men and women: the United Kingdom health and lifestyle survey. *Archives of Internal Medicine*, 170, 711–718.

Leung, R. K., Toumbourou, J. W. & Hemphill, S. A. 2014. The effect of peer influence and selection processes on adolescent alcohol use: a systematic review of longitudinal studies. *Health Psychology Review*, 8, 426–457.

Ley, S. H., Hamdy, O., Mohan, V. & Hu, F. B. 2014. Prevention and management of type 2 diabetes: dietary components and nutritional strategies. *The Lancet*, 383, 1999–2007.

Luszczynska, A. & Schwarzer, R. 2020. Changing Behavior Using Social Cognitive Theory. *In:* Hagger, M. S., Cameron, L. D., Hamilton, K., Hankonen, N. & Lintunen, T. (eds.) *The Handbook of Behavior Change*, Cambridge: Cambridge University Press.

Mackillop, J. & Ray, L. A. 2017. The etiology of addiction: a contemporary biopsychosocial approach. *Integrating Psychological and Pharmacological Treatments for Addictive Disorders*, 32–53.

Marmot, M., Allen, J., Boyce, T., Goldblatt, P. & Morrison, J. 2020. Health Equity in England: The Marmot Review 10 Years On [Online]. The Health Foundation Available: https://www.health.org.uk/publications/reports/the-marmot-review-10-years-on [Accessed].

Marmot, M., Friel, S., Bell, R., Houweling, T. A. J. & Taylor, S. 2008. Closing the gap in a generation: Health equity through action on the social determinants of health. *The Lancet*, 372, 1661–1669.

Marmot, M. G. 2010. Fair society, healthy lives: the Marmot Review: strategic review of health inequalities in England post- 2010.

Matheson, E. M., King, D. E. & Everett, C. J. 2012. Healthy lifestyle habits and mortality in overweight and obese individuals. *The Journal of the American Board of Family Medicine*, 25, 9–15.

Mccartney, G., Bartley, M., Dundas, R., Katikireddi, S. V., Mitchell, R., Popham, F., Walsh, D. & Wami, W. 2019. Theorising social class and its application to the study of health inequalities. *SSM - Population Health*, 7, 100315.

Mccartney, G., Dickie, E., Escobar, O. & Collins, C. 2021. Health inequalities, fundamental causes and power: towards the practice of good theory. *Sociology of Health & Illness*, 43, 20–39.

Miller, P. M. 2013. *Biological Research on Addiction: Comprehensive Addictive Behaviors and Disorders*, Volume *2*, Academic Press.

Mötteli, S. & Dohle, S. 2020. Egocentric social network correlates of physical activity. *Journal of Sport and Health Science*, 9, 339–344.

Mowbray, O., Quinn, A. & Cranford, J. A. 2014. Social networks and alcohol use disorders: findings from a nationally representative sample. *The American Journal of Drug and Alcohol Abuse*, 40, 181–186.

Müller, C., Paulsen, L., Bucksch, J. & Wallmann-Sperlich, B. 2024. Built and natural environment correlates of physical activity of adults living in rural areas: a systematic review. *International Journal of Behavioral Nutrition and Physical Activity*, 21, 52.

Murphy, A., Mcgowan, C., Mckee, M., Suhrcke, M. & Hanson, K. 2019. Coping with healthcare costs for chronic illness in low-income and middle-income countries: a systematic literature review. *BMJ Global Health*, 4, e001475.

Murphy, A., Palafox, B., Walli-Attaei, M., Powell-Jackson, T., Rangarajan, S., Alhabib, K. F., Calik, K. B. T., Chifamba, J., Choudhury, T. & Dagenais, G. 2020. The household economic burden of non-communicable diseases in 18 countries. *BMJ Global Health*, 5, e002040.

Nagawa, C. S., Emidio, O. M., Lapane, K. L., Houston, T. K., Barton, B. A., Faro, J. M., Blok, A. C., Orvek, E. A., Cutrona, S. L., Smith, B. M., Allison, J. J. & Sadasivam, R. S. 2020. Teamwork for smoking cessation: which smoker was willing to engage their partner? Results from a cross-sectional study. *BMC Research Notes*, 13, 344.

Ng, M., Fleming, T., Robinson, M., Thomson, B., Graetz, N., Margono, C., Mullany, E. C., Biryukov, S., Abbafati, C., Abera, S. F., Abraham, J. P., Abu-Rmeileh, N. M., Achoki, T., Albuhairan, F. S., Alemu, Z. A., Alfonso, R., Ali, M. K., Ali, R., Guzman, N. A., Ammar, W., Anwari, P., Banerjee, A., Barquera, S., Basu, S., Bennett, D. A., Bhutta, Z., Blore, J., Cabral, N., Nonato, I. C., Chang, J. C., Chowdhury, R., Courville, K. J., Criqui, M. H., Cundiff, D. K., Dabhadkar, K. C., Dandona, L., Davis, A., Dayama, A., Dharmaratne, S. D., Ding, E. L., Durrani, A. M., Esteghamati, A., Farzadfar, F., Fay, D. F., Feigin, V. L., Flaxman, A., Forouzanfar, M. H., Goto, A., Green, M. A., Gupta, R., Hafezi-Nejad, N., Hankey, G. J., Harewood, H. C., Havmoeller, R., Hay, S., Hernandez, L., Husseini, A., Idrisov, B. T., Ikeda, N., Islami, F., Jahangir, E., Jassal, S. K., Jee, S. H., Jeffreys, M., Jonas, J. B., Kabagambe, E. K., Khalifa, S. E., Kengne, A. P., Khader, Y. S., Khang, Y. H., Kim, D., Kimokoti, R. W., Kinge, J. M., Kokubo, Y., Kosen, S., Kwan, G., Lai, T., Leinsalu, M., Li, Y., Liang, X., Liu, S., Logroscino, G., Lotufo, P. A., Lu, Y., Ma, J., Mainoo, N. K., Mensah, G. A., Merriman, T. R., Mokdad, A. H., Moschandreas, J., Naghavi, M., Naheed, A., Nand, D., Narayan, K. M., Nelson, E. L., Neuhouser, M. L., Nisar, M. I., Ohkubo, T., Oti, S. O., Pedroza, A., et al. 2014. Global, regional, and national prevalence of overweight and obesity in children and adults during 1980-2013: A systematic analysis for the Global Burden of Disease Study 2013. *Lancet*, 384, 766–781.

O'connor, D. B. 2020. The future of health behaviour change interventions: opportunities for open science and personality research. *Health Psychology Review*, 14, 176–181.

Orbell, S. & Verplanken, B. 2010. The automatic component of habit in health behavior: habit as cue-contingent automaticity. *Health Psychology*, 29, 374.

Pampel, F. C., Krueger, P. M. & Denney, J. T. 2010. Socioeconomic disparities in health behaviors. *Annual Review of Sociology*, 36, 349–370.

Pepper, J. K., Squiers, L. B., Peinado, S. C., Bann, C. M., Dolina, S. D., Lynch, M. M., Nonnemaker, J. M. & Mccormack, L. A. 2019. Impact of messages about scientific uncertainty on risk perceptions and intentions to use electronic vaping products. *Addictive Behaviors*, 91, 136–140.

Petticrew, M., Maani, N., Petticrew, L., Rutter, H. & Van Schalkwyk, M. 2020. Dark nudges and sludge in big alcohol: behavioral economics, cognitive biases, and alcohol industry corporate social responsibility. *The Milbank Quarterly*, 98, 1290–1328.

Pirie, K., Peto, R., Reeves, G. K., Green, J. & Beral, V. 2013. The 21st century hazards of smoking and benefits of stopping: a prospective study of one million women in the UK. *Lancet*, 381, 133–141.

Raghavan, R., Dreibelbis, C., Kingshipp, B. L., Wong, Y. P., Abrams, B., Gernand, A. D., Rasmussen, K. M., Siega-Riz, A. M., Stang, J., Casavale, K. O., Spahn, J. M. & Stoody, E. E. 2019. Dietary patterns before and during pregnancy and birth outcomes: a systematic review. *The American Journal of Clinical Nutrition*, 109, 729s–756s.

Royal College of Physicians. 2018. Hiding in plan sight: Treating tobacco dependency in the NHS [Online]. Royal College of Physicians Available: https://www.rcp.ac.uk/media/bdnj2ykk/hiding-in-plain-sight.pdf [Accessed].

Roche, A., Kostadinov, V., Fischer, J., Nicholas, R., O'rourke, K., Pidd, K. & Trifonoff, A. 2015. Addressing inequities in alcohol consumption and related harms. *Health Promotion International*, 30, ii20–ii35.

Rochefort, C., Hoerger, M., Turiano, N. A. & Duberstein, P. 2019. Big Five personality and health in adults with and without cancer. *Journal of Health Psychology*, 24, 1494–1504.

Rogers, E. & Shoemaker, F. 1971. *Communication of Innovation*, New York: The Free Press.

Rogers, E. M., Singhal, A. & Quinlan, M. M. 2014. Diffusion of Innovations. In: *An Integrated Approach to Communication Theory and Research*, Routledge, 182–186.

Rosenquist, J. N., Murabito, J., Fowler, J. H. & Christakis, N. A. 2010. The spread of alcohol consumption behavior in a large social network. *Annals of Internal Medicine*, 152, 426–433.

Rosenstock, I. M. 1966. Why people use health services. *The Milbank Memorial Fund Quarterly*, 44, 94–127.

Rosenstock, I. M. 1974a. The health belief model and preventive health behavior. *Health Education Monographs*, 2, 354–386.

Rosenstock, I. M. 1974b. Historical origins of the health belief model. *Health Education Monographs*, 2, 328–335.

Savell, E., Gilmore, A. B., Sims, M., Mony, P. K., Koon, T., Yusoff, K., Lear, S. A., Seron, P., Ismail, N., Calik, K. B., Rosengren, A., Bahonar, A., Kumar, R., Vijayakumar, K., Kruger, A., Swidan, H., Gupta, R., Igumbor, E., Afridi, A., Rahman, O., Chifamba, J., Zatonska, K., Mohan, V., Mohan, D., Lopez-Jaramillo, P., Avezum, A., Poirier, P., Orlandini, A., Li, W., Mckee, M., Rangarajan, S., Yusuf, S. & Chow, C. K. 2015. The environmental profile of a community's health: a cross-sectional study on tobacco marketing in 16 countries. *Bulletin of the World Health Organization*, 93, 851–861g.

Serrano Fuentes, N., Rogers, A. & Portillo, M. C. 2019. Social network influences and the adoption of obesity-related behaviours in adults: a critical interpretative synthesis review. *BMC Public Health*, 19, 1178.

Serrano-Fuentes, N., Rogers, A. & Portillo, M. C. 2022. The influence of social relationships and activities on the health of adults with obesity: a qualitative study. *Health Expectations*, 25, 1892–1903.

Shield, K., Manthey, J., Rylett, M., Probst, C., Wettlaufer, A., Parry, C. D. & Rehm, J. 2020. National, regional, and global burdens of disease from 2000 to 2016 attributable to alcohol use: a comparative risk assessment study. *The Lancet Public Health*, 5, e51–e61.

Shortt, N. K., Tisch, C., Pearce, J., Mitchell, R., Richardson, E. A., Hill, S. & Collin, J. 2015. A cross-sectional analysis of the relationship between tobacco and alcohol outlet density and neighbourhood deprivation. *BMC Public Health*, 15, 1014.

Singal, A. K. & Mathurin, P. 2021. Diagnosis and treatment of alcohol-associated liver disease: a review. *JAMA*, 326, 165–176.

Smith, T. W. 2006. Personality as risk and resilience in physical health. *Current Directions in Psychological Science*, 15, 227–231.

Sontate, K. V., Rahim Kamaluddin, M., Naina Mohamed, I., Mohamed, R. M. P., Shaikh, M. F., Kamal, H. & Kumar, J. 2021. Alcohol, aggression, and violence: from public health to neuroscience. *Frontiers in Psychology*, 12, 699726.

Subramaniyan, V., Chakravarthi, S., Jegasothy, R., Seng, W. Y., Fuloria, N. K., Fuloria, S., Hazarika, I. & Das, A. 2021. Alcohol-associated liver disease: a review on its pathophysiology, diagnosis and drug therapy. *Toxicology Reports*, 8, 376–385.

Townshend, T. & Lake, A. 2017. Obesogenic environments: current evidence of the built and food environments. *Perspectives in Public Health*, 137, 38–44.

Tripathi, G. M., Misra, U. K., Kalita, J., Singh, V. K. & Tripathi, A. 2023. Effect of exercise on β-Endorphin and Its receptors in Myasthenia Gravis patients. *Molecular Neurobiology*, 60, 3010–3019.

Turiano, N. A., Hill, P. L., Graham, E. K. & Mroczek, D. K. 2018. Associations between Personality and Health Behaviors Across the Life Span. *In:* Ryff, C. D. & Krueger, R. F. (eds.) *The Oxford Handbook of Integrative Health Science*, Oxford University Press.

Umberson, D., Crosnoe, R. & Reczek, C. 2010. Social relationships and health behavior across life course. *Annual Review of Sociology*, 36, 139–157.

Vengeliene, V., Bilbao, A., Molander, A. & Spanagel, R. 2008. Neuropharmacology of alcohol addiction. *British Journal of Pharmacology*, 154, 299–315.

Verheul, R. & Van Den Brink, W. 2000. The role of personality pathology in the aetiology and treatment of substance use disorders. *Current Opinion in Psychiatry*, 13, 163–169.

Wackernah, R. C., Minnick, M. J. & Clapp, P. 2014. Alcohol use disorder: pathophysiology, effects, and pharmacologic options for treatment. *Substance Abuse and Rehabilitation*, 1–12.

Waller, P. F. 2020. Epidemiology of alcohol-related accidents and the Grand Rapids study. *Alcohol, Drugs, and Impaired Driving*, 87–103.

Wami, W., Mccartney, G., Bartley, M., Buchanan, D., Dundas, R., Katikireddi, S. V., Mitchell, R. & Walsh, D. 2020. Theory driven analysis of social class and health outcomes using UK nationally representative longitudinal data. *International Journal for Equity in Health*, 19, 193.

Watson, P., Wiers, R., Hommel, B., Ridderinkhof, K. & De Wit, S. 2016. An associative account of how the obesogenic environment biases adolescents' food choices. *Appetite*, 96, 560–571.

Weber, M. 1978. *Economy and society: An outline of interpretive sociology*, University of California press.

Weinstein, A. & Weinstein, Y. 2014. Exercise addiction- diagnosis, bio-psychological mechanisms and treatment issues. *Current Pharmaceutical Design*, 20, 4062–4069.

West, R. & Brown, J. 2013. *Theory of Addiction*, 1st Edition, Wiley.

Weyers, S., Dragano, N., Richter, M. & Bosma, H. 2010. How does socio economic position link to health behaviour? Sociological pathways and perspectives for health promotion. *Global Health Promotion*, 17, 25–33.

WHO. 2023. Commercial determinants of health [Online]. World Health Organization. Available: https://www.who.int/news-room/fact-sheets/detail/commercial-determinants-of-health [Accessed].

WHO. 2024. Physical activity [Online]. World Health Organization. Available: https://www.who.int/news-room/fact-sheets/detail/physical-activity [Accessed].

Wikler, A. 2013. *Opioid Dependence: Mechanisms and Treatment*, Springer Science & Business Media.

Williams, D. 2019. What Are the Causes of Unhealthy Behavior? In: Williams, D. M. (ed.) *Darwinian Hedonism and the Epidemic of Unhealthy Behavior*, Cambridge: Cambridge University Press.

Williams, D. & Evans, D. 2014. Current emotion research in health behaviour science. *Emotion Review.*, 6(3).

CHAPTER 13

Evidence-Based Behaviour Change Approaches

Chris Allen and Gilly Mancz
School of Health Sciences, University of Southampton, Southampton, UK

Introduction

As we have highlighted in earlier chapters, health behaviours influence health. In fact, a large part of public health provision necessarily relates to, and even depends on individuals changing behaviours that may be negatively impacting on their health. Such a focus alongside its accompanying policy, will only increase with many services reorientating care towards prevention. In fact, prevention is a fundamental aspect of most healthcare professional's roles.

This chapter will build on the previous chapter, which considered *why* people engage with behaviours they *know* might harm their health, and will explore how the social sciences have responded to and developed a range of evidence-based behaviour change approaches that have been adopted into clinical practice in a range of clinical settings, particularly within a United Kingdom context, such as motivational interviewing, and other healthy conversation skills, such as 'MECC' (Making Every Contact Count). The interventions covered in this chapter, largely seek to address behaviour change at the level of individuals, before we consider in the next chapter, behaviour change at the population level.

LEARNING OUTCOMES

By the end of this chapter, you will be able to:

- Identify the main theories that underpin behaviour change interventions that are commonly used in clinical practice.
- Recognise what individuals generally need to be able to change their health behaviours.

- Consider the evidence base for commonly used interventions, such as motivational interviewing, and other healthy conversation skills like MECC.
- Recognise the increasing importance of digital behaviour change interventions in supporting behaviour change.

A Science of Behaviour Change

> **Key Terms and Definitions**
>
> **Behaviour change techniques:** These are individual approaches to behaviour change, and often the active ingredients to more complex behaviour change interventions.
>
> **Behaviour change intervention:** An intervention that is intended to elicit behaviour change, which can involve the cessation of unhealthy behaviours or the adoption of healthy behaviours. Interventions can be in many forms and are often underpinned by behaviour change theories.
>
> **Self-efficacy:** Generally relates to an individual's belief that they can do something.

In its broadest sense, behaviour change science can be seen as any scientific study that seeks to understand individual, group and population behaviour and how we can *influence* it (Davis et al., 2015). In the context of health, this essentially relates to how we can support people to change their behaviours

Social Sciences for Healthcare Professionals, First Edition. Edited by Chris Allen.
© 2026 John Wiley & Sons Ltd. Published 2026 by John Wiley & Sons Ltd.

through our knowledge and understanding of people's contexts, and various behaviour change approaches (Davis et al., 2015). Ideally, we want to know which approaches work, who they work for and in what contexts (Michie and Johnston, 2012). Our understanding of behaviour change as a science, and the technologies that we are using to support it, has grown substantially in recent years through the efforts of a range of disciplines across the social sciences such as psychology, sociology and economics (Davis et al., 2015, Michie and Johnston, 2012, Michie et al., 2017). Such advances have the potential to help us respond to the challenges most healthcare systems are currently facing, and in turn, positively enhance individual and population health and well-being (Michie et al., 2017).

As we will explore within this chapter, behaviour change science has given us a range of behaviour change techniques that target individual behaviours. Changing established behaviour is difficult. You will have likely experienced these challenges yourself, after all, most of us have tried to change negative behaviours (such as being inactive, smoking, drinking too much, or having poor sleep hygiene) or acquire behaviours that might be health-enhancing (such as exercising more or eating a more balanced diet).

> ### Stop and Think – What Behaviour Change Techniques Are You Familiar with from Your Practice?
>
> Think about the behaviour change techniques that you are familiar with, either from your practice or from your personal life. These might include, for example, rewards, social comparison, altering your environment (making things less available – such as not having things in your fridge), prompts and reminders, self-monitoring performance, etc.
>
> - What techniques have you seen others using, or have used yourself?
> - What techniques have you, or those you know, found to be effective in supporting behaviour change? Why do you think they were effective?
> - What techniques have you, or those you know, found to be ineffective in supporting a behaviour change? Why do you think they were ineffective?

There is a significant degree of overlap between why people engage in these behaviours and why people find it tough to break them, and many of the approaches that are considered in this chapter target these. For example, convenience, habits and norms, motivation, belief, social influences, etc.

Healthcare Professionals Roles in Promoting Behaviour Change

In recognition of the challenges posed by non-communicable diseases to most healthcare systems, government policy and professional standards increasingly emphasise the importance of healthcare professionals having the required knowledge and skills to support the people they work with to change their behaviours, when the behaviours they are engaging with are potentially harmful to their health (HCPC, 2023, NHS, 2023, NMC, 2019b). In a United Kingdom context, the main professional regulators highlight the need for healthcare professionals to have the necessary knowledge and skills to support behaviour change (HCPC, 2023, NMC, 2019a). For example, the Nursing and Midwifery Council (NMC), specifically states that nurses should check (service users) understanding of the causes of health conditions, the consequence of health behaviour(s) (such as smoking, drinking, inactivity and poor diet), as well as having the knowledge and skills required to assess people's motivation and capacity to change, and where appropriate deploy individual behaviour change techniques such as motivational interviewing to support behaviour change (NMC, 2019a). Other professional standards, such as those provided by the Health and Care Professions Council (HCPC) also emphasise the importance of healthcare professionals supporting behaviour change (HCPC, 2023). In addition, behaviour change techniques have become established in clinical guidelines, such as those provided by the National Institute for Health and Care Excellence (NICE) (NICE, 2014), and professional competencies for behaviour change techniques exist (Dixon and Johnston, 2021).

Models and Theories of Behaviour Change

Many models and frameworks have been developed that attempt to explain changes in health behaviour and how these are best elicited, including some of those discussed in the previous chapter. Many of these models have gone on to underpin interventions aimed at promoting behaviour change. We will cover a few of these, notably the Transtheoretical/Stages of Change model, social cognitive theory (in relation to behaviour change), and the Behaviour Change Wheel (BCW)/Capability, Opportunity, Motivation- Behaviour (COM-B) model. These are well-known, and you might already be familiar with them. The Transtheoretical/Stages of Change model can help us consider someone's *readiness* to change, and potentially tailor support around this, whereas social cognitive theory and the more recent BCW/COM-B model, have become highly influential in the development of behaviour change interventions that consider what might be needed for someone to change. These models are summarised in distinct sections below.

Transtheoretical/Stages of Change Model

One of the most well-known models of behaviour change is the transtheoretical model, or 'stages of change' theory (Prochaska and DiClemente, 1982, Prochaska et al., 1992). The model has been used to explore the *process* of changing behaviour in the context of a range of unhealthy behaviours (Evers and Balestrieri, 2024). Whilst not without its critics (Bunton et al., 2000, Littell and Girvin, 2002), the model is still widely used, often to guide thinking about behaviour change and how ready people are to make a change, and through this tailor behaviour change techniques (some of which are discussed later in this chapter) and support to to an individual's stage of 'readiness'. Many of these stages might be recognised by you in your own attempts to change an established behaviour.

The model shown in Figure 13.1 incorporates the following broad stages, that you might see expressed slightly differently depending on the source.

There are of course notable limitations to the transtheoretical model, some of which are addressed in more recent behaviour change models, notably the BCW and social cognitive theory. Criticisms have largely focused on the lack of a scientific basis for the stages (Bunton et al., 2000, Evers and Balestrieri, 2024, Littell

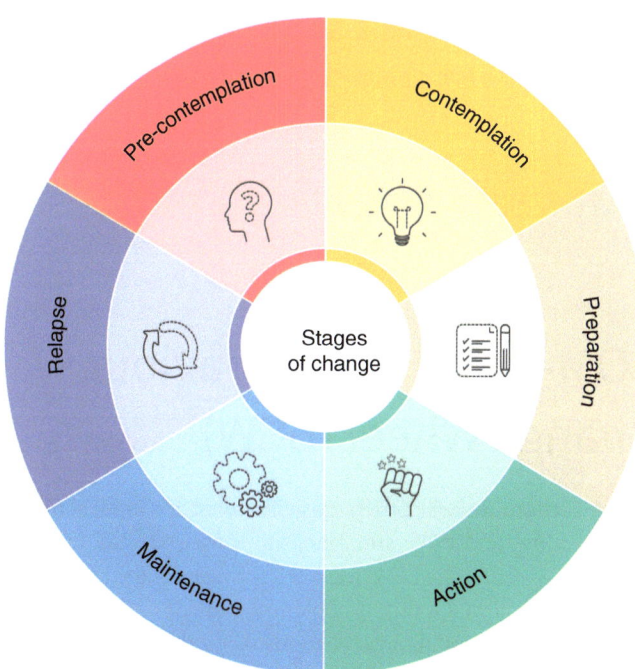

FIGURE 13.1 The Transtheoretical/stages of change model.
Source: Whale Design /Adobe Stock Photos.

and Girvin, 2002), but there are other limitations, for example, whilst a potentially useful heuristic, the model doesn't consider the full range of resources (social, economic, psychological, etc.) that may make behaviour change more or less likely. It only really considers readiness, maintenance and relapse – as opposed to specific facilitators and barriers that are increasingly being recognised as important to behaviour change outcomes.

Social Cognitive Theory

In the previous chapter, we introduced social cognitive theory as an established theory in understanding health behaviour, and in this chapter, we will build on its uses in terms of helping us understand the necessary conditions for behaviour change. As a framework, social cognitive theory has been used to underpin behaviour change interventions, including some of those that are discussed in this chapter. Previously, we introduced two key concepts that directly or indirectly influence a person's behaviours, notably, self-efficacy and outcome expectations (Bandura, 1977, Borah et al., 2024), and these, in particular, feed into how the theory has been used in behaviour change approaches.

Although both self-efficacy and outcome expectations are believed to influence our goals and our behaviours; self-efficacy is considered the primary influencing factor, as it interacts with socio-structural factors and can also directly impact on behaviours as shown in Figure 13.2 (Bandura, 1977, 2017, Beauchamp et al., 2019, Luszczynska and Schwarzer, 2020).

Perceived self-efficacy is central to human agency. It essentially means that an individual has the underpinning belief that they can shape their own lives and achieve their goals (Benight and Bandura, 2004, Szczuka et al., 2021). Low self-efficacy means little belief that things can change, leading to minimal effort to do things differently (because after all, why would you, if you believe you are going to fail anyway). Because of this, self-efficacy is recognised as one of the most important and influential predictors of behaviour change success (Szczuka et al., 2021). It is believed to be influenced by four factors: previous mastery of a behaviour, seeing someone who is similar (in terms of personal characteristics, attributes, etc.) model the behaviour, persuasion and meaningful encouragement from someone who is seen as credible (such as healthcare professionals), and emotional context, such as levels of anxiety (Bandura and Cervone, 2023, Luszczynska and Schwarzer, 2020, Schunk and Dibenedetto, 2022).

Alongside self-efficacy, outcome expectations are also important, because this relates to what an individual believes the outcome of a behaviour change will likely be. If changing a behaviour is not seen to elicit a positive, or indeed valued outcome, even with a belief that someone can change their behaviour, they are unlikely to see changing their behaviour as being particularly important ('even if I do change, the outcome will be no different', etc.).

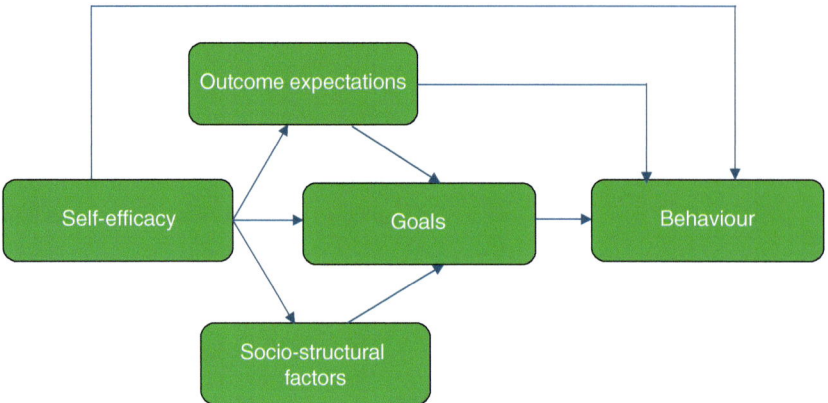

FIGURE 13.2   Social cognitive theory. **Source:** Adapted from Bandura (2012).

Outcome expectations can be broken down into three domains. These are physical, social and self-evaluative; and they relate to what an individual thinks might happen if they change their behaviour – positively or negatively (Luszczynska and Schwarzer, 2020). For example, positive expectations might include having more energy and helping to increase participation in social life. Conversely, negative expectations may include concerns that drinking less may make it harder to socialise, especially if much of the drinking happens with friends. Bandura's work suggests that when someone has high self-efficacy, they are more likely to look for positive consequences and opportunities relating to outcome expectations. Likewise, those with poor self-efficacy are more likely to look for negative consequences and barriers (i.e. reasons why they should not change their behaviour) (Bandura, 2012).

It is also recognised that it is not enough to believe you can make a change and that this change will be positive; change happens within a social context, and people may be supported, or impeded by *socio-structural factors.* These are generally the opportunities that someone might have (i.e. things that might facilitate a change) or the barriers (i.e. the things that might get in the way). Socio-structural factors include many of the aspects that we explored in Chapter 8, such as the social determinants of health, for example: people's socio-economic status, their personal network, their living and working conditions as well as the broader economic and political factors that shape these (Bandura, 2012, Luszczynska and Schwarzer, 2020).

Even with good self-efficacy, expectations that change will bring about positive outcomes, and a supportive social context, change involves *action* and a commitment to doing something, and this is where *goals* come in. Goals can be *distal* or *proximal*. Distal goals are longer-term goals. They are often seen as more challenging. Proximal goals are smaller and more achievable and can be useful in helping someone's confidence (because they can see quick success) whilst building towards their distal goals (as opposed to attempting a big goal straight away, and being unsuccessful) (Bandura and Cervone, 2023, Luszczynska and Schwarzer, 2020, Schunk and Dibenedetto, 2022). The higher a person's self-efficacy, the more likely they are to set

challenging and ambitious goals (Beauchamp et al., 2019), whereas those with very low self-efficacy may not set any at all (Luszczynska and Schwarzer, 2020).

There is now an established evidence base around the social cognitive theory that has been produced by a range of disciplines (Mantey et al., 2024). It is frequently cited in published research as the underpinning theory in behaviour change interventions, including some of those discussed in this chapter, and it has been used to target a range of unhealthy behaviours (Mantey et al., 2024). Whilst frequently used, the theory is not always applied consistently, or in its entirety, instead key elements are often researched in isolation, such as self-efficacy, or are combined with other theories, making it challenging to systematically review the theory and its evidence base as a whole (Luszczynska and Schwarzer, 2020).

This is also a challenge with behaviour change literature more generally. Behaviour change literature is broad, diverse and often messy. Recent attempts have been made to synthesise the diverse range of literature that is associated with behaviour change, into a cohesive framework, that can be used to underpin intervention design, and this has led to the development of COM-B, and the BCW.

COM-B and The Behaviour Change Wheel (BCW)

In this section, we will briefly describe what the now seminal COM-B model and BCW are. Alongside this, you may wish to explore COM-B and the BCW in more depth, and the model's creators have published a recent book, that provides a comprehensive guide to developing interventions using this model (Michie et al., 2024). COM-B and the BCW have helped guide the development and testing of behaviour change interventions, some of which, you may already be using in your practice (Michie et al., 2024).

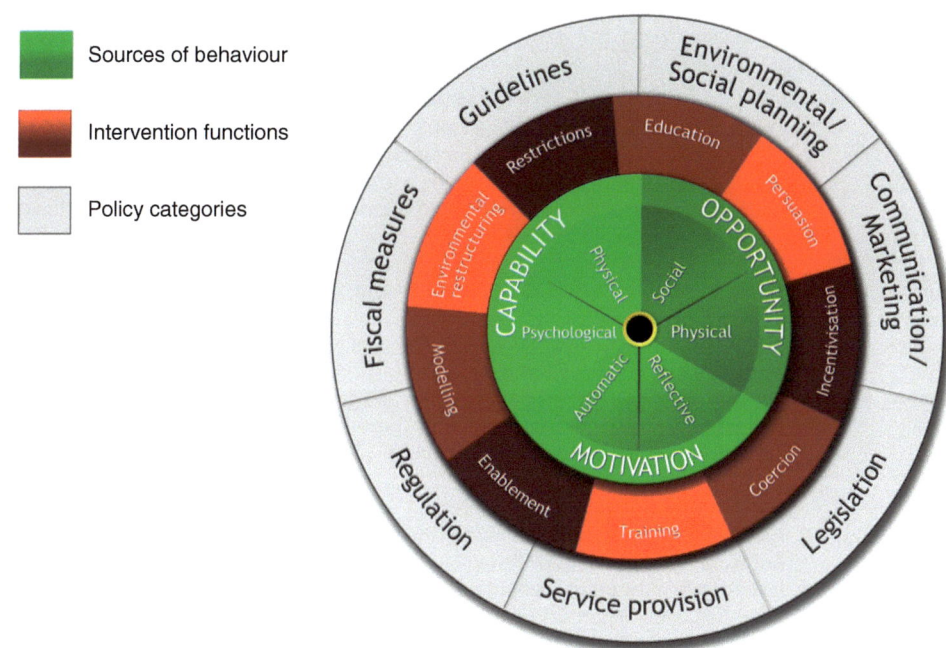

FIGURE 13.3   The behaviour change wheel (BCW). **Source:** Michie et al. (2011) / Springer Nature / CC BY 2.0.

So, what is the BCW? The BCW is a framework for developing, describing and evaluating various behaviour change interventions (Michie et al., 2024). It is essentially a step-by-step guide, presented as a 'wheel' that can be seen in Figure 13.3.

The BCW and COM-B were developed through a review of the existing frameworks, taking 19 of the most effective ones and integrating them into the holistic framework above (Michie et al., 2011). It is arguably *the* framework for considering the design and evaluation of behaviour change interventions.

The starting point of using the BCW is to consider which specific behaviours are to be targeted and in whom. Once identified, behaviour can be considered in the context of the COM-B model, helping us to consider the *causes* of the behaviour, and what may need to happen to support the person to make a change (Michie et al., 2011). The COM-B model (shown in the green section in Figure 13.3) forms the core of the BCW and includes consideration of an individual's capability (which can include their physical and psychological capabilities), as well as their opportunity (e.g. their access to resources and social

support), and their motivation. The model is useful because it encourages consideration of the broader context within which health behaviours are practised in, much of which lies outside of an individual's direct control, such as the wider social determinants of unhealthy behaviours (discussed in Chapter 8 and the previous chapter). These include the influence of our personal networks on our behaviour, cultural norms and access to material and social resources, as well as person's physical and psychological characteristics, such as their skills, knowledge, unconscious habits and impulses. This sets the model apart from other, less encompassing models, particularly those that suggest health decision-making is conscious, and deliberative (i.e. the health beliefs model, discussed in the previous chapter). It is likely that a combination of these aspects will need to be changed, for a behaviour change to happen. We can have the skills and knowledge (capability) that our behaviour is harmful to our health, but without the right motivation, or environment (opportunity), we are very unlikely to make changes or indeed sustain them over the longer term.

Stop and Think: COM-B in Action

In your practice, or in your personal life, you will have likely encountered people who have wanted to change a behaviour. This could be that they want to eat healthier, be more active, give up smoking or reduce their alcohol intake.

Pick someone whose context you know well. You should use the questions below, to help you consider whether they had

the capability, opportunity or motivation to help them change their behaviour and sustain this behaviour change over time.

Is there anything that you think might help improve their capability, opportunity or motivation, and how do you think this might impact on their being able to successfully change their behaviour(s)?

COM-B aspect	Questions that can be used to determine someone's capability, opportunity, and motivation to change
Capability (can include both physical and psychological)	1. Are they aware of what behaviour change is needed and what it will likely involve? 2. Do they understand the potential benefits of making the change or the risks of not doing so? 3. Are they confident to make the change, and do they have the required skills to do what is involved? 4. Do they have the physical strength, and the stamina to make the change and to sustain it? 5. Can they self-regulate their behaviour?
Opportunity (can include people's resources as well as their social influences)	1. To what extent is the behaviour normal amongst the people they mostly interact with (i.e. their social network)? 2. Are the people in their social networks likely to be supportive of their behaviour change? Might they also consider making a similar change? 3. Are there any social norms that influence and guide the behaviour? 4. Do they have the resources (particularly financial resources) that they need to make the change? 5. Do they have the time to make the change?
Motivation	1. To what extent is a change seen as being 'worth it'? 2. Are they likely to enjoy the change or the results the change might have on them? 3. Are there other priorities or demands that might make the change difficult? 4. Is their unhealthy behaviour influenced by any emotions, or by how they see themselves? 5. Is the behaviour a part of their normal routine?

Now that we have had the opportunity to think about people's capabilities, their opportunities and their motivations for making a behaviour change, we can consider which broad intervention types (shown in the red concentric circle in the model in Figure 13.3) might be most effective. For example, does the intervention need to address a lack of resources such as social support, does it need to address someone's capabilities (such as a lack of skills or knowledge) or does it need to address their motivation (such as through some of the techniques we discuss later in this chapter). The macro decision-making that is often needed to make the interventions in the red concentric circle possible, generally involves government action, such as the creation of guidelines, regulations, legislation, provision and planning are shown in the outer grey coloured concentric circle. We cover some of these, and the ethics around their use, in the following chapter.

Behaviour Change Techniques

Within behaviour change interventions, often sit a range of small behaviour change techniques (Michie et al., 2013). These can be considered as the active ingredients of broader interventions and often seek to encourage the discontinuation of unhealthy behaviours or to facilitate target healthy behaviours (Michie et al., 2013). In one highly influential paper, Michie et al. (2013) created a useful taxonomy of behaviour change techniques, based around consensus of what the techniques were. They did this, to create a shared language (a taxonomy), that provides clarity to those working in behaviour change as to which techniques are being used, and through homogenising the language used to describe the various techniques (e.g.

some techniques that are essentially the same thing, are referred to in multiple ways – self monitoring and daily diaries as an example), build a more coherent evidence base about what works (e.g. through increased transparency, fidelity, and reproducibility of the techniques used) (Michie et al., 2013). The taxonomy they produced, also helpfully clusters techniques that are similar to one another, for example, goals and planning, feedback and monitoring, social support, rewards, threats, etc. (Michie et al., 2013).

Behaviour Change Interventions

Behaviour change interventions are generally thought about as a range of coordinated approaches or activities that seek to elicit a change in a specific behaviour, such as harmful drinking, smoking and inactivity (Michie et al., 2011). Those interventions that are informed by theory-driven behaviour change models, are often more successful and are more likely to lead to longer-term, sustainable changes being made. However, it is acknowledged that behaviour change is a complex issue to research, and several factors impact on being able to systematically review the different theories that are available, including sometimes a lack of clear terms (discussed above), with many terms being used interchangeably, popping up in multiple different theories under slightly different guises, and a range of different concepts being highlighted as being important. This sometimes makes it challenging to identify which approaches are most effective, in who, and in what context. One potential solution is provided in the case study below.

Case Study: The Human Behaviour Change Project

The Human Behaviour-Change Project is exploring the use of Artificial Intelligence (AI) (we discuss some other novel uses of AI in Chapter 20) to inform behaviour change approaches at scale and at speed to understand what works, for who, in what context, and why (Michie et al., 2017). Essentially an ontology (or schema, something that shows the relationships between different things) of behaviour change interventions (Michie et al., 2017). The project has sought to address the challenge of making sense of a very large, rapidly expanding and increasingly diverse behaviour change literature, where things are often reported in inconsistent ways, using different language to describe the same or similar things, and often being synthesised very slowly, and inconsistently reaching into actual clinical guidelines and practice, where it can be used to support people to change their behaviours (Michie et al., 2017).

Consider the following:

- What impact do you think knowing which behaviour change approach would best meet the exact needs of those you work with?

- How might such an innovation bring about change in terms of how care is provided?

- Are there any potentially harmful impacts of using AI to guide care in this way?

There are also now several interventions that are used in clinical practice by healthcare professionals, that are underpinned by theory and have a degree of standardisation and reproducibility. We will now discuss a few examples that have relevance to your practice.

Motivational Interviewing

In this section, we will briefly describe one common approach to supporting behaviour change, which is *motivational interviewing*. Motivational interviewing was developed over 40 years ago to support people accessing alcohol intervention services to change their behaviour (Rollnick et al., 2023). Since then, it has been developed into a tool that can be used in a wide range of contexts, by a wide range of disciplines including health, psychotherapy, social care, education, etc. (Rollnick et al., 2023). Essentially motivational interviewing is a way of talking to someone about a behaviour change that strengthens their motivation and commitment to making that change happen. Miller and Rollnick (2013), whose seminal work underpins the approach, highlight the place of language in promoting change, alongside recognising the importance of collaboration, compassion and acceptance. Generally, the approach aims to empower individuals and provide them with opportunities to identify and name their own reasons for change, which is believed to increase their motivation and ability to do so. The approach recognises that individuals are experts in their own lives and social context, and that professionals need to work with, rather than do to them (Rollnick et al., 2023). Essentially, collaboration and partnership working, rather than paternalism. This is relevant because professionals often fall into the trap of the '*righting reflex*', whereby they want to support individuals to make changes to improve their health and/or well-being and inadvertently use unhelpful strategies, such as providing solutions, confronting them with the reality of the situation and/or trying to persuade them to care about the issue (Miller and Rollnick, 2013). You may have seen, or indeed engaged with this yourself in your own practice, and not realised that this might be an unhelpful way of approaching behaviour change.

The challenge for both professionals and the individuals they work with, is that the individual often knows the reasons to change (after all, as we highlighted in the previous chapter, it is uncommon for people to not know that smoking, or drinking too much, is bad for them), but people often enjoy (positive affect), or gain some other benefit from the unhealthy behaviour that they are engaged with (Rollnick et al., 2023). For this reason, when individuals are confronted with arguments to change, many individuals will consolidate their reasons not to change, arguing that they need to sustain existing behaviours (i.e. 'sustain talk' as opposed to 'change talk') (Rollnick et al., 2023). This can lead to people being unfairly labelled as 'non-compliant', 'resistant' or 'difficult', and you may have seen this, especially where appropriate behaviour change communication skills are lacking. To promote 'change talk', individuals should be encouraged to identify their reasons for change, address any challenges they may face, focus on the positives about making the change and set goals (Miller and Rollnick, 2013). To do this, motivational interviewing uses a guided communication style, that supports individuals to address their ambivalence, through evoking their own reasons to change. This approach sits in between directing and following and can be seen in Figure 13.4.

Guided communication incorporates four key skills; asking open questions (such as 'what change would you like to make?', 'How important is it for you to make that change?"), active listening which is evidenced through listening statements (such as 'I understand that you smoke more when you are with your friends'), the use of affirmations to recognise the individual's strengths (such as 'I think you have shown real strength there'), and the use of summarising, to pull together the main themes of the conversation (Rollnick et al., 2023). This approach is believed to be effective because open questions promote reflection on the reasons for change, alongside any potential challenges and how these might be overcome. Listening statements help demonstrate active listening (largely through the individual hearing their own words [rephrased] back to them). Affirmation helps

Directing:
The professional knows the solution and leads the conversation.

Guided:
The professional collaborates with the client, promotes their agency and elicits their reasons to change.

Following:
The professional follows the client's agenda and trusts them to know best.

FIGURE 13.4 Communication styles.

individuals see and appreciate where they are already doing well, and finally, an overall summary pulls together the individual's reasons for change and goals, allowing consolidation and agreement on the next steps (Rollnick et al., 2023). Generally, professionals continue to set the agenda and need to be able to appropriately challenge and offer choices. This is important, as motivational interviewing is not simply being nice or wanting to make an individual feel good (Rollnick et al., 2023). It is primarily intended to promote behaviour change.

The evidence base regarding motivational interviewing is extensive, including systematic reviews, and even systematic reviews of reviews (Frost et al., 2018). One large systematic review of systematic reviews (which included over 114 review papers covering a diverse range of behaviours including alcohol and substance misuse, inactivity, etc.– which highlights the extent to which motivational interviewing has been examined), found that studies are often low quality and tend to be short term, limiting our understanding as to how effective this approach is in bringing about long-term sustained behaviour change (Frost et al., 2018).

However, several meta-analyses have examined motivational interviewing either on its own or alongside other interventions; for example, two studies found that motivational interviewing can have significantly better outcomes than other behaviour change approaches, including in those from minoritised ethnic backgrounds (Hettema et al., 2005, Lundahl et al., 2010), with some evidence suggesting that even a single session can significantly impact on behaviour change (Eaton et al., 2012, Sagherian et al., 2016). One recent study looked at the use of motivational interviewing to reduce risky sexual behaviour in incarcerated men scheduled for release (Delaney et al., 2023). Participants were either offered one session of motivational interviewing or a didactic education session (i.e. a session where they receive one-way education, such as in a classroom). Whilst both groups were satisfied with their sessions, the men who received motivational interviewing were more likely to use condoms, more likely to have partners using contraceptives, and were more confident discussing contraception than those who instead had only didactic education (Delaney et al., 2023).

However, despite evidence that this approach can work, particularly in the short term, concern has been raised as to the lack of monitoring, and fidelity of motivational interviewing as a behaviour change intervention. In this section, we have described a very specific approach, but it is likely that what is called 'motivational interviewing' takes on many different forms and may be delivered in radically different ways, which may influence how effective it is, depending on how much approaches deviate.

Case Study: Behaviour Change Theories and Motivational Interviewing in Practice – The Family Nurse Partnership (FNP)

In Chapter 15, we explore in depth the importance of social relations, opportunities and exposures, particularly in the early years, in shaping later life health, well-being and opportunities. In this case study, we introduce one approach that can positively impact on children and their families.

The FNP is an intensive evidence-based public health program that works with vulnerable first-time young mothers and their babies (FNP, 2023c). It aims to improve outcomes and reduce inequalities experienced by young parents and their children, especially those relating to pregnancy, child health and development, and parental self-efficacy (FNP, 2023c). Supporting behaviour change through building a therapeutic

relationship and using a motivational interviewing approach is at the core of the FNP (Channon et al., 2016).

It was initially introduced in the United Kingdom in 2007, having been adapted from the US Nurse Family Partnership Programme (NFP) (FNP, 2023c, Robling et al., 2016). It is delivered by specially trained nurses and/or midwives, involves up to 64 visits that typically begin in early pregnancy, and often continue until 'graduation,' when the child is 1–2 years old (FNP, 2020, Robling et al., 2016).

FNP is underpinned by three theories: human ecology theory, attachment theory and self-efficacy theory, alongside specific behaviour change approaches, such as motivational interviewing (usually led by a nurse), and the 'New Mum Star tool,' which supports collaboration between family nurses and new parents to support behaviour change (FNP, 2020, FNP, 2023b).

To support the client in identifying their strengths and areas for development, the family nurse uses the 'New Mum Star' to identify where on the journey of change they may be for each of the nine prongs, which includes areas such as life skills, looking after their baby, and their health and wellbeing (FNP, 2020). The client and family nurse identify up to three areas to focus on, which then shapes the direction of the family nurse's work with the client regarding supporting behaviour change, alongside the delivery of the core programme content (FNP, 2020).

Being able to incorporate motivational interviewing into family nurse practice has been identified as key to family nurse engagement and the retention of clients in the programme (Channon et al., 2016, O'Brien et al., 2012). For example, research from the United States highlighted the potentially important impact of motivational interviewing skills on programme attrition (O'Brien et al., 2012). Research looking at whether motivational interviewing can be incorporated into a structured programme, rather than a standalone intervention, found that family nurses were able to deliver FNP using a consistent motivational interviewing approach, and although they did not have consistently high fidelity scores in how motivational interviewing was delivered against all measures (i.e. they adopted slightly different approaches), they did demonstrate skilful practice, alongside high levels of engagement and low levels of attrition (Channon et al., 2016).

FNP has been extensively researched and randomised controlled trials have been undertaken in England, the United States and the Netherlands, with each demonstrating positive outcomes for the child and/or parent(s), although the outcomes themselves varied within the research (Early Intervention Foundation, 2023, FNP, 2023a). The Early Intervention Foundation assesses early intervention programmes targeted at children and young people and rates the quality of the evidence base for the intervention; FNP has been rated the highest available evidence rating (4+), demonstrating positive outcomes. Although the findings of the first England RCT did not demonstrate an effect on breastfeeding rates, smoking in pregnancy or subsequent pregnancies, it did show positive effects on early child development such as language development and child cognitive development alongside increased parental self-efficacy (Robling et al., 2016). A subsequent RCT has also found positive effects on FNP children's school readiness and reading scores, alongside improved writing scores for boys (Robling et al., 2021).

Having read the case study, consider the following points:

- What kind of challenges do you think young parents face?
- How do the human ecology theory, attachment and self-efficacy inform family nurse practice and client work?
- Why do you think Family Nurses use tools, such as the New Mum's Star, to match their agenda with the parent?
- How could the evidence base for FNP and its effectiveness inform public health practice when working with other disadvantaged groups, such as those considered in Chapter 10?

Making Every Contact Count (MECC) and Healthy Conversation Skills

'Making Every Contact Count' or 'MECC', as it is oft referred to, is a brief or very brief (sometimes referred to as 'opportunist') behaviour change intervention using specific healthy conversation skills (NHS, 2016, Nichol et al., 2024a, Parchment et al., 2023a, Rodrigues et al., 2024). It has recently been expanded into conversations about the wider determinants of health (e.g. debt management, housing, etc.), and its use has now moved beyond healthcare settings (Nichol et al., 2024a, Rodrigues et al., 2024). It makes use of the unique position and everyday conversations that exist between those working in behaviour change roles, and those who may wish to make lifestyle and health behaviour changes. A recent scoping review by Parchment et al. (2023a) alongside an evaluation of implementation by Rodrigues et al. (2024) provides a useful overview of implementation, the existing evidence base for the intervention, and the potential barriers and facilitators for its use in clinical practice.

In the United Kingdom, versions of MECC are now widely used in a range of practice settings (Rodrigues et al., 2024) and are taught at universities in preregistration healthcare programmes (including on our own). It can however be delivered by anyone (Nichol et al., 2024b). As a broad approach, it draws on the COM-B model of behaviour change (Michie et al., 2011) that we discussed earlier in this chapter. Conversations typically centre around understanding behaviour change in the context of people's everyday lives (not too dissimilarly from motivational interviewing), using their own resources and potential solutions (Parchment et al., 2023a). Its justification largely follows the use of brief interventions in addressing some of the major risk factors that are amenable to change (we covered these in the previous chapter, especially smoking, high alcohol consumption, physical inactivity and diet) (Aveyard et al., 2016, DiClemente et al., 2017, Vijay et al., 2016, Whatnall et al., 2018) and is central to the United Kingdom government's agenda of tackling these behaviours (NHS, 2023, Rodrigues et al., 2024).

MECC as a broad approach is understood to be acceptable to healthcare professionals and patients (Hollis et al., 2021, Jarman et al., 2019, Parchment et al., 2023b), and research has suggested that training can increase healthcare professionals' confidence in initiating MECC and healthy conversations (Lawrence et al., 2016). Staff in particular value the approach when they see it as part of their role, and where they have organisational support to do it, but barriers are often also experienced, such as a lack of time and a lack of resources (Parchment et al., 2023a). In addition, the fleeting nature of MECC interactions (after all this is a brief intervention), lack of follow-up, and the lack of standardisation to the approach, means that evidence on its effectiveness on behaviour change is limited (Rodrigues et al., 2024). This lack of standardisation also impacts on implementation too (Rodrigues et al., 2024) and there is a push for the approach to be more standardised (Chisholm et al., 2019), with recent work seeking to reach a consensus about what 'MECC' actually is and highlighting its links with motivational interviewing (Nichol et al., 2024b).

However, one example of standardised training is the 'Healthy Conversation Skills' (HCS), developed at the University of Southampton, specifically to support health-related behaviour change (Lawrence et al., 2016). This specific version of MECC draws on aspects of the seminal social cognitive theory (discussed earlier in this chapter and in the previous chapter) (Bandura, 1986, Bandura, 1997) to support staff to have person-centred behaviour change conversations with those accessing their services, to build their motivation and empower them to change through increasing their self-efficacy, and their belief that behaviour change can be possible within their everyday context. This is largely achieved through asking open discovery questions (not dissimilar to motivational interviewing – essentially questions that get people to think and reflect on their own motivations), to help people open up about their behaviours and how they might change these (generally 'what' or 'how' questions), listening more than telling/suggesting, reflection, and SMARTER goal setting (Lawrence et al., 2016). MECC as an approach can be seen in particular in the second conversation, in the case study provided.

Case Study: MECC in Action

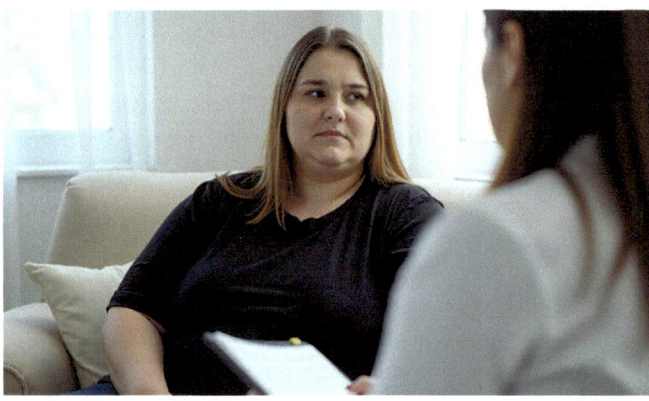

Source: D. Kaminsky/Adobe Stock Photos.

Conversation 1

Fran: Hi Jessica, I have just been reading through your notes, and I am slightly concerned about your weight, and how this might be impacting your health. I think this is an up-to-date weight we have recorded here, so I think your BMI is around about 41. I am concerned about this and how this might be affecting your health. I would like you to try and cut down on how much you are eating, and maybe consider going to the gym sometimes. Were you aware that you were overweight, and this might be having an impact on your health?

Jessica: Well, yes. I know I have put on a bit. It is just tricky, I have three young kids, and well, you know. I just don't really have the time. I tend to just eat the food that is easy to eat- just put it in the oven, once I have sorted the kids. You know how it is.

Fran: I get its difficult with kids, but I think you do need to start prioritising you. Otherwise, you might become unwell. Let's get you to the gym – shall we say you are going to go three times a week? I'll get that written in your notes, that you are going to do that. I will also refer you to the dietician.

Conversation 2

Fran: Hi Jessica, how are you feeling?

Jessica: Pretty good, all things considered. Some days are more difficult than others. It's been a tough year, what with the three kids, and managing work, on top of managing my condition.

Fran: How are you finding that, looking after the kids, whilst also having to manage all of this?

Jessica: I'm doing ok, getting there. My husband is supportive. The kids are full of energy and sometimes, I just can't keep up with them. I would like to be in a bit better shape really, so I can get a bit more involved, you know when Jack wants to kick the ball around in the garden or play tennis.

Fran: Looking at your BMI, it does look like you are overweight at the moment, I know this is tough and you are wanting to work on this. What do you think might help you get in better shape?

Jessica: My husband has talked about us all getting out on our bikes a bit more. We love the forest, and we have a bike trailer that the two youngest can go in, so they can come too. Jack is getting really good at cycling, so I think he would enjoy it to.

Having read the two versions of the conversation, we would like you to consider the following points:

- Which of the conversations involved more telling/suggesting? Was this appropriate?

- In which of the conversations is Jessica most likely to do something positive about her health?

- Why do you think Jessica is more likely to do something?

- Which of the conversations would you most like to have been on the receiving end of? Why did you choose this one?

Overall, the use of MECC and motivational interviewing techniques makes a welcome change to more paternalistic conversations, where healthcare professionals make suggestions about how people should act and live their lives, even when the context within which suggested changes should take place, are not necessarily known, or incorporated into such suggestions, and where someone's capabilities, opportunities and motivations to make a change, are not considered (as per the COM-B model). Whilst motivational interviewing and healthy conversation skills are becoming an increasingly important part of many healthcare professionals tool kits in addressing behaviour change, people's health behaviours are practised in their everyday lives, and much of this occurs without any involvement from healthcare professionals, especially where people are otherwise well, which they would largely be expected to be, with a more preventative approach. One proposed approach to meeting the behaviour change needs of populations, in a scalable and sustainable way, is to deliver behaviour change interventions digitally, such as through a smartphone application, which most people now have access to.

Digital Behaviour Change Interventions

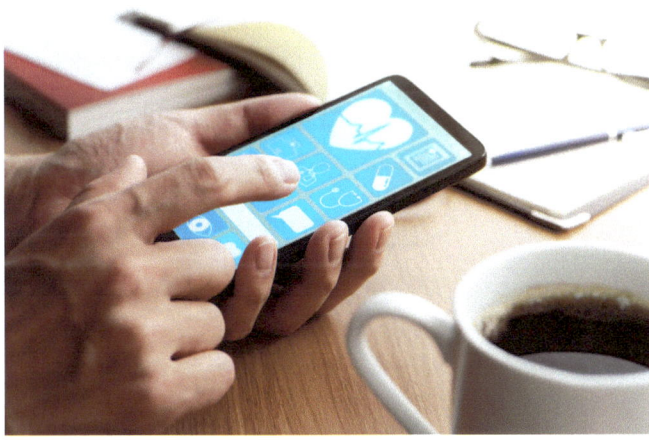

Source: Tadamichi/Adobe Stock Photos.

With the increasing ubiquity and advances of digital technologies in all aspects of everyday living, interest has grown in the potential to use a range of digitally mediated behaviour change interventions to support behaviour change (Mair et al., 2023). Behaviour change, as we have highlighted, is difficult to achieve and sustain; even in those offered a behaviour change intervention, of which only a fraction of those who might benefit surely are. Digital technologies have the potential to make behaviour change interventions available to large numbers of the population in a cost-effective, scalable and sustainable way, and largely because

of this, alongside increased concern about the impact of health behaviours on morbidity, they have been embraced with enthusiasm by academics and those working in areas promoting health behaviour change (Furness et al., 2020, Jiang et al., 2019, Li et al., 2020, Milne-Ives et al., 2020, Pal et al., 2013), with thousands of systematic reviews on digital health interventions having now been published with varying quality (Mair et al., 2023). These reviews have indicated that digital behaviour interventions may be effective in bringing about change in health behaviours (Antoun et al., 2022, Davis et al., 2020, de Leeuwerk et al., 2022, Dugas et al., 2020, Griffiths et al., 2018, Howlett et al., 2022, Schoeppe et al., 2016), as well as condition management and medication adherence for those living with chronic health conditions that require behaviour change (Fu et al., 2017, Furness et al., 2020, Pal et al., 2013). However, these are complex interventions, often composed of several behaviour change techniques, and therefore whilst change has been demonstrated, it is often less clear *exactly* which parts of these interventions are most effective and under what conditions. Whilst analysis of the various components of an intervention (e.g. goal setting, and social support) is common and seeks to identify which aspects have the greatest impacts (as well as least, or harmful impacts); our understanding of *exactly* what aspects of digital behaviour change interventions work best for *whom*, is incomplete, but expanding. One recent large narrative umbrella review (a study that analyses available meta-analysis and systematic reviews and uses these to produce an overarching narrative of what interventions have been examined, and their outcomes) (Mair et al., 2023), found that effective components of digital behaviour change interventions include:

- Credible sources and information (such as from a healthcare professional)
- Social support
- Prompts and cues
- Goal setting and action planning
- Problem-solving
- Feedback and monitoring of performance
- Graded tasks
- Human coaching
- Tailored and personalised content

In addition, it has been suggested that effective digital behaviour change interventions should seek to maximise the number of evidence-based behaviour change techniques into their design to increase the likeliness that they will be effective (Mair et al., 2023). One recent review found that social cognitive theory and the transtheoretical model (discussed above) underpin many interventions (alongside the theory of reasoned behaviour, not covered in this chapter), and may support intervention efficacy (Fielder et al., 2020).

The Limits of Individual Approaches to Behaviour Change

As we explored in the previous chapter, as well as within this chapter in relation to COM-B and the BCW, whilst people's own individual agency and choices are often significant, behaviours are always practised within social contexts that guide behaviours, and that can make it difficult to change behaviours that might be harmful. Individual approaches to behaviour change (whilst popular) can only bring about so much change. What is often more necessary is macro-level changes that promote healthier lives and healthier lifestyles for all. The limitations of focusing on individuals, their behaviour and their self-care are shown in the following quote, taken from the reflections provided in an ethnography considering the promotion of self-care in the United Kingdom, and the importance of self-care in a woman called Sharon, whose lifestyle has been brought into focus:

> 'This was reinforced by the accompanying photograph of three children, wearing baseball caps and 'hoodies', one drinking from a can of beer, against a backdrop of graffiti. There is an implicit condemnation of Sharon in the reference to 'latchkey children.' I could think of various national and community-level interventions that could potentially improve her quality of life, higher minimum wage, interventions aimed at maximising uptake of state benefits, subsidised child-care, community facilities and services that provide instrumental social support and alternative activities for their children, yet staff were guided to see the remedy for Sharon's concerns as self-care' (Jones, 2018).

This quote provides a poignant end to this chapter. Whilst individual approaches to behaviour change can be effective and are important, they do very little to address the social contexts that make certain behaviours more or less likely. By focusing on individuals, and their behaviours, we are less likely to bring about actual, just and long-lasting change in people's lives. In the next chapter, we move beyond seeking to address individual behaviours, to what steps can be taken to improve people's health (including their behaviours) at a broader population level.

Clinical Considerations

- There are a range of behaviour change techniques, and these are often the active ingredients to more complex behaviour change interventions.
- Healthcare professionals are increasingly being expected to be proficient in a range of behaviour change techniques, such as motivational interviewing and other healthy conversation skills such as MECC.
- Digital behaviour change interventions are becoming increasingly common, and will increasingly be seen within clinical practice as a way to promote behaviour change.

Conclusion

In this chapter, we have moved beyond considering why people engage in unhealthy behaviour, towards thinking of the ways that the social sciences have contributed to our understanding of how we can support people to change their behaviour. We have considered the stages of change model, social cognitive theory, and the hugely influential COM-B behaviour change model. In addition, we have highlighted the range of behaviour change techniques that provide the active ingredients for behaviour change interventions. Finally, we have shown some behaviour change approaches that are frequently used in clinical practice, such as motivational interviewing, MECC, and digital behaviour change interventions. Models that seek to address behaviour at the level of individuals do little to change the social context in which these behaviours are practised, and it is interventions at the level of populations, that we turn to in the next chapter.

References

Antoun, J., Itani, H., Alarab, N. & Elsehmawy, A. 2022. The effectiveness of combining nonmobile interventions with the use of smartphone apps with various features for weight loss: systematic review and meta-analysis. *JMIR mHealth and uHealth*, 10, e35479.

Aveyard, P., Lewis, A., Tearne, S., Hood, K., Christian-Brown, A., Adab, P., Begh, R., Jolly, K., Daley, A., Farley, A., Lycett, D., Nickless, A., Yu, L.-M., Retat, L., Webber, L., Pimpin, L. & Jebb, S. A. 2016. Screening and brief intervention for obesity in primary care: a parallel, two-arm, randomised trial. *The Lancet*, 388, 2492–2500.

Bandura, A. 1977. Self-efficacy: Toward a unifying theory of behavioral change. *Psychological Review*, 84, 191–215.

Bandura, A. 1986. *Social Foundations of Thought and Action*, Englewood Cliffs, NJ: Prentice Hall.

Bandura, A. 1997. *Self-Efficacy: The Exercise of Control*, Freeman.

Bandura, A. 2012. Cultivate Self-efficacy for Personal and Organizational Effectiveness. *In:* Locke, E. A. (ed.) *The Blackwell Handbook of Principles of Organizational Behavior*, Wiley.

Bandura, A. 2017. Cultivate Self-efficacy for Personal and Organizational Effectiveness. *In: The Blackwell Handbook of Principles of Organizational Behaviour*, Wiley.

Bandura, A. & Cervone, D. 2023. *Social Cognitive Theory: an Agentic Perspective on Human Nature*, John Wiley and Sons.

Beauchamp, M. R., Crawford, K. L. & Jackson, B. 2019. Social cognitive theory and physical activity: mechanisms of behavior change, critique, and legacy. *Psychology of Sport and Exercise*, 42, 110–117.

Benight, C. C. & Bandura, A. 2004. Social cognitive theory of posttraumatic recovery: the role of perceived self-efficacy. *Behaviour Research and Therapy*, 42, 1129–1148.

Borah, P., Lorenzano, K., Yel, E. & Austin, E. 2024. Social cognitive theory and willingness to perform recommended health behavior: the moderating role of misperceptions. *Journal of Health Communication*, 29, 49–60.

Bunton, R., Baldwin, S., Flynn, D. & Whitelaw, S. 2000. The 'stages of change' model in health promotion: science and ideology. *Critical Public Health*, 10, 55–70.

Channon, S., Bekkers, M.-J., Sanders, J., Cannings-John, R., Robertson, L., Bennert, K., Butler, C., Hood, K. & Robling, M. 2016. Motivational interviewing competencies among UK family nurse partnership nurses: a process evaluation component of the building blocks trial. *BMC Nursing*, 15, 55.

Chisholm, A., Ang-Chen, P., Peters, S., Hart, J. & Beenstock, J. 2019. Public health practitioners' views of the 'Making Every Contact Count' initiative and standards for its evaluation. *Journal of Public Health*, 41, e70–e77.

Davis, A., Sweigart, R. & Ellis, R. 2020. A systematic review of tailored mHealth interventions for physical activity promotion among adults. *Translational Behavioral Medicine*, 10, 1221–1232.

Davis, R., Campbell, R., Hildon, Z., Hobbs, L. & Michie, S. 2015. Theories of behaviour and behaviour change across the social and behavioural sciences: a scoping review. *Health Psychology Review*, 9, 323–344.

De Leeuwerk, M. E., Bor, P., Van Der Ploeg, H. P., De Groot, V., Van Der Schaaf, M. & Van Der Leeden, M. 2022. The effectiveness of physical activity interventions using activity trackers during or after inpatient care: a systematic review and meta-analysis of randomized controlled trials. *International Journal of Behavioral Nutrition and Physical Activity*, 19, 59.

Delaney, D. J., Stein, L., Bassett, S. S. & Clarke, J. G. 2023. Motivational interviewing for family planning and reducing risky sexual behavior among incarcerated men nearing release: a randomized controlled pilot study. *Psychological Services*, 20, 538.

Diclemente, C. C., Corno, C. M., Graydon, M. M., Wiprovnick, A. E. & Knoblach, D. J. 2017. Motivational interviewing, enhancement, and brief interventions over the last decade: a review of reviews of efficacy and effectiveness. *Psychology of Addictive Behaviors*, 31, 862–887.

Dixon, D. & Johnston, M. 2021. What competences are required to deliver person-person behaviour change interventions: development of a health behaviour change competency framework. *International Journal of Behavioral Medicine*, 28, 308–317.

Dugas, M., Gao, G. & Agarwal, R. 2020. Unpacking mHealth interventions: a systematic review of behavior change techniques used in randomized controlled trials assessing mHealth effectiveness. *DIGITAL HEALTH*, 6, 2055207620905411.

Early Intervention Foundation. 2023. Family Nurse Partnership [Online]. Early Intervention Foundation Available: https://www.fnp.nhs.uk/our-impact/evidence/ [Accessed].

Eaton, L. A., Huedo-Medina, T. B., Kalichman, S. C., Pellowski, J. A., Sagherian, M. J., Warren, M., Popat, A. R. & Johnson, B. T. 2012. Meta-analysis of single-session behavioral interventions to prevent sexually transmitted infections: implications for bundling prevention packages. *American Journal of Public Health*, 102, e34–e44.

Evers, K. E. & Balestrieri, S. G. 2024. The Transtheoretical Model And Stages Of Change. *In:* Glanz, K., Rimer, B. K. & Viswanath, K. (eds.) *Health Behavior: Theory, Research, and Practice*, 6th Edition, 73.

Fiedler, J., Eckert, T., Wunsch, K. & Woll, A. 2020. Key facets to build up eHealth and mHealth interventions to enhance physical activity, sedentary behavior and nutrition in healthy subjects – an umbrella review. *BMC Public Health*, 20, 1605.

FNP. 2020. FNP Adapt [Online]. The Family Nurse Partnership. Available: https://www.fnp.nhs.uk/media/1359/fnp_adapt_report_web.pdf [Accessed].

FNP. 2023a. Evidence: FNP has an internationally-recognised evidence base. [Online]. The Family Nurse Partnership. Available: https://www.fnp.nhs.uk/our-impact/evidence/ [Accessed].

FNP. 2023b. Guidebook [Online]. The Family Nurse Partnership. Available: https://www.fnp.nhs.uk/our-impact/what-fnp-delivers/ [Accessed].

FNP. 2023c. Our impact: The difference FNP makes [Online]. The Family Nurse Partnership Available: https://www.fnp.nhs.uk/our-impact/ [Accessed].

Frost, H., Campbell, P., Maxwell, M., O'carroll, R. E., Dombrowski, S. U., Williams, B., Cheyne, H., Coles, E. & Pollock, A. 2018. Effectiveness of Motivational Interviewing on adult behaviour change in health and social care settings: a systematic review of reviews. *PLoS One*, 13, e0204890.

Fu, H., Mcmahon, S. K., Gross, C. R., Adam, T. J. & Wyman, J. F. 2017. Usability and clinical efficacy of diabetes mobile applications for adults with type 2 diabetes: a systematic review. *Diabetes Research and Clinical Practice*, 131, 70–81.

Furness, K., Sarkies, M. N., Huggins, C. E., Croagh, D. & Haines, T. P. 2020. Impact of the method of delivering electronic health behavior change interventions in survivors of cancer on engagement, health behaviors, and health outcomes: systematic review and meta-analysis. *Journal of Medical Internet Research*, 22, e16112.

Griffiths, S. E., Parsons, J., Naughton, F., Fulton, E. A., Tombor, I. & Brown, K. E. 2018. Are digital interventions for smoking cessation in pregnancy effective? A systematic review and meta-analysis. *Health Psychology Review*, 12, 333–356.

HCPC. 2023. Physiotherapists: The standards of proficiency for physiotherapists. [Online]. Health & Care Professions Council. Available: https://www.hcpc-uk.org/standards/standards-of-proficiency/physiotherapists/ [Accessed].

Hettema, J., Steele, J. & Miller, W. R. 2005. Motivational interviewing. *Annual Review of Clinical Psychology*, 1, 91–111.

Hollis, J. L., Kocanda, L., Seward, K., Collins, C., Tully, B., Hunter, M., Foureur, M., Lawrence, W., Macdonald-Wicks, L. & Schumacher, T. 2021. The impact of Healthy Conversation Skills training on health professionals' barriers to having behaviour change conversations: A pre-post survey using the Theoretical Domains Framework. *BMC Health Services Research*, 21, 880.

Howlett, N., García-Iglesias, J., Bontoft, C., Breslin, G., Bartington, S., Freethy, I., Huerga-Malillos, M., Jones, J., Lloyd, N. & Marshall, T. 2022. A systematic review and behaviour change technique analysis of remotely delivered alcohol and/or substance misuse interventions for adults. *Drug and Alcohol Dependence*, 239, 109597.

Jarman, M., Adam, L., Lawrence, W., Barker, M. & Bell, R. C. 2019. Healthy conversation skills as an intervention to support healthy gestational weight gain: experience and perceptions from intervention deliverers and participants. *Patient Education and Counseling*, 102, 924–931.

Jiang, X., Ming, W.-K. & You, J. H. 2019. The cost-effectiveness of digital health interventions on the management of cardiovascular diseases: systematic review. *Journal of Medical Internet Research*, 21, e13166.

Jones, L. 2018. Pastoral power and the promotion of self-care. *Sociology of Health & Illness*, 40, 988–1004.

Lawrence, W., Black, C., Tinati, T., Cradock, S., Begum, R., Jarman, M., Pease, A., Margetts, B., Davies, J. & Inskip, H. 2016. 'Making every contact count': evaluation of the impact of an intervention to train health and social care practitioners in skills to support health behaviour change. *Journal of Health Psychology*, 21, 138–151.

Li, R., Liang, N., Bu, F. & Hesketh, T. 2020. The effectiveness of self-management of hypertension in adults using mobile health: systematic review and meta-analysis. *JMIR mHealth and uHealth*, 8, e17776.

Littell, J. H. & Girvin, H. 2002. Stages of change: A critique. *Behavior Modification*, 26, 223–273.

Lundahl, B. W., Kunz, C., Brownell, C., Tollefson, D. & Burke, B. L. 2010. A meta-analysis of motivational interviewing: twenty-five years of empirical studies. *Research on Social Work Practice*, 20, 137–160.

Luszczynska, A. & Schwarzer, R. 2020. Changing Behavior Using Social Cognitive Theory. *In:* Hagger, M., Cameron, L., Hamilton, K., Hankonen, N. & Lintunen, T. (eds.) *The Handbook of Behaviour Change*, Cambridge University Press.

Mair, J. L., Salamanca-Sanabria, A., Augsburger, M., Frese, B. F., Abend, S., Jakob, R., Kowatsch, T. & Haug, S. 2023. Effective behavior change techniques in digital health interventions for the prevention or management of noncommunicable diseases: an umbrella review. *Annals of Behavioral Medicine*, 57, 817–835.

Mantey, D., Hunt, E., Hoelscher, D. & Kelder, S. 2024. Social Cognitive Theory and Health Behaviour. *In:* Glanz, K., Rimer, B. & Viswanath, K. (eds.) *Health Behavior: Theory, Research, and Practice*, Wiley.

Michie, S., Atkins, L. & West, R. 2024. *The Behaviour Change Wheel*, Silverback publishing.

Michie, S. & Johnston, M. 2012. *Theories and techniques of behaviour change: Developing a cumulative science of behaviour change*, Taylor & Francis.

Michie, S., Richardson, M., Johnston, M., Abraham, C., Francis, J., Hardeman, W., Eccles, M. P., Cane, J. & Wood, C. E. 2013. The behavior change technique taxonomy (v1) of 93 hierarchically clustered techniques: building an international consensus for the reporting of behavior change interventions. *Annals of Behavioral Medicine*, 46, 81–95.

Michie, S., Thomas, J., Johnston, M., Aonghusa, P. M., Shawe-Taylor, J., Kelly, M. P., Deleris, L. A., Finnerty, A. N., Marques, M. M., Norris, E. & O'mara-Eves, A. & West, R. 2017. The Human Behaviour-Change Project: harnessing the power of artificial intelligence and machine learning for evidence synthesis and interpretation. *Implementation Science*, 12, 121.

Michie, S., Van Stralen, M. M. & West, R. 2011. The behaviour change wheel: a new method for characterising and designing behaviour change interventions. *Implementation Science*, 6, 42.

Miller, W. R. & Rollnick, S. 2013. *Motivational interviewing: Helping people change*, Third Edition, The Guildford Press.

Milne-Ives, M., Lam, C., De Cock, C., Van Velthoven, M. H. & Meinert, E. 2020. Mobile apps for health behavior change in physical activity, diet, drug and alcohol use, and mental health: systematic review. *JMIR mHealth and uHealth*, 8, e17046.

NHS 2016. Making every contact count (MECC): consensus statement. *Public Health England*, 201, 1–18.

NHS. 2023. NHS Long Term Workforce Plan [Online]. Available: https://www.england.nhs.uk/publication/nhs-long-term-workforce-plan/ [Accessed].

NICE. 2014. Behaviour change: individual approaches [Online]. National Institute for Health and Care Excellence (NICE). Available: https://www.nice.org.uk/guidance/ph49 [Accessed].

Nichol, B., Haighton, C., Wilson, R. & Rodrigues, A. M. 2024a. Enhancing making every contact count (MECC) training and delivery for the third and social economy (TSE) sector: a strategic behavioural analysis. *Psychology & Health*, 1–32.

Nichol, B., Kemp, E., Wilson, R., Rodrigues, A. M., Hesselgreaves, H., Robson, C. & Haighton, C. 2024b. Establishing an updated consensus on the conceptual and operational definitions of Making Every Contact Count (MECC) across experts within research and practice: an international Delphi Study. *Public Health*, 230, 29–37.

NMC. 2019a. The Code: Professional standards of practice and behaviour for nurses, midwives and nursing associates [Online]. Available: https://www.nmc.org.uk/standards/code/ [Accessed].

NMC. 2019b. Standards of proficiency for registered nurses [Online]. Nursing & Midwifery Council Available: https://www.nmc.org.uk/standards/standards-for-nurses/standards-of-proficiency-for-registered-nurses/ [Accessed].

O'brien, R. A., Moritz, P., Luckey, D. W., Mcclatchey, M. W., Ingoldsby, E. M. & Olds, D. L. 2012. Mixed methods analysis of participant attrition in the nurse-family partnership. *Prevention Science*, 13, 219–228.

Pal, K., Eastwood, S. V., Michie, S., Farmer, A. J., Barnard, M. L., Peacock, R., Wood, B., Inniss, J. D. & Murray, E. 2013. Computer-based diabetes self-management interventions for adults with type 2 diabetes mellitus. *Cochrane Database of Systematic Reviews.*.

Parchment, A., Lawrence, W., Perry, R., Rahman, E., Townsend, N., Wainwright, E. & Wainwright, D. 2023a. Making Every Contact Count and Healthy Conversation Skills as very brief or brief behaviour change interventions: a scoping review. *Journal of Public Health*, 31, 1017–1034.

Parchment, A., Lawrence, W., Rahman, E., Townsend, N., Wainwright, E. & Wainwright, D. 2023b. 'I can feel myself coming out of the rut': a brief intervention for supporting behaviour change is acceptable to patients with chronic musculoskeletal conditions. *BMC Musculoskeletal Disorders*, 24, 241.

Prochaska, J. O. & Diclemente, C. C. 1982. Transtheoretical therapy: toward a more integrative model of change. *Psychotherapy: theory, research & practice*, 19, 276.

Prochaska, J. O., Diclemente, C. C. & Norcross, J. C. 1992. In search of how people change. *Applications to addictive behaviors. Am Psychol*, 47, 1102–1114.

Robling, M., Bekkers, M.-J., Bell, K., Butler, C. C., Cannings-John, R., Channon, S., Martin, B. C., Gregory, J. W., Hood, K., Kemp, A., Kenkre, J., Montgomery, A. A., Moody, G., Owen-Jones, E., Pickett, K., Richardson, G., Roberts, Z. E. S., Ronaldson, S., Sanders, J., Stamuli, E. & Torgerson, D. 2016. Effectiveness of a nurse-led intensive home-visitation programme for first-time teenage mothers (Building Blocks): a pragmatic randomised controlled trial. *The Lancet*, 387, 146–155.

Robling, M., Lugg-Widger, F., Cannings-John, R., Sanders, J., Angel, L., Channon, S., Fitzsimmons, D., Hood, K., Kenkre, J., Moody, G., Owen-Jones, E., Pockett, R., Segrott, J. & Slater, T. 2021. The Family Nurse Partnership to reduce maltreatment and improve child health and development in young children: the BB:2–6 routine data-linkage follow-up to earlier RCT. *Public Health Research*, 9, 2.

Rodrigues, A. M., Nichol, B., Wilson, R., Charlton, C., Gibson, B., Finch, T., Haighton, C., Maniatopoulos, G., Giles, E., Harrison, D., Orange, D., Robson, C. & Harland, J. 2024. Mapping regional implementation of 'Making Every Contact Count': mixed-methods evaluation of implementation stage, strategies, barriers and facilitators of implementation. *BMJ Open*, 14, e084208.

Rollnick, S., Miller, W. R. & Butler, C. C. 2023. *Motivational Interviewing in Healthcare: Helping Patients Change Behavior*, Second Edition, The Guildford Press.

Sagherian, M. J., Huedo-Medina, T. B., Pellowski, J. A., Eaton, L. A. & Johnson, B. T. 2016. Single-session behavioral interventions for sexual risk reduction: a meta-analysis. *Annals of Behavioral Medicine*, 50, 920–934.

Schoeppe, S., Alley, S., Van Lippevelde, W., Bray, N. A., Williams, S. L., Duncan, M. J. & Vandelanotte, C. 2016. Efficacy of interventions that use apps to improve diet, physical activity and sedentary behaviour: a systematic review. *International Journal of Behavioral Nutrition and Physical Activity*, 13, 1–26.

Schunk, D. & Dibenedetto, M. 2022. Learning from a Social Cognitive Theory Perspective. *In:* Tierney, R. J., Rizvi, F. & Ercikan, K. (eds.) *International Encyclopedia of Education*, Fourth Edition.

Szczuka, Z., Banik, A., Abraham, C., Kulis, E. & Luszczynska, A. 2021. Associations between self-efficacy and sedentary behaviour: a meta-analysis. *Psychology & Health*, 36, 271–289.

Vijay, G., Wilson, E. C., Suhrcke, M., Hardeman, W. & Sutton, S. 2016. Are brief interventions to increase physical activity cost-effective? A systematic review. *British Journal of Sports Medicine*, 50, 408–417.

Whatnall, M. C., Patterson, A. J., Ashton, L. M. & Hutchesson, M. J. 2018. Effectiveness of brief nutrition interventions on dietary behaviours in adults: a systematic review. *Appetite*, 120, 335–347.

CHAPTER 14

Public Health Interventions through the Lens of the Social Sciences

Chris Allen

School of Health Sciences, University of Southampton, Southampton, UK

'Sometimes it feels like this. There I am standing by the shore of a swiftly flowing river and I hear the cry of a drowning man. So I jump into the river, put my arms around him, pull him to shore and apply artificial respiration. Just when he begins to breathe, there is another cry for help. So I jump into the river, reach him, pull him to shore, apply artificial respiration and then just as he begins to breathe, another cry for help. So back in the river again, reaching, pulling, applying, breathing and then another yell. Again and again, without end, goes the sequence. You know, I am so busy jumping in, pulling them to shore, applying artificial respiration, that I have no time to see who the hell is upstream pushing them all in' (Mckinlay, 1994, p. 509).

Introduction

Healthcare has traditionally focused on fixing people when they become unwell. However, as we have explored in the previous chapters, much of the current healthcare demand is created from health issues that in part could be avoided, such as by addressing people's health behaviour and lifestyles. In the previous two chapters, we have considered *why* people engage in unhealthy behaviours, before considering *how* individuals can be supported to change their behaviour. Focusing on individual behaviour change can only go so far in improving population health, as people's health behaviours are always practiced within a social context, which makes certain behaviour more or less likely. As we have outlined throughout this book's chapters, individuals – you and me, are far from the only people with responsibility towards health. Governments and their various institutions (such as health, education, legal and regulatory systems) play a significant role too. Generally, to change the health of populations, macro-level interventions are needed. A key question posed by this chapter is what societies should do to stop people from falling into the metaphorical river in the first place, but answering this question is not straightforward. Do we simply monitor people's unhealthy behaviour, or do we take more corrective action? If we take more corrective action, how far should we go? Is it right for governments to step in and stop people engaging in certain behaviours, or should we let people make this decision for themselves? And if we are going to intervene, what approaches work? Finally, how can we consider all of this in relation to ensuring everyone has access to the resources they need to live healthy lives, alongside our planet's health and its ability to continue to sustain life?

LEARNING OUTCOMES

By the end of this chapter, you will be able to:

- Recognise what public health is, and why it is important in addressing some of the most significant challenges healthcare systems around the world are currently facing.
- Identify the range of different social institutions that have a role and stake in public health.
- Consider some of the controversies and ethical debates that exist in relation to public health interventions.

Social Sciences for Healthcare Professionals, First Edition. Edited by Chris Allen.
© 2026 John Wiley & Sons Ltd. Published 2026 by John Wiley & Sons Ltd.

- Consider a range of different public health interventions in relation to physical activity, diet, smoking and alcohol consumption, alongside their evidence.
- Recognise the importance of whole systems approaches to public health.
- Recognise the relationship between our planet's health and the health of populations.

Upstream Prevention

> **Key Terms and Definitions**
>
> **Primary prevention:**   Taking steps to prevent someone becoming unwell in the first place.
>
> **Autonomy:**   Being able to make your own decisions, free from manipulation or coercion.
>
> **Liberty:**   Being free, without having restrictions imposed on you, in terms of how you behave and what you do.
>
> **Sin tax:**   A tax imposed on a good that is generally deemed to be harmful (i.e. a sin) as a way to curb (or disincentivise) consumption.
>
> **Nudge:**   Manipulating the decision-making environment to make it more likely that someone will make a desired choice.
>
> **Planetary health:**   The health of the planet, in which human health depends.

Aside from the harmful impact that noncommunicable diseases have on individuals and their personal networks, the way healthcare is currently provided, and the increasing drive for universal health coverage, is likely to be unsustainable in the longer term if people's unhealthy behaviours cannot be changed. There are several ways we can prevent people from falling into the river and needing to be rescued. In the context of public health, these are often broken down into primary, secondary and tertiary prevention (Goldesteen et al., 2015). These are summarised below:

Primary prevention: this generally seeks to prevent illnesses and diseases from happening in the first place, such as by promoting healthy lifestyles.

Secondary prevention: this is generally the preventative methods that are deployed to stop conditions from getting worse, or progressing, such as screening programs that can detect abnormalities (such as cancers) early on.

Tertiary prevention: largely occurs in the context of chronic illness and is largely the steps taken to prevent someone's health deteriorating further because of poor condition management, etc.

This chapter primarily focusses on primary prevention, though governments and their various institutions also have a significant role in secondary and tertiary prevention (and both are discussed throughout this book). As we have explored in the

previous chapter, individual behaviour is both leaned on as a cause of poor health and is often the target of health intervention (Danielli et al., 2023, Williams and Fullagar, 2019). However, health behaviours are not practiced in a lab and are in fact shaped by our environments, where we live, alongside a myriad number of social, economic, commercial and political influences (the wider determinants of health) (explored in Chapter 8) (Kivimäki et al., 2020, Marmot, 2010, Marmot et al., 2008, 2020). Most of these influences are shaped by governments and policies. Personal factors of course do play a role (as we explored in Chapter 12), but generally these are believed to be less significant in determining population health.

What Is Public Health?

Essentially, public health is the efforts and concern of addressing population health, which can include consideration of the aspects of our environment that contribute to poor health (Goldesteen et al., 2015, Naidoo and Wills, 2016). In Chapter 7, you were introduced to one of the pioneers of public health and epidemiology, John Snow (1813–1857), who identified the environmental causes of cholera, leading to sewage systems being overhauled, and subsequent improvements in public health. Public health is essentially a public good, as it involves the coordinated effort of governments and various other institutions to meet the needs of populations fairly and equitably. Approaches to public health are generally underpinned by science and are often creative (see, e.g. the many creative health approaches discussed in Chapter 17). Public health is not just a hard science, as it involves creativity, being able to form meaningful connections with communities, and supporting health through political influence (Goldesteen et al., 2015; Naidoo and Wills, 2016), and hence, nods to the arts and science are a common feature of many public health definitions, for example:

'The science and art of preventing disease, prolonging life and promoting health through the organized efforts and informed choices of society, organizations, public and private, communities and individuals' (Winslow, 1920).

Generally, public health is concerned with upstream activity – activities that prevent people (largely a collective or a population) from falling into the river and needing to be rescued in the first place (Goldesteen et al., 2015, Naidoo and Wills, 2016). As such, it is largely proactive (and therefore often targets those who might not think of themselves as unwell), rather than reactive, and aims to improve the health of populations often through the provision of services, and legislative frameworks to ensure that health is not left exclusively to free market forces to determine, and that those in positions of influence over health take action and conduct themselves in ways that promote health. Because of this, public health work often involves a fair bit of political work across a range of organisational contexts to promote health and address inequalities (Coggon, 2012, Lynch, 2023, Oliver, 2006). As health is determined by many things, this cannot be done in isolation and therefore, when considering public health, whilst healthcare professionals often play a leading (sometimes even political) role, most interventions require collaboration, and the efforts and contributions of a range of stakeholders, such as those involved in setting policy, those involved in operationalising this policy from the public sector (which can include health, education, legal institutions, etc.), the private sector, the community and third sector, and importantly populations themselves.

So where is this coordinating effort often focused? Whilst most of the improvements in population health have been attributed to advances in our knowledge and understanding of disease and medicine (including vaccination), most improvements in population health are largely attributable to non-medical developments (such as improvements in living and working conditions –housing, sanitation, etc.) (Bergman et al., 2018). Improvements in life expectancy through this, in line with the demographic and epidemiological transitions discussed in Chapter 7, have meant that the biggest threat to population health is now noncommunicable disease (or long-term conditions), with important research identifying links between certain behaviours (such as smoking) and certain diseases (such as cancer and cardiovascular disease) and this has resulted in a prolonged and sustained shift of public health attention towards prevention (stopping people falling in the river rather than pulling them out), largely through taking action on health behaviours and lifestyles (Bergman et al., 2018).

With health behaviours being so closely related to non-communicable disease, the extent to which individuals should be seen as responsible for their own health has been hotly debated, and for some time (Mold, 2022). Tied closely to such a discourse is a neoliberal agenda, alongside a rolling back of state involvement (i.e. austerity) in many western developed nations, that highlights that people are free to make their own choices, and are ultimately responsible for the impacts of these choices and the management of their own health (Ayo, 2012, Labonté and Stuckler, 2016, LeBesco, 2011, Mold, 2022, Vassilev et al., 2017). However, countering such a discourse is the recognition that much of a person's behaviour is determined by things that exist outside of their control, such as their living and working conditions. This raises important and complex questions about how much states can and should be involved in directing the health behaviours of their populations through public health and through public health interventions.

What Is a Public Health Intervention?

A public health intervention is simply any action that seeks to improve the health of a population (Goldesteen et al., 2015). When we consider the evidence that is important to public health, we can loosely break this down into two types:

1. The evidence for the causes of poor health (we covered this more in Chapter 7 when we introduced epidemiology as a public health science). This helps us understand the patterning and causes of ill health in populations.

2. Evidence that helps us understand how effective our attempts (or interventions) are in addressing this, such as through primary, secondary or tertiary prevention programmes.

Much of this evidence, both in relation to the causes of poor health and the best strategies to tackling public health concerns, is collected in messy everyday life. Interventions generally involve several components and are generally used in a variety of contexts, with a variety of people, who are themselves often very different. As such, evidence is rarely perfect, may often be incomplete and is very often contested. Because of this, research evidence even when strong, may not tell policymakers exactly how to proceed and there are often several ways to address the same issue (such as restricting smoking to certain age groups, curbing consumption through sin taxes, introducing smoking bans in public places, or banning smoking entirely). Additionally, interventions that benefit one group, may harm or disadvantage another (Jan et al., 2024, Kratzer et al., 2022). As a result, trade-offs and ethical debates often also exist and influence decisions. Doing something to whole populations as opposed to individuals makes many of the ethical principles (such as consent and autonomy) that underpin healthcare challenging to achieve, with many public health interventions involving at least some compromise to people's liberty and choice (e.g. a ban on smoking limits people's autonomy around smoking) (Calman, 2009). Many have experienced a recent example of this. During the COVID-19 pandemic, countries around the world mandated social distancing, and the unanticipated harms of this decision are now being widely considered (Turcotte-Tremblay et al., 2021, Kratzer et al., 2022). However, populations were given little choice. Liberty was taken from citizens across entire nations without their consent in the interests of population health and to protect those who are most vulnerable (Cameron et al., 2021). In some countries, similar liberties were taken from healthcare professionals in relation to personal decisions about vaccination, in the interest of protecting those who were most vulnerable (Bardosh et al., 2022, Giubilini et al., 2023, Olick et al., 2021). These are extreme examples of course, from an unprecedented situation, and examples that we may not see again in our lifetimes. However, other examples do exist, for example, the policy to add fluoride to water supplies to improve dental health, reduces people's choice around the consumption of fluoride, at scale and without consent (Shakeri et al., 2020). This brings us to the (bio)ethics and politics of public health.

The Political Philosophy, and (Bio)ethics of Public Health

The Harm Principle

One way of thinking about public health interventions in the context of (bio)ethics is the harm principle (Calman, 2009). First developed by philosopher John Stuart Mills (1806–1873), the harm principle is not new (Calman, 2009). It can be used to guide thinking about the extent to which it is appropriate to intervene (i.e. exerting power over another), suggesting that we should only do so, where someone's actions harm others, or to protect those who are particularly vulnerable (such as children and those lacking mental capacity) (Calman, 2009; Nuffield Bioethics Council, 2007). As just one example, we are all free to wave our fists around, provided our fists don't actually connect with (and thus harm) anyone else. Laws generally exist to prevent people and states from harming others and to prevent vulnerable people from being harmed.

Action on smoking in public places provides one salient example that fits with the harm principle. This behaviour is known to be harmful to the individuals that are engaged with it, as well as to others around them via second-hand smoke (Khan, 2022). Hence allowing smoking in private spaces, but banning smoking in public places, where this behaviour may cause harm to others. Essentially, the harm principle is concerned with people's liberty, maximising utility (i.e. benefit), choice and autonomy (Calman, 2009, Nuffield Bioethics Council, 2007). Being well informed is important here, as this allows people to be better able to make decisions about their own behaviours and understand their likely consequences (such as providing health education on diet, exercise and alcohol consumption). However, the harm principle suggests that more coercive and controlling interventions that remove choice and autonomy in those whose behaviour is not likely to harm others (such as banning smoking in private places), may threaten individual liberty (Calman, 2009, Nuffield Bioethics Council, 2007).

Nanny or Nurture?

Different societies will have different levels of tolerance towards state involvement. Decisions about how much and how governments should intervene are inherently political. Whilst a full range of views exist, these can largely be broken down into libertarian (nurture) or paternalist/collectivist (nanny) approaches (nanny vs nurture) (Calman, 2009, Nuffield Bioethics Council, 2007). Under a libertarian/individualist state, people are free to make their own way in life with little government interference. However, the state typically provides very little protection when things do go wrong. In contrast, under a collectivist state, the needs of populations are prioritised over the needs (and sometimes even to the detriment) of individuals (Calman, 2009, Nuffield Bioethics Council, 2007). Most societies have governments that sit somewhere in the middle, though often with a tendency to lean towards individualism or collectivism and where democratic processes exist, these tendencies are steered through political mandates (i.e. through democratically elected governments acting on behalf of their electorates views and what they see as most important) (Calman, 2009, Nuffield Bioethics Council, 2007).

The Stewardship Model

Stewardship generally implies a responsibility to 'look after' or 'supervise' something (Nuffield Bioethics Council, 2007). In the context of public health, it highlights the importance and responsibility of governments looking after people, primarily their health. The stewardship model is underpinned by the harm principle (Nuffield Bioethics Council, 2007).

It emphasises that action on health behaviour is often necessary to:

- Reduce the risk posed to people from the harmful behaviours of others (such as second-hand smoke).
- Address the causes of poor health, such as by creating environmental conditions (including through regulations) that are conducive to health (such as ensuring people have access to adequate shelter, sanitation, and food).
- Focus on vulnerable groups (e.g. children and those who are socially excluded).
- Support people to change their behaviour, both through providing information on health harms and through the provision of services to support behaviour change.
- Make it easier for people to live healthier lives (such as, by ensuring safe cycle lanes or reducing the financial barriers to participating in sports and exercise).
- Ensure access to healthcare as a fundamental right.
- Address the unjust, systematic difference in health outcomes (the health inequalities, discussed in Chapter 8).

Many of these also align with Mill's harm principle, for example, the protection of vulnerable groups, the provision of information to help people make their own choices, alongside attempts to increase people's freedom to live healthier lives (such as by reducing health inequalities, increasing opportunities to participate in sport and increasing access to healthcare). However, an important observation of the stewardship model is that interventions can be contentious, particularly those that are coercive, intrusive, remove choice or threaten people's values and norms (Nuffield Bioethics Council, 2007).

The Nuffield Ladder of Interventions

Using the stewardship model, the Nuffield Council (an independent body, who like other non-government organisations, informs policy and debate around issues relating to health, healthcare services and provision) created the Nuffield ladder of interventions to guide policymakers to weigh up health harms with an interventions intrusiveness (Nuffield Bioethics Council, 2007). The ladder's production involved contributions from across the social sciences (Nuffield Bioethics Council, 2007). As you can see in Table 14.1, the ladder has 8

TABLE 14.1   Nuffield Ladder of Interventions and example interventions for each rung.

Rung	Description	Examples
Eliminate choice	Laws that eliminate people's choice entirely.	• Smoking bans. • Banning drugs or other substances harmful to health. • Mandatory isolation of those with infectious diseases during pandemics. • Mandatory vaccination of healthcare workers.
Restrict choice	Laws that restrict people's choices.	• Removing or restricting certain ingredients from foods. • Restricting the sale of alcohol to certain vendors and at certain times. • Only allowing certain behaviours in certain contexts (i.e. smoking outdoors or in private).
Guide choice through disincentives	Deploying disincentives, such as sin taxes, that discourage consumption.	• Taxes on alcohol, or minimum unit (MUP) alcohol pricing to increase prices. • Taxes on cigarettes to increase prices. • Imposing a tax on drinks with high sugar content. • Congestion charges to discourage inner-city driving, particularly for those with high-emission cars.
Guide choice through incentives	Introducing incentives that promote healthier options.	• Subsidising healthy foods. • Providing or subsidising vape kits to smokers wanting to quit smoking. • Providing cycle-to-work schemes, that provide tax breaks to those purchasing a bike for commuting.
Guide choice through changing the default policy	Changing the default to the desired choice	• Changing the default policy, so that people 'opt out', rather than 'opt in' to organ donation. • Changing the default policy, so that people 'opt out', rather than 'opt in' to employee pension contributions. • Providing healthier side dishes (such as salad) as a default, but allowing people to still have the choice to change this to a less healthy option (such as cheesy chips). • Placing healthier items where people are more likely to see them in a supermarket.
Enable choice	Making it possible for people to make healthy choices	• Providing cycle lanes, so that people can cycle without concern for their safety. • Making services (such as smoking cessation services) that support behaviour change available to people locally and at suitable hours for everyone. • Creating opportunities for people to participate in sport and a range of other community-based activities (see Chapter 17). • Providing needle exchange facilities, so that people can use clean needles, whilst also accessing other forms of support.
Provide information	Providing information on the health benefits and health harms of different choices.	• Providing information on the harms of smoking, such as by displaying pictures of diseased lungs on cigarette packaging. • Providing information on the harms of alcohol consumption, such as through TV advertising. • Providing calorie and other nutritional information on food packaging and on menus. • Other public health campaigns, such as those encouraging more exercise ('This Girl Can', etc.), or increased consumption of fruit and veg.
Monitor the situation/do nothing	Monitor the situation, but do not do anything to change or influence people's behaviours.	• Monitor the situation, such as through collecting epidemiological data on current health trends. • As others have pointed out, this is far from doing 'nothing' and involves quite a lot of public health activity and coordination (Dawson 2016).

Source: Adapted from Calman (2009) / https://cdn.nuffieldbioethics.org/wp-content/uploads/Public-health-ethical-issues.pdf.

rungs, which illustrate the level and extent to which public health interventions exert influence over people's lives (Nuffield Bioethics Council, 2007). Interventions towards the top of the ladder have the biggest impact on freedoms, require the greatest justification and should therefore be reserved for tackling the greatest health threats, particularly those that negatively impact on others (such as smoking bans in public places and forced isolation during the COVID-19 pandemic). Essentially, this encourages us to think about proportionality alongside intrusiveness (Paetkau, 2024). The Nuffield Ladder of Interventions, with some example interventions for each rung, can be seen in Table 14.1.

Whilst the ladder has proved influential, critiques of the model have highlighted that it focuses too much on interventions relating to individual behaviour change (instead of, e.g. focusing on systemic factors, like the environment) (Paetkau, 2024), that it is sometimes hard to identify exactly where on the ladder an intervention falls (Dawson, 2016), and that far from reducing choice, many public health interventions actually increase a person's liberty (Griffiths and West, 2015). For example, providing someone with free access to a gym increases rather than decreases their autonomy, because they can choose to go to the gym, where they might have otherwise been unable to. In line with this, Griffiths and West (2015) and Paetkau (2024) have provided alternative models that highlight that public health interventions can both reduce and increase autonomy, and the need to focus on broader public health interventions, such as the regulation of industries, and improved public health infrastructure.

Healthy Cities

As we have explored, much of our health is determined by our lived environments, and many people around the world live in cities. People living in cities tend to have better access to healthcare, and many of those living in cities, do have better health compared to rural areas (Ezzati et al., 2018). However, significant inequalities exist within cities, and features of city living can contribute to poorer health (Danielli et al., 2023; Ezzati et al., 2018; Vlahov et al., 2007). For example, the normalisation of poor health behaviours may be in part driven by the higher density of outlets selling unhealthy food, alcohol, and tobacco in cities (Macdonald et al., 2018). Many cities also have reduced access to green and blue natural spaces, less opportunities for safe active travel (walking, cycling, etc.), and higher noise and air pollution (Danielli et al., 2023, Wight and Middleton, 2019). In addition, despite being better overall for the environment, many cities suffer from the increased impacts of global warming and poor planetary health (discussed at the end of this chapter) (Danielli et al., 2023, Wight and Middleton, 2019).

Whilst many cities provide excellent opportunities to connect with others, city living has also been associated with loneliness (see Chapter 16), and aspects of their design can contribute to people's levels of happiness (Laing, 2017, Montgomery, 2013). Because of this, there is an increasing public health interest in the creation of 'healthy cities' and '15-minute cities' through urban planning (Allam et al., 2022, Barton et al., 2015, Danielli et al., 2023, Moreno, 2024).

A recent review found 47 areas relating to health that cities were seeking to address, with most of these areas either relating to improving health or improving healthcare services, and a focus on noncommunicable disease was common, alongside some of the most frequently discussed health behaviours and associated health presentations: obesity and diet, smoking and air pollution (Danielli et al., 2023). Initiatives

mostly sought to provide education, which we know from previous chapters, may be limited and may exacerbate inequalities unless they also seek to change the context and environment of behaviours (Thomson et al., 2018, McGill et al., 2015) through other interventions including service reform and changing the physical environment to address various determinants of health (Danielli et al., 2023). An important finding is that many of these interventions currently occur in isolation (Danielli et al., 2023). Essentially, individual interventions that attempt to tackle one issue, rather than adopting a systems approach (which we discuss later in this chapter). The authors of this recent review highlight a 'Vital 5', with the four behaviours we have discussed in this, and the previous two chapters (i.e. inactivity, poor diet, smoking and drinking), being joined by planetary health (Danielli et al., 2023). It is interventions that target these that we turn too in the next section, with reference to the Nuffield ladder. Within the scope of this chapter, we cannot explore every public health intervention that exists to address these, so have focussed on a few of the most contemporary interventions that are aimed at entire populations. First, the design of cities can make physical activity more or less likely and it is this, that we turn to next.

Active Living

Greenspace and Active Transport

The relationships between greenspace, walkability, perceived neighbourhood safety and levels of physical activity in an area have been extensively studied including in systematic reviews (García de Jalón et al., 2021, Juul and Nordbø, 2023, Zare Sakhvidi et al., 2023), and the provision of greenspace is supported by the World Health Organization (WHO, 2017b). Whilst causal pathways are often difficult to determine in research like this (due to a range of other potential confounding factors), green spaces, particularly when provided in urban areas (which can be associated with stress and potentially more sedentary behaviours), may positively impact on a range of mental and physical health-related outcomes, increased rates of activity, reduced obesity prevalence and even development in children and young people (Banwell et al., 2024, García de Jalón et al., 2021, Markevych et al., 2017, McCormick, 2017, Ye et al., 2022, Zare Sakhvidi et al., 2023). Providing urban environments that promote health, especially where they also increase opportunities for active transport (such as walking and cycling, as opposed to driving, or other less active means) is an example of 'enabling choice' and may improve a population's health and wellbeing. Unsurprisingly, evidence suggests that active transport can increase overall levels of physical activity, whilst also having related benefits to the environment (Wanjau et al., 2023, Smith et al., 2017).

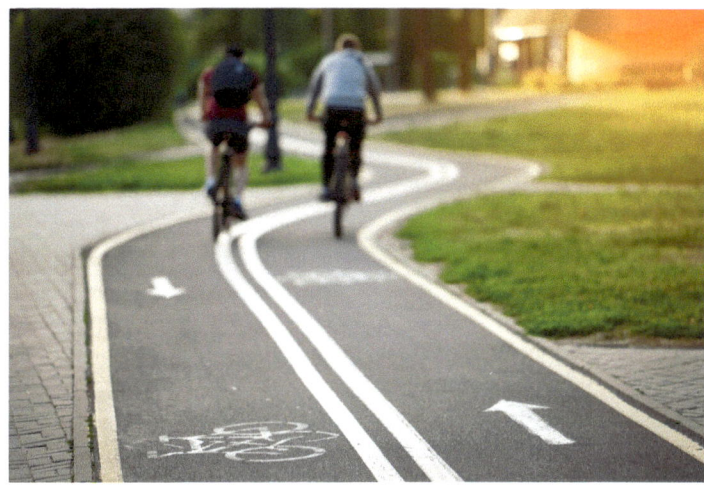

Source: Tricky Shark/Adobe Stock Photos.

Parkrun, Free Exercise Classes and Gym Memberships

As we explore further in Chapter 17, an increasing range of community and third-sector organisations (such as advocacy groups, social enterprises, faith and religious groups) have taken on an increasing role in health promotion. This has largely been led by the belief that through their local embeddedness, they are well-placed to engage with local and socially excluded groups. Park run is one local community-level intervention largely delivered through charity that you are likely familiar with. You may even participate in park runs yourself in your local community. Park run is a global charity that oversees local, often weekly (typically on Saturdays) community-based and volunteer-led 5-kilometer runs (Reece et al., 2019). These runs are free and therefore attempt to be inclusive to all in society, particularly those with lower economic means, or from socially excluded groups less likely to regularly participate in exercise. Research has highlighted that in the context of the United Kingdom, most people have a park run within 5 kilometres (an improvement in terms of accessibility from 34 kilometres reported in 2010), with areas of higher deprivation potentially being closer to organised events, than wealthier areas (Schneider et al., 2020; Smith et al. 2021).

Runs have been promoted through primary care providers (Fleming, 2019). As such, the provision of park run falls under 'enabling choice' in the Nuffield ladder as it removes some barriers to physical activity, and research has suggested that park run may reach groups that are normally poorly served (Grunseit et al., 2020). Those choosing to take part in park run, generally do so to get fit, but also to connect with others in their communities (Peterson et al., 2022). There is now some evidence that park run can improve physical health (particularly when attending regularly) and well-being, and particularly in relation to those who had previously low levels of physical activity (Grunseit et al., 2020, Peterson et al., 2022, Stevinson and Hickson, 2019). The link to health and well-being is unsurprising, as its relationship with physical activity is already well established (Farrell et al., 2014).

Less positively, research suggests that many of those who register for park run, do not attend, and this is often related to not feeling fit enough (particularly amongst women – a known determinant of initial engagement with physical activity), not having time or not being available at the set time park runs occur, as well as not having access to childcare (Reece et al., 2022). Other research has demonstrated that simply providing free exercise opportunities does not always translate into increased physical activity in those these interventions principally target (Candio et al., 2022).

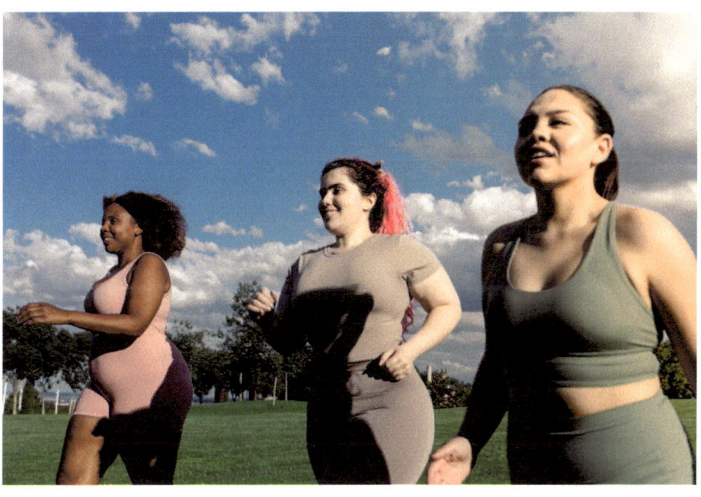

Source: Adrian Rodd/Stocksy/Adobe Stock Photos.

Diet

Calorie Information

In England, as elsewhere, most notably in America, it is now compulsory for large restaurants (generally those with multiple restaurants or many employees) to provide calorie information on menus (Kaur et al., 2022, Yeo, 2022). Research has suggested that where restaurants must display the number of calories a meal has, people may consume slightly less calories and there has been a small impact on the calorie content of meals that are offered (Colombet et al., 2024, Liu et al., 2020, Shangguan et al., 2019, Yeo, 2022, Zlatevska et al., 2018). Recent modelling of the policy impacts of calorie information highlights potential impacts on obesity and cardiovascular mortality, with the authors highlighting that greater public health improvements could be seen if the regulations were expanded to include all out-of-home food vendors (i.e. not just the large ones covered by current regulation) (Colombet et al., 2024).

Even this intervention though, which is relatively low down the Nuffield ladder of interventions (providing information), is not without controversy. First, questions have been asked as to whether calories are the right thing to display, as opposed to other types of nutritional information (sugar, fat, salt, etc.) (Yeo, 2022). Second, providing information on calories does not really fix the social or material context of high-calorie diets. It is expensive to eat healthy foods, and those with lower socio-economic means, who are more likely to be obese, are unlikely to be deterred by this information. Indeed, it has been argued that it would be far more effective to target healthier food affordability and accessibility, as well as tackling poverty (Yeo, 2022). Finally, this information has led to some experiencing 'an extra fight they didn't ask for', with those with eating disorders highlighting the potentially negative impacts of this intervention on their health and well-being (Frances et al., 2024, Polden et al., 2023).

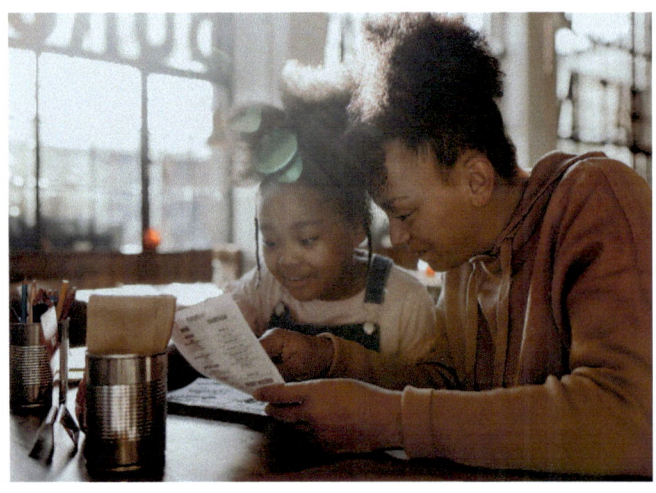

Source: Rawpixel.com/Adobe Stock Photos.

Sugar Tax and Levies

With soft drink consumption being a known contributor to the increasing prevalence of obesity and type 2 diabetes, the WHO has for a while recommended that governments implement taxes on soft drinks, particularly those that are high in sugar (WHO, 2017a). Several countries have now implemented such recommendations, including the United Kingdom, with the introduction of the Soft Drinks Industry Levy (SDIL) (Department of Health and Social Care, 2017), which was intended to both increase the cost of high-sugar drinks and incentivise the producers of soft drinks to use less sugar in their products. Revenues from the levy can be used to support wrap-around care (i.e. breakfast and after-school clubs) and increase physical activity opportunities in schools (Sutherland and Barber, 2017).

Whilst the intention of providing two tiers of taxation (one for higher and one for lower sugar contents) was intended to incentivise the drinks industry to lower the sugar content of its drinks, some of the levy has ended up being passed onto consumers (Scarborough et al., 2020). However, the introduction of the levy has reduced overall sugar purchased in soft drinks (Scarborough et al., 2020, Rogers et al., 2023b). Research has highlighted positive impacts including reduced levels of obesity in children, with greater reductions being seen in those living in more deprived areas, particularly girls (Rogers et al., 2023a).

Smoking

Swap to Stop

Whilst the exact harms of vaping are not fully understood, it is generally believed that vaping is significantly less harmful than tobacco smoking (Khan, 2022). Because of this, vaping has been explored as a potentially effective tool in supporting smoking cessation, including in the United Kingdom, where vape starter kits have been provided to smokers, alongside behavioural support (Khan, 2022).

Smoking Bans and Smoke-Free Generations

In a UK context, the majority of 18–24-year-olds, and just over 46% of all people feel the government's actions on smoking are not enough (Khan, 2022). Research suggests that bans on smoking in public places have improved smoking prevalence and population health outcomes (Callinan et al., 2010; Faber et al., 2017; Frazer et al., 2016; Strassman et al., 2023) and have improved the occupational health of those working in hospitality previously exposed to significant second-hand smoke (Callinan et al., 2010, Frazer et al., 2016, Goodman et al., 2007, Menzies et al., 2006). In addition, there has been a denormalisation of smoking behaviours (Hoek et al., 2022), in part through this legislation and reduced peer influence (Hamilton et al., 2008). Evidence suggests increasing bans to all public places (parks, beaches, etc.) and some private spaces (such as cars) can have an even greater impact on health outcomes, including through further denormalising smoking (Laverty et al., 2021, Painter, 2019, Radó et al., 2021), and such legislation has been sporadically adopted around the world (Johns et al., 2013, Levy et al., 2017, Painter, 2019). Importantly, research has suggested the public (and particularly non-smokers and ex-smokers) are generally supportive of public smoking bans, especially in places frequented by children, as well as in cars (Boderie et al., 2023). Outright banning of smoking, until relatively recently, has been uncommon. There is one notable exception. In 2004, Bhutan became the first country to outright ban the sale of tobacco (Aneja and Gopal, 2023, Givel, 2011, Tamil Selvan et al., 2024). However, this ban has since been lifted in 2021, through concern that movement across borders to purchase tobacco in other countries might increase rates of COVID-19 transmission (Aneja and Gopal, 2023, Givel, 2011, Tamil Selvan et al., 2024).

Many countries have now set out tobacco 'endgame' targets, which seek to make tobacco obsolete through reductions/ eliminations of tobacco smoking prevalence (typically to less than 5%) by a given year (McDaniel et al., 2016, Moon et al., 2018, Tamil Selvan et al., 2024), and such ambitions are arguably most likely to be realised in countries with relatively low smoking prevalence, alongside robust smoking control measures and available smoking cessation support (Tamil Selvan et al., 2024). A recent scoping review clustered countries on how 'endgame' ready they were (based on tobacco control and prevalence levels) (Tamil Selvan et al., 2024). Twenty-eight countries were 'endgame ready', with a further 48 countries being 'almost endgame ready' (Tamil Selvan et al., 2024). Most countries with endgame targets have adopted a range of strategies (such as smoke-free legislation, plain packets, taxes and providing support) (Tamil Selvan et al., 2024).

In 2023, following the Khan review, the UK Government put forward legislation to ensure future smoke-free generations (Balogun, 2024, Khan, 2022). The legislation means anyone under the age of 15 (as of 2023) will never be able to legally smoke tobacco in the United Kingdom, arguably ushing in UK tobacco's 'end game'. Similar legislation had been introduced elsewhere, for example, in New Zealand (before being controversially scrapped by a new government) (Mao, 2023), and other countries are considering similar steps (Tamil Selvan et al., 2024).

Drinking

Minimum Unit Pricing (MUP) of Alcohol

Interventions aimed at reducing harmful alcohol consumption have often targeted alcohol's affordability through various 'sin taxes'. As with tobacco consumption, an important consideration here is price elasticity. Price elasticity simply means the amount a price change is likely to change patterns of consumption (Clements et al., 2022). Where prices influence consumption a lot (lowering price leading to greater consumption, increasing price leading to reduced consumption, etc.), prices are said to be elastic, likewise where prices do not have much influence over consumption (as is often the case with addictions), prices are said to be inelastic. Alcohol price and consumption is relatively inelastic (Clements et al., 2022).

Minimum unit pricing (MUP) is one approach that seeks to reduce levels of harmful alcohol consumption (Maharaj et al., 2023). MUP targets the heaviest and most vulnerable drinkers, who typically consume the cheapest, strongest (in terms of strength) and largest (in terms of volume) available alcoholic beverages (Black et al., 2011). By targeting the cost per unit of alcohol, it is the strongest, cheapest, largest beverages whose cost changes most significantly, whilst less strong alternatives are either hardly affected or not affected at all.

Stop and Think: Know Your Units (and How MUP Affects Price)

The current MUP for alcohol in Scotland, one of the nations to implement a minimum unit, is 65p per unit of alcohol (Scottish Government, 2024). As a healthcare professional, it is important to understand alcohol units, how they are calculated and the potential impact of MUP on alcohol costs. This will also help you understand if someone's daily glass of wine is problematic or not (as glasses of wine can vary significantly in terms of volume and strength).

You can work out the number of units an alcoholic drink has relatively easily. Essentially, all you need to do is multiply the total volume of the drink (in ml) by its abbreviation (expressed as a percentage) and then divide the result by 1,000. So, for example, a 700 ml bottle of whisky, with an abbreviation of 40% would be 28 units per bottle.

700x40 = 28,000

28,000/1000 = 28 units.

Now let's consider the impact of introducing a MUP in England would have on the cost (and therefore potential desirability of three different alcoholic drinks in the below example).

	High strength, high volume, cheap cider	4 cans of medium-strength beer sold in a shop	A pint of medium-strength beer served in a pub
Volume	2500 ml	440 ml x 4 (1,760 ml)	568 ml
Abv (%)	7.5	4.4	4.4
Number of units	18.75	7.74	2.5
Current price	£5.25	£5.65	£6.00
Minimum price under 65p MUP (and % increase)	£12.19 (+132.19%)	£5.03	£1.63

In the above example, the current costs of some drinks have been provided. As you can see, a 4-can pack of medium strength beer is completely unaffected by the introduction of MUP, as the retail price is currently higher than the MUP. The same can also be said for a pint of medium strength beer sold in a pub. In fact, the beer sold in a pub is £4.37 more than the MUP price. What is clear though, is that the price of low cost, high strength, high volume alcohol would increase substantially following an introduction of MUP, with this drink actually increasing by over 132%! As we will go on to consider, research has shown MUP to be effective.

You can find your own drinks and compare the impact the MUP has on sale price, using the grid provided.

	Drink 1	Drink 2	Drink 3
Volume			
Abv (%)			
Number of units			
Current price			
Minimum price under 65p MUP (and % increase)			

In the context of Scotland, recent research has highlighted that the introduction of MUP has resulted in decreased alcohol sales (Giles et al., 2024), reduced alcohol-related harms, including significant reductions in deaths and hospitalisations wholly attributable to alcohol consumption, particularly in the most deprived areas, and particularly in men (Wyper et al., 2023).

Getting Rid of the Pint!

It is not just governments that can take action to curb alcohol consumption. In England, beer is generally served in either a pint or half-pint measure (Mantzari et al., 2024a). Recent research explored the impact of removing the option of a pint (but allowing smaller measurements such as half pints) on the volume of beer sold in pubs (Mantzari et al., 2024a). The researchers found that removing the pint option was associated with a 10% reduction in the volume of beer sold in participating pubs (Mantzari et al., 2024a). Similar findings have been found in the context of wine, when removing the largest service size (250 ml), the volume of wine that licensed premises sold decreased by around 8% (Mantzari et al., 2024b).

Nudging and Liberal Paternalism

'Nudging' or 'liberal paternalism', which was made well-known by Thaler and Sunstein's (2009) popular book (*Nudge: Improving Decisions About Health, Wealth and Happiness*), emerged through work across the social sciences, including behavioural economics, social psychology and political science. Nudging generally involves the deliberate manipulation of the decision-making environment (this is sometimes referred to as 'choice architecture') to 'nudge' people into desired ways of behaving (for themselves, as well as for society) (Thaler and Sunstein, 2009). A typology of nudges now exists (Hollands et al., 2017) and includes for example providing less healthy options further away from where people are likely to see them, and reducing portion sizes (as in the research on pints discussed previously), or appearance. Essentially nudges can be broken down into 'placement' (where things are placed) and 'properties' (appearance, etc.). With nudging, people retain their choice (e.g. they can still choose the cheesy fries, if they so wish), but the design of the environment is intended to steer them towards making the right one (having plain rice or a salad instead) (Thaler and Sunstein, 2009). Nudging is believed to work because human judgements tend to be fast, and often automatic and unconscious (sometimes referred to as 'system 1' thinking, in contrast to slower and more deliberative 'system 2' thinking (Kahneman, 2012)).

Being able to think fast and unconsciously, frees up the cognitive capacity to focus on tasks that require greater cognition, but it does leave us vulnerable to making the odd mistake, and this cognitive process can be exploited through nudges and choice architecture (Thaler and Sunstein, 2009). Nudging has been examined as an intervention for a range of health-related behaviours, including, for example, food consumption (Marcano-Olivier et al., 2019, Pandey et al., 2023) and vaccine uptake (Reñosa et al., 2021, Johansen et al., 2023). Because nudging people to be healthier is relatively inexpensive and un-invasive, it has become popular with researchers, public health professionals, governments and policymakers as one intervention to improve health (Halpern, 2015, Marteau et al., 2011).

Nudging is not without ethical concerns. For example, is it right that the environment is manipulated in such a way as to coerce people's behaviour(s), without their knowledge, and without their consent? Probably. But the arguments here are complex. For example, no environment is value- and manipulation-free. People will always be influenced by something (Thaler and Sunstein, 2009). Not putting healthy products at eye level in a supermarket, and instead putting unhealthy products in their place (as is often done to maximise profit) still involves influencing behaviour, but this time negatively. Foodstuffs, after all, must be displayed somewhere. If you decide to do neither, or just randomly assign where food is displayed, healthy food might be displayed in areas that promote their consumption in some stores, but not in others, leading to inequalities. On balance, most would want to be manipulated in this way, if it led to them making healthier choices, but nudges can also be aggressive and can encourage unhealthy behaviours too.

More recently sludges have been defined alongside nudges – these are essentially the man-made processes that make it deliberately difficult to do something or to challenge the status quo (Sunstein, 2022, Thaler, 2018). This unnecessary 'sludge' then 'nudges' behaviours. 'Sludge' can be used to steer positive behaviours, such as making it more difficult to buy something harmful such as a firearm, but they can also be deployed in ways that are harmful, such as preventing people from applying for benefits they are entitled to, or making people confirm they have read an impossibly long list of information before providing their consent, as well as over-burdensome referral pathways, such as having to see multiple different people in order to access needed mental health support (Sunstein, 2022, Thaler, 2018).

Case Study: Dark Nudges, Sludges and Big Alcohol's Corporate Social Responsibility Healthwashing

Companies are known to use behavioural economics to exploit our cognitive biases, making us make poor choices (such as gambling and drinking), in much the same way as nudges are used to promote healthy choices (Fortier et al., 2024, Petticrew et al., 2020, Schüll, 2012). In Chapter 12, the concept of the commercial determinants of health and corporate social responsibility is introduced.

Recent research into alcohol industry-sponsored corporate social responsibility bodies (often industry-sponsored charities) has highlighted the use of dark nudges and sludges to create an illusion of health messaging, whilst simultaneously nudging consumption (Petticrew et al., 2020). These methods create the illusion that these large companies are 'doing their bit' (Babor and Robaina, 2013), whilst simultaneously promoting consumption (Petticrew et al., 2020). In their study. Petticrew et al. (2020) found that this 'health information' is essentially designed to fail, is often 'cherry picked', tends to emphasise uncertainty about health-related harms and is often designed in such a way as to hide important information. This is done by placing key information in places less likely to be seen, diluting key messages by providing sludges in the form of lots of distracting information (including lesser health risks), or using colourways that are difficult to see. Other deployed strategies include priming, stimulating and normalising alcohol consumption by displaying health advice about consumption alongside illustrations of people clearly enjoying alcohol with friends (an example of 'social proof' or 'normalisation'), or highlighting the norm of drinking on certain days (such as New Year's Eve) (Maani Hessari et al., 2019, Petticrew et al., 2020).

For UK readers, next time you pick up a bottle of wine in the shop, have a look at the pregnancy logo that is often used to indicate that pregnant women should stop drinking. Sometimes it is absent. But importantly, take note of what colour the cross is. Often it is not red, a colour that is synonymous with danger and the need to stop (which would be a rather obvious colour to use). Grey/black is common, but it has even been green, a colour that is synonymous with 'go ahead'. This is a dark nudge (Petticrew et al., 2020). Generally, red means stop, green means go, and this mismatch (a 'stimulus incompatibility') makes cognitive processing challenging, resulting in important warnings being missed (Petticrew et al., 2020).

A Whole Systems Approach to Public Health

In the United Kingdom, the government has committed to a programme of 'Levelling Up', to help improve the lives of those living in the poorest communities, so that outcomes and opportunities are more on par with other parts of the country (Liddle et al., 2022). A recent rapid review provides a useful evidence-based framework for tackling inequalities, particularly using a whole systems levelling up approach (Davey et al., 2022). The authors highlighted the importance of:

Health by default initiatives: The authors found consistent evidence of the value of guiding choice through incentives (such as subsidising healthy food) and disincentives (such as sin taxes on unhealthy foods) to reduce health inequalities (Davey et al., 2022). Providing people with the resources they need to live healthy lifestyles (i.e. enabling choice in the Nuffield ladder) can also have significant impacts on health outcomes.

Longer term multi-sector action: People's social and lived environments, as we have shown, influence their health in several ways. A key finding of this review was that taking action to address one particular issue (such as housing), can only be minimally effective if other social stressors (such as a lack of cash) are not also simultaneously tackled (Davey et al., 2022, Gibson et al., 2011). Hence, as the review on healthy cities presented earlier in this chapter found, one intervention, tackling one issue is unlikely to be effective (Danielli et al., 2023), and intensive interventions, address multiple barriers to healthier lifestyles and are supported by several settings (because people are not static), are more likely to work (Davey et al., 2022). Sustainable funding is also needed, to ensure barriers to participation (such as financial) do not reappear when funding runs out (Williams and Fullagar, 2019).

Locally designed interventions: To be most effective, interventions should fit the local contexts in which they are delivered. Making use of the local community can help sustain behaviour change (such as those relating to physical activity) over time (Davey et al., 2022). Making health easier to access, through, for example, extended access hours, can also increase people's opportunities to make healthier choices, such as increasing ease of access to local vaccination programmes (Davey et al., 2022).

Targeting disadvantaged communities: Targeting an entire population through universal programmes may exacerbate inequalities. Interventions are often most effective when they target specific groups, rather than whole populations (Davey et al., 2022).

Matching of resources to needs: Increasing the proportion of funding to specific areas of need can be effective in reducing health inequalities, whilst also addressing mortality that is amenable to healthcare (Barr et al., 2014, Davey et al., 2022) (Figure 14.1).

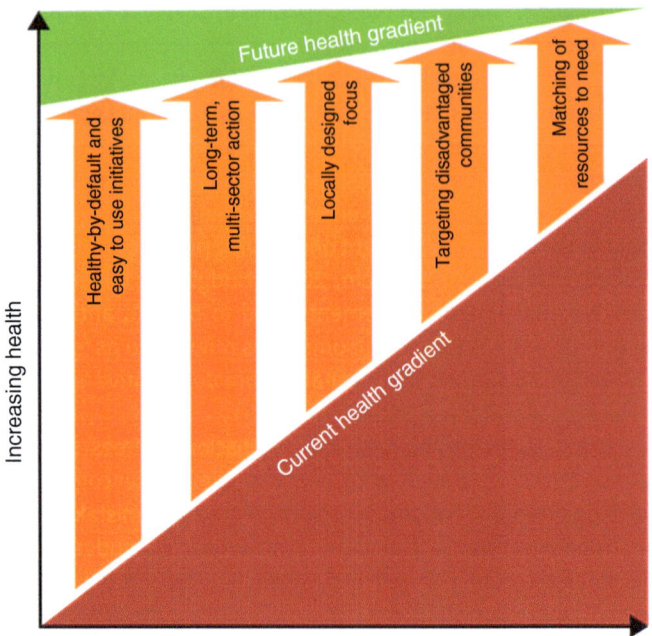

FIGURE 14.1 Levelling up health, using a whole systems approach. **Source:** Davey et al. (2022) / Elsevier / CC BY 4.0.

Population and Planetary Health

Increasingly, as we highlighted in the context of healthy cities, population health must be discussed alongside planetary health (the health of our planet). The impact humans are having on planetary health has accelerated, particularly over the last century (Raworth, 2017, 2018). There are now signs that we have significantly and potentially also irreversibly harmed our planet and its future ability to sustain health (Raworth, 2017, 2018). Our planet's health is intrinsically linked to our own health and well-being, and poor planetary health is disproportionately felt by some of society's most vulnerable people and groups (Millward-Hopkins and Oswald, 2023, Raworth, 2017, 2018). One useful way to consider population health in the context of planetary health is through using a doughnut (yes, really). Doughnut economics was first put forward by Professor Kate Raworth as a framework for considering social needs such as global health, inequality and justice, alongside the needs of our planet (Raworth, 2017, 2018). Essentially, it is a framework that helps inform policy and sustainable development (Raworth, 2017, 2018). It is called a doughnut because as you can see in Figure 14.2, the model's main concentric circles give it an appearance of a doughnut.

Looking at the model, you will see two concentric radar-like circles that can highlight either an 'overshoot' of our planets 'ecological ceiling' (essentially how much harm our planet can tolerate across a range of different domains), and a 'shortfall' of our 'social foundation' (Raworth, 2017, 2018).

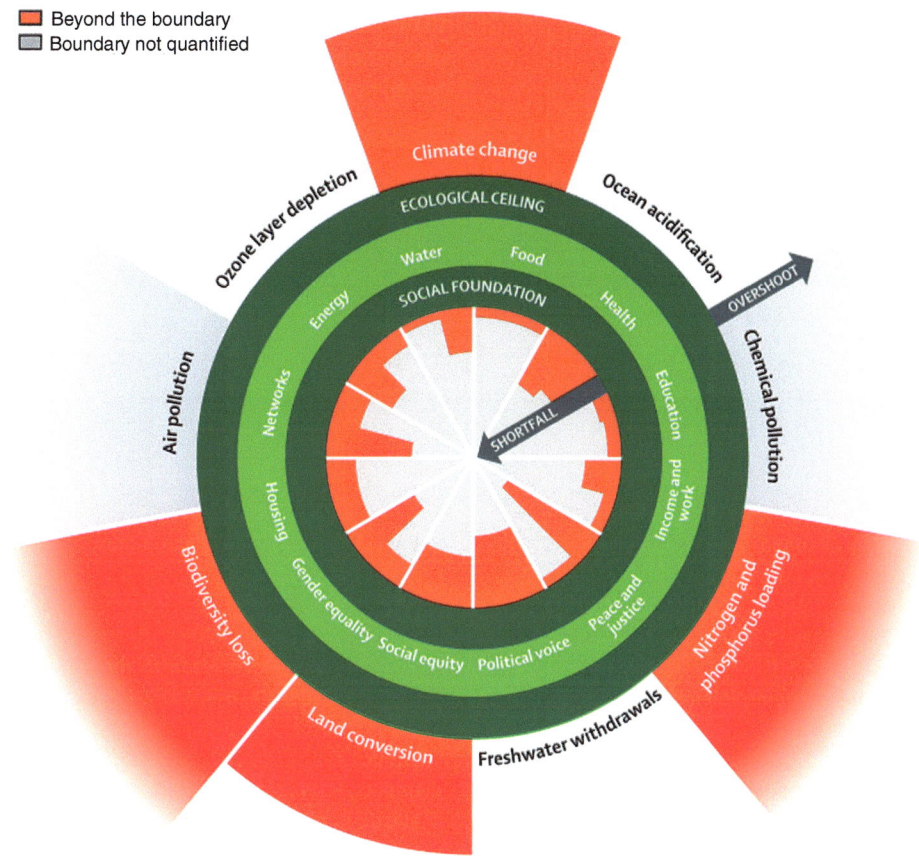

Beyond the boundary
Boundary not quantified

FIGURE 14.2 The doughnut used to consider shortfalls in the social foundation, and overshoots in our planet's ecological ceiling.
Source: Raworth (2017) / Elsevier / CC BY 4.0.

The social foundation essentially represents the things all those in a society need to live happy, healthy and valued lives (Raworth, 2017, 2018). Any overshoot of the ecological ceiling represents planetary strain, and any shortfall of the social foundation represents potential human suffering (Raworth, 2017, 2018). The safe and just place for our planet, and for all those our planet supports, is within the space between these concentric circles (Raworth, 2017, 2018). However, large proportions of the world's population currently fall well short of the agreed minimum standards for human living, including in relation to access to adequate nutrition, housing and healthcare (WHO, 2024). Alongside this social shortfall, are significant planetary overshoots, including in relation to climate change and biodiversity loss (Raworth, 2017, 2018). And importantly these overshoots and shortfalls are not equally created or experienced. For example, some countries contribute to overshoots more than others, shortfalls in the social foundation are unequally experienced, and the impacts of poor planetary health disproportionately affect some of the planets' most vulnerable populations (Millward-Hopkins and Oswald, 2023, WHO, 2024).

Clinical Considerations

- Public health typically involves upstream efforts intended to prevent people from becoming unwell in the first place.
- There are a range of different public health interventions aimed at targeting some of the most common unhealthy behaviours, such as smoking, poor diet, inactivity and harmful alcohol consumption.
- Often several interventions exist for the same issue, and it is important to consider which interventions are most effective, alongside their potential levels of intrusion on individuals and populations.
- It is possible to use nudges to support people to make healthier decisions, whilst retaining their autonomy to make less healthy choices if they wish.
- Our social environment is linked to our health and our health behaviours.
- The impact of worsening planetary health will be felt more severely by more vulnerable communities.

Conclusion

This chapter has moved beyond the individual approaches taken to behaviour change in the previous two chapters, to consider behaviour change at the level of populations. This chapter has expanded on previous discussions relating to public health and inequalities, including some of the debates and controversies that exist around how much governments should be involved in steering the behaviour of their citizens. You have been introduced to the Nuffield ladder of interventions as one way to consider the proportionality of an intervention's intrusion, alongside the risks posed by different health behaviours, such as smoking, drinking, inactivity and poor diet. You have also been introduced to some contemporary interventions, that seek to address these at the level of populations. Finally, we have highlighted the importance of planetary health and population health, alongside the unequal impacts of worsening planetary health on societies' most vulnerable groups.

References

Allam, Z., Nieuwenhuijsen, M., Chabaud, D. & Moreno, C. 2022. The 15-minute city offers a new framework for sustainability, liveability, and health. *The Lancet Planetary Health*, 6, e181–e183.

Aneja, K. & Gopal, S. 2023. Bhutan reverses sales ban on tobacco. BMJ Tobacco Control Blog.

Ayo, N. 2012. Understanding health promotion in a neoliberal climate and the making of health conscious citizens. *Critical Public Health*, 22, 99–105.

Babor, T. F. & Robaina, K. 2013. Public health, academic medicine, and the alcohol industry's corporate social responsibility activities. *American Journal of Public Health*, 103, 206–214.

Balogun, B. 2024. Tobacco and Vapes Bill [Online]. House of Commons Library UK Parliament Available: https://commonslibrary.parliament.uk/research-briefings/cbp-9992/ [Accessed].

Banwell, N., Michel, S. & Senn, N. 2024. Greenspaces and Health: scoping review of studies in Europe. *Public Health Reviews*, 45, 1606863.

Bardosh, K., De Figueiredo, A., Gur-Arie, R., Jamrozik, E., Doidge, J., Lemmens, T., Keshavjee, S., Graham, J. E. & Baral, S. 2022. The unintended consequences of COVID-19 vaccine policy: Why mandates, passports and restrictions may cause more harm than good. *BMJ Global Health*, 7, e008684.

Barr, B., Bambra, C. & Whitehead, M. 2014. The impact of NHS resource allocation policy on health inequalities in England 2001-11: longitudinal ecological study. *BMJ*, 348.

Barton, H., Thompson, S., Burgess, S. & Grant, M. 2015. *The Routledge Handbook of Planning for Health and Well-Being*, Routledge.

Bergman, B. P., Laing, F., Chandler, A. S. & Calman, K. C. 2018. Witnessing history: a personal view of half a century in public health. *The Journal of the Royal College of Physicians of Edinburgh*, 48, 181–191.

Black, H., Gill, J. & Chick, J. 2011. The price of a drink: levels of consumption and price paid per unit of alcohol by Edinburgh's ill drinkers with a comparison to wider alcohol sales in Scotland. *Addiction*, 106, 729–736.

Boderie, N. W., Sheikh, A., Lo, E., Sheikh, A., Burdorf, A., Van Lenthe, F. J., Mölenberg, F. J. M. & Been, J. V. 2023. Public support for smoke-free policies in outdoor areas and (semi-)private places: a systematic review and meta-analysis. *eClinicalMedicine*, 59.

Callinan, J., Clarke, A., Doherty, K. & Kelleher, C. 2010. Legislative smoking bans for reducing secondhand smoke exposure, smoking prevalence, and tobacco consumption. *Cochrane Database of Systematic Reviews.*, 4.

Calman, K. 2009. Beyond the 'nanny state': stewardship and public health. *Public Health*, 123, e6–e10.

Cameron, J., Williams, B., Ragonnet, R., Marais, B., Trauer, J. & Savulescu, J. 2021. Ethics of selective restriction of liberty in a pandemic. *Journal of Medical Ethics*, 47, 553.

Candio, P., Meads, D., Hill, A. J. & Bojke, L. 2022. Does providing everyone with free-of-charge organised exercise opportunities work in public health? *Health Policy*, 126, 129–142.

Clements, K. W., Mariano, M. J. M., Verikios, G. & Wong, B. 2022. How elastic is alcohol consumption? *Economic Analysis and Policy*, 76, 568–581.

Coggon, J. 2012. *What makes health public? A critical evaluation of Moral, Legal, and Political Claims in Public Health*, Cambridge University Press.

Colombet, Z., Robinson, E., Kypridemos, C., Jones, A. & O'flaherty, M. 2024. Effect of calorie labelling in the out-of-home food sector on adult obesity prevalence, cardiovascular mortality, and social inequalities in England: a modelling study. *The Lancet Public Health*, 9, e178–e185.

Conrad, P. 2005. *The sociology of health and illness*, Macmillan.

Danielli, S., Ashrafian, H. & Darzi, A. 2023. Healthy city: global systematic scoping review of city initiatives to improve health with policy recommendations. *BMC Public Health*, 23, 1277.

Davey, F., Mcgowan, V., Birch, J., Kuhn, I., Lahiri, A., Gkiouleka, A., Arora, A., Sowden, S., Bambra, C. & Ford, J. 2022. Levelling up health: a practical, evidence-based framework for reducing health inequalities. *Public Health in Practice*, 4, 100322.

Dawson, A. J. 2016. Snakes and ladders: state interventions and the place of liberty in public health policy. *Public Health Ethics.*, 42, 510–513.

Department Of Health And Social Care. 2017. Policy paper: Childhood obesity: a plan for action [Online]. UK Government: Department of Health & Social Care Available: https://www.gov.uk/government/publications/childhood-obesity-a-plan-for-action/childhood-obesity-a-plan-for-action [Accessed].

Ezzati, M., Webster, C. J., Doyle, Y. G., Rashid, S., Owusu, G. & Leung, G. M. 2018. Cities for global health. *BMJ*, 363, k3794.

Faber, T., Kumar, A., Mackenbach, J. P., Millett, C., Basu, S., Sheikh, A. & Been, J. V. 2017. Effect of tobacco control policies on perinatal and child health: a systematic review and meta-analysis. *The Lancet Public Health*, 2, e420–e437.

Farrell, L., Hollingsworth, B., Propper, C. & Shields, M. A. 2014. The socioeconomic gradient in physical inactivity: evidence from one million adults in England. *Social Science & Medicine*, 123, 55–63.

Fleming, J. 2019. Parkrun: increasing physical activity in primary care. *The British Journal of General Practice*, 69, 483–484.

Fortier, M., Audette-Chapdelaine, S., Auger, A. M. & Brodeur, M. 2024. Nudge theory and gambling: a scoping review. *Frontiers in Public Health*, 12, 1377183.

Frances, T., O'neill, K. & Newman, K. 2024. 'An extra fight I didn't ask for': a qualitative survey exploring the impact of calories on menus for people with experience of eating disorders. *British Journal of Health Psychology*, 29, 20–36.

Frazer, K., Callinan, J. E., Mchugh, J., Van Baarsel, S., Clarke, A., Doherty, K. & Kelleher, C. 2016. Legislative smoking bans for reducing harms from secondhand smoke exposure, smoking prevalence and tobacco consumption. *Cochrane Database of Systematic Reviews.* .

García De Jalón, S., Chiabai, A., Quiroga, S., Suárez, C., Ščasný, M., Máca, V., Zvěřinová, I., Marques, S., Craveiro, D. & Taylor, T. 2021. The influence of urban greenspaces on people's physical activity: a population-based study in Spain. *Landscape and Urban Planning*, 215, 104229.

Gibson, M., Petticrew, M., Bambra, C., Sowden, A. J., Wright, K. E. & Whitehead, M. 2011. Housing and health inequalities: a synthesis of systematic reviews of interventions aimed at different pathways linking housing and health. *Health & Place*, 17, 175–184.

Giles, L., Mackay, D., Richardson, E., Lewsey, J., Robinson, M. & Beeston, C. 2024. Evaluating the impact of minimum unit pricing (MUP) on alcohol sales after 3 years of implementation in Scotland: a controlled interrupted time-series study. *Addiction*, 119, 1378–1386.

Giubilini, A., Savulescu, J., Pugh, J. & Wilkinson, D. 2023. Vaccine mandates for healthcare workers beyond COVID-19. *Journal of Medical Ethics*, 49, 211.

Givel, M. S. 2011. History of Bhutan's prohibition of cigarettes: implications for neo-prohibitionists and their critics. *International Journal of Drug Policy*, 22, 306–310.

Goldesteen, D., Goldsteen, K. & Dwelle, T. 2015. *Introduction to Public Health, Promises and Practices* Springer Publishing Company.

Goodman, P., Agnew, M., Mccaffrey, M., Paul, G. & Clancy, L. 2007. Effects of the Irish smoking ban on respiratory health of bar workers and air quality in Dublin pubs. *American Journal of Respiratory and Critical Care Medicine*, 175, 840–845.

Griffiths, P. E. & West, C. 2015. A balanced intervention ladder: promoting autonomy through public health action. *Public Health*, 129, 1092–1098.

Grunseit, A. C., Richards, J., Reece, L., Bauman, A. & Merom, D. 2020. Evidence on the reach and impact of the social physical activity phenomenon parkrun: a scoping review. *Preventive Medicine Reports*, 20, 101231.

Halpern, D. 2015. *Inside the Nudge Unit: How Small Changes Can Make a Big Difference*, WH Allen.

Hamilton, W. L., Biener, L. & Brennan, R. T. 2008. Do local tobacco regulations influence perceived smoking norms? Evidence from adult and youth surveys in Massachusetts. *Health Education Research*, 23, 709–722.

Hoek, J., Edwards, R. & Waa, A. 2022. From social accessory to societal disapproval: smoking, social norms and tobacco endgames. *Tobacco Control*, 31, 358.

Hollands, G. J., Bignardi, G., Johnston, M., Kelly, M. P., Ogilvie, D., Petticrew, M., Prestwich, A., Shemilt, I., Sutton, S. & Marteau, T. M. 2017. The TIPPME intervention typology for changing environments to change behaviour. *Nature Human Behaviour*, 1, 1–9.

Jan, M. S., Renke, L. B., Ani, M., Kathryn, O. & Eva, A. R. 2024. Development of an overarching framework for anticipating and assessing adverse and other unintended consequences of public health interventions (CONSEQUENT): a best-fit framework synthesis. *BMJ Public Health*, 2, e000209.

Johansen, N. D., Vaduganathan, M., Bhatt, A. S., Lee, S. G., Modin, D., Claggett, B. L., Dueger, E. L., Samson, S. I., Loiacono, M. M., Køber, L., Solomon, S. D., Sivapalan, P., Jensen, J. U. S., Martel, C. J.-M., Valentiner-Branth, P., Krause, T. G. & Biering-Sørensen, T. 2023. Electronic nudges to increase influenza vaccination uptake in Denmark: a nationwide, pragmatic, registry-based, randomised implementation trial. *The Lancet*, 401, 1103–1114.

Johns, M., Coady, M. H., Chan, C. A., Farley, S. M. & Kansagra, S. M. 2013. Evaluating New York City's smoke-free parks and beaches law: a critical multiplist approach to assessing behavioral impact. *American Journal of Community Psychology*, 51, 254–263.

Juul, V. & Nordbø, E. C. A. 2023. Examining activity-friendly neighborhoods in the Norwegian context: green space and walkability in relation to physical activity and the moderating role of perceived safety. *BMC Public Health*, 23, 259.

Kahneman, D. 2012. *Thinking, Fast and Slow*: Penguin.

Kaur, A., Briggs, A., Adams, J. & Rayner, M. 2022. New calorie labelling regulations in England. *BMJ*, 377, o1079.

Khan, J. 2022. The Khan review: Making smoking obsolete. Gov.UK: UK Government. Available online at: https://assets.publishing.service.gov.uk/media/62a0c3f38fa8f503921c159f/khan-review-making-smoking-obsolete.pdf.

Kivimäki, M., Batty, G. D., Pentti, J., Shipley, M. J., Sipilä, P. N., Nyberg, S. T., Suominen, S. B., Oksanen, T., Stenholm, S., Virtanen, M., Marmot, M. G., Singh-Manoux, A., Brunner, E. J., Lindbohm, J. V., Ferrie, J. E. & Vahtera, J. 2020. Association between socioeconomic status and the development of mental and physical health conditions in adulthood: a multi-cohort study. *The Lancet Public Health*, 5, e140–e149.

Kratzer, S., Pfadenhauer, L. M., Biallas, R. L., Featherstone, R., Klinger, C., Movsisyan, A., Rabe, J. E., Stadelmaier, J., Rehfuess, E., Wabnitz, K., et al. 2022. Unintended consequences of measures implemented in the school setting to contain the COVID-19 pandemic: a scoping review. *Cochrane Database of Systematic Reviews*, 6, CD015397.

Labonté, R. & Stuckler, D. 2016. The rise of neoliberalism: how bad economics imperils health and what to do about it. *Journal of Epidemiology and Community Health*, 70, 312.

Laing, O. 2017. *The Lonely City: Adventures in the Art of Being Alone*, Canongate Books.

Laverty, A. A., Filippidis, F. T., Been, J. V., Campbell, F., Cheeseman, H. & Hopkinson, N. S. 2021. Smoke-free vehicles: impact of legislation on child smoke exposure across three countries. *European Respiratory Journal*, 58.

Lebesco, K. 2011. Neoliberalism, public health, and the moral perils of fatness. *Critical Public Health*, 21, 153–164.

Levy, D. E., Adams, I. F. & Adamkiewicz, G. 2017. Delivering on the promise of smoke-free public housing. *American Journal of Public Health*, 107, 380–383.

Liddle, J., Shutt, J. & Addidle, G. 2022. Levelling up the United Kingdom? A useful mantra but too little substance or delivery? *Local Economy: The Journal of the Local Economy Policy Unit.*, 37(1–2).

Liu, J., Mozaffarian, D., Sy, S., Lee, Y., Wilde, P. E., Abrahams-Gessel, S., Gaziano, T., Micha, R. & Project, F. P. 2020. Health and economic impacts of the national menu calorie labeling law in the United States: a microsimulation study. *Circulation: Cardiovascular Quality and Outcomes*, 13, e006313.

Lynch, J. 2023. The political economy of health: bringing political science in. *Annual Review of Political Science*, 26, 389–410.

Maani Hessari, N., Van Schalkwyk, M. C., Thomas, S. & Petticrew, M. 2019. *Alcohol Industry CSR Organisations: What Can Their Twitter Activity Tell Us about Their Independence and Their Priorities? A Comparative Analysis:* Int J Environ Res Public Health, 16.

Macdonald, L., Olsen, J. R., Shortt, N. K. & Ellaway, A. 2018. Do 'environmental bads' such as alcohol, fast food, tobacco, and gambling outlets cluster and co-locate in more deprived areas in Glasgow City, Scotland? *Health & Place*, 51, 224–231.

Maharaj, T., Angus, C., Fitzgerald, N., Allen, K., Stewart, S., Machale, S. & Ryan, J. D. 2023. Impact of minimum unit pricing on alcohol-related hospital outcomes: systematic review. *BMJ Open*, 13, e065220.

Mantzari, E., Hollands, G. J., Law, M., Couturier, D.-L. & Marteau, T. M. 2024a. Impact on beer sales of removing the pint serving size: an A-B-A reversal trial in pubs, bars, and restaurants in England. *PLoS Medicine*, 21, e1004442.

Mantzari, E., Ventsel, M., Pechey, E., Lee, I., Pilling, M. A., Hollands, G. J. & Marteau, T. M. 2024b. Impact on wine sales of removing the largest serving size by the glass: an A-B-A reversal trial in 21 pubs, bars, and restaurants in England. *PLoS Medicine*, 21, e1004313.

Mao, F. 2023. New Zealand smoking ban: Health experts criticise new governments shock reveal [Online]. BBC: BBC. Available: https://www.bbc.co.uk/news/world-asia-67540190 [Accessed].

Marcano-Olivier, M., Pearson, R., Ruparell, A., Horne, P. J., Viktor, S. & Erjavec, M. 2019. A low-cost Behavioural Nudge and choice architecture intervention targeting school lunches increases children's consumption of fruit: a cluster randomised trial. *International Journal of Behavioral Nutrition and Physical Activity*, 16, 1–9.

Markevych, I., Schoierer, J., Hartig, T., Chudnovsky, A., Hystad, P., Dzhambov, A. M., De Vries, S., Triguero-Mas, M., Brauer, M. & Nieuwenhuijsen, M. J. 2017. Exploring pathways linking greenspace to health: theoretical and methodological guidance. *Environmental Research*, 158, 301–317.

Marmot, M., Allen, J., Boyce, T., Goldblatt, P. & Morrison, J. 2020. Health Equity in England: The Marmot Review 10 Years On [Online]. The Health Foundation Available: https://www.health.org.uk/publications/reports/the-marmot-review-10-years-on [Accessed].

Marmot, M., Friel, S., Bell, R., Houweling, T. A. J. & Taylor, S. 2008. Closing the gap in a generation: health equity through action on the social determinants of health. *The Lancet*, 372, 1661–1669.

Marmot, M. G. 2010. Fair society, healthy lives: The Marmot Review: Strategic review of health inequalities in England post- 2010.

Marteau, T. M., Ogilvie, D., Roland, M., Suhrcke, M. & Kelly, M. P. 2011. Judging nudging: can nudging improve population health? *BMJ*, 342.

Mccormick, R. 2017. Does access to green space impact the mental well-being of children: a systematic review. *Journal of Pediatric Nursing*, 37, 3–7.

Mcdaniel, P. A., Smith, E. A. & Malone, R. E. 2016. The tobacco endgame: a qualitative review and synthesis. *Tobacco Control*, 25, 594–604.

Mcgill, R., Anwar, E., Orton, L., Bromley, H., Lloyd-Williams, F., O'flaherty, M., Taylor-Robinson, D., Guzman-Castillo, M., Gillespie, D. & Moreira, P. 2015. Are interventions to promote healthy eating equally effective for all? Systematic review of socioeconomic inequalities in impact. *BMC Public Health*, 15, 1–15.

Mckinlay, J. B. 1994. A case for refocussing upstream: The political economy of illness. *In:* Conrad, P. & Kern, R. (eds.) *The Sociology of Health and Illness: Critical Perspectives*, 4th Edition, New York.

Menzies, D., Nair, A., Williamson, P. A., Schembri, S., Al-Khairalla, M. Z. H., Barnes, M., Fardon, T. C., Mcfarlane, L., Magee, G. J. & Lipworth, B. J. 2006. Respiratory symptoms, pulmonary function, and markers of inflammation among bar workers before and after a legislative ban on smoking in public places. *JAMA*, 296, 1742–1748.

Millward-Hopkins, J. & Oswald, Y. 2023. Reducing global inequality to secure human wellbeing and climate safety: a modelling study. *The Lancet Planetary Health*, 7, e147–e154.

Mold, A. 2022. Publics and their health: 50 years of continuity and change. *Journal of Public Health*, 44, i17–i22.

Montgomery, C. 2013. *Happy City: Transforming Our Lives Through Urban Design*, Penguin UK.

Moon, G., Barnett, R., Pearce, J., Thompson, L. & Twigg, L. 2018. The tobacco endgame: the neglected role of place and environment. *Health & Place*, 53, 271–278.

Moreno, C. 2024. *The 15- Minute City*, Wiley.

Naidoo, J. & Wills, J. 2016. *Foundations for Health Promotion*, Elsevier.

Nuffield Bioethics Council 2007. *Public health: Ethical Issues*, London: Nuffield Council on Bioethics. Available online at: https://cdn.nuffieldbioethics.org/wp-content/uploads/Public-health-ethical-issues.pdf.

Olick, R. S., Shaw, J. & Yang, Y. T. 2021. Ethical Issues in Mandating COVID-19 Vaccination for Health Care Personnel. *Mayo Clinic Proceedings*, 96, 2958–2962.

Oliver, T. R. 2006. The politics of public health policy. *Annual Review of Public Health*, 27, 195–233.

Painter, K. 2019. Outdoor smoking: fair or foul? *BMJ*, 366.

Pandey, S., Olsen, A., Perez-Cueto, F. J. A. & Thomsen, M. 2023. Nudging toward sustainable food consumption at university canteens: a systematic review and meta-analysis. *Journal of Nutrition Education and Behavior*, 55, 894–904.

Paetkau, T. 2024. Ladders and stairs: how the intervention ladder focuses blame on individuals and obscures systemic failings and interventions. *Journal of Medical Ethics.*, 50(10).

Peterson, B., Withers, B., Hawke, F., Spink, M., Callister, R. & Chuter, V. 2022. Outcomes of participation in parkrun, and factors influencing why and how often individuals participate: a systematic review of quantitative studies. *Journal of Sports Sciences*, 40, 1486–1499.

Petticrew, M., Maani, N., Petticrew, L., Rutter, H. & Van Schalkwyk, M. 2020. Dark nudges and sludge in big alcohol: behavioral economics, cognitive biases, and alcohol industry corporate social responsibility. *The Milbank Quarterly*, 98, 1290–1328.

Polden, M., Robinson, E. & Jones, A. 2023. Assessing public perception and awareness of UK mandatory calorie labeling in the out-of-home sector: using Twitter and Google trends data. *Obesity Science & Practice*, 9, 459–467.

Radó, M. K., Mölenberg, F. J., Westenberg, L. E., Sheikh, A., Millett, C., Burdorf, A., Van Lenthe, F. J. & Been, J. V. 2021. Effect of smoke-free policies in outdoor areas and private places on children's tobacco smoke exposure and respiratory health: a systematic review and meta-analysis. *The Lancet Public Health*, 6, e566–e578.

Raworth, K. 2017. A Doughnut for the Anthropocene: humanity's compass in the 21st century. *The Lancet Planetary Health*, 1, e48–e49.

Raworth, K. 2018. *Doughnut Economics: Seven Ways to Think Like a 21st-Century Economist*, Penguin.

Reece, L. J., Owen, K., Graney, M., Jackson, C., Shields, M., Turner, G. & Wellington, C. 2022. Barriers to initiating and maintaining participation in parkrun. *BMC Public Health*, 22, 83.

Reece, L. J., Quirk, H., Wellington, C., Haake, S. J. & Wilson, F. 2019. Bright Spots, physical activity investments that work: Parkrun; a global initiative striving for healthier and happier communities. *British Journal of Sports Medicine*, 53, 326–327.

Reñosa, M. D. C., Landicho, J., Wachinger, J., Dalglish, S. L., Bärnighausen, K., Bärnighausen, T. & Mcmahon, S. A. 2021. Nudging toward vaccination: a systematic review. *BMJ Global Health*, 6, e006237.

Rogers, N. T., Cummins, S., Forde, H., Jones, C. P., Mytton, O., Rutter, H., Sharp, S. J., Theis, D., White, M. & Adams, J. 2023a. Associations between trajectories of obesity prevalence in English primary school children and the UK soft drinks industry levy: an interrupted time series analysis of surveillance data. *PLoS Medicine*, 20, e1004160.

Rogers, N. T., Pell, D., Mytton, O. T., Penney, T. L., Briggs, A., Cummins, S., Jones, C., Rayner, M., Rutter, H., Scarborough, P., Sharp, S., Smith, R., White, M. & Adams, J. 2023b. Changes in soft drinks purchased by British households associated with the UK soft drinks industry levy: a controlled interrupted time series analysis. *BMJ Open*, 13, e077059.

Scarborough, P., Adhikari, V., Harrington, R. A., Elhussein, A., Briggs, A., Rayner, M., Adams, J., Cummins, S., Penney, T. & White, M. 2020. Impact of the announcement and implementation of the UK Soft Drinks Industry Levy on sugar content, price, product size and number of available soft drinks in the UK, 2015-19: a controlled interrupted time series analysis. *PLoS Medicine*, 17, e1003025.

Schneider, P. P., Smith, R. A., Bullas, A. M., Quirk, H., Bayley, T., Haake, S. J., Brennan, A. & Goyder, E. 2020. Multiple deprivation and geographic distance to community physical activity events — achieving equitable access to parkrun in England. *Public Health*, 189, 48–53.

Schüll, N. D. 2012. *Addiction by design: Machine gambling in Las Vegas*, Princeton University Press.

Scottish Government. 2024. Minimum unit pricing for alcohol in Scotland [Online]. Scottish Government Available: https://www.mygov.scot/minimum-unit-pricing [Accessed].

Shakeri, A., Adanty, C. & Kugathasan, H. 2020. Revisiting the Ethical framework governing Water Fluoridation and Food Fortification. *Voices in Bioethics*, 6.

Shangguan, S., Afshin, A., Shulkin, M., Ma, W., Marsden, D., Smith, J., Saheb-Kashaf, M., Shi, P., Micha, R. & Imamura, F. 2019. A meta-analysis of food labeling effects on consumer diet behaviors and industry practices. *American Journal of Preventive Medicine*, 56, 300–314.

Smith, M., Hosking, J., Woodward, A., Witten, K., Macmillan, A., Field, A., Baas, P. & Mackie, H. 2017. Systematic literature review of built environment effects on physical activity and active transport – an update and new findings on health equity. *International Journal of Behavioral Nutrition and Physical Activity*, 14, 158.

Smith, R. A., Schneider, P. P., Cosulich, R., Quirk, H., Bullas, A. M., Haake, S. J. & Goyder, E. 2021. Socioeconomic inequalities in distance and participation in a community-based running and walking activity. A longitudinal ecological student of parkrun 2010 to 2019. *Health & Place.*, 71.

Stevinson, C. & Hickson, M. 2019. Changes in physical activity, weight and wellbeing outcomes among attendees of a weekly mass participation event: a prospective 12-month study. *Journal of Public Health*, 41, 807–814.

Strassman, A., Colak, Y., Serra-Burriel, M., Nordestgaard, B., Turk, A., Afzal, S. & Puhan, M. 2023. Nationwide indoor smoking ban and impact on smoking behaviour and lung function: a two-population natural experiment. *Thorax*, 78, 144–150.

Sunstein, C. R. 2022. Sludge Audits. *Behavioural Public Policy*, 6, 654–673.

Sutherland, N. & Barber, S. 2017. Allocation of funding from the soft drinks industry levy for sports in schools [Online]. House of Commons Library UK Parliament. Available: https://commonslibrary.parliament.uk/research-briefings/cdp-2017-0006/ [Accessed].

Tamil Selvan, S., Yeo, X. X. & Van Der Eijk, Y. 2024. Which countries are ready for a tobacco endgame? A scoping review and cluster analysis. *The Lancet Global Health*, 12, e1049–e1058.

Thaler, R. & Sunstein, C. 2009. *Nudge: Improving decisions about health, wealth and happiness*, Penguin.

Thaler, R. H. 2018. Nudge, not sludge. *Science*, 361, 431. American Association for the Advancement of Science. Available online at: https://www.science.org/doi/10.1126/science.aau9241.

Thomson, K., Hillier-Brown, F., Todd, A., Mcnamara, C., Huijts, T. & Bambra, C. 2018. The effects of public health policies on health inequalities in high-income countries: an umbrella review. *BMC Public Health*, 18, 1–21.

Turcotte-Tremblay, A.-M., Gali Gali, I. A. & Ridde, V. 2021. The unintended consequences of COVID-19 mitigation measures matter: practical guidance for investigating them. *BMC Medical Research Methodology*, 21, 28.

Vassilev, I., Rogers, A., Todorova, E., Kennedy, A. & Roukova, P. 2017. The articulation of neoliberalism: narratives of experience of chronic illness management in Bulgaria and the UK. *Sociology of Health & Illness*, 39, 349–364.

Vlahov, D., Freudenberg, N., Proietti, F., Ompad, D., Quinn, A., Nandi, V. & Galea, S. 2007. Urban as a determinant of health. *Journal of Urban Health*, 84, i16–i26.

Wanjau, M. N., Dalugoda, Y., Oberai, M., Möller, H., Standen, C., Haigh, F., Milat, A., Lucas, P. & Veerman, J. L. 2023. Does active transport displace other physical activity? A systematic review of the evidence. *Journal of Transport & Health*, 31, 101631.

WHO. 2017a. Taxes on sugary drinks: Why do it? [Online]. The World Health Organization. Available: https://iris.who.int/bitstream/handle/10665/260253/WHO-NMH-PND-16.5Rev.1-eng.pdf [Accessed].

WHO 2017b. Urban green spaces: A brief for action. Available online at: https://www.who.int/europe/publications/i/item/9789289052498.

WHO 2024. World Health Statistics 2024: Monitoring Health for the SDGs, Sustainable Development Goals.

Wight, J. & Middleton, J. 2019. Climate change: the greatest public health threat of the century. *BMJ*, 365.

Williams, O. & Fullagar, S. 2019. Lifestyle drift and the phenomenon of 'citizen shift' in contemporary UK health policy. *Sociology of Health & Illness*, 41, 20–35.

Winslow, C. E. 1920. The untilled fields of public health. *Science*, 51, 23–33.

Wyper, G. M. A., Mackay, D. F., Fraser, C., Lewsey, J., Robinson, M., Beeston, C. & Giles, L. 2023. Evaluating the impact of alcohol minimum unit pricing on deaths and hospitalisations in Scotland: a controlled interrupted time series study. *The Lancet*, 401, 1361–1370.

Ye, T., Yu, P., Wen, B., Yang, Z., Huang, W., Guo, Y., Abramson, M. J. & Li, S. 2022. Greenspace and health outcomes in children and adolescents: a systematic review. *Environmental Pollution*, 314, 120193.

Yeo, G. S. H. 2022. Is calorie labelling on menus the solution to obesity? *Nature Reviews Endocrinology*, 18, 453–454.

Zare Sakhvidi, M. J., Mehrparvar, A. H., Zare Sakhvidi, F. & Dadvand, P. 2023. Greenspace and health, wellbeing, physical activity, and development in children and adolescents: An overview of the systematic reviews. *Current Opinion in Environmental Science & Health*, 32, 100445.

Zlatevska, N., Neumann, N. & Dubelaar, C. 2018. Mandatory calorie disclosure: a comprehensive analysis of its effect on consumers and retailers. *Journal of Retailing*, 94, 89–101.

PART 4

Social and Community Networks, Loneliness, and Social Prescribing

CHAPTER 15

Understanding Support Networks and Influence Across the Life Course

Chris Allen[1], Jasmine Snowden[1], Janine Hall[2], and Ellen Kitson-Reynolds[1]

[1] *School of Health Sciences, University of Southampton, Southampton, UK*
[2] *School of Health and Social Wellbeing, University of the West of England, Bristol, UK*

Introduction

This chapter explores the impact of people's 'personal networks', sometimes called 'social networks', and how they shape health through their influence and their support across the life course. It draws upon research examining the life course perspective and health behaviour, alongside consideration of the importance of different types of support during different life stages, and in response to people's changing needs. As you have explored earlier in this book, health behaviours, such as our diet, whether we smoke, how active or sedentary we are and how much alcohol we consume, are often related to people's physical and social environments across the life course. As covered elsewhere in this book, most notably in chapters 8–11, people's material advantages and disadvantages often relate to the opportunities they have, which in turn, relate to their overall health and well-being.

A large part of this chapter considers network advantages (and indeed disadvantages) – what the people around you can do for you (and what you might be able to do for them) and importantly, how this relates to our health and our well-being. Whilst access to healthcare services and healthcare professionals remain important when people become unwell, much of the support people get, and the influences of this support on their health outcomes and life chances, comes from their connections with various strong (such as close family and friends) and weaker (such as acquittances and work colleagues)

ties. It is therefore people's personal networks across the life course that is the focus of this chapter.

This chapter covers the life course approach, life course epidemiology and social networks. These areas are increasingly being weaved together but are substantial in their own rights, each with their own comprehensive literature. To further consolidate your reading of this chapter, we recommend Alwin et al. (2018) as a comprehensive overview of social networks across the life course, alongside Wagner et al.'s (2024) paper on life course epidemiology.

LEARNING OUTCOMES

By the end of this chapter, you will be able to:

- Recognise the importance of the life course in determining health outcomes.
- Recognise how various events and exposures, as well as accumulated advantages and disadvantages across the life course, influence health outcomes.
- Recognise the value of strong and weak social ties in providing different types of support across the life course.
- Recognise the role of social ties in influencing health behaviours across the life course.

Social Sciences for Healthcare Professionals, First Edition. Edited by Chris Allen.
© 2026 John Wiley & Sons Ltd. Published 2026 by John Wiley & Sons Ltd.

The Life Course Perspective

> ### Key Terms and Definitions
>
> **Social/personal network:** Generally, refers to a person's total contacts, including their weak and strong ties.
>
> **Strong ties:** Generally, family or kin ties. Ties that people are particularly close to and that are particularly enduring.
>
> **Weak ties:** Acquaintances, and other less intimate ties, that are still recognised as being important in providing various types of support.
>
> **Social capital:** Generally refers to the social resources that are shared between people within a network.

We briefly introduced you to the life course perspective in chapter 8, as one way to consider health inequalities. Whilst some older studies used methods similar to the life course approach, interest in the life course was arguably introduced by a now seminal cohort study, that sought to understand the long-term health impacts of the Great Depression (Elder, 2018) and since then, there has been a rising interest and recognition of the life course, which allows us to take a long view of human development by recognising the impact of earlier years on later years (Halfon et al., 2014, Shanahan et al., 2016, Wagner et al., 2024). As an approach, it has been adopted by the World Health Organisation, amongst others (Beard et al., 2016, WHO, 2018) and has been utilised across the social and medical sciences, for example, sociology, psychology, gerontology, political science, economics and epidemiology (Elder et al., 2003, Elder, 2018, Kuh et al., 2003, Mayer, 2009, Shanahan et al., 2016, Wagner et al., 2024).

You will be familiar with some of the biologically and socially created age-graded life stages that are discussed in this chapter. These represent a continuum of development across the life course. Movement between these life stages and the events and exposures of individual people's lives, often shape outcomes and the lives people have (Kendig and Nazroo, 2016, Pavalko and Caputo, 2013). A lack of support, influence and engagement in unhealthy behaviours, reduced opportunities in education and the labour market, as well as negative life events and exposures can have a deleterious impact on our future health and opportunities across the different stages of life (Bartley, 2017, Elovainio et al., 2016, Umberson et al., 2010, Whitley et al., 2014). This is sometimes referred to as accumulated advantage[1] (or inversely, disadvantage) (Bartley, 2017, Dannefer, 2003, Merton, 1988). Our experiences in each stage of

the life course do not necessarily determine our experiences in subsequent stages. People can, for example, have particularly negative experiences in adolescence, that do not result in reduced opportunities and success in early adulthood, particularly in societies with good social mobility. However, research has highlighted that there often is a connection between the life course stages.

The different stages of life that are discussed in this chapter are of course not clear cut, and there is increasing diversity in the activities that people do throughout different stages of their life, especially through increased longevity (discussed in chapter 7). For example, norms around when people access education, and when people leave full-time employment differ in different societies and are subject to constant revision. As examples, increased longevity is resulting in increased interest in university study for older people, and through this, age-friendly university initiatives have emerged (Montepare et al., 2020). Aswell as this, there is variance in the extent to which different individuals and groups choose to work beyond the state retirement age (Zaccagni et al., 2024). Other roles in the life course are also changing or becoming more important. For example, increased longevity, alongside changes in gendered norms relating to work particularly in western industrialised societies, may have created a larger role for intergenerational child rearing (Di Gessa et al., 2020, Herlofson and Hagestad, 2012).

Health across the life course is not necessarily predetermined for all, especially at the level of individuals. People can be very healthy in later life, and likewise, people can become chronically unwell in early life and have to manage this across their life course. Whilst we need to be cautious about making inferences about people's health, and what things people do during different stages of the life course, particularly in relation to stereotyping later life (Ramírez and Palacios-Espinosa, 2016), these biologically, socially and institutionally defined age categories are useful in considering our life course and what support we typically need in different stages of life, as well as considering how events and exposures through different stages of our lives might support, or have a negative impact later on (Alwin, 2012, Kohli, 2007). Life stages are often punctuated by life events – some of these events are normative, things that are commonly experienced during certain stages, such as movement through education, entry into work, marriage, parenthood and retirement (Alwin, 2012). Less predictable events can also happen that can significantly impact people's networks and the material and social resources that they have available to them, such as bereavement (especially in earlier life, when it is less expected), divorce and forced or voluntary migration (Infurna and Mayer, 2019, Wrzus et al., 2013). These events shape our social ties and can involve gaining, as well as losing the different types of support that these contacts provide across the life course (Wrzus et al., 2013).

Adopting a life course perspective allows us to consider patterns of advantages and disadvantages that move with individuals and their networks, as they age, and how these impact on later life outcomes. This perspective assumes that

---

[1] The sociologist Robert Merton (1988), who we introduced you to earlier in this book, highlighted that accumulated advantage can help those with training, who are well located and who have ample access to resources, gain further advantage throughout the life course, in such a way as the gap between the 'haves' and the 'have nots' widens.

our lives and our unique personal circumstances are shaped and influenced by life events that can be both intended and unintended. It recognises that all of our lives have a historical context; what a person has access to now, and what they can experience now, will in part be determined by the things (both positive and negative) that have happened in earlier stages of life, including things that happened even before they were born (Mayer, 2003, Zacher and Froidevaux, 2021).

We can think of the life course approach through the following principles:

- Lifespan development (human development is continuous)
- Agency (whilst people may be constrained by their environment, resources and historical contexts, they can influence their own lives)
- Time (all of our life courses are influenced by historical contexts)
- Timing (events and exposures can have different impacts depending on when they are experienced in the life course)
- **Linked lives (We are all connected to others. We do not experience life on our own. Others influence the lives we lead).**

(Elder Jr and Shanahan, 2007)

There is a growing body of research examining the life course. This work is often necessarily longitudinal (work that follows individuals, or cohorts, and records their outcomes for a long period of time) and has become an increasingly important way to understand the early life opportunities that are potentially protective, as well as the events and exposures that are potentially harmful (Wagner et al., 2024). This has informed public health interventions that when initiated in earlier life stages may benefit later life outcomes (Livingston et al., 2020, Olsen et al., 2016, Russ et al., 2022, Woods-Townsend et al., 2021).

'Linked Lives': What Are Personal Networks and Why Are They Relevant to Health?

For a while now, the value of social connections has been recognised as shaping individual outcomes and opportunities. Durkheim's seminal work on suicide, which we discussed in chapter 4, demonstrated a connection between social integration and the risk of suicide in a population (Durkheim, 2005). In the period since then, other seminal work has demonstrated a relationship between the number of social contacts someone has with mortality and morbidity (Berkman and Syme, 1979, Holt-Lunstad et al., 2010, House et al., 1982). Other research has considered the material and social resources that are gained through people and groups and their relevance to health (Thoits, 2011). Social ties and personal networks can provide a diverse range of support that can help people navigate everyday

needs, such as accessing and being successful in employment (Castilla et al., 2013), supporting with childcare (Gage-Bouchard, 2017), and promoting health and helping when unwell (Derose and Varda, 2009, Koetsenruijter et al., 2016, Smith and Christakis, 2008, Vassilev et al., 2014). Larger, more diverse networks are generally seen as being better placed to provide a range of support, compared to smaller ones (Webster et al., 2022).

The support that we can gain that may help us in life, and that can help us in poor health, can be considered a form of social capital. Whilst there is a lack of a unifying definition for social capital (Kawachi et al., 2008), as a broad concept, it refers to the resources, influences and social support that people can access through their personal networks (Coleman, 1988, Eriksson, 2011, Lin, 2002). There are different types of support and you will often see these broken down into:

- Instrumental (such as doing something practical for someone like cleaning)
- Emotional (such as supporting someone when they are upset)
- Informational (such as providing someone with useful information, including health-related information)
- Material/financial support (such as helping someone with money or providing other types of material resources).

A person's personal network, specifically, their position within it, and who they have access to, influences the types of support and resources they can access.

Generally, in the context of health, you will have likely considered mostly the role of strong ties – often close family (largely kin). After all, in your roles as healthcare professionals, these are often the people you are most likely to see and speak to. Whilst these are clearly important to people, since the early seminal work of Granovetter (1973), the importance of weak ties (such as friends, acquaintances and work colleagues) has been increasingly recognised (Huxhold et al., 2020, Rogers et al., 2014, Small, 2013). Whilst they often do different things for us than what strong ties typically do, and by their nature are more fragile, weak ties can greatly diversify the range of resources, useful information and emotional support that are available to someone by extending people's reach to resources beyond what they have available to them in intimate networks (Huxhold et al., 2020, Rogers et al., 2014). In fact, those with a higher proportion of kin compared to less formal ties, tend to be less socially active and tend to receive less support, and networks are becoming increasingly friend-focused (Suanet and Antonucci, 2017). However, those who are physically or mentally unwell across the life course, generally experience reductions to their social network size, due to having less time and energy to build and maintain weaker network ties, alongside people's changing attitudes towards them (Cornwell, 2009, Haas et al., 2010, Northcott et al., 2016, Perry and Pescosolido, 2012).

Personal networks can also be highly influential over behaviours (Fletcher et al., 2011, Macdonald-Wallis et al., 2012, Sawka et al., 2013), promoting healthy, as well as unhealthy behaviours such as binge drinking (Villalonga-Olives et al., 2020) and smoking (Christakis and Fowler, 2008). Research including Christakis and Fowler's now seminal Framingham Heart study have highlighted a process of contagion, whereby social networks influence ideas, norms and behaviours about health (Christakis and Fowler, 2013, Heijmans et al., 2017). Influences like this are often involuntary. If your friends smoke, this influences your own behaviour, and consequently, you are more likely to smoke yourself (Christakis and Fowler, 2008). Conversely, studies also show that people generally give up unhealthy behaviours together (Christakis and Fowler, 2008), and as a result, interventions that seek to change behaviours through social networks have become increasingly common (Hunter et al., 2019).

Whilst life course and social networks have been studied for some time in relation to health, they have rarely been studied together[2] (Alwin et al., 2018, Vacchiano et al., 2024). After all, it is challenging to collect large social network data, and then track network changes, and potentially relevant health outcomes across a life course. But increasingly it is being recognised as important to consider the life course and networks together, because people's life course transitions impact on their networks, and vice versa. At the same time, many life events are stressful and the buffering thesis suggests that networks can provide support to help people through them (Praharso et al., 2017).

Life transitions, such as getting married, moving area, getting a new job or retiring, are often network transitions too, as they influence the number and quality of people's social ties and in turn, what resources people can access, and the choices they can make (Alwin et al., 2018, Hollstein, 2023, Landes and Settersten, 2019, Lin and Marin, 2022, Marsden, 2018, Settersten, 2015, Settersten et al., 2024). In one large meta-analysis, the size of social networks was seen to vary across the life course – peaking in adolescence, and early adulthood, then gradually reducing throughout the rest of the life course, often punctuated by life events and a focus on maintaining closer mostly family and kin relationships to meet emotional needs (Wrzus et al., 2013). Other more recent work has also suggested that weaker ties are more subject to change and loss over time (Fischer and Offer, 2020, Lin and Marin, 2022). Changing social contexts across the life course affects the ties we have, and the relevance of different network members changes, in response to different needs (Min et al., 2022, Mollenhorst et al., 2014). Of course, there is diversity in what major life events happen to people, when these happen, and the resultant impact these events have on people's networks and their available support (Lin and Marin, 2022).

Family ties are often seen as most important in early and later life, and the value and influence of different family members changes across the life course with the importance of parents in early life, shifting to romantic partners in adult and later life. In most cultures, family relations differ from other types of ties in that people often see them as an obligation and therefore they are more stable over time. Indeed, kinship bias, and the importance placed on maintaining familial ties, likely has a biological and evolutionary basis – you are more likely to support those who might pass on your genes (Dunbar, 2021). However, it is worth noting though that there is considerable diversity in how different types of ties are seen by different people and this varies across cultures, and the concept of 'family' is a social, as well as a biological construct (Sanner et al., 2021). Societies differ in their orientations towards individualism[3] and collectivism[4] and in many societies people now marry less, marry later, divorce more, have less children, move more often, and live alone more (Antonucci and Wong, 2010). Therefore, increasingly people live and are supported by non-traditional family structures and contexts.

Preconception and Maternity

Stop and Think: Support and Influence in Preconception and Maternity

Before reading the following section, please reflect on the following questions in the context of people you have provided care to, or who you may provide care to in the future, who might be considering having a baby or who may be pregnant.

- In what ways might support from personal networks be important during preconception and maternity?
- Who is likely to provide support, and what types of support at they likely to provide?
- What impact, if any, do you think a lack of support in this stage in the life course might have?
- How might those within someone's personal network impact on their behaviour, and what impact might this have on their health, as well as the health of their child?

Pregnancy is a period characterised by biological changes to a woman's body in preparation for parenthood (Hodgkinson et al., 2014, Orchard et al., 2023, Sahrakorpi et al., 2017). For many women, this is an emotionally sensitive time that is accompanied by changes in their physical appearance, their social groups and

---

[2] Whilst life course research has been able to trace the health outcomes of individuals overtime through large population-based cohort studies (Power et al., 2013), data and studies that look at health outcomes alongside personal networks across the life course are less common. There are studies that have used longitudinal ego-network data, such as the UC Social Network Study (UCNets) – to show the relevance of social networks and their change across the life course (Weiss et al., 2022). However, social network studies have tended to be a snapshot in time, whereas life course studies, as we have highlighted as necessarily longitudinal (Vacchiano et al., 2024).

[3] Where there is an expectation that people will largely support themselves and will not be reliant on others.

[4] Where there is an expectation that people will support others.

roles, identities, employment and their life more generally (Klobučar, 2016, Matley, 2020, Prinds et al., 2014, Saxbe et al., 2018). The health behaviours and support women[5] (and birthing people) receive prior to, during their pregnancy and the period immediately after, are vitally important for their own health and the health of their child (Al-Mutawtah et al., 2023, Asselmann et al., 2020, Bedaso et al., 2021, Bedaso et al., 2023, Bernardi and Klärner, 2014, Ekström-Bergström et al., 2022, Oakley, 2018, Sigurdardottir et al., 2017, Stephenson et al., 2018, Żyrek et al., 2024).

Health behaviours adopted prior to, maintained or initiated during pregnancy can impact on later life outcomes for mother and baby (Stephenson et al., 2018), and social networks can be a strong influence on health-enhancing behaviours such as breast-feeding, as well as health-damaging behaviours such as smoking and alcohol consumption (Carlin et al., 2021, Ortega-García et al., 2020, Rockliffe et al., 2021). Harmful health behaviours during pregnancy are linked to socio-economic status and network influences, with those from disadvantaged groups being more likely to have previously engaged with and continue to engage in behaviours that are harmful to themselves and to their baby (Bonello et al., 2023). Perceived social support during pregnancy is associated with increased adoption of healthy behaviours (Fathnezhad-Kazemi et al., 2021), whilst those experiencing perinatal stress, where social support may be lacking, may be more likely to engage in unhealthy behaviours such as drinking and smoking that are known to negatively impact birth and future health outcomes (Beijers et al., 2014). Such behaviours can impact future outcomes such as hypertension, even before conception (Bruin et al., 2010, Fleming et al., 2018). Barker's foetal programming hypothesis highlights the relevance of health behaviours to the prenatal environment, to later life health outcomes. The hypothesis suggests that a baby's body undergoes in utero programming in response to, for example, maternal nutrition, which impacts physiology and metabolism, and as a result, may shape future health outcomes such as cardiovascular disease (Gluckman and Hanson, 2006, Kwon and Kim, 2017, Barker, 2004).

Beyond their influence on behaviours, the way families function, their resources and the support that expectant mothers have available to them, may buffer (i.e. protect against) some of the negative stressors that are experienced by women and their partners (Bedaso et al., 2023, Divney et al., 2012), and the social support that expectant mothers can access have been shown to perform a 'buffering' effect for perinatal stress and a number of maternal conditions (Dunkel Schetter, 2011, Giesbrecht et al., 2013), whilst improving physical and mental health and well-being (Bedaso et al., 2021, Bedaso et al., 2023, Taylor et al., 2022). As with other stages, pregnant women typically draw various types of support from a range of people and groups to meet their changing needs (Hinton et al., 2023, Żyrek et al., 2024). Individual social needs differ for all pregnant women, regardless of whether they are having universal care (i.e. in a United Kingdon context, care that every pregnant woman can receive), or whether they have additional care needs. It is recognised that appropriate support contributes to well-being in relatively uneventful pregnancies (Carter and Guittar, 2014), as well as in those at higher risk (East et al., 2019, Hinton et al., 2023). Where social support is lacking, women are more at risk of developing mental health issues, as well as experiencing poor birth outcomes and low birth weight babies (Dunkel Schetter, 2011, Wang et al., 2013).

Recent research has shown that expectant mothers evaluate the support that is provided in their networks, as part of their 'nesting' preparation (Hinton et al., 2023). Recognising increased and new support needs, expectant mothers and their partners may start to consider the importance of the various types of support from different people within their personal network (Entsieh and Hallström, 2016, Hinton et al., 2023, Weiss et al., 2022). This might include some consideration as to who they know that also has experience of pregnancy, birth and post-birth, who may be able to provide unique insights and perspectives (Al-Mutawtah et al., 2023, Lubker Cornish and Roberts Dobie, 2018).

Whilst the role and expectancy of support from partners varies across cultures, research has suggested that those without a partner, are more likely to report lower social support (Peter et al., 2016). When available, partners are typically seen as providing high degrees of social support to expectant mothers (Al-Mutawtah et al., 2023, Battulga et al., 2021, Hinton et al., 2023, Rini et al., 2006), and perceived partner support may improve birth outcomes (Stapleton et al., 2012). Partners can also support women to change behaviours that are unhealthy (Rockliffe et al., 2021). Whilst for many women, partners are a solid and dependable source of support, for some, they may negatively influence health behaviours (Rockliffe et al., 2021) and can also elicit varying levels of dissatisfaction, and physical and emotional abuse, all of which can negatively impact birth outcomes (Hill et al., 2016, Jonsdottir et al., 2017, Nesari et al., 2018). Importantly, research has highlighted that partners are better placed to provide support when they are well-supported themselves (Bäckström et al., 2021).

The First 1,000 Days and Childhood

Stop and Think: The First 1,000 Days and Childhood

Before reading the following section, please reflect on the following questions in the context of a child you have either provided care for, or who you may provide care to in the future.

- In what ways might support from personal networks be important during childhood, particularly up until the age of 2?

---

[5] For clarity, women and mothers are used to represent women and birthing people throughout this chapter.

- Who is likely to provide support, and what types of support at they likely to provide?
- Is there anything that might impact on these people's ability to provide the support that is needed at this stage in the life course?
- What impact, if any, do you think a lack of support in this stage in the life course might have?
- How might those within someone's personal network impact on their behaviours, and what impact might this have on their health?

Childhood, followed by adolescence, is characterised by the child's gradual transition from the home to society which involves the necessary biological, emotional and psychological changes that are needed to thrive (Keenan et al., 2016). There is now a significant body of evidence that highlights 'the long arm of childhood'. Children who are well supported and have healthy early years, are more likely to go on to experience healthy later life (Haas, 2008, Hayward and Gorman, 2004, Likhar and Patil, 2022, Marmot, 2010). In particular, the first 1,000 days (covering the period from a woman's pregnancy, some of which is covered above, through to the child's second birthday) are now recognised as being highly significant to a child's physical, cognitive, social, emotional and behavioural development, which impacts upon their future health, as well as their related future social and economic prospects (Blake-Lamb et al., 2016, Epure et al., 2020, Hanson and Green, 2022, Wagner et al., 2024).

At the very start of life, especially in a Western context, it is common for a new-born baby's social network to primarily consist of their parent(s) or primary caregiver(s), who ultimately shape the child's exposures, resources, nutrition, behaviours, environment, relationships and primary socialisation, which can significantly shape development, future health and opportunities (Likhar and Patil, 2022, Pears et al., 2007, UK Government, 2019). The parent or caregivers' physical and mental health, their health behaviours (including unhealthy coping strategies), the nature of their relationships (such as any conflict or domestic violence), their education, their style of parenting and the decisions they make about their child's health (e.g. decisions relating to vaccination) all impact on the child's development, their health and future health behaviours (Bellis et al., 2019, Gowda and Dempsey, 2013, UK Government, 2019). Exposure to stress, and in particular adverse childhood experiences, during this stage can also negatively impact on a child's development and can impact on their future physical and mental health and social and economic prospects (Bellis et al., 2019). Negative impacts can even cascade into future generations, for example, we know that children are more likely to be exposed to adverse

experiences and trauma, where their parents also experienced these in their childhood (Armfield et al., 2021).

You may already be familiar with John Bowlby's (1907–1990), and Mary Ainsworth's (1913–1999) now seminal work on attachment theory, which has been useful in considering the impact of the quality of a child's relationship with caregivers on their development and future outcomes (Antonucci et al., 2019). The quality of the parent(s) or caregiver(s) relationship with the child is vitally important in ensuring that the child can form a secure attachment, with secure attachments positively influencing development, and later life social skills, and insecure attachments relating to negative outcomes that can cascade throughout the later stages of the life course and may result in negative social and emotional responses in later life stages that are guided by the thoughts, feelings and expectations of relationships (Fraley and Roisman, 2015, Raby et al., 2015).

The environments parents can provide for their children are influenced by their own social and material resources. The transition to parenthood is tough, with new parents facing a changing identity, alongside new practical, emotional and financial pressures that can be challenging to individuals and their relationships with others. Socioeconomic position can play a role in how well parent(s) and caregiver(s) are equipped to deal with such changes, because it influences the types of social and material resources, they themselves have, and through this, the environment and support that they can provide to their children. Personal networks can be an important resource to new parents and may have a role in reducing parenting stress, influencing the quality of care that new parents can provide and the total resources they have to provide it (Parkes et al., 2015).

Despite the importance of personal networks, the number of ties (particularly friends and acquaintances) new parents have available to them often decreases during the transition to parenthood (Kalmijn, 2012). This decrease often occurs alongside a greater closeness and reliance on immediate kin (Lin and Marin, 2022) though there maybe efforts to connect with, or strengthen relationships with similarly aged families (Weiss et al., 2022).

Whilst recognising the wider networks that exist for caregivers and their relevance, the child's own personal network of primary contacts is typically quite small. As children age, and through their gradual transition into society through exposure to education, and social and community groups, their networks begin to increase and diversify. As the saying goes, it really does take a village to raise a child (Reupert et al., 2022). Alongside the child's network expanding beyond the home, there is a greater number of people shaping the resources that a child has available to them, their experiences and their influences, as extended family, family friends, local communities, their own friends, clubs and activities and their schools become increasingly important to their current and future development, health behaviours and health outcomes (Marmot, 2010).

Adolescence and Emerging Adulthood

Stop and Think: Adolescence

Before reading the following section, reflect on the following questions in the context of an adolescent you have provided care for, or who you might provide care to in the future.

- In what ways might support from personal networks be important during adolescence?
- How might life transitions impact on the support that is available in adolescence?
- Who is likely to provide support, and what types of support at they likely to provide?
- Is there anything that might impact on these people's ability to provide the support that is needed at this stage in the life course?
- What impact, if any, do you think a lack of support in this stage in the life course might have?
- How might those within someone's personal network impact on their behaviour, and what impact might this have on their health?

Exactly what age constitutes adolescence and emerging adulthood is debated, with some highlighting that early onset of puberty, alongside the recognition of the biological and social skills development that continues well into a person's 20s, as well as the shifting of life course role transitions such as marriage and parenthood into later young adulthood, may suggest that this life stage encapsulates a rather broad age range of 10–24 (Sawyer et al., 2018). Our adolescent years provide the platform for our adult working lives and, by their very nature, are characterised by transitions such as moving rapidly between different educational institutions (e.g. college, then higher education), starting employment, moving out of the family home, finding a life partner/getting married and becoming a parent. During these years, networks have a significant impact on supporting young people to adjust to such changes, how they cope with life's stressors, the social and material resources that they are able to draw from, their educational attainment and their health behaviours; all of which can impact on later life outcomes and opportunities (Benner et al., 2021, Steiner et al., 2019). During adolescence and emerging adulthood relationships with parents remain important, particularly in relation to development, and equipping young people with the healthy coping skills, resilience and relational skills needed in later life stages (Delgado et al., 2022, Kingston et al., 2023,

Peng et al., 2021). At the same time, the harmful health behaviours of parents can result in adolescents adopting similar behaviours, which has life course impacts (Rossow et al., 2016).

Relationships with parents can be strained by adolescence, as they are renegotiated whilst young people continue to develop their own identity and seek greater levels of autonomy and independence outside of their home (Branje, 2018). Increasing independence and autonomy often means that adolescents experience a rapid expansion and increasing diversification of their personal network, as they have a greater ability to connect with an increasing range of ties (including those online) to meet their needs beyond their family and their immediate neighbourhood and community (Dunbar, 2021, Weiss et al., 2022, Wrzus et al., 2013). At this stage in the life course, networks are typically composed of a diverse mix of strong (such as family) and weaker ties (such as less close friends gained through education, sports and social organisations) (Blum et al., 2022). High-quality friendships may be especially important in facilitating identity development in adolescence and, alongside first romantic and sexual partners, are seen as being particularly important in adolescence and emergent adulthood as a source for well-being and development, and may better equip individuals to manage such relationships later in life (Branje et al., 2021, Johnson et al., 2011, Shulman and Connolly, 2013, Xia et al., 2018).

These new types of relationships also play a crucial role in health behaviours. As children age, and especially as they hit adolescence, they have a greater say in the health-enhancing (such as physical activity and following a healthy diet) and health-damaging (such as smoking, taking illegal drugs, drinking harmful levels of alcohol, and having unprotected sex) behaviours that they follow. Indeed, it has been suggested that as much as 70% of preventable deaths relate to risks and the genesis of health-harming behaviours initiated during a person's adolescence (Sawyer et al., 2012) and this is a period in which the adoption of harmful coping strategies and poor habits may also first emerge that have the potential to extend into later life stages (Zaso et al., 2023). Such strategies are more common in those experiencing adverse events and social stress (Kort-Butler, 2009, Zaso et al., 2023).

Adolescence is also a period that is often associated with engagement in high-risk behaviours, that can have a detrimental impact on health and well-being across the life course (Romer, 2010). There is a social and biological basis to the higher-risk behaviours more frequently seen in adolescence. Changes in the brain's socio-emotional system may increase reward-seeking, and high-risk behaviour, particularly in the presence of peers who carry significant influence (Albert et al., 2013, Steinberg, 2008). The extent to which individuals are exposed to unhealthy or risk-taking behaviours can related to socio-economic status (Aschengrau et al., 2021). Individuals who are exposed to people in their networks, especially highly influential people who engage in unhealthy behaviours such as drinking excess alcohol, smoking or using recreational drugs, are more likely to also engage in this behaviour themselves (Kreager and Haynie, 2011, Ivaniushina and Titkova, 2021). As one example of the harmful impact this can have on later life stages, adolescent drinking is associated with higher risks of developing dependence and other problems later on (McCambridge et al., 2011, Sjödin et al., 2024).

As with earlier years, education in adolescence continues to be an important determinant of future outcomes (Johnson et al., 2011, Zajacova and Lawrence, 2018). Research consistently links educational attainment to positive health outcomes (Zajacova and Lawrence, 2018). Educational opportunities can be disrupted in adolescence in several ways, for example, through poor physical and mental health and through pregnancy. Teenage pregnancy is more common in the daughters of those who were themselves teenage mums (Meade et al., 2008) and is associated with reduced education and other opportunities (Kane et al., 2013), reduced social network size (Ellis-Sloan and Tamplin, 2019) and stigma (SmithBattle, 2020), which can reduce the material and social resources that are available, with such disadvantages accumulating, and having a significant impact on later life opportunities (Hadley, 2020). Interestingly, those teenage mums with large friendship networks are more likely to continue in education than those who are more socially isolated (Humberstone, 2018) highlighting the protective influence of personal networks.

Being in poor physical health in adolescence is a less common experience than it is for most of the rest of the life course, and therefore the impacts of poor health on personal biographies and identity formation can be quite significant (Wicks et al., 2019). Adolescents in poor health may find it hard to build and maintain social networks, specifically weak ties, and as a result, typically have smaller networks than their peers (Haas et al., 2010). Poor health is known to impact on engagement with education and, as a result, is linked to poor education attainment, especially in those who are chronically unwell and who require increasing healthcare (Champaloux and Young, 2015, Lum et al., 2017). Additionally, it is common for mental health issues that people struggle with throughout their lives, to emerge during adolescence (Kessler et al., 2005).

Working Age Adult Life

Stop and Think: In Working Age Adult Life

Before reading the following section, reflect on the following questions in the context of someone who is of working age and who you have provided care for, or who you might provide care to in the future.

- In what ways might support from personal networks be important during working age adult life?
- How might life transitions impact on the support that is available in working age adult life?
- Who is likely to provide support, and what types of support at they likely to provide?
- Is there anything that might impact on these people's ability to provide the support that is needed at this stage in the life course?
- What impact, if any, do you think a lack of support in this stage in the life course might have?
- How might those within someone's personal network impact on their behaviour, and what impact might this have on their health?

Social and economic opportunities within working age are highly influenced by accumulated advantages and disadvantages in earlier life stages. As with earlier stages in the life course, socio-economic status, social networks and health behaviours in this stage of the life course, lay the foundations for healthy aging in later life (Wagner et al., 2024). The behaviours of others, particularly those who people are close to, can influence and shape the behaviours of working-age people, as with the other life course stages, and these behaviours can result in better (if the behaviours are health-enhancing) or poorer (if the behaviours are health-harming) later life health (Lau-Barraco and Linden, 2014, Neighbors et al., 2019, Wagner et al., 2024). Even in this stage of the life course, where people arguably have the greatest level of functional capability, personal network support remains highly relevant, including in particular to those with chronic illness, or who are living with impairment(s) (Emerson et al., 2021).

During working-age adult life, an individual's personal network can experience significant turnover (or 'churn'). This is often in relation to weak ties specifically, which can be advantageous, as less relevant ties can be replaced by those deemed to be more useful (Hollstein, 2023, Weiss et al., 2022). Younger adult networks are less established than older adult networks, and therefore this 'churn' of ties is more likely (Carmichael et al., 2015). After peaking in early adulthood, personal networks generally begin to shrink, largely through the loss of weaker ties. This is largely through the impact of life events, greater selectivity in ties, and a general decrease in the time available to tend to such a large social network (Weiss et al., 2022, Wrzus et al., 2013). Interactions with our strong ties generally increase though, highlighting increased efforts being directed towards maintaining relationships with those seen as being most important (Weiss et al., 2022, Wrzus et al., 2013). In our working lives, we might have fewer total contacts, but the contacts we do have, we are generally closer to and have more in common with (i.e. we are more selective) (Völker, 2022).

There are of course life events that have a significant impact on working-age people's personal networks. Partnering, or more formally marriage, can influence network size. However, recent research suggests that changes might not be as significant as they once were, due to people being less dislocated from their previous pre-marriage networks[6] and partners often being embedded within the same network prior to getting married (Weiss et al., 2022). We know that partners can be a strong influence on health behaviours. Couples tend to follow similar health behaviours (Franks et al., 2012, Meyler et al., 2007), and whilst causality is hard to determine,[7] marriage has been linked to improved health outcomes (Lindström et al., 2024) and a reduction in some unhealthy behaviours (Keenan et al., 2017), though research has also suggested that married people weigh more, and are less likely to engage in physical activity (Keenan et al., 2017, The and Gordon-Larsen, 2009).

Whilst those getting married, do not generally intend to get divorced, divorce in Western industrialised societies is relatively common (Wilcox, 2009). Divorce can lead to significant stress, may reduce a person's overall standard of living through reducing access to social and material resources, can create situations of co-parenting, and potentially reduce wanted access to children, etc. Whilst many cope well after a divorce, and for some divorce may actually increase well-being (especially if relationships are abusive or strained), it can negatively impact on health (Bourassa et al., 2019, Pellón-Elexpuru et al., 2024, Sbarra, 2015). The impacts of divorce are likely to vary by gender, socio-economic status and health behaviours (Pellón-Elexpuru et al., 2024). A recent meta-analysis found that childless unemployed women with lower educational attainment were most likely to experience poor health following a divorce, alongside those engaging in poor health behaviours (alcohol consumption, inactivity, etc.) (Pellón-Elexpuru et al., 2024). Where marriage may promote healthy behaviour, research has suggested that people can adopt unhealthy behaviours to cope with the stress of divorce (Bourassa et al., 2019).

The nature of our employment can also influence our networks. Employment itself is a unique stressor at this stage of the life course. We highlighted the importance of well-paid, secure and meaningful employment as a social determinant of health in chapter 8. The nature of employment, including how stimulating it is, is recognised as being a factor in later life health outcomes (Kivimäki et al., 2021). In addition, occupational changes can influence our networks in several ways. Firstly, our work environments provide a source of weak ties. Changing employment is often related to a turnover in weak ties, with old work friends and acquaintances being replaced by new ones (Wrzus et al., 2013). What work we do, and the hours that we work can also have an influence on the weak ties that we can secure outside of work, and how embedded we can become in our local communities (Cornwell and Warburton, 2014). Those whose work patterns involve working unsocial hours in the evening and at night are invariably less socially connected than those who work more sociable shift patterns (Cornwell and Warburton, 2014).

Retirement and Later Life

> ## Stop and Think: Support and Influence in Retirement and Late Life
>
> Before reading the following section, please reflect on the following questions in the context of an older person you have provided care for, or who you might provide care to in the future.
>
> - In what ways might support from personal networks be important after retirement and during later life?
> - How might life transitions impact on the support that is available to older people?
> - Who is likely to provide support, and what types of support are they likely to provide?
> - Is there anything that might impact on these people's ability to provide the support that is needed at this stage in the life course?
> - What impact, if any, do you think a lack of support in this stage in the life course might have?
> - How might those within someone's personal network impact on their behaviours, and what impact might this have on their health?

Much of the life course literature relating to later life, highlights the importance of earlier years, and life course socio-economic status in laying the foundations for healthy aging or 'aging well' (Haas, 2008, Lu et al., 2023, Marden et al., 2017, Power et al., 2013, Wagner et al., 2022). This life stage is essentially the destination for the accumulated advantages and disadvantages we have discussed in the earlier life stages – much of which has an impact on whether someone reaches later life, and if they do, how healthy they are in it. In chapter 8, we explored that as we age our risk of poor health quite significantly increases. Indeed, we often see later life as a period characterised by reduced functional, cognitive and physical ability and an increased need for various types of support (Raymond et al., 2021). Whilst for those able to 'age well', any decline is not as substantial as the negative stereotypes about aging might suggest (Shafiq et al., 2023), there is an empirical and biological basis that highlights that advancing old age can bring about cognitive and physical decline, with significant differences in healthy life expectancy being related to differences in socio-economic status and inequalities across the life course (Marmot, 2010, Wagner et al., 2022, Wagner et al., 2024).

Networks during this stage, largely relate to decisions and opportunities taken in earlier stages of life, that now in

---

[6] Which traditionally for women, might have been an entirely different network – this is still largely the case in many cultures.

[7] After all, you cannot randomise people to marriage. Marriage is related to socioeconomic status, and healthier people may be more likely to get married in the first place.

particular significantly shape what support someone has available to them. For example, the decision to get married, and to stay married, relates to the availability of spousal or partner support, which is particularly relevant in later life (van Tilburg and Suanet, 2018). Likewise, older adults with available children may be able to secure support, that their childless peers cannot, though the impact of this on health appears to vary between countries (Quashie et al., 2019).

As with other life course stages, personal networks often provide social and economic resources, therefore unsurprisingly, personal networks and connectedness are vital to successful aging (Roth, 2020b). In later life, those with the strongest networks of support generally do better, experiencing longer healthier lives, with less cognitive decline than their less-connected peers (Cornwell and Waite, 2009, O'Rourke and Sidani, 2017, Zahodne et al., 2019). Whilst earlier life course events are clearly important, key events can also happen within this stage, that can influence a person's network size and composition. Later life in general is associated with a reduction in some ties, but as with earlier adulthood, this decreasing network mostly relates to a reduction in the number of weaker social ties (Wrzus et al., 2013), with kin relationships being significantly more resilient to change over time (Lin and Marin, 2022), highlighting a focus on maintaining relationships that are perceived as being most important. However, this can be influenced by events in later life. Whilst retirement itself (a normative event at this stage in the life course) may bring about reductions in network size, this is not fully understood. Contact with co-workers might reduce (Van Tilburg, 2003), though more recent evidence suggests co-worker contact is often maintained post-retirement (Cozijnsen et al., 2010, Fletcher, 2014, Webster et al., 2022), which may become more common with access to others being increasingly mediated through the internet. Even where they are lost, weak-tie co-workers may be replaced with new ties, due to the greater amount of time those who have recently retired may have, and their ability to reach out to people based on shared interests and passions outside of work. As with other life course stages, weak ties and friends in particular are generally seen as an important form of support and well-being in later life (Huxhold et al., 2014, Huxhold et al., 2020). In later life, those with more diverse networks generally fare better than those with less diverse support (Ellwardt et al., 2017)

Other later life events following retirement, such as changes to health, reductions in physical and cognitive capabilities, becoming a carer, having a partner admitted to long-term care, residential mobility, and bereavement can all influence who is available, how readily available they are and what support they are likely to be able to provide (Gillespie and Fokkema, 2024, Teo, 2023). Some are unfortunate in that they experience negative events such as bereavement, or ill health and reduced capabilities before they reach old age, and where this is the case, this can have a particularly significant impact on network size and composition, which is likely to also reduce the availability of later life social and economic resources (Cornwell and Schafer, 2016, Roth, 2020a, Roth, 2020b).

Whilst bereavement can occur at any stage in the life course, spousal death, and the loss of people who are close, is particularly common in later life (Cornwell and Laumann, 2018). The loss of a spouse, in particular, is generally accompanied by a reduction in personal network size, due not only to the loss of support from the spouse or partner, and those more closely associated with them, but also potentially the distancing of friends, family and acquittances that can arise through the temporary withdraw from social interactions that can occur through the grieving process, and people's needs to adjust to new routines and roles (Naef et al., 2013).

Those recently bereaved have a higher risk of mortality themselves, a phenomenon that has come to be known as 'widowhood mortality' or the 'widowhood effect' (Cornwell and Qu, 2024, Dabergott, 2022). It is not fully understood why this happens, and there are several explanations for this – for example, increased stress, grief and the sudden loss of spousal support (Dabergott, 2022). Personal network influence on health behaviour across the life course provides another possible explanation. It is common for spouses to share similar characteristics (birds of a feather flock together, etc.) and through social influence on one another, follow similar health-related behaviours and lifestyles – recent bereavement might in itself cause increased mortality in the surviving spouse, but may also reflect the impact of a couple's shared characteristics, behaviours and exposures across the life course, influencing each partners longevity (Dabergott, 2022).

Clinical Considerations

- Social ties influence health in several ways, the most relevant being access to resources and support, and influence on health behaviours. Such influences are present across the life course.

- Certain events and exposures across the life course influence the support people have available to them.

- People accumulate advantages and disadvantages across the life course, with poor health in later life, often relating to events and exposures in earlier life.

- Public health interventions often target early years, through the recognition of their influence on later life health outcomes.

Conclusion

In this chapter, we have introduced you to the life course approach, life course epidemiology and 'personal', or 'social' networks and highlighted their relevance to health across lives various stages. We have used this to fully unpack the accumulated advantages and disadvantages that are often experienced across the life course, and how these can be used to explain the different health outcomes that are observed during different life course stages, that relate to previous events and exposures. We have unpacked the relevance of support and behaviours, across different stages of the life course, from preconception through to later life and used these to help you consider different outcomes. Along the way, we have encouraged you to think about the different types of support that are relevant in different life stages, and who is likely to provide this type of support. In this chapter, we have viewed the impact of support, and how our networks influence our health behaviours. In the next chapter, we move beyond this, to consider the impact of a perceived lack of support, which is commonly referred to as loneliness.

References

Al-Mutawtah, M., Campbell, E., Kubis, H.-P. & Erjavec, M. 2023. Women's experiences of social support during pregnancy: a qualitative systematic review. *BMC Pregnancy and Childbirth*, 23, 782.

Albert, D., Chein, J. & Steinberg, L. 2013. Peer Influences on adolescent decision making. *Current Directions in Psychological Science*, 22, 114–120.

Alwin, D. F. 2012. Integrating varieties of life course concepts. *The Journals of Gerontology. Series B, Psychological Sciences and Social Sciences*, 67, 206–220.

Alwin, D. F., Felmlee, D. H. & Kreager, D. A. 2018. Social networks and the life course. *In:* Alwin, D. F., Felmlee, D. H. & Kreager, D. A. (eds.) *Integrating the Development of Human Lives and Social Relational Networks*, S. l.: Springer.

Antonucci, T. C., Ajrouch, K. J., Webster, N. J. & Zahodne, L. B. 2019. Social relations across the life span: scientific advances, emerging issues, and future challenges. *Annual Review of Developmental Psychology*, 1, 313–336.

Antonucci, T. C. & Wong, K. M. 2010. Public health and the aging family. *Public Health Reviews*, 32, 512–531.

Armfield, J. M., Gnanamanickam, E. S., Johnston, D. W., Preen, D. B., Brown, D. S., Nguyen, H. & Segal, L. 2021. Intergenerational transmission of child maltreatment in South Australia, 1986–2017: a retrospective cohort study. *The Lancet Public Health*, 6, e450–e461.

Aschengrau, A., Grippo, A. & Winter, M. R. 2021. Influence of family and community socioeconomic status on the risk of adolescent drug use. *Substance Use & Misuse*, 56, 577–587.

Asselmann, E., Kunas, S. L., Wittchen, H. U. & Martini, J. 2020. Maternal personality, social support, and changes in depressive, anxiety, and stress symptoms during pregnancy and after delivery: a prospective-longitudinal study. *PLoS One*, 15, e0237609.

Bäckström, C., Larsson, T. & Thorstensson, S. 2021. How partners of pregnant women use their social networks when preparing for childbirth and parenthood: a qualitative study. *Nordic Journal of Nursing Research*, 41, 25–33.

Bartley, M. 2017. *Health Inequality: An Introduction to Concepts Theories and Methods*, Cambridge Polity.

Barker, D. (2004). The Developmental Origins of Adult Disease. *Journal of the American College of Nutrition*, 23, 588S-595S. https://doi.org/10.1080/07315724.2004.10719428

Battulga, B., Benjamin, M. R., Chen, H. & Bat-Enkh, E. 2021. The impact of social support and pregnancy on subjective well-being: a systematic review. *Frontiers in Psychology*, 12, 710858.

Beard, J. R., Officer, A., De Carvalho, I. A., Sadana, R., Pot, A. M., Michel, J. P., Lloyd-Sherlock, P., Epping-Jordan, J. E., Peeters, G., Mahanani, W. R., Thiyagarajan, J. A. & Chatterji, S. 2016. The world report on ageing and health: a policy framework for healthy ageing. *Lancet*, 387, 2145–2154.

Bedaso, A., Adams, J., Peng, W. & Sibbritt, D. 2021. The relationship between social support and mental health problems during pregnancy: a systematic review and meta-analysis. *Reproductive Health*, 18, 162.

Bedaso, A., Adams, J., Peng, W. & Sibbritt, D. 2023. The direct and mediating effect of social support on health-related quality of life during pregnancy among Australian women. *BMC Pregnancy and Childbirth*, 23, 372.

Beijers, C., Ormel, J., Meijer, J. L., Verbeek, T., Bockting, C. L. & Burger, H. 2014. Stressful events and continued smoking and continued alcohol consumption during mid-pregnancy. *PLoS One*, 9, e86359.

Bellis, M. A., Hughes, K., Ford, K., Ramos Rodriguez, G., Sethi, D. & Passmore, J. 2019. Life course health consequences and associated annual costs of adverse childhood experiences across Europe and North America: a systematic review and meta-analysis. *The Lancet Public Health*, 4, e517–e528.

Benner, A. D., Chen, S., Mistry, R. S. & Shen, Y. 2021. Life course transitions and educational trajectories: examining adolescents who fall off track academically. *Journal of Youth and Adolescence*, 50, 1068–1080.

Berkman, L. F. & Syme, S. L. 1979. Social networks, host resistance, and mortality: a nine-year follow-up study of Alameda County residents. *American Journal of Epidemiology*, 109, 186–204.

Bernardi, L. & Klärner, A. 2014. Social networks and fertility. *Demographic Research*, 30, 641–670.

Blake-Lamb, T. L., Locks, L. M., Perkins, M. E., Baidal, J. A. W., Cheng, E. R. & Taveras, E. M. 2016. Interventions for childhood obesity in the first 1,000 days a systematic review. *American Journal of Preventive Medicine*, 50, 780–789.

Blum, R. W., Lai, J., Martinez, M. & Jessee, C. 2022. Adolescent connectedness: cornerstone for health and wellbeing. *BMJ*, 379, e069213.

Bonello, K., Figoni, H., Blanchard, E., Vignier, N., Avenin, G., Melchior, M., Cadwallader, J.-S., Chastang, J. & Ibanez, G. 2023. Prevalence of smoking during pregnancy and associated social inequalities in developed countries over the 1995–2020 period: a systematic review. *Paediatric and Perinatal Epidemiology*, 37, 555–565.

Bourassa, K. J., Ruiz, J. M. & Sbarra, D. A. 2019. Smoking and physical activity explain the increased mortality risk following marital separation and divorce: evidence from the English longitudinal study of ageing. *Annals of Behavioral Medicine*, 53, 255–266.

Branje, S. 2018. Development of parent–adolescent relationships: conflict interactions as a mechanism of change. *Child Development Perspectives*, 12, 171–176.

Branje, S., De Moor, E. L., Spitzer, J. & Becht, A. I. 2021. Dynamics of identity development in adolescence: a decade in review. *Journal of Research on Adolescence*, 31, 908–927.

Bruin, J. E., Gerstein, H. C. & Holloway, A. C. 2010. Long-term consequences of fetal and neonatal nicotine exposure: a critical review. *Toxicological Sciences*, 116, 364–374.

Carlin, R. F., Cornwell, B., Mathews, A., Wang, J., Cheng, Y. I., Yan, X., Fu, L. Y. & Moon, R. Y. 2021. Impact of personal social network types on breastfeeding practices in United States-born black and white women. *Breastfeeding Medicine*, 16, 807–813.

Carmichael, C. L., Reis, H. T. & Duberstein, P. R. 2015. In your 20s it's quantity, in your 30s it's quality: the prognostic value of social activity across 30 years of adulthood. *Psychology and Aging*, 30, 95.

Carter, S. K. & Guittar, S. G. 2014. Emotion work among pregnant and birthing women. *Midwifery*, 30, 1021–1028.

Castilla, E. J., Lan, G. J. & Rissing, B. A. 2013. Social networks and employment: mechanisms (part 1). *Sociology Compass*, 7, 999–1012.

Champaloux, S. W. & Young, D. R. 2015. Childhood chronic health conditions and educational attainment: a social ecological approach. *Journal of Adolescent Health*, 56, 98–105.

Christakis, N. A. & Fowler, J. H. 2008. The collective dynamics of smoking in a large social network. *New England Journal of Medicine*, 358, 2249–2258.

Christakis, N. A. & Fowler, J. H. 2013. Social contagion theory: examining dynamic social networks and human behavior. *Statistics in Medicine*, 32, 556–577.

Coleman, J. S. 1988. Social capital in the creation of human capital. *American Journal of Sociology*, 94, S95–S120.

Cornwell, B. 2009. Good health and the bridging of structural holes. *Social Networks*, 31, 92–103.

Cornwell, B. & Laumann, E. O. 2018. Structure by Death: Social Network Replenishment in the Wake of Confidant Loss. *In:* Alwin, D. F., Felmlee, D. H. & Kreager, D. A. (eds.) *Social Networks and the Life Course: Integrating the Development of Human Lives and Social Relational Networks*, Springer.

Cornwell, B. & Qu, T. 2024. "I love you to death": social networks and the widowhood effect on mortality. *Journal of Health and Social Behavior*, 65, 273–291.

Cornwell, B. & Schafer, M. H. 2016. Social Networks in Later Life. *In:* George, L. K. & Ferraro, K. F. (eds.) *Handbook of Aging and the Social Sciences*, Elsevier.

Cornwell, B. & Warburton, E. 2014. Work schedules and community ties. *Work and Occupations*, 41, 139–174.

Cornwell, E. Y. & Waite, L. J. 2009. Social disconnectedness, perceived isolation, and health among older adults. *Journal of Health and Social Behavior*, 50, 31–48.

Cozijnsen, R., Stevens, N. L. & Van Tilburg, T. G. 2010. Maintaining work-related personal ties following retirement. *Personal Relationships*, 17, 345–356.

Dabergott, F. 2022. The gendered widowhood effect and social mortality gap. *Population Studies*, 76, 295–307.

Dannefer, D. 2003. Cumulative advantage/disadvantage and the life course: cross-fertilizing age and social science theory. *The Journals of Gerontology: Series B*, 58, S327–S337.

Delgado, E., Serna, C., Martínez, I. & Cruise, E. 2022. Parental attachment and peer relationships in adolescence: a systematic review. *International Journal of Environmental Research and Public Health*, 19, 1064.

Derose, K. P. & Varda, D. M. 2009. Social capital and health care access: a systematic review. *Medical Care Research and Review*, 66, 272–306.

Di Gessa, G., Zaninotto, P. & Glaser, K. 2020. Looking after grandchildren: gender differences in 'when,' 'what,' and 'why': evidence from the English longitudinal study of ageing. *Demographic Research*, 43, 1545–1562.

Divney, A. A., Sipsma, H., Gordon, D., Niccolai, L., Magriples, U. & Kershaw, T. 2012. Depression during pregnancy among young couples: the effect of personal and partner experiences of stressors and the buffering effects of social relationships. *Journal of Pediatric and Adolescent Gynecology*, 25, 201–207.

Dunbar, R. 2021. *Friends: Understanding the Power of Our Most Important Relationships*, Little, Brown.

Dunkel Schetter, C. 2011. Psychological science on pregnancy: stress processes, biopsychosocial models, and emerging research issues. *Annual Review of Psychology*, 62, 531–558.

Durkheim, E. 2005. *Suicide: A Study in Sociology*, Routledge.

East, C. E., Biro, M. A., Fredericks, S. & Lau, R. 2019. Support during pregnancy for women at increased risk of low birthweight babies. *Cochrane Database of Systematic Reviews*, 4.

Ekström-Bergström, A., Thorstensson, S. & Bäckström, C. 2022. The concept, importance and values of support during childbearing and breastfeeding - a discourse paper. *Nursing Open*, 9, 156–167.

Elder, G. H. 2018. *Children of the Great Depression*, Routledge.

Elder, G. H., Johnson, M. K. & Crosnoe, R. 2003. *The Emergence and Development of Life Course Theory*, Springer.

Elder, G. H., Jr. & Shanahan, M. J. 2007. The Life Course and Human Development. *In:* Lerner, R. M. & Damon, W. (eds.) *Handbook of Child Psychology*, Volume 1, Wiley.

Ellis-Sloan, K. & Tamplin, A. 2019. Teenage mothers and social isolation: the role of friendship as protection against relational exclusion. *Social Policy and Society*, 18, 203–218.

Ellwardt, L., Aartsen, M. & Van Tilburg, T. 2017. Types of non-kin networks and their association with survival in late adulthood: a latent class approach. *The Journals of Gerontology. Series B, Psychological Sciences and Social Sciences*, 72, 694–705.

Elovainio, M., Rosenström, T., Hakulinen, C., Pulkki-Råback, L., Mullola, S., Jokela, M., Josefsson, K., Raitakari, O. T. & Keltikangas-Järvinen, L. 2016. Educational attainment and health transitions over the life course: testing the potential mechanisms. *Journal of Public Health*, 38, e254–e262.

Emerson, E., Fortune, N., Llewellyn, G. & Stancliffe, R. 2021. Loneliness, social support, social isolation and wellbeing among working age adults with and without disability: cross-sectional study. *Disability and Health Journal*, 14, 100965.

Entsieh, A. A. & Hallström, I. K. 2016. First-time parents' prenatal needs for early parenthood preparation-A systematic review and meta-synthesis of qualitative literature. *Midwifery*, 39, 1–11.

Epure, A. M., Rios-Leyvraz, M., Anker, D., Di Bernardo, S., Da Costa, B. R., Chiolero, A. & Sekarski, N. 2020. Risk factors during first 1,000 days of life for carotid intima-media thickness in infants, children, and adolescents: a systematic review with meta-analyses. *PLoS Medicine*, 17, e1003414.

Eriksson, M. 2011. Social capital and health--implications for health promotion. *Global Health Action*, 4, 5611.

Fathnezhad-Kazemi, A., Aslani, A. & Hajian, S. 2021. Association between perceived social support and health-promoting lifestyle in pregnant women: a cross-sectional study. *Journal of Caring Sciences*, 10, 96–102.

Fischer, C. S. & Offer, S. 2020. Who is dropped and why? Methodological and substantive accounts for network loss. *Social Networks*, 61, 78–86.

Fleming, T. P., Watkins, A. J., Velazquez, M. A., Mathers, J. C., Prentice, A. M., Stephenson, J., Barker, M., Saffery, R., Yajnik, C. S. & Eckert, J. J.

2018. Origins of lifetime health around the time of conception: causes and consequences. *The Lancet*, 391, 1842–1852.

Fletcher, A., Bonell, C. & Sorhaindo, A. 2011. You are what your friends eat: systematic review of social network analyses of young people's eating behaviours and bodyweight. *Journal of Epidemiology and Community Health*, 65, 548–555.

Fletcher, J. M. 2014. Late life transitions and social networks: the case of retirement. *Economics Letters*, 125, 459–462.

Fraley, R. C. & Roisman, G. I. 2015. Do early caregiving experiences leave an enduring or transient mark on developmental adaptation? *Current Opinion in Psychology*, 1, 101–106.

Franks, M. M., Shields, C. G., Lim, E., Sands, L. P., Mobley, S. & Boushey, C. J. 2012. I will if you will: similarity in married partners' readiness to change health risk behaviors. *Health Education & Behavior*, 39, 324–331.

Gage-Bouchard, E. A. 2017. Social support, flexible resources, and health care navigation. *Social Science & Medicine*, 190, 111–118.

Giesbrecht, G. F., Poole, J. C., Letourneau, N., Campbell, T. & Kaplan, B. J. 2013. The buffering effect of social support on hypothalamic-pituitary-adrenal axis function during pregnancy. *Psychosomatic Medicine*, 75, 856–862.

Gillespie, B. J. & Fokkema, T. 2024. Life events, social conditions and residential mobility among older adults. *Population, Space and Place*, 30, e2706.

Gluckman, P. D. & Hanson, M. A. 2006. The Developmental Origins of Health and Disease. *In:* Wintour, E. M. & Owens, J. A. (eds.) *Early Life Origins of Health and Disease*, 1–7.

Gowda, C. & Dempsey, A. F. 2013. The rise (and fall?) of parental vaccine hesitancy. *Human Vaccines & Immunotherapeutics*, 9, 1755–1762.

Granovetter, M. S. 1973. The strength of weak ties. *American Journal of Sociology*, 78, 1360–1380.

Haas, S. 2008. Trajectories of functional health: the 'long arm' of childhood health and socioeconomic factors. *Social Science & Medicine*, 66, 849–861.

Haas, S. A., Schaefer, D. R. & Kornienko, O. 2010. Health and the structure of adolescent social networks. *Journal of Health and Social Behavior*, 51, 424–439.

Hadley, A. 2020. Teenage pregnancy: strategies for prevention. *Obstetrics, Gynaecology and Reproductive Medicine*, 30, 387–394.

Halfon, N., Larson, K., Lu, M., Tullis, E. & Russ, S. 2014. Lifecourse health development: past, present and future. *Maternal and Child Health Journal*, 18, 344–365.

Hanson, M. & Green, L. 2022. *What Makes a Person? Secrets of Our First 1,000 Days*, Cambridge: Cambridge University Press.

Hayward, M. D. & Gorman, B. K. 2004. The long arm of childhood: the influence of early-life social conditions on men's mortality. *Demography*, 41, 87–107.

Heijmans, N., Van Lieshout, J. & Wensing, M. 2017. Social network composition of vascular patients and its associations with health behavior and clinical risk factors. *PLoS One*, 12, e0185341.

Herlofson, K. & Hagestad, G. O. 2012. Transformations in the Role of Grandparents Across Welfare States. *In:* Arber, S. & Timonen, V. (eds.) *Contemporary Grandparenting: Changing Family Relationships in Global Contexts*, Policy Press.

Hill, A., Pallitto, C., Mccleary-Sills, J. & Garcia-Moreno, C. 2016. A systematic review and meta-analysis of intimate partner violence during pregnancy and selected birth outcomes. *International Journal of Gynecology & Obstetrics*, 133, 269–276.

Hinton, L., Dumelow, C., Hodgkinson, J., Montgomery, C., Martin, A., Allen, C., Tucker, K., Green, M. E., Wilson, H., Mcmanus, R. J.,

Chappell, L. C. & Band, R. 2023. 'Nesting networks': women's experiences of social network support in high-risk pregnancy. *Midwifery*, 120, 103622.

Hodgkinson, E. L., Smith, D. M. & Wittkowski, A. 2014. Women's experiences of their pregnancy and postpartum body image: a systematic review and meta-synthesis. *BMC Pregnancy and Childbirth*, 14, 330.

Hollstein, B. 2023. Personal network dynamics across the life course: a relationship-related structural approach. *Advances in Life Course Research*, 58, 100567.

Holt-Lunstad, J., Smith, T. B. & Layton, J. B. 2010. Social relationships and mortality risk: a meta-analytic review. *PLoS Medicine*, 7, e1000316.

House, J. S., Robbins, C. & Metzner, H. L. 1982. The association of social relationships and activities with mortality: prospective evidence from the Tecumseh community health study. *American Journal of Epidemiology*, 116, 123–140.

Humberstone, E. 2018. Social networks and educational attainment among adolescents experiencing pregnancy. *Socius*, 4, 2378023118803803.

Hunter, R. F., De La Haye, K., Murray, J. M., Badham, J., Valente, T. W., Clarke, M. & Kee, F. 2019. Social network interventions for health behaviours and outcomes: a systematic review and meta-analysis. *PLoS Medicine*, 16, e1002890.

Huxhold, O., Fiori, K. L., Webster, N. J. & Antonucci, T. C. 2020. The strength of weaker ties: an underexplored resource for maintaining emotional well-being in later life. *The Journals of Gerontology: Series B*, 75, 1433–1442.

Huxhold, O., Miche, M. & Schüz, B. 2014. Benefits of having friends in older ages: differential effects of informal social activities on well-being in middle-aged and older adults. *The Journals of Gerontology. Series B, Psychological Sciences and Social Sciences*, 69, 366–375.

Infurna, F. J. & Mayer, A. 2019. Repeated bereavement takes its toll on subjective well-being. *Innovation in Aging*, 3, igz047.

Ivaniushina, V. & Titkova, V. 2021. Peer influence in adolescent drinking behavior: a meta-analysis of stochastic actor-based modeling studies. *PLoS One*, 16, e0250169.

Johnson, M. K., Crosnoe, R. & Elder, G. H., Jr. 2011. Insights on adolescence from a life course perspective. *Journal of Research on Adolescence*, 21, 273–280.

Jonsdottir, S. S., Thome, M., Steingrimsdottir, T., Lydsdottir, L. B., Sigurdsson, J. F., Olafsdottir, H. & Swahnberg, K. 2017. Partner relationship, social support and perinatal distress among pregnant Icelandic women. *Women and Birth*, 30, e46–e55.

Kalmijn, M. 2012. Longitudinal analyses of the effects of age, marriage, and parenthood on social contacts and support. *Advances in Life Course Research*, 17, 177–190.

Kane, J. B., Morgan, S. P., Harris, K. M. & Guilkey, D. K. 2013. The educational consequences of teen childbearing. *Demography*, 50, 2129–2150.

Kawachi, I., Subramanian, S. V. & Kim, D. 2008. *Social Capital and Health: A Decade of Progress and Beyond*, Springer.

Keenan, K., Ploubidis, G. B., Silverwood, R. J. & Grundy, E. 2017. Lifecourse partnership history and midlife health behaviours in a population-based birth cohort. *Journal of Epidemiology and Community Health*, 71, 232–238.

Keenan, T., Evans, S. & Crowley, K. 2016. *An introduction to Child Development*, Third Edition, Sage.

Kendig, H. & Nazroo, J. 2016. Life course influences on inequalities in later life: comparative perspectives. *Journal of Population Ageing*, 9, 1–7.

Kessler, R. C., Berglund, P., Demler, O., Jin, R., Merikangas, K. R. & Walters, E. E. 2005. Lifetime prevalence and age-of-onset distributions of DSM-IV disorders in the national comorbidity survey replication. *Archives of General Psychiatry*, 62, 593–602.

Kingston, J. L., Ellett, L., Thompson, E. C., Gaudiano, B. A. & Krkovic, K. 2023. A child–parent dyad study on adolescent paranoia and the influence of adverse life events, bullying, parenting stress, and family support. *Schizophrenia Bulletin*, 49, 1486–1493.

Kivimäki, M., Walker, K. A., Pentti, J., Nyberg, S. T., Mars, N., Vahtera, J., Suominen, S. B., Lallukka, T., Rahkonen, O. & Pietiläinen, O. 2021. Cognitive stimulation in the workplace, plasma proteins, and risk of dementia: three analyses of population cohort studies. *BMJ*, 374, n1804.

Klobučar, N. R. 2016. The role of spirituality in transition to parenthood: qualitative research using transformative learning theory. *Journal of Religion and Health*, 55, 1345–1358.

Koetsenruijter, J., Van Eikelenboom, N., Van Lieshout, J., Vassilev, I., Lionis, C., Todorova, E., Portillo, M. C., Foss, C., Serrano Gil, M., Roukova, P., Angelaki, A., Mujika, A., Knutsen, I. R., Rogers, A. & Wensing, M. 2016. Social support and self-management capabilities in diabetes patients: an international observational study. *Patient Education and Counseling*, 99, 638–643.

Kohli, M. 2007. The institutionalization of the life course: looking back to look ahead. *Research in Human Development*, 4, 253–271.

Kort-Butler, L. A. 2009. Coping styles and sex differences in depressive symptoms and delinquent behavior. *Journal of Youth and Adolescence*, 38, 122–136.

Kreager, D. A. & Haynie, D. L. 2011. Dangerous liaisons? Dating and drinking diffusion in adolescent peer networks. *American Sociological Review*, 76, 737–763.

Kuh, D., Ben-Shlomo, Y., Lynch, J., Hallqvist, J. & Power, C. 2003. Life course epidemiology. *Journal of Epidemiology and Community Health*, 57, 778–783.

Kwon, E. J. & Kim, Y. J. 2017. What is fetal programming?: A lifetime health is under the control of in utero health. *Obstetrics & Gynecology Science*, 60, 506–519.

Landes, S. D. & Settersten, R. A., Jr. 2019. The inseparability of human agency and linked lives. *Advances in Life Course Research*, 42, 100306.

Lau-Barraco, C. & Linden, A. N. 2014. Drinking buddies: who are they and when do they matter? *Addiction Research & Theory*, 22, 57–67.

Likhar, A. & Patil, M. S. 2022. Importance of maternal nutrition in the first 1,000 days of life and its effects on child development: a narrative review. *Cureus*, 14, e30083.

Lin, C. Z. & Marin, A. 2022. When life happens: a multidimensional approach to studying the effects of major life events on relationship change. *Advances in Life Course Research*, 54, 100501.

Lin, N. 2002. *Social Capital: A Theory of Social Structure and Action*, Cambridge University Press.

Lindström, M., Pirouzifard, M., Rosvall, M. & Fridh, M. 2024. Marital status and cause-specific mortality: a population-based prospective cohort study in southern Sweden. *Preventive Medicine Reports*, 37, 102542.

Livingston, G., Huntley, J., Sommerlad, A., Ames, D., Ballard, C., Banerjee, S., Brayne, C., Burns, A., Cohen-Mansfield, J. & Cooper, C. 2020. Dementia prevention, intervention, and care: 2020 report of the lancet commission. *The Lancet*, 396, 413–446.

Lu, N., Nie, P. & Siette, J. 2023. The roots of healthy aging: investigating the link between early-life and childhood experiences and later-life health. *BMC Geriatrics*, 23, 639.

Lubker Cornish, D. & Roberts Dobie, S. 2018. Social support in the "fourth trimester": a qualitative analysis of women at 1 month and 3 months postpartum. *The Journal of Perinatal Education*, 27, 233–242.

Lum, A., Wakefield, C., Donnan, B., Burns, M., Fardell, J. & Marshall, G. 2017. Understanding the school experiences of children and adolescents with serious chronic illness: a systematic meta-review. *Child: Care, Health and Development*, 43, 645–662.

Macdonald-Wallis, K., Jago, R. & Sterne, J. A. 2012. Social network analysis of childhood and youth physical activity: a systematic review. *American Journal of Preventive Medicine*, 43, 636–642.

Marden, J. R., Tchetgen Tchetgen, E. J., Kawachi, I. & Glymour, M. M. 2017. Contribution of socioeconomic status at 3 life-course periods to late-life memory function and decline: early and late predictors of dementia risk. *American Journal of Epidemiology*, 186, 805–814.

Marmot, M. G. 2010. *Fair Society, Healthy Lives: The Marmot Review: Strategic Review of Health Inequalities in England Post-2010*, Institute of Health Equity.

Marsden, P. V. 2018. Life Course Events and Network Composition. *In:* Alwin, D. F., Felmlee, D. H. & Kreager, D. A. (eds.) *Social Networks and the Life Course: Integrating the Development of Human Lives and Social Relational Networks*, 89–113.

Matley, D. 2020. "I miss my old life": regretting motherhood on Mumsnet. *Discourse, Context & Media*, 37, 100417.

Mayer, K. U. 2003. The Sociology of the Life Course and Lifespan Psychology: Diverging or Converging Pathways? In: Staudinger, U. M. & Lindenberger, U. (eds.) *Understanding Human Development: Dialogues with Lifespan Psychology*, Springer.

Mayer, K. U. 2009. New directions in life course research. *Annual Review of Sociology*, 35, 413–433.

Mccambridge, J., Mcalaney, J. & Rowe, R. 2011. Adult consequences of late adolescent alcohol consumption: a systematic review of cohort studies. *PLoS Medicine*, 8, e1000413.

Meade, C. S., Kershaw, T. S. & Ickovics, J. R. 2008. The intergenerational cycle of teenage motherhood: an ecological approach. *Health Psychology*, 27, 419–429.

Merton, R. K. 1988. The Matthew effect in science, II: cumulative advantage and the symbolism of intellectual property. *Isis*, 79, 606–623.

Meyler, D., Stimpson, J. P. & Peek, M. K. 2007. Health concordance within couples: a systematic review. *Social Science & Medicine*, 64, 2297–2310.

Min, J., Johnson, M. D., Anderson, J. R. & Yurkiw, J. 2022. Support exchanges between adult children and their parents across life transitions. *Journal of Marriage and Family*, 84, 367–392.

Mollenhorst, G., Volker, B. & Flap, H. 2014. Changes in personal relationships: how social contexts affect the emergence and discontinuation of relationships. *Social Networks*, 37, 65–80.

Montepare, J. M., Farah, K. S., Bloom, S. F. & Tauriac, J. 2020. Age-friendly universities (AFU): possibilities and power in campus connections. *Gerontology & Geriatrics Education*, 41, 273–280.

Naef, R., Ward, R., Mahrer-Imhof, R. & Grande, G. 2013. Characteristics of the bereavement experience of older persons after spousal loss: an integrative review. *International Journal of Nursing Studies*, 50, 1108–1121.

Neighbors, C., Krieger, H., Rodriguez, L. M., Rinker, D. V. & Lembo, J. M. 2019. Social identity and drinking: dissecting social networks and implications for novel interventions. *Journal of Prevention & Intervention in the Community*, 47, 259–273.

Nesari, M., Olson, J. K., Vandermeer, B., Slater, L. & Olson, D. M. 2018. Does a maternal history of abuse before pregnancy affect pregnancy outcomes? A systematic review with meta-analysis. *BMC Pregnancy and Childbirth*, 18, 404.

Northcott, S., Moss, B., Harrison, K. & Hilari, K. 2016. A systematic review of the impact of stroke on social support and social networks: associated factors and patterns of change. *Clinical Rehabilitation*, 30, 811–831.

O'rourke, H. M. & Sidani, S. 2017. Definition, determinants, and outcomes of social connectedness for older adults: a scoping review. *Journal of Gerontological Nursing*, 43, 43–52.

Oakley, A. 2018. *Social Support and Motherhood (Reissue): The Natural History of a Research Project*, Policy Press.

Olsen, M. H., Angell, S. Y., Asma, S., Boutouyrie, P., Burger, D., Chirinos, J. A., Damasceno, A., Delles, C., Gimenez-Roqueplo, A.-P. & Hering, D. 2016. A call to action and a lifecourse strategy to address the global burden of raised blood pressure on current and future generations: the lancet commission on hypertension. *The Lancet*, 388, 2665–2712.

Orchard, E. R., Rutherford, H. J., Holmes, A. J. & Jamadar, S. D. 2023. Matrescence: lifetime impact of motherhood on cognition and the brain. *Trends in Cognitive Sciences*, 27, 302–316.

Ortega-García, J. A., López-Hernández, F. A., Azurmendi Funes, M. L., Sánchez Sauco, M. F. & Ramis, R. 2020. My partner and my neighbourhood: The built environment and social networks' impact on alcohol consumption during early pregnancy. *Health & Place*, 61, 102239.

Parkes, A., Sweeting, H. & Wight, D. 2015. Parenting stress and parent support among mothers with high and low education. *Journal of Family Psychology*, 29, 907–918.

Pavalko, E. K. & Caputo, J. 2013. Social inequality and health across the life course. *American Behavioral Scientist*, 57, 1040–1056.

Pears, K., Capaldi, D. M. & Owen, L. D. 2007. Substance use risk across three generations: the roles of parent discipline practices and inhibitory control. *Psychology of Addictive Behaviors*, 21, 373.

Pellón-Elexpuru, I., Van Dijk, R., Van Der Valk, I., Martínez-Pampliega, A., Molleda, A. & Cormenzana, S. 2024. Divorce and physical health: a three-level meta-analysis. *Social Science & Medicine*, 352, 117005.

Peng, B., Hu, N., Yu, H., Xiao, H. & Luo, J. 2021. Parenting style and adolescent mental health: the chain mediating effects of self-esteem and psychological inflexibility. *Frontiers in Psychology*, 12, 738170.

Perry, B. L. & Pescosolido, B. A. 2012. Social network dynamics and biographical disruption: the case of "first-timers" with mental illness. *American Journal of Sociology*, 118, 134–175.

Peter, P. J., De Mola, C. L., De Matos, M. B., Coelho, F. M., Pinheiro, K. A., Da Silva, R. A., Castelli, R. D., Pinheiro, R. T. & Quevedo, L. A. 2016. Association between perceived social support and anxiety in pregnant adolescents. *Revista Brasileira de Psiquiatria*, 39, 21–27.

Power, C., Kuh, D. & Morton, S. 2013. From developmental origins of adult disease to life course research on adult disease and aging: insights from birth cohort studies. *Annual Review of Public Health*, 34, 7–28.

Praharso, N. F., Tear, M. J. & Cruwys, T. 2017. Stressful life transitions and wellbeing: a comparison of the stress buffering hypothesis and the social identity model of identity change. *Psychiatry Research*, 247, 265–275.

Prinds, C., Hvidt, N. C., Mogensen, O. & Buus, N. 2014. Making existential meaning in transition to motherhood—a scoping review. *Midwifery*, 30, 733–741.

Quashie, N. T., Arpino, B., Antczak, R. & Mair, C. A. 2019. Childlessness and health among older adults: variation across five outcomes and 20 countries. *The Journals of Gerontology: Series B*, 76, 348–359.

Raby, K. L., Roisman, G. I., Fraley, R. C. & Simpson, J. A. 2015. The enduring predictive significance of early maternal sensitivity: social and academic competence through age 32 years. *Child Development*, 86, 695–708.

Ramírez, L. & Palacios-Espinosa, X. 2016. Stereotypes about old age, social support, aging anxiety and evaluations of one's own health. *Journal of Social Issues*, 72, 47–68.

Raymond, A., Bazeer, N., Barclay, C., Krelle, H., Omar, I., Tallack, C. & Kelly, E. 2021. *Real Centre Our Aging Population: How Ageing Affects Health and Care Need in England*, The Health Foundation.

Reupert, A., Straussner, S. L., Weimand, B. & Maybery, D. 2022. It takes a village to raise a child: understanding and expanding the concept of the "village". *Frontiers in Public Health*, 10, 756066.

Rini, C., Schetter, C. D., Hobel, C. J., Glynn, L. M. & Sandman, C. A. 2006. Effective social support: antecedents and consequences of partner support during pregnancy. *Personal Relationships*, 13, 207–229.

Rockliffe, L., Peters, S., Heazell, A. E. P. & Smith, D. M. 2021. Factors influencing health behaviour change during pregnancy: a systematic review and meta-synthesis. *Health Psychology Review*, 15, 613–632.

Rogers, A., Brooks, H., Vassilev, I., Kennedy, A., Blickem, C. & Reeves, D. 2014. Why less may be more: a mixed methods study of the work and relatedness of 'weak ties' in supporting long-term condition self-management. *Implementation Science*, 9, 19.

Romer, D. 2010. Adolescent risk taking, impulsivity, and brain development: implications for prevention. *Developmental Psychobiology*, 52, 263–276.

Rossow, I., Keating, P., Felix, L. & Mccambridge, J. 2016. Does parental drinking influence children's drinking? A systematic review of prospective cohort studies. *Addiction*, 111, 204–217.

Roth, A. R. 2020a. Informal caregiving and network turnover among older adults. *The Journals of Gerontology. Series B, Psychological Sciences and Social Sciences*, 75, 1538–1547.

Roth, A. R. 2020b. Social networks and health in later life: a state of the literature. *Sociology of Health & Illness*, 42, 1642–1656.

Russ, S. A., Hotez, E., Berghaus, M., Hoover, C., Verbiest, S., Schor, E. L. & Halfon, N. 2022. Building a life course intervention research framework. *Pediatrics*, 149, e2021053509E.

Sahrakorpi, N., Koivusalo, S. B., Stach-Lempinen, B., Eriksson, J. G., Kautiainen, H. & Roine, R. P. 2017. "The burden of pregnancy"; heavier for the heaviest? The changes in health related quality of life (HRQ oL) assessed by the 15D instrument during pregnancy and postpartum in different body mass index groups: a longitudinal survey. *Acta Obstetricia et Gynecologica Scandinavica*, 96, 352–358.

Sanner, C., Ganong, L. & Coleman, M. 2021. Families are socially constructed: pragmatic implications for researchers. *Journal of Family Issues*, 42, 422–444.

Sawka, K. J., Mccormack, G. R., Nettel-Aguirre, A., Hawe, P. & Doyle-Baker, P. K. 2013. Friendship networks and physical activity and sedentary behavior among youth: a systematized review. *International Journal of Behavioral Nutrition and Physical Activity*, 10, 130.

Sawyer, S. M., Afifi, R. A., Bearinger, L. H., Blakemore, S.-J., Dick, B., Ezeh, A. C. & Patton, G. C. 2012. Adolescence: a foundation for future health. *The Lancet*, 379, 1630–1640.

Sawyer, S. M., Azzopardi, P. S., Wickremarathne, D. & Patton, G. C. 2018. The age of adolescence. *The Lancet Child & Adolescent Health*, 2, 223–228.

Saxbe, D., Rossin-Slater, M. & Goldenberg, D. 2018. The transition to parenthood as a critical window for adult health. *The American Psychologist*, 73, 1190–1200.

Sbarra, D. A. 2015. Divorce and health: current trends and future directions. *Psychosomatic Medicine*, 77, 227–236.

Settersten, R. A., Jr. 2015. Relationships in time and the life course: the significance of linked lives. *Research in Human Development*, 12, 217–223.

Settersten, R. A., Hollstein, B. & Mcelvaine, K. K. 2024. "Unlinked lives": elaboration of a concept and its significance for the life course. *Advances in Life Course Research*, 59, 100583.

Shafiq, S., Haith-Cooper, M., Hawkins, R. & Parveen, S. 2023. What are lay UK public perceptions of frailty: a scoping review. *Age and Ageing*, 52.

Shanahan, M. J., Mortimer, J. T. & Kirkpatrick Johnson, M. 2016. Introduction: Life Course Studies – Trends, Challenges, and Future Directions. *In:* Shanahan, M. J., Mortimer, J. T. & Kirkpatrick Johnson, M. (eds.) *Handbook of the Life Course: Volume II*, Cham: Springer International Publishing.

Shulman, S. & Connolly, J. 2013. The challenge of romantic relationships in emerging adulthood: reconceptualization of the field. *Emerging Adulthood*, 1, 27–39.

Sigurdardottir, V. L., Gamble, J., Gudmundsdottir, B., Kristjansdottir, H., Sveinsdottir, H. & Gottfredsdottir, H. 2017. The predictive role of support in the birth experience: a longitudinal cohort study. *Women and Birth*, 30, 450–459.

Sjödin, L., Raninen, J. & Larm, P. 2024. Early drinking onset and subsequent alcohol use in late adolescence: a longitudinal study of drinking patterns. *Journal of Adolescent Health*, 74, 1225–1230.

Small, M. L. 2013. Weak ties and the core discussion network: why people regularly discuss important matters with unimportant alters. *Social Networks*, 35, 470–483.

Smith, K. P. & Christakis, N. A. 2008. Social networks and health. *Annual Review of Sociology*, 34, 405–429.

Smithbattle, L. 2020. Walking on eggshells: an update on the stigmatizing of teen mothers. *MCN: American Journal of Maternal Child Nursing*, 45, 322–327.

Stapleton, L. R., Schetter, C. D., Westling, E., Rini, C., Glynn, L. M., Hobel, C. J. & Sandman, C. A. 2012. Perceived partner support in pregnancy predicts lower maternal and infant distress. *Journal of Family Psychology*, 26, 453–463.

Steinberg, L. 2008. A social neuroscience perspective on adolescent risk-taking. *Developmental Review*, 28, 78–106.

Steiner, R. J., Sheremenko, G., Lesesne, C., Dittus, P. J., Sieving, R. E. & Ethier, K. A. 2019. Adolescent connectedness and adult health outcomes. *Pediatrics*, 144.

Stephenson, J., Heslehurst, N., Hall, J., Schoenaker, D. A., Hutchinson, J., Cade, J. E., Poston, L., Barrett, G., Crozier, S. R. & Barker, M. 2018. Before the beginning: nutrition and lifestyle in the preconception period and its importance for future health. *The Lancet*, 391, 1830–1841.

Suanet, B. & Antonucci, T. C. 2017. Cohort differences in received social support in later life: the role of network type. *The Journals of Gerontology. Series B, Psychological Sciences and Social Sciences*, 72, 706–715.

Taylor, B. L., Nath, S., Sokolova, A. Y., Lewis, G., Howard, L. M., Johnson, S. & Sweeney, A. 2022. The relationship between social support in pregnancy and postnatal depression. *Social Psychiatry and Psychiatric Epidemiology*, 57, 1435–1444.

Teo, H. 2023. The impact of a partner's nursing home admission on individuals' mental well-being. *Social Science & Medicine*, 327, 115941.

The, N. S. & Gordon-Larsen, P. 2009. Entry into romantic partnership is associated with obesity. *Obesity (Silver Spring)*, 17, 1441–1447.

Thoits, P. A. 2011. Mechanisms linking social ties and support to physical and mental health. *Journal of Health and Social Behavior*, 52, 145–161.

UK Government. 2019. First 1000 days of life [Online]. UK Government. Available: https://publications.parliament.uk/pa/cm201719/cm select/cmhealth/1496/149603.htm#_idTextAnchor000 [Accessed].

Umberson, D., Crosnoe, R. & Reczek, C. 2010. Social relationships and health behavior across life course. *Annual Review of Sociology*, 36, 139–157.

Vacchiano, M., Hollstein, B., Settersten, R. A. & Spini, D. 2024. Networked lives: probing the influence of social networks on the life course. *Advances in Life Course Research*, 59, 100590.

Van Tilburg, T. 2003. Consequences of men's retirement for the continuation of work-related personal relationships. *Ageing International*, 28, 345–358.

Van Tilburg, T. G. & Suanet, B. 2018. Unmarried older people: are they socially better off today? *The Journals of Gerontology: Series B*, 74, 1463–1473.

Vassilev, I., Rogers, A., Kennedy, A. & Koetsenruijter, J. 2014. The influence of social networks on self-management support: a metasynthesis. *BMC Public Health*, 14, 719.

Villalonga-Olives, E., Almansa, J., Shaya, F. & Kawachi, I. 2020. Perceived social capital and binge drinking in older adults: the health and retirement study, US data from 2006–2014. *Drug and Alcohol Dependence*, 214, 108099.

Völker, B. 2022. 'Birds of a feather' - forever? Homogeneity in adult friendship networks through the life course. *Advances in Life Course Research*, 53, 100498.

Wagner, C., Carmeli, C., Chiolero, A. & Cullati, S. 2022. Life course socioeconomic conditions and multimorbidity in old age – a scoping review. *Ageing Research Reviews*, 78, 101630.

Wagner, C., Carmeli, C., Jackisch, J., Kivimäki, M., Van Der Linden, B. W. A., Cullati, S. & Chiolero, A. 2024. Life course epidemiology and public health. *The Lancet Public Health*, 9, e261–e269.

Wang, P., Liou, S.-R. & Cheng, C.-Y. 2013. Prediction of maternal quality of life on preterm birth and low birthweight: a longitudinal study. *BMC Pregnancy and Childbirth*, 13, 124.

Webster, N. J., Antonucci, T. C. & Ajrouch, K. J. 2022. Linked lives and convoys of social relations. *Advances in Life Course Research*, 54, 100502.

Weiss, J., Lawton, L. E. & Fischer, C. S. 2022. Life course transitions and changes in network ties among younger and older adults. *Advances in Life Course Research*, 52, 100478.

Whitley, E., Batty, G. D., Hunt, K., Popham, F. & Benzeval, M. 2014. The role of health behaviours across the life course in the socioeconomic patterning of all-cause mortality: the west of Scotland twenty-07 prospective cohort study. *Annals of Behavioral Medicine*, 47, 148–157.

WHO 2018. *The Life-Course Approach: From Theory to Practice. Case Stories From Two Small Countries in Europe*, World Health Organization.

Wicks, S., Berger, Z. & Camic, P. M. 2019. It's how I am … it's what I am … it's a part of who I am: a narrative exploration of the impact of adolescent-onset chronic illness on identity formation in young people. *Clinical Child Psychology and Psychiatry*, 24, 40–52.

Wilcox, W. B. 2009. The evolution of divorce. *National Affairs*, 1, 81–94.

Woods-Townsend, K., Hardy-Johnson, P., Bagust, L., Barker, M., Davey, H., Griffiths, J., Grace, M., Lawrence, W., Lovelock, D., Hanson, M.,

Godfrey, K. M. & Inskip, H. 2021. A cluster-randomised controlled trial of the LifeLab education intervention to improve health literacy in adolescents. *PLoS One*, 16, e0250545.

Wrzus, C., Hänel, M., Wagner, J. & Neyer, F. J. 2013. Social network changes and life events across the life span: a meta-analysis. *Psychological Bulletin*, 139, 53.

Xia, M., Fosco, G. M., Lippold, M. A. & Feinberg, M. E. 2018. A developmental perspective on young adult romantic relationships: examining family and individual factors in adolescence. *Journal of Youth and Adolescence*, 47, 1499–1516.

Zaccagni, S., Sigsgaard, A. M., Vrangbaek, K. & Noermark, L. P. 2024. Who continues to work after retirement age? *BMC Public Health*, 24, 692.

Zacher, H. & Froidevaux, A. 2021. Life stage, lifespan, and life course perspectives on vocational behavior and development: a theoretical framework, review, and research agenda. *Journal of Vocational Behavior*, 126, 103476.

Zahodne, L. B., Ajrouch, K. J., Sharifian, N. & Antonucci, T. C. 2019. Social relations and age-related change in memory. *Psychology and Aging*, 34, 751–765.

Zajacova, A. & Lawrence, E. M. 2018. The relationship between education and health: reducing disparities through a contextual approach. *Annual Review of Public Health*, 39, 273–289.

Zaso, M. J., Read, J. P. & Colder, C. R. 2023. Coping-motivated escalations in adolescent alcohol problems following early adversity. *Psychology of Addictive Behaviors*, 37, 331–340.

Żyrek, J., Klimek, M., Apanasewicz, A., Ciochoń, A., Danel, D. P., Marcinkowska, U. M., Mijas, M., Ziomkiewicz, A. & Galbarczyk, A. 2024. Social support during pregnancy and the risk of postpartum depression in Polish women: a prospective study. *Scientific Reports*, 14, 6906.

CHAPTER 16

Social Isolation and Loneliness in Contemporary Society

Chris Allen

School of Health Sciences, University of Southampton, Southampton, UK

Introduction

As we explored in the previous chapter, there is an increased awareness and understanding of the value of quality social connections to our health and well-being. When these are absent or less than a person desires, this can lead to people experiencing loneliness. With increasing recognition of the impact of loneliness on both health and general well-being, loneliness as a concept and an experience is increasingly being recognised as a contemporary public health issue.

You are likely very aware that aspects of contemporary society, especially in western developed countries, contribute to social isolation and loneliness throughout the life course, and we will have the opportunity in this chapter to critically look at how society may contribute to rising social isolation and the experience of loneliness. In fact, loneliness provides an interesting case study for how societies impact on our health and well-being, as well as the dynamic interplay between our biology (including our evolutionary biology), our psychology and our society, and this chapter draws from many of the earlier chapters in this book, particularly in highlighting the impact of the social determinants of health, social exclusion and global demographic and epidemiological transitions.

Concern around loneliness has led to a now large and continuously expanding evidence base that allows us to know more about who is most affected, why these people are most affected and what the likely impact of loneliness is in terms of their health and well-being. Our knowledge of how lonely people can be best supported is also growing, and this evidence is drawn on to provide an overview of some potentially effective ways of supporting those experiencing loneliness.

LEARNING OUTCOMES

By the end of this chapter, you will be able to:

- Recognise social isolation and loneliness, how they overlap, as well as how they are distinct concepts and experiences.
- Recognise the complex social factors that result in social isolation and loneliness within societies.
- Understand the range of physical, mental and social health impacts of social isolation.
- Consider some of the interventions that are being used to address the public health issue of loneliness.

Social Isolation and Loneliness

> **Key Terms and Definitions**
>
> **Social isolation:** An objective measure of a lack of social contact.
>
> **Loneliness:** A negative experience and emotion caused by a mismatch in the levels of desired social contact and the actual social contact someone has.

As a species, alongside our primate relatives, we have evolved to need and feel safest when connected with others (Cacioppo et al., 2015, Eisenberger, 2012). Humans connecting with one

Social Sciences for Healthcare Professionals, First Edition. Edited by Chris Allen.
© 2026 John Wiley & Sons Ltd. Published 2026 by John Wiley & Sons Ltd.

another has proved the catalyst for societies functioning the way that they do, and even the most primitive hunter-gatherer communities, once seen as having relatively limited social contact beyond their immediate nomadic group, are now recognised as being highly social (Hill et al., 2014). We are hard-wired to connect with and rely on one another. When social contact is lacking, this can lead to us becoming unwell, and social isolation and loneliness are increasingly being recognised as public health issues that have a negative impact on people and communities (Cacioppo and Cacioppo, 2018, Holt-Lunstad, 2018, Leigh-Hunt et al., 2017). In fact, the impact of loneliness on health is potentially so severe that research has identified that it has a similar impact on mortality to cigarette smoking and a greater impact than obesity and inactivity (Holt-Lunstad et al., 2010, Holt-Lunstad et al., 2015). Increasing concern around loneliness as both a social and health issue has led to the creation of a minister for loneliness in countries such as the United Kingdom and Japan (Pimlott, 2018, UK Government, 2021b), as well as governments publishing specific strategies highlighting intentions to address loneliness (UK Government, 2018), and the emergence of charities and advocacy groups with a specific or secondary focus of addressing the issue of loneliness and inclusion (e.g. the National Academy for Social Prescribing [NASP], Campaign to End Loneliness, etc.), and many of the charities advocating for the needs of at-risk groups releasing position statements, such as AGE UK (Age UK, 2019). In addition, action has also involved the creation of 'tackling loneliness networks' (UK Government, 2021a), alongside the rolling out of national programmes, such as social prescribing (covered in the next chapter), with the specific intention of addressing social isolation (NHS, 2019). Whilst people have always had the potential to be socially isolated, and through this, experience loneliness – COVID-19, and the associated macro-level factors such as social distancing that was mandated in countries around the world, alongside the economic challenges and increased unemployment that the pandemic caused, further highlighted the challenges posed by these issues (Banerjee and Rai, 2020, Hwang et al., 2020, Li and Wang, 2020, Kirkland et al., 2023). With such potentially severe impacts on health, alongside the significant pain, suffering and accumulated disadvantages that those who are lonely face, it is perhaps unsurprising that loneliness may increase healthcare utilisation (Beutel et al., 2017, Christiansen et al., 2023, Gerst-Emerson and Jayawardhana, 2015, Smith and Victor, 2022) and may carry a significant economic cost to society (Casal et al., 2024, Michaelson et al., 2017, Mihalopoulos et al., 2020).

Loneliness lacks a clear definition (Park et al., 2020) and academics have argued that rather than seeing loneliness as a binary lonely/not lonely concept, experiences of loneliness are likely far more nuanced, and may differ depending on levels of isolation, whether people live alone and whether they have health or other issues that might make life more challenging (Smith and Victor, 2019, Yanguas et al., 2018). Different subtypes of loneliness have also been proposed, such as 'emotional

loneliness[1]' and 'social loneliness[2]' (Dahlberg and McKee, 2014, Weiss, 1975). However, generally, social isolation and loneliness are distinct, and whilst related (and believed to carry similar risks to health and well-being), they are largely seen as different, as both concepts and as personal experiences.

Social isolation is an *objective* measure of a lack of interaction with other people. It is *objective* because it can be measured. We can count the number of social contacts a person has, and how long and how frequently they are in contact with them. Variables that relate to social isolation, such as living alone, and spending an increased amount of time spent alone have increased in many societies, especially those that are more individualistic,[3] as opposed to collectivist[4] (Anttila et al., 2020, Bühler and Nikitin, 2020, Drewelies et al., 2019).

Loneliness on the other hand is a pervasive and distressing negative emotion or experience; seminal definitions point towards a mismatch between someone's desired and actual social relationships (Hawkley and Cacioppo, 2010, Perlman and Peplau, 1981, Peplau and Perlman, 1982). Loneliness and social isolation are therefore related, but conceptually distinct. Loneliness tends to arise from a lack of meaningful social contact with other people as well as where someone is lacking a level of social contact that they want. This is an important point, as people can in fact have lots of social contacts, but still experience feelings of loneliness.

Whilst there are objective ways that loneliness can be measured (such as validated scales, some of which are discussed later), **loneliness** is essentially a *subjective* experience and an emotional response to someone's social situation. To varying degrees, loneliness is something we can likely all recognise, as from time to time, we all experience it. For many, loneliness is a largely transient experience; it comes and goes, usually in response to how connected we feel at a given point in time. Whilst experiences can be similar, exactly how it is experienced, and the perceived causes and consequences can differ from person to person, but many of those experiencing significant loneliness report that it is painful (Eisenberger, 2012). Observations linking social pain with physical pain date back to some seminal thinkers in psychology, including Sigmund Freud (1856–1939) (Freud, 2003). In the same way as physical pain[5] can protect us from danger (e.g. by making us remove our hand from a heat source), and being hungry or thirsty prompts us to eat and drink, social pain may in fact be evolutionarily useful, in prompting us to seek out new connections or to re-establish existing ones that may be fading (Hawkley and Capitanio, 2015). In primitive times,

---

[1] Essentially the absence of close intimate relationships – relationships are lacking (Dahlberg and McKee, 2014, Weiss, 1975).

[2] Essentially lacking a stable social network- relationships are absent (Dahlberg and McKee, 2014, Weiss, 1975).

[3] Where there is an expectation that people will largely support themselves and will not be reliant on others.

[4] Where there is an expectation that people will support others.

[5] Research has suggested that when we feel social pain, the same neural processes are activated as when we feel physical pain (Eisenberger, 2012).

social exclusion was very risky, and therefore, such a response may increase the chances of survival, by motivating people to take action when socially isolated (Eisenberger, 2012).

In this chapter, we will mostly consider the impact of loneliness that is chronic or severe, where it is persistent enough to result in recurrent negative thoughts, sensations and behaviours that may negatively impact on people's ability to maintain existing relationships or create new ones (Hawkley and Cacioppo, 2010) as well as negatively impacting on physical and mental health (Holt-Lunstad et al., 2015, Ong et al., 2016). Whether we experience chronic loneliness such as this, is determined by many factors, for example, research has suggested genetic contributions to loneliness, and that loneliness is trait like, with some of us being predisposed to needing more contact (Mund et al., 2020, Spithoven et al., 2019), and the connectedness, values and norms of a society, may also play a role. These aspects will be considered next.

Who Is Affected, Where and Why?

The social context of loneliness is complex and not fully understood (Luhmann et al., 2023). For a variety of reasons, as we will later explore, it is challenging to gain precise rates of loneliness in a population. From a global perspective, there are gaps in what we know. For example, whilst loneliness exists at a problematic level across the globe; a lack of robust data makes it hard to understand the extent of the issue in low-and middle-income countries, in particular (Surkalim et al., 2022). Where data exists, it demonstrates that rates are different in different countries (Luhmann et al., 2023, Surkalim et al., 2022). Some of this variance is likely because of the different ways of collecting data on loneliness, but societies contribute to population and individual experiences of loneliness in different ways.

Global Loneliness Trends

In western industrialised nations, loneliness may affect as much as one-third of the population (Cacioppo and Cacioppo, 2018). In the context of Europe, recent survey findings highlight that at least one-third of respondents were lonely at least sometimes, with 13% experiencing loneliness most of the time (European Commission, 2023). However, even within regions, there is often significant variation in loneliness prevalence between and within countries (Surkalim et al., 2022).

Differences are likely down to not just how data has been collected, but also society itself, which can influence people's experiences of loneliness, in the living and working conditions that it sets, as well as the expectations that are placed on relationships and what others can and should be doing for you. For example, levels of social integration may be important (de Jong Gierveld and Tesch-Römer, 2012), as to are the societal norms around marriage and divorce, which have shifted over time, changing the value that may be placed on partners and in particular married support (Luhmann et al., 2023, Ortiz-Ospina and Roser, 2024, van Tilburg et al., 2015). This is complex and will likely relate to the quality of individual relationships – for example, spousal support might not always be helpful and may in fact reduce someone's contacts outside of that relationship. A country's loneliness prevalence is likely also influenced by other factors, for example, income differences between citizens of different countries, whether a society is more orientated towards collectivism or individualism, as well as the demographics, with countries with a higher proportion of older people, particularly those who have never married or who live alone, potentially experiencing higher rates (Barreto et al., 2021, Fokkema et al., 2012, Hansen and Slagsvold, 2016, Luhmann et al., 2023).

How relationships are generally seen in a society can also impact on loneliness, because it may influence people's expectations for relationships and for how much closeness people *should* experience. This is a reason why academics have attempted to unpick differences in loneliness based on how individualistic or collectivist different societies are. However, drawing clear distinctions between individualism/collectivism is challenging, as this essentially simplifies a country's norms into two disparate binary types (i.e. collectivist/individualist) (Wong et al., 2018). Certainly, different cultures ascribe different values and meanings to social relationships, but the extent to which these orientations influence loneliness is unclear, and loneliness may be influenced by both individualism and collectivism via different pathways (Heu et al., 2019, Lykes and Kemmelmeier, 2014, Schermer et al., 2023). For example, especially in western and developed countries, as well as elsewhere, there has been a transition towards individualism and reduced expectations placed on family ties (Wong et al., 2018), which may invariably shift what is expected from others in terms of 'normal' and expected levels of contact and closeness. In individualistic societies, ties may be less strong, and people may invest less time and resources in building and maintaining these (Luhmann et al., 2023). People may place less of an expectancy on others, and therefore, where support is lacking, this might not feel particularly abnormal. However, with ties being seen as more important in collectivist societies, their absence may be felt especially strongly, as too might living alone (which is less common in collectivist societies). Both may be less socially accepted and potentially result in stigmatising processes (explored in chapter 9) when people do not have this support (Barreto et al., 2022, Heu et al., 2019, Kerr and Stanley, 2021). Such expectations, alongside fear of being negatively evaluated by others, may result in loneliness being underreported in societies that are characterised by collectivism (Luhmann et al., 2023). In addition, simply being within a group, does not necessarily mean people can extract support from relationships, and relationships can be a source of threat, strain and frustration. Where such negative connections are experienced, collectivist societies generally have more restrictive norms about who people should be close to (i.e. the traditional family unit), which may influence loneliness, as it is then harder/potentially less socially acceptable for individuals to withdraw themselves or disinvest in difficult relationships to meet their social needs elsewhere (Heu et al., 2019). This may be more possible in individualist societies, and in many societies, the concept of 'family' is increasingly becoming more inclusive, meaning it can incorporate, for example, close friends, who people are not biologically related to. This has the potential to give people, particularly in individualist, less restrictive societies, greater freedom to connect with others, when the social needs are not being met by traditional family set ups (Sanner et al., 2021).

The availability and dispersion of employment, and the norms around how far people are willing and able to travel for work, as well as migration and forced displacement, can also influence loneliness. For example, societies with higher levels of mobility may experience loneliness at greater rates (especially where integration is challenging), than societies where it is more common to reside within a less transient community, where people stay put and have mostly been there all their lives (Delaruelle, 2023). Ease of integration is complex, but research has suggested that first generations experience more loneliness than do second-generation migrants (who have the benefit of increased access to others who are similar) and that migrants experience more loneliness where communities are unwelcoming (Delaruelle, 2023).

Personal Characteristics of Loneliness

Variation in the prevalence of loneliness within countries is also common, and this is likely related to differences in individuals and their living situations. Loneliness is best considered as being multi-causal. At an individual level, people's personal characteristics and personality traits (especially the 'big five[6]') may impact on loneliness. With the exception of 'openness to experience', these traits affect risk, albeit through likely different pathways, for example, extraversion, agreeableness and conscientiousness, likely reduce risks of loneliness, whilst neuroticism, likely increases a person's risk (Buecker et al., 2020b).

Other work has looked at individual capacities to deal with social isolation when it occurs. Cacioppo and Patrick (2008), in their book on loneliness, highlight three interrelated factors that contribute to our ability to deal with isolation when it occurs. These are:

- How vulnerable we are to social disconnection?
- How well we can self-regulate our emotions, particularly those associated with feeling alone?
- What our expectations of social interaction are and how do we make sense of our interactions?

As well as this, there are of course many contextual factors that influence people's ability to form and maintain meaningful social relationships. The social connections that people have available to them, particularly having access to and living with a spouse, living with other people and having a large personal network and frequent high-quality contact with members, reduce one's risk of loneliness (Böger and Huxhold, 2020, Cohen-Mansfield et al., 2016, Dahlberg et al., 2022, Hawkley et al., 2008).

Loneliness and Age

Whilst many factors can contribute to increased risks of loneliness, and therefore it can impact on anyone, there are certain groups in which loneliness is potentially more commonly experienced. These include younger and older people, with a suggested 'double peak' being seen in early adulthood (i.e. before 30) and early later life (i.e. around about 60) (Lasgaard et al., 2016, Luhmann and Hawkley, 2016, Victor and Yang, 2012). Research tends to suggest lower levels in mid-life (albeit with lots of contextual caveats – employment, status, health, disability, etc.) (Luhmann and Hawkley, 2016); though some contrasting evidence has suggested that middle-aged people experience more loneliness than older ages (Barreto et al., 2021).

An enduring stereotype (see chapter 9) of loneliness is that it is something primarily experienced by isolated and frail older people. Whilst studies have highlighted that older adults may be at higher risk of loneliness, this likely relates to their increased risk of being socially isolated and living alone, being widowed and having reduced physical and cognitive capabilities, limiting the opportunities for some older people to maintain contacts beyond the home, and actively seek and gain new connections. However, recent research in the context of the European Union has highlighted that the prevalence of loneliness may actually decrease as people age (European Commission, 2023); so again, the picture isn't entirely clear. Because loneliness is conceptualised as differences between social contact and desired social contact, possible explanations include older people anticipating a reduction in social network size in later life (through for example, the death of people in their social networks), and therefore not experiencing as significant a mismatch between desired and actual social contact (Cornwell and Waite, 2009).

In the context of younger people, loneliness may present a particular risk to those undergoing various life course transitions (a key feature in this stage of the life course some of which were discussed in the previous chapter), such as moving away for education (or moving to a different school, college or university than their friends) and moving into or away for employment.

Loneliness and Inequality

Loneliness is more common in those already facing disadvantage in other ways, and some of these relationships are likely to be bi-directional. For example, those from lower socio-economic groups, those who are unemployed, those who are physically or mentally unwell, or who have a disability, and those experiencing social exclusion, are more likely to experience

---

[6] Traits are commonly studied in social psychology. What is commonly referred to as the 'big 5 personality traits' include extraversion, neuroticism, openness to experience, conscientiousness, and agreeableness (Buecker et al., 2020a,b).

loneliness (Anderssen et al., 2020, Buczak-Stec et al., 2023, Cotterell et al., 2024, Dahlberg et al., 2022, Delaruelle, 2023, Emerson et al., 2021, Hughes et al., 2023, Lasgaard et al., 2016, Macdonald et al., 2018, Matthews et al., 2019, Morrish and Medina-Lara, 2021). The influence of unemployment, for example, is likely bi-directional. Unemployment has been found to significantly increase the likelihood of someone experiencing loneliness, but being lonely, is likely to also increase the likelihood of someone becoming unemployed (Morrish and Medina-Lara, 2021). All these factors have the potential to decrease the levels of material and social resources that are available to someone, alongside differences relating to the area itself, such as a neighbourhood's specific characteristics, that may promote or act as a barrier to social connectedness.

Loneliness and the Lived Environment

The built environment or 'human-made-space(s)', are the areas where we live, work, socialise and play in daily, as well as the surrounding environments (natural and built) (Roof and Oleru, 2008). The built environment's impact on health and sustainability has become an important feature of discussions around health and well-being promotion (discussed in chapter 14) and includes, for example, ensuring accessibility, provision of greenspace, and safe and green transport options (such as cycle lanes) (Boniface et al., 2015, Giles-Corti et al., 2022). Alongside this, is an increased recognition that features of the built environment can act as a barrier and a facilitator of social connection (Boniface et al., 2015, McGrath and Reavey, 2018).

In one recent review, aspects of the built environment with relevance to loneliness included an area's infrastructure such as transport including safe cycling, walking routes, etc., internet infrastructure, common and public spaces that are well distributed and accessible, healthcare access, high-quality and roomy housing (to allow for entertaining), general services, and local social and community centres, as well as an area's attractiveness and general upkeep, perceived safety and access to natural green spaces (Bower et al., 2023). The provision of safety nets to prevent people from becoming displaced (such as affordable rent) was also highlighted as important (Bower et al., 2023). With so many features potentially influencing isolation and loneliness, it is hard to isolate which aspects are most significant, and all of these aspects of the built environment are both created by and influence broader social and economic factors, alongside individual experiences, needs, practices and values (Bower et al., 2023). In summary though, it is certainly prudent to design the urban environments in ways that promote social inclusion.

Digital Communication Technology and Loneliness

Digital communication may both exacerbate and alleviate loneliness (Lim et al., 2020). It is hard to determine if loneliness causes increased social media use or if increased social media use causes loneliness, as causal pathways are unclear. Studies have highlighted that increased social media use is associated with loneliness (Bonsaksen et al., 2023), whilst others have highlighted that experiencing loneliness can lead to increased use of social media, which may displace offline interactions (Nowland et al., 2018). The rapid and increasing importance of digital communication platforms such as social media, instant messaging services and smartphone communication applications creates new ways of reaching out, but also new ways of distancing ourselves from one another (especially where some might prefer to connect at a distance). Existing research has highlighted the potentially negative impact excessive screen time has on mental health (Twenge and Campbell, 2018), but there is also plenty of evidence of people using it to combat loneliness and extend their sociability beyond those who are physically proximate, especially in instances where it is not actually possible or appropriate to meet people in person (Boyd, 2014).

How Is Loneliness Measured?

Whilst loneliness is a subjective feeling, there are several ways in which this can be objectively measured, using a range of validated scales. This is the gold standard for capturing loneliness in surveys (Osborn et al., 2018). Commonly used scales include the De Jong Gierveld (DJG) 11-item scale (de Jong-Gierveld and van Tilbury, 1999) and the University of California Los Angeles (UCLA) 20-item scale (Russell et al., 1980), with shorter versions of these scales also existing; which is particularly useful if they are included in very large surveys,[7] seeking to capture large amounts of data, often beyond just loneliness. Both are self-reported scales.

What Are the Health Impacts of Loneliness?

Whilst loneliness as a public health issue was highlighted earlier in this chapter, in this section, the specific health impacts on chronic loneliness will be unpacked in more depth. Here, we are considering chronic loneliness – loneliness that is pervasive, rather than simply transient (that comes and goes). Loneliness such as this is now known to negatively impact on physical, mental and social health (Holt-Lunstad et al., 2010, Leigh-Hunt et al., 2017, Ong et al., 2016, Park et al., 2020, Petitte et al., 2015, Wang et al., 2023). However, whilst loneliness is associated with particularly poor health outcomes, it is relevant to

---

[7] Because the number of questions included in these surveys, puts a premium on any further questions- surveys with fewer questions, are less burdensome, and therefore more likely to be completed.

highlight that many of the risk factors for loneliness are in themselves risk factors for a range of physical and mental health conditions, such as social isolation, low socio-economic status, disability and pre-existing health conditions (Emerson et al., 2021, Smith et al., 2021), making it hard to unpick how much is attributable to loneliness itself, vs the other factors we know relate to poor health. To help guide understanding as to the varied impacts of loneliness on health, the next section is broken down into physical, mental and social health in discrete sections below, mirroring the WHO's definition of health (introduced to you in chapter 3).

Physical Health

Research conducted during the COVID-19 pandemic (which provided an opportunity for natural experimental methods to be used[8]), highlighted that significant negative physiological and behavioural consequences can stem from even a temporary lack of social contact (Aknin et al., 2022, Buecker et al., 2020a, Groarke et al., 2020, Hwang et al., 2020, Luchetti et al., 2020). This work builds on earlier seminal work that has highlighted significant associations between various degrees of social isolation including living alone, subjective loneliness, and network size (i.e. the number of social contacts a person has) with all-cause mortality (Elovainio et al., 2017, Holt-Lunstad et al., 2010, Holt-Lunstad et al., 2015, Nyqvist et al., 2014).

Research to date has highlighted that much of impact of loneliness on physical health stems from its impact on biological mechanisms, such as increased inflammatory and stress biomarkers, which has an adverse impact on the cardiovascular system (including increased blood pressure as part of a stress response), as well as immune and endocrine system functioning (also related to a stress response), and deleterious health behaviours (largely through a lack of self-care and coping strategies) (Ford et al., 2006, Glaser and Kiecolt-Glaser, 2005, Hawkley and Capitanio, 2015, Kiecolt-Glaser et al., 2010, Loucks et al., 2006, Park et al., 2020, Shankar et al., 2011, Yang et al., 2013), and its impact on sleep, which is believed to be of poorer quality and therefore less restorative (Cacioppo et al., 2002, Griffin et al., 2020, Smith et al., 2012), alongside changes to an individual's brain – specifically the levels of grey and white matter, as well as changes to the pre-frontal cortex (the social bit of the brain) (Cacioppo et al., 2014, Lam et al., 2021, Spreng et al., 2020), making us more susceptible to disease, accelerating aging and increasing our risk of early mortality and morbidity (Holt-Lunstad and Smith, 2016, Lara et al., 2019a, Lara et al., 2019b, Rico-Uribe et al., 2018, Salinas et al., 2022, Valtorta et al., 2016, Zhou et al., 2018).

---

[8] Mandated restrictions on social contact were common in most high-income countries. Ordinarily, it would be highly unethical to restrict whole populations in this way, simply to see the impact of isolation on health and well-being.

Unhealthy Behaviours

We tend to follow more unhealthy behaviours when we are socially isolated as well as potentially when we are lonely (Hawkley and Cacioppo, 2010, Kobayashi and Steptoe, 2018, Lauder et al., 2006, Shankar et al., 2011, Stickley et al., 2013), and as we have shown in previous chapters, these can lead to increased mortality and morbidity. The negative psychological impact of loneliness may result in people being more likely to drink too much alcohol, smoke, overeat and follow a poor diet, as well as exercise less (Dyal and Valente, 2015, Shankar et al., 2011, Stickley et al., 2013). These behaviours may be engaged with as a coping strategy to mask the social pain brought about by loneliness, alongside the reduced self-regulation that loneliness can bring; and once people are following these potentially harmful behaviours, reduced social contact limits opportunities to be exposed to healthier norms – essentially reducing access to the regulation of behaviours from others, alongside reducing access to those who might support behaviour change (Berkman et al., 2000, Gallant, 2013, Rosenquist et al., 2010, Tucker, 2002).

It is worth highlighting that studies demonstrating associations between loneliness (as distinct from social isolation) tend to use cross-sectional methods (i.e. a snapshot in time), but when longitudinal methods have been used, social isolation has been shown to be a stronger predictor of poor health behaviours than loneliness, though loneliness does relate to smoking (Kobayashi and Steptoe, 2018). There is also the possibility that health behaviours, such as smoking and problematic drinking may themselves result in people becoming more isolated and pushed to the periphery of their social networks (Christakis and Fowler, 2008, Kobayashi and Steptoe, 2018).

Mental Health

Whilst a recent review demonstrated that loneliness has the potential to impact on a range of health outcomes, the most significant impacts were on mental health, alongside general well-being (Park et al., 2020). Research consistently links loneliness and isolation to increased risk of a range of mental health presentations including depression (Beutel et al., 2017, Cacioppo et al., 2006, Cacioppo et al., 2010, Courtin and Knapp, 2017, Cruwys et al., 2013, Erzen and Çikrikci, 2018, Ge et al., 2017, Lee et al., 2021, Park et al., 2020) and anxiety (Beutel et al., 2017, Maes et al., 2019, Park et al., 2020), alongside severe mental ill health (Badcock et al., 2020, Ludwig et al., 2020) and suicide/suicidal ideation (Beutel et al., 2017, McClelland et al., 2020).

In the context of mental health, research including systematic reviews has highlighted that in those with depression, schizophrenia, bipolar disorder and anxiety disorders, loneliness predicts poorer mental health outcomes (Wang et al., 2018). But loneliness and mental health can and generally is recognised as being reciprocal and bi-directional (Cacioppo et al., 2006, Cacioppo et al., 2010). By this, we mean that poor mental health can exacerbate loneliness, and loneliness can exacerbate poor mental health.

Reduced Social Contact

Because loneliness can influence how people think and feel about themselves and can result in reduced executive function from the brain's frontal lobe, it can, rather paradoxically, result in people becoming further isolated (Cacioppo and Patrick, 2008, Ong et al., 2016, Tao et al., 2022). There are several reasons why those feeling lonely might find it harder to connect with others. First, whilst loneliness does not lower our social skills, it can influence how we see social interactions, as well as our confidence, motivation and our ability to use these skills to make meaningful contact with others (Cacioppo and Patrick, 2008). This can impact on people's confidence and the motivation they need to make meaningful social contact with others (Cacioppo and Patrick, 2008). Second, when we are lonely, our altered perceptions of threat can lead to us becoming more acutely aware and hypervigilant of social signals (Hawkley and Cacioppo, 2010). This hypervigilance can lead to the release of hormones and chemicals that can influence our emotions, and through these, our behaviours (Cacioppo et al., 2016). When we are hypervigilant, we can misinterpret and react more negatively to the cues from our social interactions, leading us to see threats that are not there (Cacioppo and Patrick, 2008). Finally, feeling socially excluded

can result in poorer self-regulation and poorer self-care (Baumeister et al., 2005). As we explored in earlier chapters, how we look is important to how others evaluate us. Those experiencing loneliness, especially where they are avoiding social interaction with others, may have less energy to complete even basic daily tasks and may take less pride in how they look (Cacioppo and Patrick, 2008). Negative feelings about oneself, reduced self-esteem and self-efficacy, and concern about the perceptions of others can result in pessimistic expectations of social contact, and this, in turn, can lead to cognitive shortcuts that make it more likely that social cues are misinterpreted as negative evaluative judgments (Cacioppo et al., 2016). Feeling excluded can also make us more difficult to be around, and this can place a strain on those relationships that are maintained, whilst also decreasing the likeliness of new connections from being formed (Cacioppo et al., 2016). Overtime, this complex and slightly paradoxical behaviour, in which individuals feel negatively about themselves, are concerned about social contact and potential negative evaluations of others, and when contact is actually made, misinterpret benign social cues, can result in a 'downwards spiral of loneliness' that negatively impacts on existing relationships, whilst also making new and needed connections less likely (Cacioppo and Patrick, 2008).

Case Study – Middle-Aged and Divorced

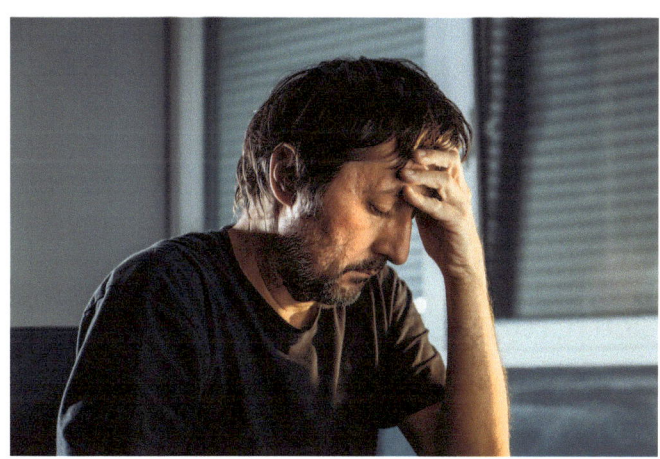

Source: Bits and Splits/Adobe Stock Photos.

Richard is a 48-year-old man who lives alone in a small apartment, having recently divorced his wife Elaine, after what seemed like years of growing apart.

This is not really where Richard wanted to be with his life and relationships, approaching his 50th year, emotionally shattered and having to rebuild his life and career, whilst living alone in a dinky apartment in a new city miles away from anyone he knows. Richard's adult children are now all grown up,

are fully independent and have dispersed all over the country, with one of his sons now living in Australia, on the other side of the planet.

Richard was well connected before his divorce, receiving social and emotional support from a diverse and wide range of ties, including family, friends, acquittances, etc., many of whom he shared valued activities with, such as sports (five-a-side football mostly).

Whilst he is still in contact with those he knows back home through WhatsApp and Facebook, it is not the same as seeing them in person, and he is less able to materially benefit from these relationships to (such as being lent household equipment). Locally, he has very few people he can call in a favour from – further worsening his feelings of isolation and vulnerability.

His new work colleagues have invited him out a few times. He has spent the odd evening with them, but they are generally much younger and seem immature. Some of their 'banter' he has not appreciated – particularly around his divorce, and this has put him on edge when he is with them. He had started online dating, as he knows his ex-wife also has, but has not actually been on any dates and is highly fearful of rejection – so eventually he ended up cancelling his account.

Richard is not sleeping well and often feels fatigued, he is drinking more and is eating irregularly, with his mealtimes no longer structured through work and his evening family meal. Most of what he eats is processed, high in fat and prepared in the microwave. He does little exercise, lacking the motivation to do so, and without having access to his previous five-a-side team, he has begun to put on weight.

After reviewing Richard's case study, you might want to consider the following:

- What aspects of Richard's circumstances might have contributed to his experiences of loneliness?
- What aspects of society may have contributed to Richard's experiences of loneliness?
- To what extent are Richard's perceptions about relationships at this stage in the life course, impacting his experience of loneliness?
- How can Richard's social inclusion in his new community be supported?

What Interventions Have Been Considered?

The stigma attached to loneliness can make it challenging for people to talk about their experiences with it, potentially limiting their access to relevant and much-needed support and social contact (Barreto et al., 2022, Kerr and Stanley, 2021). Currently, there is a gap in healthcare provision in relation to screening to identify and address loneliness as part of routine clinical care, though screening tools are beginning to emerge that may in time help identify those needing support so that appropriate interventions can be offered (Park et al., 2020).

The literature on interventions to address loneliness is growing, alongside the number of possible approaches, that generally look either at addressing social skills and maladaptive responses to loneliness (such as the downwards spiral discussed earlier) or at increasing someone's opportunities to connect and form meaningful connections with others (Masi et al., 2011), and there are now several reviews, including those concentrating on interventions at specific target populations (i.e. older people, younger people, etc.) (Bessaha et al., 2020, Eccles and Qualter, 2021, Hickin et al., 2021, Hoang et al., 2022, Masi et al., 2011, Patil and Braun, 2024). No approach is likely to meet the needs of all those who are lonely, and it is generally recognised that approaches to tackling loneliness in individuals, should be tailored to an individual's needs, the person's unique experience of loneliness and their challenges (routes to social exclusion, proximity and lack of contact with others, mobility issues, social anxiety, etc.) (Park et al., 2020).

Approaches to loneliness often centre around breaking the unhelpful patterns of behaviour that can be triggered in those experiencing loneliness, such as Making Every Contact Count (MECC) one of the healthy conversation skills we introduced you to in chapter 13 (which may help people talk about loneliness), and CBT, including that delivered online (that might help challenge negative thoughts) and other interventions such as counselling, and even reminiscence therapy, that may target coping strategies and potentially modify individual emotions and behaviours (Hickin et al., 2021, Hoang et al., 2022, Käll et al., 2020, Mann et al., 2017). However, addressing negative thoughts and behaviours may only be effective, if people have opportunities to connect with people in meaningful ways

(Mann et al., 2017) and there are an increasing number of interventions that seek to address this, including network interventions (Band et al., 2019, Ellis et al., 2020, Ellis et al., 2022), as well as increasing social prescribing and creative health approaches (covered in detail in the following chapter).

As we have highlighted, where those who are disadvantaged in other ways are more likely to experience loneliness, action at the level of public policy and broader population-level interventions that seek to address risk factors of loneliness, such as taking action on poverty, unemployment and social exclusion, likely also have a key part to play in terms of prevention (Mann et al., 2017).

Clinical Considerations

- Loneliness is multi-causal and can be present even with those who have lots of social contact.
- Loneliness is a public health issue and has the potential to cause significant physical and mental ill health. The risks posed by chronic loneliness are similar to the risks of other known health harms, such as tobacco smoking and obesity.
- There are various interventions that are being used to address the issue of loneliness, including CBT, as well as interventions that seek to increase the number and quality of people's social connections, such as social prescribing.

Conclusion

This chapter has provided an overview of social isolation and loneliness, highlighting them as distinct, but related and overlapping concepts that can have a significant impact on health and well-being. Increasingly, loneliness is being seen as a public health issue, due to the increased understanding of its deleterious impact on mortality and morbidity. We have highlighted the individual and social causes of loneliness and provided a summary as to how loneliness can be measured, using commonly used scales that allow for a subjective experience to be objectively captured. The health and social impacts of loneliness have also been summarised, before an overview of some of the interventions that have been considered to help alleviate loneliness in individuals and the community.

References

Age UK. 2019. Policy position paper: loneliness (England) [Online]. AGE UK. Available: https://www.ageuk.org.uk/globalassets/age-uk/documents/policy-positions/health-and-wellbeing/ppp_loneliness_and_isolation_uk.pdf [Accessed].

Aknin, L. B., De Neve, J. E., Dunn, E. W., Fancourt, D. E., Goldberg, E., Helliwell, J. F., Jones, S. P., Karam, E., Layard, R., Lyubomirsky, S., Rzepa, A., Saxena, S., Thornton, E. M., Vanderweele, T. J., Whillans, A. V., Zaki, J., Karadag, O. & Ben Amor, Y. 2022. Mental health during the first year of the COVID-19 Pandemic: a review and recommendations for Moving Forward. *Perspectives on Psychological Science*, 17, 915–936.

Anderssen, N., Sivertsen, B., Lønning, K. J. & Malterud, K. 2020. Life satisfaction and mental health among transgender students in Norway. *BMC Public Health*, 20, 138.

Anttila, T., Selander, K. & Oinas, T. 2020. Disconnected lives: trends in time spent alone in Finland. *Social Indicators Research*, 150, 711–730.

Badcock, J. C., Adery, L. H. & Park, S. 2020. Loneliness in psychosis: a practical review and critique for clinicians. *Clinical Psychology: Science and Practice*, 27, e12345.

Band, R., Ewings, S., Cheetham-Blake, T., Ellis, J., Breheny, K., Vassilev, I., Portillo, M. C., Yardley, L., Blickem, C., Kandiyali, R., Culliford, D. & Rogers, A. 2019. Study protocol for 'the project about loneliness and social networks (PALS)': a pragmatic, randomised trial comparing a facilitated social network intervention (genie) with a wait-list control for lonely and socially isolated people. *BMJ Open*, 9, e028718.

Banerjee, D. & Rai, M. 2020. Social isolation in Covid-19: the impact of loneliness. *International Journal of Social Psychiatry*, 66, 525–527.

Barreto, M., Victor, C., Hammond, C., Eccles, A., Richins, M. T. & Qualter, P. 2021. Loneliness around the world: age, gender, and cultural differences in loneliness. *Personality and Individual Differences*, 169, 110066.

Barreto, M., Van Breen, J., Victor, C., Hammond, C., Eccles, A., Richins, M. T. & Qualter, P. 2022. Exploring the nature and variation of the stigma associated with loneliness. *Journal of Social and Personal Relationships*, 39, 2658–2679.

Baumeister, R. F., Dewall, C. N., Ciarocco, N. J. & Twenge, J. M. 2005. Social exclusion impairs self-regulation. *Journal of Personality and Social Psychology*, 88, 589–604.

Berkman, L. F., Glass, T., Brissette, I. & Seeman, T. E. 2000. From social integration to health: Durkheim in the new millennium. *Social Science & Medicine*, 51, 843–857.

Bessaha, M. L., Sabbath, E. L., Morris, Z., Malik, S., Scheinfeld, L. & Saragossi, J. 2020. A systematic review of loneliness interventions among non-elderly adults. *Clinical Social Work Journal*, 48, 110–125.

Beutel, M. E., Klein, E. M., Brähler, E., Reiner, I., Jünger, C., Michal, M., Wiltink, J., Wild, P. S., Münzel, T., Lackner, K. J. & Tibubos, A. N. 2017. Loneliness in the general population: prevalence, determinants and relations to mental health. *BMC Psychiatry*, 17, 97.

Böger, A. & Huxhold, O. 2020. The changing relationship between partnership status and loneliness: effects related to aging and historical time. *The Journals of Gerontology. Series B, Psychological Sciences and Social Sciences*, 75, 1423–1432.

Boniface, S., Scantlebury, R., Watkins, S. & Mindell, J. 2015. Health implications of transport: evidence of effects of transport on social interactions. *Journal of Transport & Health*, 2, 441–446.

Bonsaksen, T., Ruffolo, M., Price, D., Leung, J., Thygesen, H., Lamph, G., Kabelenga, I. & Geirdal, A. 2023. Associations between social media use and loneliness in a cross-national population: do motives for social media use matter? *Health Psychology and Behavioral Medicine*, 11, 2158089.

Bower, M., Kent, J., Patulny, R., Green, O., Mcgrath, L., Teesson, L., Jamalishahni, T., Sandison, H. & Rugel, E. 2023. The impact of the built environment on loneliness: a systematic review and narrative synthesis. *Health & Place*, 79, 102962.

Boyd, D. 2014. *It's Complicated: The Social Lives of Networked Teens*, Yale University Press.

Buczak-Stec, E., König, H. H. & Hajek, A. 2023. Sexual orientation and psychosocial factors in terms of loneliness and subjective well-being in later life. *Gerontologist*, 63, 338–349.

Buecker, S., Horstmann, K. T., Krasko, J., Kritzler, S., Terwiel, S., Kaiser, T. & Luhmann, M. 2020a. Changes in daily loneliness for German residents during the first four weeks of the COVID-19 pandemic. *Social Science & Medicine*, 265, 113541.

Buecker, S., Maes, M., Denissen, J. J. A. & Luhmann, M. 2020b. Loneliness and the big five personality traits: a meta-analysis. *European Journal of Personality*, 34, 8–28.

Bühler, J. L. & Nikitin, J. 2020. Sociohistorical context and adult social development: new directions for 21st century research. *The American Psychologist*, 75, 457–469.

Cacioppo, J. T. & Cacioppo, S. 2018. The growing problem of loneliness. *Lancet*, 391, 426.

Cacioppo, J. & Patrick, W. 2008. *Loneliness: Human Nature and the Need for Social Connection*, New York: W.W. Norton and Company.

Cacioppo, J. T., Hawkley, L. C., Berntson, G. G., Ernst, J. M., Gibbs, A. C., Stickgold, R. & Hobson, J. A. 2002. Do lonely days invade the nights? Potential social modulation of sleep efficiency. *Psychological Science*, 13, 384–387.

Cacioppo, J. T., Hughes, M. E., Waite, L. J., Hawkley, L. C. & Thisted, R. A. 2006. Loneliness as a specific risk factor for depressive symptoms: cross-sectional and longitudinal analyses. *Psychology and Aging*, 21, 140–151.

Cacioppo, J. T., Hawkley, L. C. & Thisted, R. A. 2010. Perceived social isolation makes me sad: 5-year cross-lagged analyses of loneliness and depressive symptomatology in the Chicago health, aging, and social relations study. *Psychology and Aging*, 25, 453–463.

Cacioppo, S., Capitanio, J. P. & Cacioppo, J. T. 2014. Toward a neurology of loneliness. *Psychological Bulletin*, 140, 1464–1504.

Cacioppo, J. T., Cacioppo, S., Cole, S. W., Capitanio, J. P., Goossens, L. & Boomsma, D. I. 2015. Loneliness across phylogeny and a call for comparative studies and animal models. *Perspectives on Psychological Science*, 10, 202–212.

Cacioppo, S., Bangee, M., Balogh, S., Cardenas-Iniguez, C., Qualter, P. & Cacioppo, J. T. 2016. Loneliness and implicit attention to social threat: a high-performance electrical neuroimaging study. *Cognitive Neuroscience*, 7, 138–159.

Casal, B., Rodríguez-Miguez, E. & Rivera, B. 2024. The societal cost of 'unwanted' loneliness in Spain. *The European Journal of Health Economics*.

Christakis, N. A. & Fowler, J. H. 2008. The collective dynamics of smoking in a large social network. *The New England Journal of Medicine*, 358, 2249–2258.

Christiansen, J., Pedersen, S. S., Andersen, C. M., Qualter, P., Lund, R. & Lasgaard, M. 2023. Loneliness, social isolation, and healthcare utilization in the general population. *Health Psychology*, 42, 63–72.

Cohen-Mansfield, J., Hazan, H., Lerman, Y. & Shalom, V. 2016. Correlates and predictors of loneliness in older-adults: a review of quantitative results informed by qualitative insights. *International Psychogeriatrics*, 28, 557–576.

Cornwell, E. Y. & Waite, L. J. 2009. Social disconnectedness, perceived isolation, and health among older adults. *Journal of Health and Social Behavior*, 50, 31–48.

Cotterell, N., Buffel, T., Nazroo, J. & Qualter, P. 2024. Loneliness among older ethnic minority people: exploring the role of structural disadvantage and place using a co-research methodology. *Ethnic and Racial Studies*, 1–23.

Courtin, E. & Knapp, M. 2017. Social isolation, loneliness and health in old age: a scoping review. *Health & Social Care in the Community*, 25, 799–812.

Cruwys, T., Dingle, G. A., Haslam, C., Haslam, S. A., Jetten, J. & Morton, T. A. 2013. Social group memberships protect against future depression, alleviate depression symptoms and prevent depression relapse. *Social Science & Medicine*, 98, 179–186.

Dahlberg, L. & Mckee, K. J. 2014. Correlates of social and emotional loneliness in older people: evidence from an English community study. *Aging & Mental Health*, 18, 504–514.

Dahlberg, L., Mckee, K. J., Frank, A. & Naseer, M. 2022. A systematic review of longitudinal risk factors for loneliness in older adults. *Aging & Mental Health*, 26, 225–249.

De Jong Gierveld, J. & Tesch-Römer, C. 2012. Loneliness in old age in Eastern and Western European societies: theoretical perspectives. *European Journal of Ageing*, 9, 285–295.

De Jong-Gierveld, J. & Van Tilbury, T. 1999. *Manual of the loneliness scale* [Online]. Methoden en technieken. [Accessed].

Delaruelle, K. 2023. Migration-related inequalities in loneliness across age groups: a cross-national comparative study in Europe. *European Journal of Ageing*, 20, 35.

Drewelies, J., Huxhold, O. & Gerstorf, D. 2019. The role of historical change for adult development and aging: towards a theoretical framework about the how and the why. *Psychology and Aging*, 34, 1021–1039.

Dyal, S. R. & Valente, T. W. 2015. A systematic review of loneliness and smoking: small effects, big implications. *Substance Use & Misuse*, 50, 1697–1716.

Eccles, A. M. & Qualter, P. 2021. Review: alleviating loneliness in young people - a meta-analysis of interventions. *Child and Adolescent Mental Health*, 26, 17–33.

Eisenberger, N. I. 2012. The pain of social disconnection: examining the shared neural underpinnings of physical and social pain. *Nature Reviews Neuroscience*, 13, 421–434.

Ellis, J., Band, R., Kinsella, K., Cheetham-Blake, T., James, E., Ewings, S. & Rogers, A. 2020. Optimising and profiling pre-implementation contexts to create and implement a public health network intervention for tackling loneliness. *Implementation Science*, 15, 35.

Ellis, J., Kinsella, K., James, E., Cheetham-Blake, T., Lambrou, M., Ciccognani, A., Rogers, A. & Band, R. 2022. Examining the optimal factors that promote implementation and sustainability of a network intervention to alleviate loneliness in community contexts. *Health & Social Care in the Community*, 30, e4144–e4154.

Elovainio, M., Hakulinen, C., Pulkki-Råback, L., Virtanen, M., Josefsson, K., Jokela, M., Vahtera, J. & Kivimäki, M. 2017. Contribution of risk factors to excess mortality in isolated and lonely individuals: an analysis of data from the UK Biobank cohort study. *The Lancet Public Health*, 2, e260–e266.

Emerson, E., Fortune, N., Llewellyn, G. & Stancliffe, R. 2021. Loneliness, social support, social isolation and wellbeing among working age adults with and without disability: cross-sectional study. *Disability and Health Journal*, 14, 100965.

Erzen, E. & Çikrikci, Ö. 2018. The effect of loneliness on depression: a meta-analysis. *The International Journal of Social Psychiatry*, 64, 427–435.

European Commission 2023. Loneliness and social connectedness: insights from a new EU-wide survey. Available online at: https://publications.jrc.ec.europa.eu/repository/handle/JRC133351.

Fokkema, T., De Jong Gierveld, J. & Dykstra, P. A. 2012. Cross-national differences in older adult loneliness. *The Journal of Psychology*, 146, 201–228.

Ford, E. S., Loucks, E. B. & Berkman, L. F. 2006. Social integration and concentrations of C-reactive protein among US adults. *Annals of Epidemiology*, 16, 78–84.

Freud, S. 2003. *Beyond the Pleasure Principle*, Penguin Modern Classics.

Gallant, M. P. 2013. Social Networks, Social Support, and Health-Related Behavior. *In:* Martin, L. R. & Dimatteo, M. R. (eds.) *The Oxford Handbook of Health Communication, Behavior Change, and Treatment Adherence*, Oxford University Press.

Ge, L., Yap, C. W., Ong, R. & Heng, B. H. 2017. Social isolation, loneliness and their relationships with depressive symptoms: a population-based study. *PLoS One*, 12, e0182145.

Gerst-Emerson, K. & Jayawardhana, J. 2015. Loneliness as a public health issue: the impact of loneliness on health care utilization among older adults. *American Journal of Public Health*, 105, 1013–1019.

Giles-Corti, B., Moudon, A. V., Lowe, M., Adlakha, D., Cerin, E., Boeing, G., Higgs, C., Arundel, J., Liu, S. & Hinckson, E. 2022. Creating healthy and sustainable cities: what gets measured, gets done. *The Lancet Global Health*, 10, e782–e785.

Glaser, R. & Kiecolt-Glaser, J. K. 2005. Stress-induced immune dysfunction: implications for health. *Nature Reviews Immunology*, 5, 243–251.

Griffin, S. C., Williams, A. B., Ravyts, S. G., Mladen, S. N. & Rybarczyk, B. D. 2020. Loneliness and sleep: a systematic review and meta-analysis. *Health Psychology Open*, 7, 2055102920913235.

Groarke, J. M., Berry, E., Graham-Wisener, L., Mckenna-Plumley, P. E., Mcglinchey, E. & Armour, C. 2020. Loneliness in the UK during the COVID-19 pandemic: cross-sectional results from the COVID-19 psychological wellbeing study. *PLoS One*, 15, e0239698.

Hansen, T. & Slagsvold, B. 2016. Late-life loneliness in 11 European countries: results from the generations and gender survey. *Social Indicators Research*, 129, 445–464.

Hawkley, L. C. & Cacioppo, J. T. 2010. Loneliness matters: a theoretical and empirical review of consequences and mechanisms. *Annals of Behavioral Medicine*, 40, 218–227.

Hawkley, L. C. & Capitanio, J. P. 2015. Perceived social isolation, evolutionary fitness and health outcomes: a lifespan approach. *Philosophical Transactions of the Royal Society of London. Series B, Biological Sciences*, 370.

Hawkley, L. C., Hughes, M. E., Waite, L. J., Masi, C. M., Thisted, R. A. & Cacioppo, J. T. 2008. From social structural factors to perceptions of relationship quality and loneliness: the Chicago health, aging, and social relations study. *The Journals of Gerontology. Series B, Psychological Sciences and Social Sciences*, 63, S375–S384.

Heu, L. C., Van Zomeren, M. & Hansen, N. 2019. Lonely alone or lonely together? A cultural-psychological examination of individualism–collectivism and loneliness in five European countries. *Personality and Social Psychology Bulletin*, 45, 780–793.

Hickin, N., Käll, A., Shafran, R., Sutcliffe, S., Manzotti, G. & Langan, D. 2021. The effectiveness of psychological interventions for loneliness: a systematic review and meta-analysis. *Clinical Psychology Review*, 88, 102066.

Hill, K. R., Wood, B. M., Baggio, J., Hurtado, A. M. & Boyd, R. T. 2014. Hunter-gatherer inter-band interaction rates: implications for cumulative culture. *PLoS One*, 9, e102806.

Hoang, P., King, J. A., Moore, S., Moore, K., Reich, K., Sidhu, H., Tan, C. V., Whaley, C. & Mcmillan, J. 2022. Interventions associated with reduced loneliness and social isolation in older adults: a systematic review and meta-analysis. *JAMA Network Open*, 5, e2236676.

Holt-Lunstad, J. 2018. The potential public health relevance of social isolation and loneliness: prevalence, epidemiology, and risk factors. *Public Policy & Aging Report*, 27, 127–130.

Holt-Lunstad, J. & Smith, T. B. 2016. Loneliness and social isolation as risk factors for CVD: implications for evidence-based patient care and scientific inquiry. *Heart*, 102, 987–989.

Holt-Lunstad, J., Smith, T. B. & Layton, J. B. 2010. Social relationships and mortality risk: a meta-analytic review. *PLoS Medicine*, 7, e1000316.

Holt-Lunstad, J., Smith, T. B., Baker, M., Harris, T. & Stephenson, D. 2015. Loneliness and social isolation as risk factors for mortality: a meta-analytic review. *Perspectives on Psychological Science*, 10, 227–237.

Hughes, M., Lyons, A., Alba, B., Waling, A., Minichiello, V., Fredriksen-Goldsen, K., Barrett, C., Savage, T., Blanchard, M. & Edmonds, S. 2023. Predictors of loneliness among older lesbian and gay people. *Journal of Homosexuality*, 70, 917–937.

Hwang, T. J., Rabheru, K., Peisah, C., Reichman, W. & Ikeda, M. 2020. Loneliness and social isolation during the COVID-19 pandemic. *International Psychogeriatrics*, 32, 1217–1220.

Käll, A., Jägholm, S., Hesser, H., Andersson, F., Mathaldi, A., Norkvist, B. T., Shafran, R. & Andersson, G. 2020. Internet-based cognitive behavior therapy for loneliness: a pilot randomized controlled trial. *Behavior Therapy*, 51, 54–68.

Kerr, N. A. & Stanley, T. B. 2021. Revisiting the social stigma of loneliness. *Personality and Individual Differences*, 171, 110482.

Kiecolt-Glaser, J. K., Gouin, J. P. & Hantsoo, L. 2010. Close relationships, inflammation, and health. *Neuroscience and Biobehavioral Reviews*, 35, 33–38.

Kirkland, S. A., Griffith, L. E., Oz, U. E., Thompson, M., Wister, A., Kadowaki, L., Basta, N. E., Mcmillan, J., Wolfson, C., Raina, P., Anderson, L., Balion, C., Costa, A., Asada, Y., Cossette, B., Levasseur, M., Hofer, S., Paterson, T., Hogan, D., liu-Ambrose, T., Menec, V., St. John, P., Mugford, G., Gao, Z., Taler, V., Davidson, P., Cosco, T. & On Behalf of the Canadian Longitudinal Study on Aging, T 2023. Increased prevalence of loneliness and associated risk factors during the COVID-19 pandemic: findings from the Canadian longitudinal study on aging (CLSA). *BMC Public Health*, 23, 872.

Kobayashi, L. C. & Steptoe, A. 2018. Social isolation, loneliness, and health behaviors at older ages: longitudinal cohort study. *Annals of Behavioral Medicine*, 52, 582–593.

Lam, J. A., Murray, E. R., Yu, K. E., Ramsey, M., Nguyen, T. T., Mishra, J., Martis, B., Thomas, M. L. & Lee, E. E. 2021. Neurobiology of loneliness: a systematic review. *Neuropsychopharmacology*, 46, 1873–1887.

Lara, E., Caballero, F. F., Rico-Uribe, L. A., Olaya, B., Haro, J. M., Ayuso-Mateos, J. L. & Miret, M. 2019a. Are loneliness and social isolation associated with cognitive decline? *International Journal of Geriatric Psychiatry*, 34, 1613–1622.

Lara, E., Martín-María, N., De La Torre-Luque, A., Koyanagi, A., Vancampfort, D., Izquierdo, A. & Miret, M. 2019b. Does loneliness contribute to mild cognitive impairment and dementia? A systematic review and meta-analysis of longitudinal studies. *Ageing Research Reviews*, 52, 7–16.

Lasgaard, M., Friis, K. & Shevlin, M. 2016. "Where are all the lonely people?" A population-based study of high-risk groups across the life span. *Social Psychiatry and Psychiatric Epidemiology*, 51, 1373–1384.

Lauder, W., Mummery, K., Jones, M. & Caperchione, C. 2006. A comparison of health behaviours in lonely and non-lonely populations. *Psychology, Health & Medicine*, 11, 233–245.

Lee, S. L., Pearce, E., Ajnakina, O., Johnson, S., Lewis, G., Mann, F., Pitman, A., Solmi, F., Sommerlad, A., Steptoe, A., Tymoszuk, U. & Lewis, G. 2021. The association between loneliness and depressive symptoms among adults aged 50 years and older: a 12-year population-based cohort study. *The Lancet Psychiatry*, 8, 48–57.

Leigh-Hunt, N., Bagguley, D., Bash, K., Turner, V., Turnbull, S., Valtorta, N. & Caan, W. 2017. An overview of systematic reviews on the public health consequences of social isolation and loneliness. *Public Health*, 152, 157–171.

Li, L. Z. & Wang, S. 2020. Prevalence and predictors of general psychiatric disorders and loneliness during COVID-19 in the United Kingdom. *Psychiatry Research*, 291, 113267.

Lim, M. H., Eres, R. & Vasan, S. 2020. Understanding loneliness in the twenty-first century: an update on correlates, risk factors, and potential solutions. *Social Psychiatry and Psychiatric Epidemiology*, 55, 793–810.

Loucks, E. B., Sullivan, L. M., D'agostino, R. B., Sr., Larson, M. G., Berkman, L. F. & Benjamin, E. J. 2006. Social networks and inflammatory markers in the Framingham heart study. *Journal of Biosocial Science*, 38, 835–842.

Luchetti, M., Lee, J. H., Aschwanden, D., Sesker, A., Strickhouser, J. E., Terracciano, A. & Sutin, A. R. 2020. The trajectory of loneliness in response to COVID-19. *The American Psychologist*, 75, 897–908.

Ludwig, K. A., Nye, L. N., Simmons, G. L., Jarskog, L. F., Pinkham, A. E., Harvey, P. D. & Penn, D. L. 2020. Correlates of loneliness among persons with psychotic disorders. *Social Psychiatry and Psychiatric Epidemiology*, 55, 549–559.

Luhmann, M. & Hawkley, L. C. 2016. Age differences in loneliness from late adolescence to oldest old age. *Developmental Psychology*, 52, 943–959.

Luhmann, M., Buecker, S. & Rüsberg, M. 2023. Loneliness across time and space. *Nature Reviews Psychology*, 2, 9–23.

Lykes, V. A. & Kemmelmeier, M. 2014. What predicts loneliness? Cultural difference between individualistic and collectivistic societies in Europe. *Journal of Cross-Cultural Psychology*, 45, 468–490.

Macdonald, S. J., Deacon, L., Nixon, J., Akintola, A., Gillingham, A., Kent, J., Ellis, G., Mathews, D., Ismail, A., Sullivan, S., Dore, S. & Highmore, L. 2018. 'The invisible enemy': disability, loneliness and isolation. *Disability & Society*, 33, 1138–1159.

Maes, M., Nelemans, S. A., Danneel, S., Fernández-Castilla, B., Van Den Noortgate, W., Goossens, L. & Vanhalst, J. 2019. Loneliness and social anxiety across childhood and adolescence: multilevel meta-analyses of cross-sectional and longitudinal associations. *Developmental Psychology*, 55, 1548–1565.

Mann, F., Bone, J. K., Lloyd-Evans, B., Frerichs, J., Pinfold, V., Ma, R., Wang, J. & Johnson, S. 2017. A life less lonely: the state of the art in interventions to reduce loneliness in people with mental health problems. *Social Psychiatry and Psychiatric Epidemiology*, 52, 627–638.

Masi, C. M., Chen, H.-Y., Hawkley, L. C. & Cacioppo, J. T. 2011. A meta-analysis of interventions to reduce loneliness. *Personality and Social Psychology Review*, 15, 219–266.

Matthews, T., Danese, A., Caspi, A., Fisher, H. L., Goldman-Mellor, S., Kepa, A., Moffitt, T. E., Odgers, C. L. & Arseneault, L. 2019. Lonely young adults in modern Britain: findings from an epidemiological cohort study. *Psychological Medicine*, 49, 268–277.

Mcclelland, H., Evans, J. J., Nowland, R., Ferguson, E. & O'connor, R. C. 2020. Loneliness as a predictor of suicidal ideation and behaviour: a systematic review and meta-analysis of prospective studies. *Journal of Affective Disorders*, 274, 880–896.

Mcgrath, L. & Reavey, P. 2018. *The Handbook of Mental Health and Space: Community and Clinical Applications*, Routledge.

Michaelson, J., Jeffrey, K. & Abdallah, S. 2017. The cost of loneliness to UK employers [Online]. New Economics Foundation Available: https://neweconomics.org/2017/02/cost-loneliness-uk-employers [Accessed].

Mihalopoulos, C., Le, L. K.-D., Chatterton, M. L., Bucholc, J., Holt-Lunstad, J., Lim, M. H. & Engel, L. 2020. The economic costs of loneliness: a review of cost-of-illness and economic evaluation studies. *Social Psychiatry and Psychiatric Epidemiology*, 55, 823–836.

Morrish, N. & Medina-Lara, A. 2021. Does unemployment lead to greater levels of loneliness? A systematic review. *Social Science & Medicine*, 287, 114339.

Mund, M., Freuding, M. M., Möbius, K., Horn, N. & Neyer, F. J. 2020. The stability and change of loneliness across the life span: a meta-analysis of longitudinal studies. *Personality and Social Psychology Review*, 24, 24–52.

NHS. 2019. The NHS long term plan [Online]. NHS. Available: https://www.longtermplan.nhs.uk/publication/nhs-long-term-plan/ [Accessed].

Nowland, R., Necka, E. A. & Cacioppo, J. T. 2018. Loneliness and social internet use: pathways to reconnection in a digital world? *Perspectives on Psychological Science*, 13, 70–87.

Nyqvist, F., Pape, B., Pellfolk, T., Forsman, A. K. & Wahlbeck, K. 2014. Structural and cognitive aspects of social capital and all-cause mortality: a meta-analysis of cohort studies. *Social Indicators Research*, 116, 545–566.

Ong, A. D., Uchino, B. N. & Wethington, E. 2016. Loneliness and health in older adults: a mini-review and synthesis. *Gerontology*, 62, 443–449.

Ortiz-Ospina, E. & Roser, M. 2024. Marriages and divorces [Online]. Our world in data Available: https://ourworldindata.org/marriages-and-divorces [Accessed].

Osborn, C. Y., Hassell, C., Martin, G. & Cochrane, A. 2018. Testing of loneliness questions in surveys [Online]. Office of National Statistics Available: https://www.ons.gov.uk/peoplepopulationandcommunity/wellbeing/compendium/nationalmeasurementofloneliness/2018/testingoflonelinessquestionsinsurveys [Accessed].

Park, C., Majeed, A., Gill, H., Tamura, J., Ho, R. C., Mansur, R. B., Nasri, F., Lee, Y., Rosenblat, J. D., Wong, E. & Mcintyre, R. S. 2020. The effect of loneliness on distinct health outcomes: a comprehensive review and meta-analysis. *Psychiatry Research*, 294, 113514.

Patil, U. & Braun, K. L. 2024. Interventions for loneliness in older adults: a systematic review of reviews. *Frontiers in Public Health*, 12, 1427605.

Peplau, L. & Perlman, D. 1982. Perspectives on loneliness. *In:* Peplau, L. & Perlman, D. (eds.) *Loneliness: A Sourcebook of Current Theory, Research and Therapy*, New York: Wiley.

Perlman, D. & Peplau, L. 1981. Toward a Social Psychology of Loneliness Personal Relationships 3. *In:* Gilmour, R. & Duck, S. (eds.) *Personal Relationships in Disorder*, Volume 3, London: Academic Press, 31–56.

Petitte, T., Mallow, J., Barnes, E., Petrone, A., Barr, T. & Theeke, L. 2015. A systematic review of loneliness and common chronic physical conditions in adults. *The Open Psychology Journal*, 8, 113–132.

Pimlott, N. 2018. The ministry of loneliness. *Canadian Family Physician*, 64, 166.

Rico-Uribe, L. A., Caballero, F. F., Martín-María, N., Cabello, M., Ayuso-Mateos, J. L. & Miret, M. 2018. Association of loneliness with all-cause mortality: a meta-analysis. *PLoS One*, 13, e0190033.

Roof, K. & Oleru, N. 2008. Public health: Seattle and King County's push for the built environment. *Journal of Environmental Health*, 71, 24–27.

Rosenquist, J. N., Murabito, J., Fowler, J. H. & Christakis, N. A. 2010. The spread of alcohol consumption behavior in a large social network. *Annals of Internal Medicine*, 152, 426–433, w141.

Russell, D., Peplau, L. A. & Cutrona, C. E. 1980. The revised UCLA loneliness scale: concurrent and discriminant validity evidence. *Journal of Personality and Social Psychology*, 39, 472.

Salinas, J., Beiser, A. S., Samra, J. K. & O'donnell, A., Decarli, C. S., Gonzales, M. M., Aparicio, H. J. & Seshadri, S. 2022. Association of loneliness with 10-year dementia risk and early markers of vulnerability for neurocognitive decline. *Neurology*, 98, e1337–e1348.

Sanner, C., Ganong, L. & Coleman, M. 2021. Families are socially constructed: pragmatic implications for researchers. *Journal of Family Issues*, 42, 422–444.

Schermer, J. A., Branković, M., Čekrlija, Đ., Macdonald, K. B., Park, J., Papazova, E., Volkodav, T., Iliško, D., Wlodarczyk, A., Kwiatkowska, M. M., Rogoza, R., Oviedo-Trespalacios, O., Ha, T. T. K., Kowalski, C. M., Malik, S., Lins, S., Navarro-Carrillo, G., Aquino, S. D., Doroszuk, M., Riđić, O., Pylat, N., Özsoy, E., Tan, C.-S., Mamuti, A., Ardi, R., Jukić, T., Uslu, O., Buelvas, L. M., Liik, K. & Kruger, G. 2023. Loneliness and vertical and horizontal collectivism and individualism: a multinational study. *Current Research in Behavioral Sciences*, 4, 100105.

Shankar, A., Mcmunn, A., Banks, J. & Steptoe, A. 2011. Loneliness, social isolation, and behavioral and biological health indicators in older adults. *Health Psychology*, 30, 377–385.

Smith, K. J. & Victor, C. 2019. Typologies of loneliness, living alone and social isolation, and their associations with physical and mental health. *Ageing and Society*, 39, 1709–1730.

Smith, K. J. & Victor, C. 2022. The association of loneliness with health and social care utilization in older adults in the general population: a systematic review. *The Gerontologist*, 62, e578–e596.

Smith, S. S., Kozak, N. & Sullivan, K. A. 2012. An investigation of the relationship between subjective sleep quality, loneliness and mood in an Australian sample: can daily routine explain the links? *The International Journal of Social Psychiatry*, 58, 166–171.

Smith, R. W., Barnes, I., Green, J., Reeves, G. K., Beral, V. & Floud, S. 2021. Social isolation and risk of heart disease and stroke: analysis of two large UK prospective studies. *The Lancet Public Health*, 6, e232–e239.

Spithoven, A. W., Cacioppo, S., Goossens, L. & Cacioppo, J. T. 2019. Genetic contributions to loneliness and their relevance to the evolutionary theory of loneliness. *Perspectives on Psychological Science*, 14, 376–396.

Spreng, R. N., Dimas, E., Mwilambwe-Tshilobo, L., Dagher, A., Koellinger, P., Nave, G., Ong, A., Kernbach, J. M., Wiecki, T. V., Ge, T., Li, Y., Holmes, A. J., Yeo, B. T. T., Turner, G. R., Dunbar, R. I. M. & Bzdok, D. 2020. The default network of the human brain is associated with perceived social isolation. *Nature Communications*, 11, 6393.

Stickley, A., Koyanagi, A., Roberts, B., Richardson, E., Abbott, P., Tumanov, S. & Mckee, M. 2013. Loneliness: its correlates and association with health behaviours and outcomes in nine countries of the former Soviet Union. *PLoS One*, 8, e67978.

Surkalim, D. L., Luo, M., Eres, R., Gebel, K., Buskirk, J. V., Bauman, A. & Ding, D. 2022. The prevalence of loneliness across 113 countries: systematic review and meta-analysis. *BMJ*, 376, e067068.

Tao, Q., Akhter-Khan, S. C., Ang, T. F. A., Decarli, C., Alosco, M. L., Mez, J., Killiany, R., Devine, S., Rokach, A., Itchapurapu, I. S., Zhang, X., Lunetta, K. L., Steffens, D. C., Farrer, L. A., Greve, D. N., Au, R. & Qiu, W. Q. 2022. Different loneliness types, cognitive function, and brain structure in midlife: findings from the Framingham heart study. *eClinicalMedicine*, 53.

Tucker, J. S. 2002. Health-related social control within older adults' relationships. *The Journals of Gerontology: Series B*, 57, P387–P395.

Twenge, J. M. & Campbell, W. K. 2018. Associations between screen time and lower psychological well-being among children and adolescents: evidence from a population-based study. *Preventive Medicine Reports*, 12, 271–283.

UK Government. 2018. A connected society: a strategy for tackling loneliness [Online]. UK Government. Available: https://www.gov.uk/government/publications/a-connected-society-a-strategy-for-tackling-loneliness [Accessed].

UK Government. 2021a. Emerging together the talking loneliness network action plan [Online]. Available: https://www.gov.uk/government/publications/emerging-together-the-tackling-loneliness-network-action-plan [Accessed].

UK Government. 2021b. Joint message from the UK and Japanese loneliness ministers [Online]. UK Government Available: https://www.gov.uk/government/news/joint-message-from-the-uk-and-japanese-loneliness-ministers [Accessed].

Valtorta, N. K., Kanaan, M., Gilbody, S., Ronzi, S. & Hanratty, B. 2016. Loneliness and social isolation as risk factors for coronary heart disease and stroke: systematic review and meta-analysis of longitudinal observational studies. *Heart*, 102, 1009.

Van Tilburg, T. G., Aartsen, M. J. & Van Der Pas, S. 2015. Loneliness after divorce: a cohort comparison among Dutch young-old adults. *European Sociological Review*, 31, 243–252.

Victor, C. R. & Yang, K. 2012. The prevalence of loneliness among adults: a case study of the United Kingdom. *The Journal of Psychology*, 146, 85–104.

Wang, J., Mann, F., Lloyd-Evans, B., Ma, R. & Johnson, S. 2018. Associations between loneliness and perceived social support and outcomes of mental health problems: a systematic review. *BMC Psychiatry*, 18, 156.

Wang, F., Gao, Y., Han, Z., Yu, Y., Long, Z., Jiang, X., Wu, Y., Pei, B., Cao, Y., Ye, J., Wang, M. & Zhao, Y. 2023. A systematic review and meta-analysis of 90 cohort studies of social isolation, loneliness and mortality. *Nature Human Behaviour*, 7, 1307–1319.

Weiss, R. 1975. *Loneliness: The Experience of Emotional and Social Isolation*, MIT press.

Wong, Y. J., Wang, S.-Y. & Klann, E. 2018. The emperor with no clothes: a critique of collectivism and individualism. *Archives of Scientific Psychology*, 6, 251–260.

Yang, Y. C., Mcclintock, M. K., Kozloski, M. & Li, T. 2013. Social isolation and adult mortality: the role of chronic inflammation and sex differences. *Journal of Health and Social Behavior*, 54, 183–203.

Yanguas, J., Pinazo-Henandis, S. & Tarazona-Santabalbina, F. J. 2018. The complexity of loneliness. *Acta Biomed*, 89, 302–314.

Zhou, Z., Wang, P. & Fang, Y. 2018. Loneliness and the risk of dementia among older Chinese adults: gender differences. *Aging & Mental Health*, 22, 519–525.

CHAPTER 17

Social Prescribing and Health and Well-Being

Louise Baxter[1] and Chris Allen[2]

[1] *Faculty of Arts and Humanities, University College London, London, UK*
[2] *School of Health Sciences, University of Southampton, Southampton, UK*

Introduction

We know that there are substantial differences in health outcomes for different groups of people in society. In chapter 8 you had the opportunity to consider some of the explanations for such differences. How long we can expect to live, mirrors the 'social gradient' – with life expectancy being shorter in more deprived areas. The significant shifts in poor health that have occurred due to demographic and epidemiological transitions in western and developed countries have resulted in people increasingly living with one or more complex long-term condition; those who are poorest face the greatest burdens and outcomes of these.

In line with our increased understanding of the social determinants of health, healthcare encounters now often involve discussions of social issues and the social determinants of health, such as unemployment. In addition, as we outlined in the previous chapter, the relevance of social connections and the negative impact of social isolation and loneliness on health is now increasingly recognised. However, healthcare professionals are often less prepared to address these issues, rather than the specific illnesses and diseases which have traditionally been the focus of their training and professional development.

Because our health outcomes originate in and are shaped by our social circumstances, including the situations we are born into and in which we live, there has been an increasing focus on improving the social circumstances that negatively influence health. Recognition of these determinants has led to important questions being raised about how best to support populations to live well, especially where the underlying causes of ill health are social, rather than medical, and are typically experienced unequally. In this chapter, we will examine creative health, and the contemporary use of social prescribing initiatives to address such issues.

LEARNING OUTCOMES

By the end of this chapter, you will be able to:

- Understand what creative health is and be able to recognise some common approaches that have been taken to addressing health using creative health approaches.
- Understand what social prescribing is, including the role of the social prescribing link worker.
- Recognise some of the challenges as well as potential benefits that exist in relation to social prescribing and the use of community resources to promote health.

Social Sciences for Healthcare Professionals, First Edition. Edited by Chris Allen.
© 2026 John Wiley & Sons Ltd. Published 2026 by John Wiley & Sons Ltd.

Creative Health and Health Inequalities

Key Terms and Definitions

Creative health: The creative approaches that are taken to improve the health and well-being of populations.

Social prescribing: An approach that connects people to a range of community groups and activities that may promote general health and well-being.

Social prescribing link worker: A new role within the UK health system. Social prescribing link workers provide support to individuals relating to social prescribing, including working with them to identify appropriate community groups and supporting engagement with these.

It is estimated that socio-economic factors are the largest predictor of health outcomes (Hood et al., 2016), and we know that a significant number of primary care visits, and time spent in these consultations involves discussions related to socio-economic factors such as unemployment, financial worries, and relationship problems (Caper and Plunkett, 2015, Parkinson and Buttrick, 2015). In the United Kingdom in particular, healthcare professionals, researchers and policymakers are increasingly looking for creative ways to address the social circumstances that lead to poorer health outcomes. In 2017, the All-Party Parliamentary Group for Arts in Health (APPGA) published the first 'Creative Health Review' which made 10 recommendations, including the establishment of a National Centre for Creative Health (NCCH) (https://ncch.org.uk/) that would be responsible for disseminating research, informing policy and delivering on the vision for creative health (APPGA, 2017). Importantly, the report reviewed the increasing evidence base for the role of arts in health and the possibility of developing their role in health for addressing some of the impacts of the social determinants of health on health inequalities (see the All Party Parliamentary Group on Arts, Health and Wellbeing's 'Creative Health Review' for more details).

Since then, consideration of 'Creative Health' has come to encompass the potential benefits to health of arts, culture, heritage and nature, and this is reflected in the NCCH definition of creative health, highlighting it as the 'creative approaches and activities which have benefits for our health and well-being'.

Activities can include but are not limited to:

- Visual and performing arts
- Arts and crafts
- Film and literature
- Cooking
- Creative activities in nature

- And other creative and innovative ways to approach health and care services (APPGA, 2023).

We have included examples from some of these areas below, alongside some of the associated evidence base.

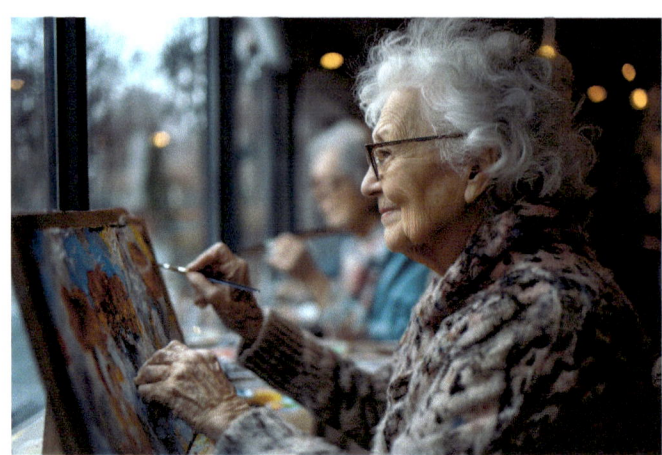

Source: Harvinder/Adobe Stock Photos.

Heritage and Museum-Based Activities

It is recognised that the health outcomes of those able to access and engage with community assets such as museums and libraries are generally better than those who either lack access or are unable to engage with such assets (Munford et al., 2017). Engagement with a range of local community assets has been shown to have a number of health benefits, including reduced dementia risk in later life as one example (Fancourt et al., 2020).

Museums are a community-based asset. Their social value has been promoted around the world, leading to an increased interest in their potential health benefits from researchers, policymakers and healthcare professionals (Chatterjee, 2019). Museum and heritage-based creative health solutions have been used to support older people, those with mental ill health, those with dementia, cancer, those who have survived a stroke, as well as those with a physical disability (Camic et al., 2019, Camic et al., 2021, Morse et al., 2023, Sharma and Lee, 2020, Thomson et al., 2011, Thomson et al., 2012a, Thomson et al., 2012b, Thomson et al., 2018, Todd et al., 2017). They are believed to be salutogenic because they support engagement, learning and social connectivity (Thomson et al., 2018, Todd et al., 2017), with these potentially health-related benefits being delivered in a non-stigmatising way, using what is already available and accessible in people's local communities (Camic and Chatterjee, 2013).

Whilst the evidence base is still developing, the evidence that exists does suggest that such programmes may be useful in promoting physical and mental health, as well as general well-being in those accessing such programmes. In a recent rapid review, heritage and culture-based prescription was found to be beneficial for participant's physical and mental health across the reviewed literature (Mughal et al., 2022). Research has highlighted that museum-based programmes can improve people's psychological well-being, whilst helping people learn useful skills and feel more connected to their communities and others (Liou et al., 2021, Thomson et al., 2018, Thomson et al., 2020). Object handling, both inside and outside museum settings, may also be beneficial to well-being (Camic et al., 2021, Thomson et al., 2012b, Thomson and Chatterjee, 2016). However, the existing evidence is unable to tell us exactly how these programmes work to promote health and well-being (Mughal et al., 2022). It is possible that being able to look at and engage with objects, helps engage people's senses such as touch, and that this may bring about positive emotions that may ignite people's imaginations and curiosity – especially through allowing people to consider their social traditions, culture and heritage, and that of their society (Mughal et al., 2022). Other potentially salutogenic (i.e. health enhancing) aspects of such programmes include their promotion of activity, and social interaction. Both of which are recognised as being associated with positive biopsychosocial outcomes such as reduced loneliness, better coping strategies, less stress and adoption of healthier behaviours.

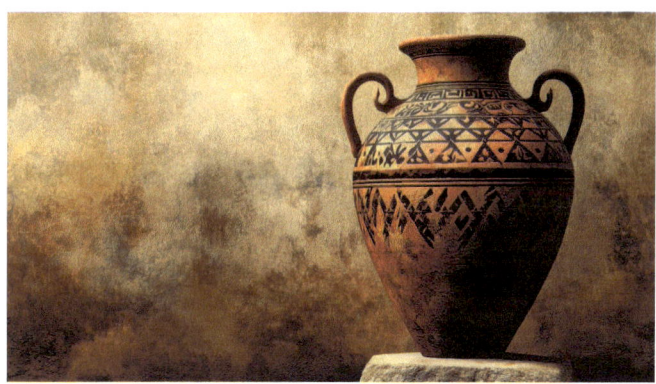

Source: javier/Adobe Stock Photos.

Physical Activity – Football Fans in Training (FFIT)

As we have explored elsewhere in this book, obesity, which has been described as a pandemic, alongside physical inactivity, is a known contributor to poor health outcomes worldwide (GBD Obesity Collaborators, 2017, Katzmarzyk et al., 2022). In the United Kingdom, rates of both have been increasing and are a particular problem for men (NHS, 2021, Office for Health Improvement and Disparities, 2024). Men are considered a particularly hard-to-reach group, especially in the context of behaviour change interventions (Zwolinsky et al., 2013). Various gendered interventions have been deployed that provide creative solutions to men's health, particularly in relation to physical activity, which it has been suggested men may more likely engage with, compared to other types of behaviour

change interventions (Bottorff et al., 2015). In the United Kingdom, football (or soccer as it is known in some other countries – notably America) is arguably the nation's most popular sport. There are several examples of using football to promote physical activity and education around health-related behaviours. A now seminal programme in Scotland, that occurred through a collaboration between several universities and the Scottish Football Association is known as 'Football Fans in Training' (FFIT) (Wyke et al., 2015). The programme was developed using behaviour change theory and participative peer-supported learning (see chapters 12–13) as a way of incentivising overweight men to engage in weight management. Sessions were hosted at local professional football clubs (another example of making use of local community assets) and provided participants with health education, particularly around diet, alongside activity sessions that provided exclusive access to the clubs' facilities (Wyke et al., 2015). Similar programmes have been deployed in England (Pringle et al., 2013), as well as in Europe through the EuroFIT programme, which targeted unhealthy behaviour in men through 4 countries and 15 professional football clubs (Wyke et al., 2019).

These programmes have been evaluated in randomised controlled trials, and whilst some have demonstrated relatively similar outcomes to other non-gendered weight loss programmes (e.g. Hunt et al. [2014]), others have suggested they may better promote increased levels of physical activity in their participants than other activity-based interventions (Wyke et al., 2019). The programmes are generally relatively inexpensive to deliver, enjoyable and effective in helping participants lose weight, as well as making positive changes to their behaviours relating to diet, alcohol consumption and activity levels (Hunt et al., 2014, Wyke et al., 2015, Wyke et al., 2019). Additionally, longitudinal evidence suggests some improvements can be sustained by participants (Gray et al., 2018). In particular, these programmes may be particularly effective at reaching those at highest risk, and whilst often being more likely to be attended by those from higher status groups, can reach those with lower socio-economic status too (Hunt et al., 2014, Wyke et al., 2015, Wyke et al., 2019).

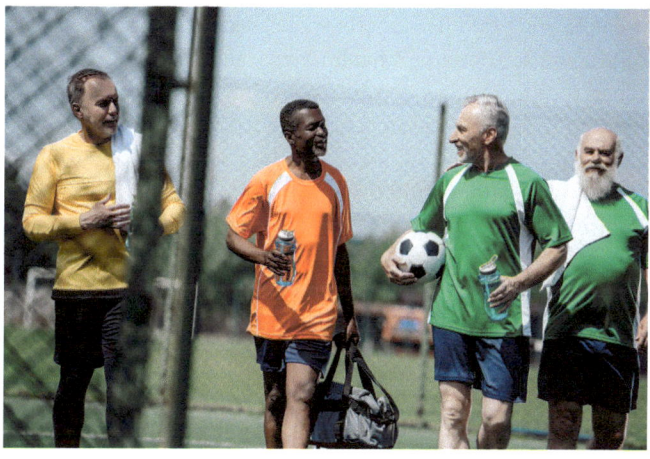

Source: LIGHTFIELD STUDIOS/Adobe Stock Photos.

Nature – Blue Care Interventions

'Nature-based therapies' make use of natural ecosystems to bring about health benefits for those with or without a specific health need (Joschko et al., 2023). Water and nature more generally provide an environmental backdrop for activities that are potentially salutogenic (Foley and Kistemann, 2015). A large amount of the planet's population lives near open water (even as much as a third) and this poses both a threat in terms of global warming (Neumann et al., 2015) and a potential opportunity for people to reconnect with nature and in particular blue spaces (Bell et al., 2015, Grellier et al., 2017). In fact, studies have even suggested that the coast is an underappreciated public health resource and that efforts to help people reconnect with nature represent important upstream health promotion (Maller et al., 2006, White et al., 2014).

A recent systematic review of 'blue care' initiatives examined the role of a range of 'planned' water-based activities, including canoeing and kayaking, dragon boat racing, fly-fishing, sailing, surfing and scuba-diving on 'outdoor natural surface water' such as rivers, lakes and the sea with the specific aim of promoting individual health and well-being (Britton et al., 2020). Of the included activities in the review, surfing in particular has a growing evidence base (Armitano et al., 2015, Caddick et al., 2015, Gibbs et al., 2022, Godfrey et al., 2015), and organisations such as the 'International Surf Therapy Organisation' (ITSO) have been established to support its growth. In the case of the review, these interventions typically aimed to support people's reablement, mental health, and general well-being in young people (Godfrey et al., 2015), and service veterans (Caddick et al., 2015). As is the challenge with evaluating creative health interventions using systematic approaches, the included studies involved very different interventions, different dosing (i.e. different amounts of the activity being prescribed), different participants, and used very different outcome measures, with some considering the extent to which participants were able to connect with nature, and some specifically looking at health and well-being related outcomes, albeit, normally only for the duration of the programmes or immediately pre- and post intervention (Britton et al., 2020).

The lack of similarity between the included studies makes it challenging to draw concrete conclusions about the benefits of blue care to people's health and well-being. As with other types of intervention of this nature, high-quality evidence is hard to achieve. Research falling outside of this review, for example, Costello et al. (2019) (in the context of ocean swimming) have demonstrated positive impacts, including potentially on healthy aging.

Authors such as Britton et al. (2020) have pointed out some similarities between blue and green care interventions, with both activities posing implementation challenges. Whilst formal organisations are now established that support such activities (the International Surf Therapy Organisation (ITSO) (ntlsurftherapy .org) and the Wave Project (www.waveproject. co.uk) as two notable examples), recent research has highlighted that smaller initiatives in particular, face challenges including

personal and environmental barriers, access to adequate resources including funding (funding is often short term and related to 'start up'), safety, quality assurance, governance and training (Juster-Horsfield and Bell, 2022). The nature of activities that occur in open water (i.e. fluctuating depth, water hazards such as tides, dangerous currents, and hidden underwater objects) means these are inherently riskier than most other creative health approaches.

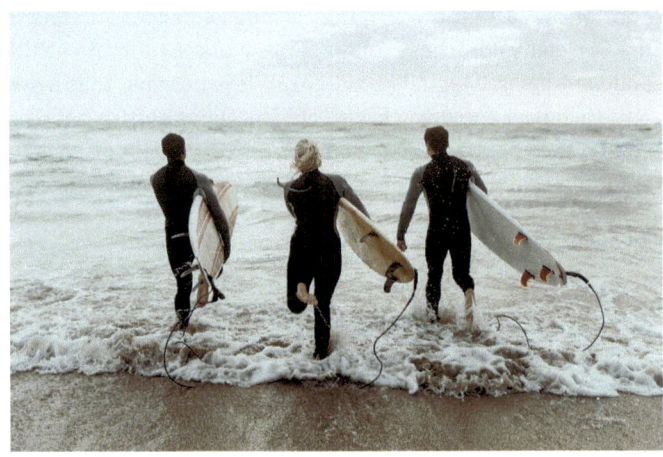

Source: rawpixel.com/Adobe Stock Photos.

What Is Social Prescribing?

Alongside this broader development of research and practice around different creative solutions for addressing the social determinants of health and inequalities, there has been a growing concern for understanding how we can connect those who might benefit from these interventions to what is on offer in the communities in which they live, and who should be responsible for facilitating these connections. Connecting people who have sought medical care to activities and social support in the wider community which might help to address underlying social factors, is broadly known as 'social prescribing' (sometimes also referred to as 'community referral' (Chatterjee et al., 2018). Social prescribing is a method of care delivery that links patients to non-medical services and interventions in their communities, to support their health and well-being, by helping patients address their emotional, practical or social needs, such as those that may be socially isolated or live with long-term health conditions (Chatterjee et al., 2018, Fixsen et al., 2020). As a process, social prescribing can link people to the types of creative health activities, interventions and organisations that are available in their communities and that might be supportive, alongside other services that target specific social determinants, such as housing or benefits support (Husk et al., 2020).

Husk et al. (2020) in a recent realist review outlined four possible social prescribing routes through primary care and these were:

1. Signposting to various activities, through the provision of information, often in the form of a leaflet, from a primary healthcare worker

2. Direct referral from primary care to an activity

3. Referral to the activity via a link worker

4. Holistic approaches, where the health professional conducting the primary care consultation refers to a link worker, and from there to social, community or cultural activities, with ongoing relational support being provided by the link worker (Husk et al., 2020).

The provision of social prescribing link workers (discussed more below) and social prescribing pathways within primary care, as well as other organisations within local communities such as charities and community groups, can be used to connect individuals to supportive resources and groups that may help address the social disadvantage that people can experience, such as a lack of engagement and social contact with those in their community.

What Is a Social Prescribing Link Worker?

Whilst other social prescribing pathways exist, in the current UK context, social prescribing link workers are predominantly employed and funded through the NHS. These roles are often funded through individual Primary Care Networks[1] (PCN) in response to the 2019 NHS Long Term Plan (Howarth and Burns, 2019, Husk et al., 2020). At present social prescribing link workers are generally based in a GP[2] practice, or within community health organisations (Sandhu et al., 2022). They work with those referred to them to identify what their concerns are, what they think might be affecting or causing their health condition and what steps they would like to take to address these. This is known as a 'what matters to me' conversation and contrasts the more traditional biomedical approach, which might instead focus on 'what is the matter with me' (Howarth and Burns, 2019). Generally, these initial conversations last around an hour, with the focus being largely on an individual's concerns, but most importantly their personal strengths (their assets). These might be from individuals themselves, from within their social networks, or from within their wider community (Howarth and Burns, 2019). The role of the SPLW takes social prescribing beyond signposting people to services (e.g. in the first and second pathways outlined above in the summary of Husk's review). Generally, link workers continue to see those who have been referred to them several times, helping them to develop a plan and agree a set of actions to address their concerns (Howarth and Burns, 2019). This may also involve the link worker attending services with them, to offer

support or help with attendance or arranging peer support (Rothe and Heiss, 2022). In placing individuals at the centre of decisions about their health, providing them with opportunities to consider their strengths and supporting their access to relevant network and community resources, this approach seeks to support individuals to alleviate some of the material and social disadvantages that impact on their health and well-being (Howarth and Burns, 2019).

Does Social Prescribing Work?

Social prescribing seeks to support people using the resources that often already exist in their communities. For such an intervention to be effective, healthcare professionals and those being referred through social prescribing, need to understand the potential benefits and believe that the referral will have the desired impact (Aughterson et al., 2020, Husk et al., 2020). Whilst community referral has existed for some time (Grant et al., 2000, Polley et al., 2017), within a UK context, the use of 'social prescribing' through specialist 'link workers' is relatively new (Polley et al., 2017). However, with the approach being increasingly deployed, we are beginning to understand more about how these pathways may work and who they might work for.

In particular, recent research has highlighted that social prescribing programmes may be effective in reducing anxiety and loneliness, as well as increasing mental well-being (Cooper et al., 2022, Morton et al., 2015, Napierala et al., 2022, Vidovic et al., 2021, Wakefield et al., 2022, Woodall et al., 2018). For example, Dingle and colleagues' recent work found improvements in both loneliness (see previous chapter) and social trust, and small improvements in well-being and social anxiety after an 8-week social prescribing intervention (Dingle et al., 2024). In addition, Kellezi and colleagues found evidence that social prescribing programmes might facilitate social belonging, which may address the negative impact of loneliness in those with chronic illnesses and which may in turn reduce healthcare utilisation (Kellezi et al., 2019).

However, several systematic reviews have found that evidence of the positive impact of social prescribing may be limited by the design of existing studies. For example, Napierala et al. (2022) report that positive effects were often observed in studies that analysed outcomes over a short period of time, but that similar findings were less visible when studies used longitudinal methods that allowed longer-term effects to be observed. This is reflected in some of the challenges in evaluating complex interventions and programmes that involve multiple component parts, such as social prescribing, and that are themselves aimed at meeting the needs of those with complex needs. Even in the examples we have provided here, there is a lack of homogeneity between different social prescribing programmes, and the range of activities that they may refer people to. For example, different programmes may offer varying levels of personalisation and co-design, be delivered by different roles and

---

[1] In the United Kingdom, the NHS Long Term Plan (2019) led to the creation of primary care networks (PCNs). A primary care network brings together several General Practices to work in partnership. The potential impact of such networks is that they might offer improved access to different services and might better help integrate primary care, with wider health and community services.

[2] In the United Kingdom, General Practices generally provide the gateway to NHS services, treat acute and chronic illness, as well as provide health education and advice across the life course.

may be delivered in varying locations, using different referral methods and to groups with potentially very different needs. This can make it difficult to evaluate social prescribing 'like for like', using standardised methods (such as those seen in trials for medical interventions), that allow for studies to be compared (as most interventions are not exactly the same) and there is a lack of standardisation to how programmes are evaluated, with different methods and outcome measures being used (Ayorinde et al., 2024). For example, in the evaluation of social prescribing carried out by Dingle et al. (2024), described above, those experiencing loneliness were not randomised for ethical and design reasons, which led in turn to the composition of the two comparator groups (social prescribing vs treatment as usual) being different (Dingle et al., 2024). It has been suggested that employing other methods and developing programme theories (as is the case in realist evaluation discussed in chapter 2) will help us to understand what aspects of social prescribing work, what groups of people it might work for, and in what particular contexts, and that this will lead to more robust understanding of *how* social prescribing works (Bertotti et al., 2018). Research that has used this approach has been able to demonstrate that improvements for participants in well-being outcomes are linked to the different stages of the social prescribing pathway working together effectively, from the GP referral, through to the quality of the interaction with the social prescribing link worker, and lastly, the interaction between the participant and the voluntary or community groups and activities they are referred to (Bertotti et al., 2018). A specific mechanism reflecting the role of the link worker in supporting the referral process is highlighted in the review by Husk et al. (2020), as well as the work of Bertotti et al. (2018).

The Role of the 'Social Prescribing Link Worker'

Whilst the social prescribing link worker role is relatively new, 'referral facilitators', performing a relatively similar role, have been found in an RCT to be effective in reducing people's anxiety, improving their quality of life and perceived health status and improving their ability to carry out everyday activities, despite not reducing levels of depression or perceptions of social support (Grant et al., 2000). The role of the social prescribing link worker has been identified as fundamental to the success of social prescribing, with the link worker's communication and relational skills being emphasised as important in building trust (Wildman et al., 2019). The evidence base for the role highlights their importance to the referral process and ultimately how successful social prescribing is in connecting health services and those who access them to local communities (Aughterson et al., 2020, Rothe and Heiss, 2022), and in turn, how effective they are in improving health outcomes (Bertotti et al., 2018). As a relatively new role within healthcare systems, the link worker role is increasingly carrying more responsibility

and is demanding and complex, yet lacks regulation, education or training standards (Rothe and Heiss, 2022). In addition, funding cuts to the voluntary and community sectors that link workers' support participants to access, create situations of increasing uncertainty that link workers must be able to effectively navigate and understand (Aughterson et al., 2020). Work has highlighted the need for link workers to be supported in a number of ways, including being given adequate time to support service users effectively, being offered training to cope with the demands of the role and having opportunities for career progression (Rhodes and Bell, 2021, Wildman et al., 2019).

The Role of the Voluntary and Community Sector

Earlier in this chapter, we highlighted that there is an increasing evidence base for the effectiveness of many of the community-based services and activities that social prescribing programmes refer to (e.g. Museums on Prescription, Football Fans In Training, and Blue Care Interventions). The sector is, along with the link workers, a key factor in the implementation and success of social prescribing pathways – as they provide the activities that people are referred to, however, how these work within social prescribing programmes, rather than simply as stand-alone activities, needs to be carefully considered (Baxter and Fancourt, 2020, Bertotti et al., 2018).

Whilst the voluntary, community and social enterprise sectors are vital to social prescribing programmes, public sector cuts and insecure longer-term funding streams mean that many groups and activities that link workers can support people to access, are unable to sustain themselves in the long term (Baxter and Fancourt, 2020, Rothe and Heiss, 2022). Those that are able to continue, may be placed under additional demand, which in turn then threatens their longer-term sustainability (Bertotti et al., 2018, Rothe and Heiss, 2022). Hence, the lack of sustainable funding for the sector that delivers the support and activities that service users are referred to, is also a barrier to community organisations making existing activities available through social prescribing programmes (Baxter and Fancourt, 2020). In addition, community and voluntary sector organisations have identified challenges such as lacking understanding of social prescribing and NHS commissioning landscapes, a lack of training and skills in supporting participants with potentially challenging health issues or circumstances, and differences in the technical language of the health and cultural sectors – which make it difficult for them to accept referrals through social prescribing programmes (Baxter and Fancourt, 2020, Juster-Horsfield and Bell, 2022). These challenges may make it difficult for such organisations to create sustainable and truly salutogenic encounters, and such services are also at risk of being overburdened by the volume of referrals being made (Juster-Horsfield and Bell, 2022).

How Social Prescribing Is Experienced by Those Accessing Support

Of course, the benefits of social prescribing in addressing health inequalities also depend on those most in need of this support being able to access it. Our understanding of the experiences of and access to social prescribing is developing, but we do already have some early insights. As we highlighted in chapter 8, there are gendered differences in healthcare utilisation, and social prescribing appears to be no different. For example, we know that more women than men currently access social prescribing – both in terms of being referred to social prescribing and then accepting the referral (Khan et al., 2023). Whilst the way primary care data is recorded can make it challenging to look at age-related differences, research shows that despite NHS England's aim for social prescribing to be an 'all age' offer, there are gaps in both provision and referral rates for younger people (Khan et al., 2023). In response to this, work is increasingly exploring how social prescribing might better meet the needs of and benefit young people, who are themselves also exposed to the social circumstances that social prescribing seeks to address (Fancourt et al., 2023, Hayes et al., 2023).

A key challenge for participants in engaging with social prescribing is in the availability and accessibility of community and voluntary organisations that deliver activities or services. Participants have reported that a key motivation for participation, is the belief that it will help with their health (Husk et al., 2020). However, access can often be a challenge, especially for those lacking material resources through structural inequality and multiple forms of disadvantage that make the cost of the activity, or the cost of getting to the activity (for example, through public transport) too expensive (Baxter et al., 2022, Husk et al., 2020). This is a particularly important factor when considered alongside financial difficulties and disadvantages as key social determinants of mental health (Allen et al., 2014).

Those who have been referred to social prescribing programmes are generally positive about their experiences – reporting positive relationships with social prescribing staff, and the amount of time they were able to give them, as well as valuing the extent to which care was tailored around their specific needs (Kellezi et al., 2019). A key aspect of their positive feelings towards the social prescribing programme was how they felt listened to and heard by those they worked with, in particular the support the link worker provided to help them attend specific groups that helped them become more socially connected, through building and sustaining links to these groups (Kellezi et al., 2019). This is supported by evidence that those with lived experience of mental ill health would feel more able to attend social groups to support their recovery if there was some support to attend (Baxter et al., 2022), which in turn suggests that the holistic model of social prescribing outlined earlier in this chapter, is the most likely to be engaged with by participants (Husk et al., 2020).

A need for positive group experience has also been identified as important to participants (Baxter et al., 2022, Kellezi et al., 2019). Where groups are unwelcoming, or less well suited to a participant's needs, people may have less positive experiences of such programmes and are less likely to engage with their referral. These are important considerations as social prescribing programmes and creative health interventions often aim to address issues such as loneliness and fatigue, where participants may need to expend significant effort to attend sessions.

More information on the evidence base for Social Prescribing is available at the National Academy for Social Prescribing website (www.nasp.org).

> ### Clinical Considerations
>
> - Social prescribing primarily aims to address the social causes of poor health.
> - Social prescribing is likely to become increasingly important in supporting people to live healthy and fulfilling lives.
> - There are challenges to creating a robust evidence base for social prescribing, due to the range of different activities that people can be referred to and the range of different ways these have been evaluated.
> - As healthcare professionals, it is important to be aware of social prescribing, and the process of social prescribing, including the role of the social prescribing link worker.

Conclusion

Increased awareness of the impact of social disadvantage on health outcomes has resulted in an increased interest in how such differences can be addressed using creative health interventions. In this chapter, we reviewed some examples of creative health interventions such as culture (specifically heritage-based interventions and object handling), fitness (specifically Football Fans in Training, but also aspects of Blue Care) and nature-based interventions (specifically Blue Care) and considered the developing evidence base for these, alongside some of the challenges that exist in terms of creating an evidence base for a range of different creative health approaches. We also explored how people can be connected to these activities, through our exploration of social prescribing. In considering social prescribing, we have provided an overview of the evidence for social prescribing, what we know about who is likely to benefit from social prescribing, and how this is experienced. We have also examined the relatively new role of social prescribing link workers, and how they may support social prescribing referrals to those who may benefit from a range of different community-based creative health approaches.

References

Allen, J., Balfour, R., Bell, R. & Marmot, M. 2014. Social determinants of mental health. *International Review of Psychiatry*, 26, 392–407.

APPGA 2017. Creative Health: The Arts for Health and Wellbeing: Short Report. All-Party Parliamentary Group on Arts, Health and Wellbeing Inquiry.

APPGA. 2023. Creative health review [Online]. National Centre for Creative Health. Available: https://ncch.org.uk/creative-health-review [Accessed].

Armitano, C. N., Clapham, E. D., Lamont, L. S. & Audette, J. G. 2015. Benefits of surfing for children with disabilities: a pilot study. *Palaestra*, 29(3).

Aughterson, H., Baxter, L. & Fancourt, D. 2020. Social prescribing for individuals with mental health problems: a qualitative study of barriers and enablers experienced by general practitioners. *BMC Family Practice*, 21, 194.

Ayorinde, A., Grove, A., Ghosh, I., Harlock, J., Meehan, E., Tyldesley-Marshall, N., Briggs, A., Clarke, A. & Al-Khudairy, L. 2024. What is the best way to evaluate social prescribing? A qualitative feasibility assessment for a national impact evaluation study in England. *Journal of Health Services Research & Policy*, 29, 111–121.

Baxter, L. & Fancourt, D. 2020. What are the barriers to, and enablers of, working with people with lived experience of mental illness amongst community and voluntary sector organisations? A qualitative study. *PLoS One*, 15, e0235334.

Baxter, L., Burton, A. & Fancourt, D. 2022. Community and cultural engagement for people with lived experience of mental health conditions: what are the barriers and enablers? *BMC Psychology*, 10, 71.

Bell, S. L., Phoenix, C., Lovell, R. & Wheeler, B. W. 2015. Seeking everyday wellbeing: the coast as a therapeutic landscape. *Social Science & Medicine*, 142, 56–67.

Bertotti, M., Frostick, C., Hutt, P., Sohanpal, R. & Carnes, D. 2018. A realist evaluation of social prescribing: an exploration into the context and mechanisms underpinning a pathway linking primary care with the voluntary sector. *Primary Health Care Research & Development*, 19, 232–245.

Bottorff, J. L., Seaton, C. L., Johnson, S. T., Caperchione, C. M., Oliffe, J. L., More, K., Jaffer-Hirji, H. & Tillotson, S. M. 2015. An updated review of interventions that include promotion of physical activity for adult men. *Sports Medicine*, 45, 775–800.

Britton, E., Kindermann, G., Domegan, C. & Carlin, C. 2020. Blue care: a systematic review of blue space interventions for health and wellbeing. *Health Promotion International*, 35, 50–69.

Caddick, N., Smith, B. & Phoenix, C. 2015. The effects of surfing and the natural environment on the well-being of combat veterans. *Qualitative Health Research*, 25, 76–86.

Camic, P. M. & Chatterjee, H. J. 2013. Museums and art galleries as partners for public health interventions. *Perspectives in Public Health*, 133, 66–71.

Camic, P. M., Hulbert, S. & Kimmel, J. 2019. Museum object handling: a health-promoting community-based activity for dementia care. *Journal of Health Psychology*, 24, 787–798.

Camic, P. M., Dickens, L., Zeilig, H. & Strohmaier, S. 2021. Subjective wellbeing in people living with dementia: exploring processes of multiple object handling sessions in a museum setting. *Wellcome Open Research*, 6, 96.

Caper, K. & Plunkett, J. 2015. A very general practice: How much time do GPs spend on issues other than health? https://www.citizensadvice.org.uk/Global/CitizensAdvice/Public%20services%20publications/CitizensAdvice_AVeryGeneralPractice_May2015.pdf.

Chatterjee, H. 2019. Partnership for Health: The Role of Cultural and Natural Assets in Public Health. *In:* O'Neill, M. & Hooper, G. (eds.) *Connecting Museums*, Routledge. https://www.taylorfrancis.com/books/edit/10.4324/9781351036184/connecting-museums-mark-neill-glenn-hooper?refId=d699a632-54d1-4773-9828-4e060428b5b6&context=ubx.

Chatterjee, H. J., Camic, P. M., Lockyer, B. & Thomson, L. J. M. 2018. Non-clinical community interventions: a systematised review of social prescribing schemes. *Arts & Health*, 10, 97–123.

Cooper, M., Avery, L., Scott, J., Ashley, K., Jordan, C., Errington, L. & Flynn, D. 2022. Effectiveness and active ingredients of social prescribing interventions targeting mental health: a systematic review. *BMJ Open*, 12, e060214.

Costello, L., Mcdermott, M.-L., Patel, P. & Dare, J. 2019. 'A lot better than medicine' - self-organised ocean swimming groups as facilitators for healthy ageing. *Health & Place*, 60, 102212.

Dingle, G. A., Sharman, L. S., Hayes, S., Haslam, C., Cruwys, T., Jetten, J., Haslam, S. A., Mcnamara, N., Chua, D., Baker, J. R. & Johnson, T. 2024. A controlled evaluation of social prescribing on loneliness for adults in Queensland: 8-week outcomes. *Frontiers in Psychology*, 15, 1359855.

Fancourt, D., Steptoe, A. & Cadar, D. 2020. Community engagement and dementia risk: time-to-event analyses from a national cohort study. *Journal of Epidemiology and Community Health*, 74, 71–77.

Fancourt, D., Burton, A., Bu, F., Deighton, J., Turner, R., Wright, J., Bradbury, A., Tibber, M., Talwar, S. & Hayes, D. 2023. Wellbeing while waiting evaluating social prescribing in CAMHS: study protocol for a hybrid type II implementation-effectiveness study. *BMC Psychiatry*, 23, 328.

Fixsen, A., Seers, H., Polley, M. & Robins, J. 2020. Applying critical systems thinking to social prescribing: a relational model of stakeholder "buy-in". *BMC Health Services Research*, 20, 580.

Foley, R. & Kistemann, T. 2015. Blue space geographies: enabling health in place. *Health & Place*, 35, 157–165.

GBD Obesity Collaborators 2017. Health effects of overweight and obesity in 195 countries over 25 years. *New England Journal of Medicine*, 377, 13–27.

Gibbs, K., Wilkie, L., Jarman, J., Barker-Smith, A., Kemp, A. H. & Fisher, Z. 2022. Riding the wave into wellbeing: a qualitative evaluation of surf therapy for individuals living with acquired brain injury. *PLoS One*, 17, e0266388.

Godfrey, C., Devine-Wright, H. & Taylor, J. 2015. The positive impact of structured surfing courses on the wellbeing of vulnerable young people. *Community Practitioner*, 88, 26–29.

Grant, C., Goodenough, T., Harvey, I. & Hine, C. 2000. A randomised controlled trial and economic evaluation of a referrals facilitator between primary care and the voluntary sector. *BMJ*, 320, 419–423.

Gray, C. M., Wyke, S., Zhang, R., Anderson, A. S., Barry, S., Boyer, N., Brennan, G., Briggs, A., Bunn, C. & Donnachie, C. 2018. Long-term weight loss trajectories following participation in a randomised controlled trial of a weight management programme for men delivered through professional football clubs: a longitudinal cohort study and economic evaluation. *International Journal of Behavioral Nutrition and Physical Activity*, 15, 1–13.

Grellier, J., White, M. P., Albin, M., Bell, S., Elliott, L. R., Gascón, M., Gualdi, S., Mancini, L., Nieuwenhuijsen, M. J., Sarigiannis, D. A., Van Den Bosch, M., Wolf, T., Wuijts, S. & Fleming, L. E. 2017. BlueHealth: a study programme protocol for mapping and quantifying the potential benefits to public health and well-being from Europe's blue spaces. *BMJ Open*, 7, e016188.

Hayes, D., Jarvis-Beesley, P., Mitchell, D., Polley, M., Husk, K. & Collaborative., O. B. O. T. N. A. P 2023. *The Impact of Social Prescribing on Children and Young People's Mental Health and Wellbeing*, London: National Academy for Social Prescribing.

Hood, C. M., Gennuso, K. P., Swain, G. R. & Catlin, B. B. 2016. County health rankings: relationships between determinant factors and health outcomes. *American Journal of Preventive Medicine*, 50, 129–135.

Howarth, M. & Burns, L. 2019. Social prescribing in practice: community-centred approaches. *Practice Nursing*, 30, 338–341.

Hunt, K., Wyke, S., Gray, C. M., Anderson, A. S., Brady, A., Bunn, C., Donnan, P. T., Fenwick, E., Grieve, E., Leishman, J., Miller, E., Mutrie, N., Rauchhaus, P., White, A. & Treweek, S. 2014. A gender-sensitised weight loss and healthy living programme for overweight and obese men delivered by Scottish premier league football clubs (FFIT): a pragmatic randomised controlled trial. *Lancet*, 383, 1211–1221.

Husk, K., Blockley, K., Lovell, R., Bethel, A., Lang, I., Byng, R. & Garside, R. 2020. What approaches to social prescribing work, for whom, and in what circumstances? A realist review. *Health & Social Care in the Community*, 28, 309–324.

Joschko, L., Pálsdóttir, A. M., Grahn, P. & Hinse, M. 2023. Nature-based therapy in individuals with mental health disorders, with a focus on mental well-being and connectedness to nature-a pilot study. *International Journal of Environmental Research and Public Health*, 20.

Juster-Horsfield, H. H. & Bell, S. L. 2022. Supporting 'blue care' through outdoor water-based activities: practitioner perspectives. *Qualitative Research in Sport, Exercise and Health*, 14, 137–150.

Katzmarzyk, P. T., Friedenreich, C., Shiroma, E. J. & Lee, I.-M. 2022. Physical inactivity and non-communicable disease burden in low-income, middle-income and high-income countries. *British Journal of Sports Medicine*, 56, 101–106.

Kellezi, B., Wakefield, J. R. H., Stevenson, C., Mcnamara, N., Mair, E., Bowe, M., Wilson, I. & Halder, M. M. 2019. The social cure of social prescribing: a mixed-methods study on the benefits of social connectedness on quality and effectiveness of care provision. *BMJ Open*, 9, e033137.

Khan, K., Al-Izzi, R., Montasem, A., Gordon, C., Brown, H. & Goldthorpe, J. 2023. The feasibility of identifying health inequalities in social prescribing referrals and declines using primary care patient records. *NIHR Open Research*, 3, 1.

Liou, K. T., Boas, R., Murphy, S., Leung, P., Boas, S., Card, A. & Asgary, R. 2021. Addressing psychosocial stressors through a community-academic partnership between a museum and a federally qualified health center: a qualitative study. *Journal of Health Care for the Poor and Underserved*, 32, 767–782.

Maller, C., Townsend, M., Pryor, A., Brown, P. & St Leger, L. 2006. Healthy nature healthy people: 'contact with nature' as an upstream health promotion intervention for populations. *Health Promotion International*, 21, 45–54.

Morse, N., Thomson, L. J., Elsden, E., Rogers, H. & Chatterjee, H. J. 2023. Exploring the potential of creative museum-led activities to support stroke In-patient rehabilitation and wellbeing: a pilot mixed-methods study. *Arts & Health*, 15, 135–152.

Morton, L., Ferguson, M. & Baty, F. 2015. Improving wellbeing and self-efficacy by social prescription. *Public Health*, 129, 286–289.

Mughal, R., Polley, M., Sabey, A. & Chatterjee, H. 2022. *How Arts, Heritage and Culture can Support Health and Wellbeing Through Social Prescribing*, NASP.

Munford, L. A., Sidaway, M., Blakemore, A., Sutton, M. & Bower, P. 2017. Associations of participation in community assets with health-related quality of life and healthcare usage: a cross-sectional study of older people in the community. *BMJ Open*, 7, e012374.

Napierala, H., Krüger, K., Kuschick, D., Heintze, C., Herrmann, W. J. & Holzinger, F. 2022. Social prescribing: systematic review of the effectiveness of psychosocial community referral interventions in primary care. *International Journal of Integrated Care*, 22, 11.

Neumann, B., Vafeidis, A. T., Zimmermann, J. & Nicholls, R. J. 2015. Future coastal population growth and exposure to sea-level rise and coastal flooding - a global assessment. *PLoS One*, 10, e0118571.

NHS 2021. Statistics on Obesity, Physical Activity, and Diet, England 2021.

Office for Health Improvement and Disparities. 2024. Obesity profile: short statistical commentary May 2024 [Online]. Office for Health Improvement and Disparities. Available: https://www.gov.uk/government/statistics/update-to-the-obesity-profile-on-fingertips/obesity-profile-short-statistical-commentary-may-2024#:~:text=In%202022%20to%202023%2C%20the,%25)%20and%20women%20(26.2%25). [Accessed].

Parkinson, A. & Buttrick, J. 2015. *The Role of Advice Services in Health Outcomes: Evidence Review and Mapping Study*, The Low Commission: Advice Services Alliance. Available online at: https://www.thelegaleducationfoundation.org/wp-content/uploads/2015/06/Role-of-Advice-Services-in-Health-Outcomes.pdf.

Polley, M., Fleming, J., Anfilogoff, T. & Carpenter, A. 2017. *Making Sense of Social Prescribing*, University of Westminster. Available online at: https://westminsterresearch.westminster.ac.uk/item/q1v77/making-sense-of-social-prescribing.

Pringle, A., Zwolinsky, S., Mckenna, J., Daly-Smith, A., Robertson, S. & White, A. 2013. Effect of a national programme of men's health delivered in English premier league football clubs. *Public Health*, 127, 18–26.

Rhodes, J. & Bell, S. 2021. "It sounded a lot simpler on the job description": a qualitative study exploring the role of social prescribing link workers and their training and support needs (2020). *Health & Social Care in the Community*, 29, e338–e347.

Rothe, D. & Heiss, R. 2022. Link workers, activities and target groups in social prescribing: a literature review. *Journal of Integrated Care*, 30, 1–11.

Sandhu, S., Lian, T., Drake, C., Moffatt, S., Wildman, J. & Wildman, J. 2022. Intervention components of link worker social prescribing programmes: a scoping review. *Health & Social Care in the Community*, 30, e3761–e3774.

Sharma, M. & Lee, A. 2020. Dementia-friendly heritage settings: a research review. *International Journal of Building Pathology and Adaptation*, 38, 279–310.

Thomson, L. J. & Chatterjee, H. J. 2016. Well-being with objects: evaluating a museum object-handling intervention for older adults in health care settings. *Journal of Applied Gerontology*, 35, 349–362.

Thomson, L. J., Ander, E. E., Menon, U., Lanceley, A. & Chatterjee, H. J. 2011. Evaluating the therapeutic effects of museum object handling with hospital patients: a review and initial trial of well-being measures. *Journal of Applied Arts & Health*, 2, 37–56.

Thomson, L. J., Ander, E. E., Menon, U., Lanceley, A. & Chatterjee, H. J. 2012a. Enhancing cancer patient well-being with a nonpharmacological, heritage-focused intervention. *Journal of Pain and Symptom Management*, 44, 731–740.

Thomson, L. J., Ander, E. E., Menon, U., Lanceley, A. & Chatterjee, H. J. 2012b. Quantitative evidence for wellbeing benefits from a heritage-in-health intervention with hospital patients. *International Journal of Art Therapy*, 17, 63–79.

Thomson, L. J., Lockyer, B., Camic, P. M. & Chatterjee, H. J. 2018. Effects of a museum-based social prescription intervention on quantitative measures of psychological wellbeing in older adults. *Perspectives in Public Health*, 138, 28–38.

Thomson, L. J., Morse, N., Elsden, E. & Chatterjee, H. J. 2020. Art, nature and mental health: assessing the biopsychosocial effects of a 'creative green prescription' museum programme involving horticulture, artmaking and collections. *Perspectives in Public Health*, 140, 277–285.

Todd, C., Camic, P. M., Lockyer, B., Thomson, L. J. M. & Chatterjee, H. J. 2017. Museum-based programs for socially isolated older adults: understanding what works. *Health & Place*, 48, 47–55.

Vidovic, D., Reinhardt, G. Y. & Hammerton, C. 2021. Can social prescribing foster individual and community well-being? A systematic review of the evidence. *International Journal of Environmental Research and Public Health*, 18(10), 5276.

Wakefield, J. R. H., Kellezi, B., Stevenson, C., Mcnamara, N., Bowe, M., Wilson, I., Halder, M. M. & Mair, E. 2022. Social prescribing as 'social cure': a longitudinal study of the health benefits of social connectedness within a social prescribing pathway. *Journal of Health Psychology*, 27, 386–396.

White, M. P., Wheeler, B. W., Herbert, S., Alcock, I. & Depledge, M. H. 2014. Coastal proximity and physical activity: is the coast an under-appreciated public health resource? *Preventive Medicine*, 69, 135–140.

Wildman, J. M., Moffatt, S., Penn, L. & O'brien, N., Steer, M. & Hill, C. 2019. Link workers' perspectives on factors enabling and preventing client engagement with social prescribing. *Health & Social Care in the Community*, 27, 991–998.

Woodall, J., Trigwell, J., Bunyan, A.-M., Raine, G., Eaton, V., Davis, J., Hancock, L., Cunningham, M. & Wilkinson, S. 2018. Understanding the effectiveness and mechanisms of a social prescribing service: a mixed method analysis. *BMC Health Services Research*, 18, 604.

Wyke, S., Hunt, K., Gray, C. M., Fenwick, E., Bunn, C., Donnan, P. T., Rauchhaus, P., Mutrie, N., Anderson, A. S., Boyer, N., Brady, A., Grieve, E., White, A., Ferrell, C., Hindle, E. & Treweek, S. 2015. Public Health Research. *In: Football Fans in Training (FFIT): A Randomised Controlled Trial of a Gender-Sensitised Weight Loss and Healthy Living Programme for Men – End of Study Report*, Southampton (UK): NIHR Journals Library. https://www.ncbi.nlm.nih.gov/books/NBK273998/pdf/Bookshelf_NBK273998.pdf. Copyright © Queen's Printer and Controller of HMSO. 2015. This work was produced by Wyke et al. under the terms of a commissioning contract issued by the Secretary of State for Health. This issue may be freely reproduced for the purposes of private research and study and extracts (or indeed, the full report) may be included in professional journals provided that suitable acknowledgement is made and the reproduction is not associated with any form of advertising. Applications for commercial reproduction should be addressed to: NIHR Journals Library, National Institute for Health Research, Evaluation, Trials and Studies Coordinating Centre, Alpha House, University of Southampton Science Park, Southampton SO16 7NS, UK.

Wyke, S., Bunn, C., Andersen, E., Silva, M. N., Van Nassau, F., Mcskimming, P., Kolovos, S., Gill, J. M. R., Gray, C. M., Hunt, K., Anderson, A. S., Bosmans, J., Jelsma, J. G. M., Kean, S., Lemyre, N., Loudon, D. W., Macaulay, L., Maxwell, D. J., Mcconnachie, A., Mutrie, N., Nijhuis-Van Der Sanden, M., Pereira, H. V., Philpott, M., Roberts, G. C., Rooksby, J., Røynesdal, Ø. B., Sattar, N., Sørensen, M., Teixeira, P. J., Treweek, S., Van Achterberg, T., Van De Glind, I., Van Mechelen, W. & Van Der Ploeg, H. P. 2019. The effect of a programme to improve men's sedentary time and physical activity: the European fans in training (EuroFIT) randomised controlled trial. *PLoS Medicine*, 16, e1002736.

Zwolinsky, S., Mckenna, J., Pringle, A., Daly-Smith, A., Robertson, S. & White, A. 2013. Optimizing lifestyles for men regarded as 'hard-to-reach' through top-flight football/soccer clubs. *Health Education Research*, 28, 405–413.

PART 5

Leading Safe and Effective Care in Increasingly Changing Healthcare Systems

Leading Safe and Effective Healthcare Teams: Leadership, Management and Complexity

Matt Flynn and Chris Allen

School of Health Sciences, University of Southampton, Southampton, UK

Introduction

The chapters so far have highlighted the importance of delivering care in a socially sensitive and equitable way, to ensure that the needs of those accessing care are adequately met. Leadership, and specifically team leadership, play an important part in creating environments of care able to achieve this. In the following two chapters, we will consider healthcare's complex adaptive systems in the context of leadership and teamwork. In this first chapter, we will explore what effective and inclusive leadership and management in healthcare is. To do this, we will explore what is known about the various ways that leadership and management operate within a healthcare context, through the work of social sciences, including organisational studies. We will also explore the impact of any specific leader or leadership style, and how a leader's actions can inspire or demotivate individuals and groups.

Certain behaviours can create opportunities for integration, but they can also create isolation, leaving team members feeling undervalued and unheard, and potentially even leading to unsafe situations. We will start by considering the context of leadership. Leadership is made necessary by the increasingly complex care environments that are now common in most healthcare systems. To fully understand the work systems within which leaders operate, we will briefly introduce you to complexity, systems thinking, human factors and ergonomics.

LEARNING OUTCOMES

By the end of this chapter, you will be able to:

- Understand the importance of designing work systems around the needs of staff and patients, to ensure safe and effective care.
- Understand the impact of leadership and management in healthcare, and why both are important.
- Consider the different ways leadership has been considered, including healthcare specifically.

Complexity and Contemporary Healthcare

> **Key Terms and Definitions**
>
> **Complex adaptive systems:** Are characterised by dynamic interactions between different parts of a complex system. The impact of actions, such as making a change to one part of the system, cannot always be fully anticipated within these systems.

Social Sciences for Healthcare Professionals, First Edition. Edited by Chris Allen.
© 2026 John Wiley & Sons Ltd. Published 2026 by John Wiley & Sons Ltd.

> **Human factors/ergonomics:** Ergonomics is a scientific discipline that is concerned with understanding human interactions within systems, recognising that humans are fallible (i.e. they make mistakes) and that work systems should be designed with this in mind.
>
> **Leadership:** Influencing the behaviour of individuals and groups, usually towards a goal or goal accomplishment.
>
> **Management:** Generally, relates to managing a set of human and/or non-human resources, within an organisational context.

For a while now, healthcare has been recognised as increasingly complex and constantly evolving (Holmes et al., 2017, Plsek and Greenhalgh, 2001). We have already shown evidence of this throughout this book, both in terms of the different professionals that are involved in care (chapter 6), as well as the recognition of the increasingly diverse and complex needs of patients themselves throughout the life course (chapter 7) and the increasing recognition of wider determinants of health (chapter 8). Many factors are now understood to contribute to health and subsequently increase the complexity of care. In addition, as we explore in more depth in chapter 20, new innovations are influencing how care is provided, and whilst technology can be an enabler, it can also further increase the complexity of the socio-technical systems in which care is typically provided (Carayon et al., 2020). All these factors, alongside others, have and continue to require staff to work collaboratively and be adaptive to change, as the resilience of healthcare systems around the world is continuously tested (Belrhiti et al., 2018, Carayon et al., 2020, Salas et al., 2018b). This also increases the need for teamwork (discussed in the next chapter), as well as the importance of healthcare leaders to be able to support themselves, and their teams to adapt to and embrace situations of near-constant change and complexity (Belrhiti et al., 2018, Dinh et al., 2020, Shuffler and Carter, 2018).

Leadership can influence care across different levels of society, with some degree of overlap (i.e. micro, meso and macro levels – see chapter 2). For example, an encounter between individual team members can be influenced by the environments that leaders and colleagues co-create, as well as the direction the leader sets. Likewise, how responsive care environments are to people's needs, and how sensitively they respond to them can be significantly influenced by leader behaviours, and the direction they set, including what is prioritised and what is not. These micro-level interactions are shaped and constrained by the policies and procedures of the care environment, which can be influenced by leadership behaviours at different levels of the organisation, and even broader national policy at the macro level, which can influence how care is thought about and delivered – what is prioritised and what is not. Leaders can influence care across healthcare systems, and when things go wrong, it is often the 'leaders' and 'leadership' that is called into question and argued to be deficient.

Complex Systems: When Things Go Wrong

In the context of the United Kingdom, several recent reviews have highlighted significant shortcomings in patient safety and care. These include the Report of the Mid Staffordshire NHS Foundation Trust Public Enquiry (Francis, 2013) and the independent review of maternity services of Shrewsbury and Telford Hospital NHS Trust, often referred to as the Ockenden review (Ockenden, 2022). Lord Francis, in the report into the documented failings of Mid Staffordshire, highlighted significant shortcomings in care that occurred within a complex system (Francis, 2013).

The issues that were seen, could not be attributed to any one individual. Certainly, there were individuals, including those in positions of power and influence who could have done better. But Francis rightly pointed out that 'when examining what went wrong in the case of a systems failure as complex as that surrounding the events in Stafford, the temptation of offering up scapegoats is a dangerous one which must be resisted' (Francis, 2013). Whilst no one individual was blamed, the role of poor leadership was highlighted throughout the report (Francis, 2013). It should be recognised that healthcare leadership, as with other organisational contexts, is often seen as a panacea, or magic catch-all remedy for improvement. Essentially, if we only had more, or better leaders, maybe everything would work better. Yet even the most inspiring and capable leaders are required to work within complex multi-team systems that can limit their positive impact and dilute their influence (Salas et al., 2018a, Shuffler and Carter, 2018).

The Francis report highlighted the challenges relating to inadequate staffing levels and other, broader, system influences commonly faced by healthcare professionals. It recognised that when things go wrong, it is generally the case that the root cause is multifaceted, and the result of complex interactions within an increasingly complex socio-technical healthcare system (Belrhiti et al., 2018, Carayon et al., 2020, Holden et al., 2013).

Human Factors and Ergonomics

Since the Institute of Medicine (IOM) in the United States of America (USA) published its now seminal review of human factors in healthcare, interest has grown significantly, largely because of its recognised impact on care quality and safety (IOM, 2000). Historically, when things have gone wrong in healthcare, there have been efforts to understand the 'root cause' of the issue. Often this root cause has been identified as an individual, who for whatever reason, either deliberately or accidentally did something that was 'wrong' or created the opportunity or environment that led to patient harm occurring. However, the reality is that most incidents that occur in practice, are not the sole result of any single person's actions or omissions. Humans make mistakes. All the time in fact. But with adequate work systems, these mistakes should not lead to harm. For example, in the context of human factors, comparisons are often drawn with aviation (Kapur et al., 2016). When a pilot makes a mistake, the work system is generally designed in such a way that any impact on people is limited (crashes are uncommon – planes do not generally fall out of the sky following a simple act or omission). This is through the recognition that people are fallible, they make mistakes and by only focusing on individuals, we fail to make more resilient work systems, where inevitable human mistakes are less costly (IOM, 2000). We can train healthcare professionals who have made mistakes, but other healthcare professionals will continue to make the same mistake if we do not fix the underlying issues with the work systems that allow harm to occur (Carayon et al., 2020, IOM, 2000, Kapur et al., 2016). Work systems that are appropriately designed and consider human fallibility are safer systems (Carayon et al., 2006, Carayon et al., 2020, Holden et al., 2013, Reason, 1990). 'Human Factors' and 'Ergonomics' are two approaches that focus on the relationship between humans, their environment, equipment and capabilities, with a view to reducing opportunities for error and improving care quality and safety.

When unpicking incidents, accidents and issues related to patient safety, several models are used to allow us to explore the root cause and help us better consider work systems and how they influence care quality and particularly safety (Carayon et al., 2006, Carayon et al., 2014, Carayon et al., 2020, Donabedian, 1988, Holden et al., 2013, Reason, 1990). These models can help us to reorientate our approach when things *do* go wrong and work with healthcare teams to design and put in place better systems that reduce the likeliness of similar issues arising in the future to other individuals and groups. Two notable models that we will discuss further are Reason's seminal Swiss Cheese Model (Reason, 1990) and the Systems Engineering Initiative of Patient Safety (SEIPS) models, of which there are now three versions, reflecting how thinking has evolved in this area (Carayon et al., 2006, Carayon et al., 2020, Holden et al., 2013). We will now expand on these.

Reasons Swiss Cheese Model (Theory of Active and Latent Failures)

The theory of active and latent failures first proposed by James Reason (1938–2025) provides the underpinnings of the Swiss Cheese Model (Reason, 2000). Like the SEIPS models, which we will go on to discuss, the model recognises the complex socio-technical systems within which errors often occur. Whilst there are multiple layers to the model (e.g. unsafe acts, preconditions, supervisory factors), most discussed are active failures (the acts or omissions of individuals) and latent conditions (essentially the latent unsafe conditions or holes in the Swiss cheese) (Wiegmann et al., 2022). The model highlights that people's acts or omissions should have only a limited impact on outcomes if

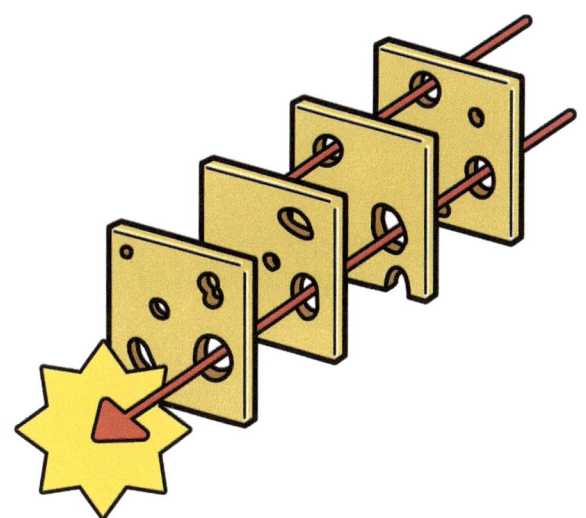

FIGURE 18.1   Reason's Swiss Cheese Model. **Source:** sasami018 / Adobe Stock Photos.

adequate work systems are in place to prevent their impact (Wiegmann et al., 2022). For example, in a closed loop medication administration system, nurses are alerted when they scan the wrong patient's ID (Holden et al., 2013, Spataru et al., 2024). Though the nurse has made an error, the work system is safe enough to prevent harm from happening. Incidents occur when active failures can move through the latent conditions (essentially vulnerabilities in the work system). You can think of this as passing through the holes of a Swiss cheese as shown in Figure 18.1.

As a model, it is commonly used to guide root cause analysis when something goes wrong, helping to identify holes in the system and steering attempts to close these (turning the Swiss cheese into a solid wedge of cheese with no vulnerabilities instead) (Wiegmann et al., 2022). Whilst a useful and thought-provoking heuristic, the model is simplistic and reactive. Rather than using a model such as the Swiss cheese model to identify latent issues and fix these, it is more proactive to design work systems around the needs of individuals, work teams and patients themselves. The SEIPS models can help us do this – and these all highlight people as central to systems thinking – reinforcing that systems should be designed with their capabilities and limitations in mind (Holden et al., 2013).

The Systems Engineering Initiative of Patient Safety (SEIPS) Models

First created in 2006, and now in its third iteration, the Systems Engineering Initiative for Patient Safety (SEIPS) model provides a comprehensive overview of work systems, and how they contribute to outcomes including patient safety (Carayon et al., 2006, Carayon et al., 2020, Holden et al., 2013). It is designed through the perspectives of human factors and ergonomics, placing 'person(s)' (individual

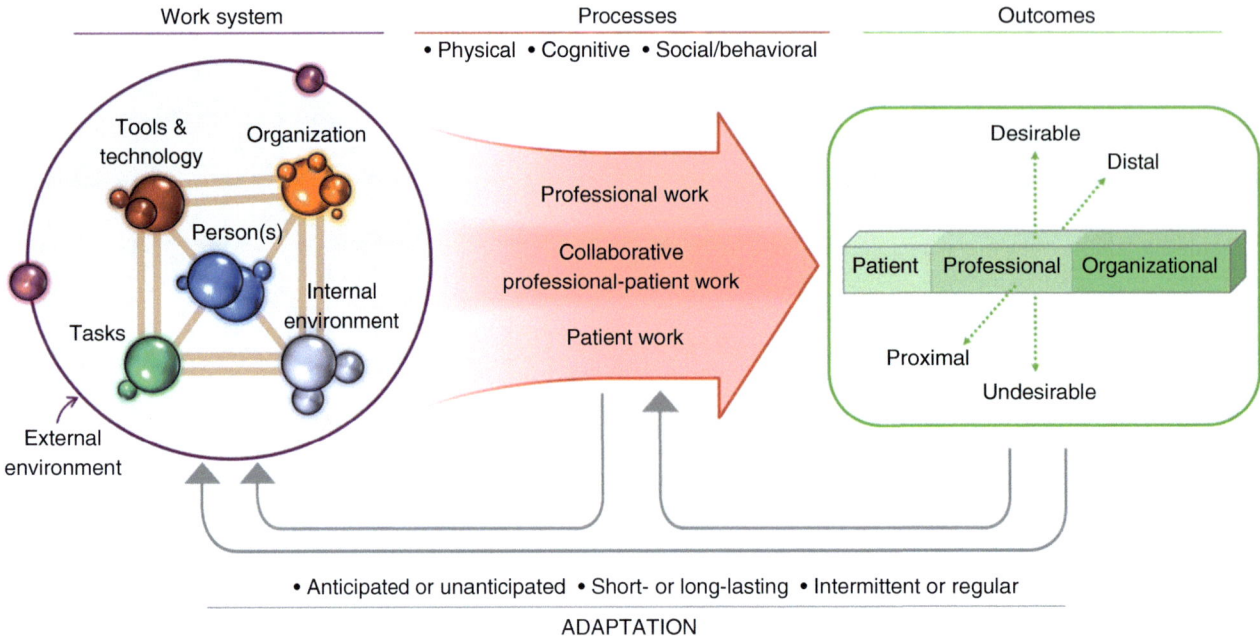

FIGURE 18.2 The SEIPS 2.0 model. **Source:** Holden et al., (2013) / with permission of Taylor & Francis Group.

healthcare professionals, healthcare teams or patients) at the model's centre and emphasising that work systems must be designed to promote quality, safety and well-being (including for healthcare workers) (Carayon et al., 2020, Holden et al., 2013). The model evolved from the Donabedian Structure-Process-Outcome (SPO) model, and both are examples of systems models (Carayon et al., 2020, Donabedian, 1988). The second iteration of the SEIPS model is shown in Figure 18.2.

Within the SEIPS models, the '**work system**' is composed of the person(s), task, tools and technologies (which we will expand upon in chapter 20), environment and organisational conditions, which influence and interact with one another, and through these influences and interactions produce different outcomes (such as quality and safety) depending on how effective or not the work system is. Whilst what exactly is included within the work system has evolved across the three versions of SEIPS, ensuring the model remains contemporary, the fundamental aspects of the work system have remained intact (Carayon et al., 2006, Carayon et al., 2020, Holden et al., 2013).

Let us focus on the **person** and the **environment** of this work system, and how these interact with the other aspects:

The person: Deliberately placed in the centre of the model. This could be you as a healthcare professional. Or even a patient or someone accessing care, as they are increasingly recognised as doing much of the health-related work (emphasised in SEIPS 2.0 and 3.0) (Carayon et al., 2020, Holden et al., 2013). It could even be a healthcare team or group of people. Importantly, a systems approach

recognises that this person interacts with *tools and technologies*, to do various health-related *tasks* (which can vary in terms of their complexity).

The environment: The *tasks* that people carry out, and the *tools and technologies* (which can vary in terms of their usability and accessibility, etc.) that they use to do them, are nested within an *environment*. Environmental conditions (such as noise and poor lighting) can make the completion of tasks trickier. In addition, work environments in which these *tasks* are carried out are also influenced by various *organisational conditions* (such as culture, teamwork, leadership, power distances and hierarchy, psychological safety, and technical infrastructure). The external environment is also relevant, as various macro-level social, economic and political influences can shape micro and meso-level work systems (Holden et al., 2013).

The SEIPS models serve to highlight just how much goes on within a socio-technical system, and the importance of working with people, tasks, technologies and organisational conditions, to create care environments that are safe, and that meet people's needs (Carayon et al., 2006, Carayon et al., 2020, Holden et al., 2013). We will return to the most recent iteration of SEIPS (3.0) towards the end of this chapter. However, all these models highlight the important role of people in creating work systems that are safe and effective, and leadership and management play a vitally important role in creating and maintaining such systems, especially through their influence on organisational conditions, as well as through their influence, vision, control and coordination of resources and work-related tasks.

What Is Leadership and How Is It Different to Management?

Often used interchangeably, leadership and management are different but related concepts (Fennell, 2021). Leadership has been described as a choice, not a rank (Sinek, 2017). So, if we see leadership as a choice, rather than a rank or something that is tied to power, status or hierarchy, then presumably anyone can choose to be a leader. However, within a healthcare context, a traditional perspective of a healthcare 'leader' refers to a person in 'charge'. This person was often in a position of authority and is responsible for directing and managing teams, to ensure that high-quality care is provided and overarching organisational goals are achieved. This position is something many of you will still be familiar with. Leadership is often assumed to relate to specific roles (such as ward leader/manager) that may also involve aspects that relate to management, such as operational oversight, and the management of human and non-human resources (equipment, finances, etc.) (Bennett and James, 2022, Fennell, 2021). Whilst management and leadership do clearly share some overlapping features, they are different and draw on fundamentally different approaches and systems. For example, managers operate within a framework of policies and procedures, essentially, the tools of bureaucracy (Gopee and Galloway, 2017, Northouse, 2022). In contrast, a leader's main tool or 'currency' is their influence, which they can use to engage, motivate and inspire others (Gopee and Galloway, 2017, Northouse, 2022).

Because anyone can influence, it can be argued that anyone can be a leader provided they have a vision of what needs to be achieved and can inspire others to be invested in it too (Fennell, 2021, Gopee and Galloway, 2017, Kouzes and Posner, 1995). Leadership is sometimes associated with status and authority, but you don't need these to lead (Fennell, 2021). Where management roles have inherent links with hierarchy and authority, leadership is more about role modelling and inspiring others through actions, creating shared visions that people can ascribe to and engage with; and eliciting followership by making people feel valued, and that their contributions are important (Fennel, 2021, Gopee and Galloway, 2017, Northouse, 2022). Leadership influence can be so strong that others may also be inspired to lead, strengthening the team and increasing the likelihood of achieving overarching visions (Gopee and Galloway, 2017, Northouse, 2022). However, leaders can also inspire people to do disruptive or harmful things, and whilst important in terms of motivating teams towards goal accomplishment, is not without risks, especially if the goal is counter to the needs of the team, the organisation, or even society.

Stop and Think: What Does a Healthcare Leader Look Like?

You are encouraged to read the following two case studies and reflect on the below questions that relate to them.

Case Study One

Steve works on a ward and has identified a small area of outdoor space that he believes could be better utilised as a garden area, full of flowers, vegetables and a bug hotel. Initially self-funding some small pot plants and a few bags of compost, he goes to work.

Within six weeks, he has a small budget to purchase the things that he needs to create his outdoor space. He also has three patients who were interested in what he was doing and begun to help him daily to maintain the upkeep of the space.

Within six months, he has created a garden project, involving a variety of patients, that has achieved organisational acknowledgement for his work. He is now the main point of contact for five other green spaces being developed in his original project blueprint.

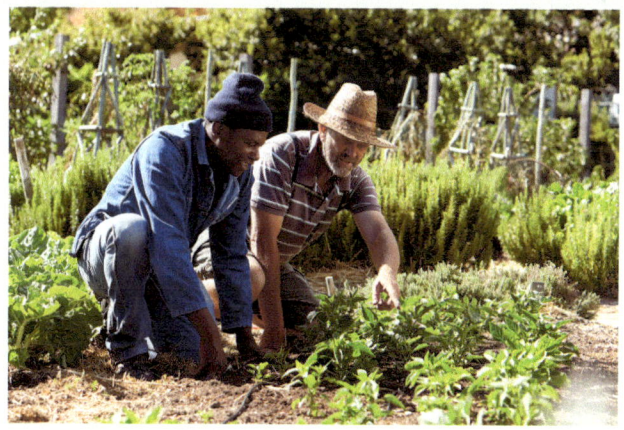

Source: Monkey Business/Adobe Stock Photos.

Case Study Two

Helen has worked within the organisation for the last 14 years. In that time she has seen several managers come and go. Having worked there for so long, she understands all the roles in the team, and the work environment. This has led to other staff, especially those who are new approaching her for advice or guidance.

Helen is happy with the shifts that she does, believing that she has done her fair share of unsociable hours over the years. She works one day during the week and then on a Saturday and Sunday, largely for the unsociable hours extra pay this gets her.

When Kirsty, a new manager joins the unit, she calls a meeting to highlight several changes including changes to shifts and working patterns to promote an equitable distribution of shifts. However, within two weeks of this meeting, Kirsty begins to recognise she has a significant challenge in developing relationships with the unit's staff. She notices an increased reluctance to engage in her proposed changes, and staff increasingly engaging with Helen as their main source of information, guidance and support.

Consider both case studies and the impact of Steve and Helen. Would you consider Steve, Helen or Kirsty to be a leader? What elements of leadership can you identify?

You might also wish to consider the following:

- What leadership qualities did Steve demonstrate in identifying and acting on the opportunity to create an outdoor garden space?
- Do you think Steve had intended to become a leader?
- How might the length of time an individual has worked within a team, as seen with Helen, affect leadership dynamics and the reception of new leaders?
- In what ways does the informal leadership that Helen showed, affect the formal leadership structures and decision-making of the unit?
- What role did followership play in the two cases?

Leadership can be thought of as both a social construct and a social process (Lord et al., 2017). As a construct, it goes beyond any individual and their ability to inspire or motivate, as the expectations of a leader, and even to an extent who can easily lead is influenced by society. For example, some people have traditionally been far more likely to be put forward into roles (such as white men or those with very high intellect) in which they have more potential to influence and inspire others (Lord et al., 2017, Stanley, 2022). This is not to say that those falling outside of these groups cannot lead, as they absolutely can, but they do have barriers in the form of social stereotypes (which are themselves shaped by culture, norms, values and beliefs) relating to leadership that may make it harder for them to have that opportunity in the first place. In addition, people's understanding of leadership and leaders, and what is expected of them, are based on their own lived experience, as well as societal norms and values around leadership and how it is seen (Northouse, 2022). Similarly, leadership can be thought of as a social process; essentially a social relationship that emerges between leaders and their followers (Fennel, 2021, Lord et al., 2017, Monzani and Van Dick, 2020). Leadership requires relational work – leaders must build and maintain ties with others, identifying their strengths and potential contributions, to ensure they can maximise collaboration through communication and at times, the further diffusion and distribution of leadership within a group (Fennel, 2021, Lord et al., 2017, Monzani and Van Dick, 2020, Northouse, 2022).

A significant amount of literature has been written about leadership in healthcare contexts (see Wu et al., 2024 for one recent overview), and we cannot cover it all in the scope of this chapter. Whilst no universally agreed definition exists, most point towards leadership being a process rooted in an ability to influence others, towards the attainment of an agreed goal or vision (Fennell, 2021, Gopee and Galloway, 2017, Northouse, 2022).

As we have discussed, leadership and management are often pitched against each other and do share some overlap,

especially where leaders are also in management or supervisory roles (Bennett and James, 2022, Fennel, 2021, Gopee and Galloway, 2017, Northouse, 2022). However, it is important to emphasise that leadership is not better than management or vice versa (Bennett and James, 2022, Gopee and Galloway, 2017). Both are integral to achieving organisational

Stop and Think: Leadership or Management?

From the information previously provided, consider the table below and confirm whether you believe they relate to management or leadership. Do they fit neatly into one or the other? Could some fit into both or is there a distinct difference?

Task	Management	Leadership
Create a vision		
Allocate resources		
Motivate stakeholders (including team members)		
Plan		
Welcome risk		
Explain procedures and monitor these		
Utilise stakeholder (including team members) strengths		
Inspire engagement		
Manage performance		

goals, including in healthcare (Bennett and James, 2022, Gopee and Galloway, 2017). Organisations are often reliant on management and bureaucratic processes to ensure care is delivered safely and effectively, and that employers have rules and procedures that they can follow to guide their working practices (Bennett and James, 2022, Gopee and Galloway, 2017).

Another fundamental difference between leaders and managers is the different influences, uses and impacts of power. There are different forms of power, which are used by managers and leaders. Some different types of power are summarised in Table 18.1.

TABLE 18.1   Different types of power.

Reward power	Reward power generally relates to the ability to provide rewards to people. Usually, these are financial rewards, but they can also be in the form of other things, such as time, favours or anything that is deemed to be valuable to the recipient (essentially, the 'carrot').
Punishment, authoritarian or coercive power	This relates to the ability to create fear, through actual, implied or perceived threats, and can be related to job security, progression or similarly the loss of something meaningful to the recipient (essentially, the 'stick' to reward powers 'carrot')
Legitimate power	This relates to the power that someone has bestowed on them, based on their rank or based on their role within an organisation.
Expert power	When we have specific knowledge or expertise, we can be described as having 'expert power'. This is because with have a credible voice, especially in discussions that relate to our area of expertise. This power is context specific. For example, a healthcare professional has less expert power than a mechanic in a car garage.
Referent or charismatic power	You will have likely encountered very charismatic people who are easy to follow. Their charisma gives them the power to motivate and inspire others. Charisma is often discussed in the context of leadership, particularly transformational leadership (discussed later).
Resource power	This can sometimes be harder to see but generally relates to someone being able to control access to needed resources, such as budgets, or physical resources, such as equipment (e.g. the ward manager that refuses to let hybrid team members care for patients off the ward, using the wards IV pumps) (Sanford et al., 2024), as well as, having power over rosters and working patterns.
Informational power	The power that is gained through being 'in the know'. This power relates to having access to information that others might need and being able to control who gets access to it. This information can relate to other colleagues, as well as planned changes to working practices, or commercially sensitive or confidential information.

Source: Adapted from James, AH and Bennett, CL. (2022).

> **Stop and Think: What Types of Power Do You Regularly Encounter in Your Work?**
>
> Consider your current circumstances, are you aware of the types of power that you regularly encounter but have not been able to previously identify them, using the taxonomy provided in Table 18.1? You might want to think about this in the current role that you have, but you might also find it useful to reflect on previous roles. You might want to reflect on the following:
>
> - Who controls the hours you work?
> - How do you access information?
> - Who makes decisions regarding your role, wages or time off?
> - What power do you have to influence these factors?

What Makes a Leader?

So far, we have outlined why leadership is important, highlighted how it is different to management and given you some sense of how valuable good leadership and management are to healthcare delivery. Now, we turn to leaders, who they are and what they do. First, we consider people's own behaviours, and how well they can lead themselves, as this ultimately influences how well-placed they are to lead others.

Self-Leadership and Emotional Intelligence

Rather than seeing leadership as simply influencing others, the concept of self-leadership captures our ability to influence and motivate ourselves (Stewart et al., 2019). Related to how well we can lead ourselves is the concept of emotional intelligence (of which there are many definitions), which is important to leaders and leadership behaviours, because it relates to how well we know and subsequently handle ourselves, and the relationships we are able to form with others, such as patients and team members. The seminal work of Daniel Goleman (1998) highlights the following aspects of emotional intelligence:

Self-awareness: This involves understanding how you feel, and how your own emotions might impact on you and those you work with. Being unaware of your emotions, and how they influence your own behaviours and judgments can influence your decision-making and might lead to you reacting in ways that don't align with your values and how you want to behave. Being self-aware, also means you can reflect and work on your own strengths, weaknesses, and biases (covered in chapter 9), acting on and improving on limitations.

Self-regulation: *Being self-aware, especially in the context of your own emotions and how they influence what you do, is arguably a prerequisite to self-regulation, which is the ability to recognise and control behaviours that might negatively impact on yourself, and those that you work with. People who can self-regulate themselves well, are more likely to influence and instil confidence in others.*

Motivation: *Understanding what motivates yourself and what might motivate others.*

Empathy: *Being able to recognise and respond appropriately to the feelings and concerns of others. Essentially, how well someone can put themselves into someone else's position and understand their emotions.*

Social skills: Good social skills help with building and managing relationships. This can involve taking action to manage the emotions of others within a team, resolving conflict, building motivation and inspiring others.

Once people can appropriately lead themselves (i.e. their internal leadership), they are in a better position to lead and positively influence the actions of others. There are a range of ways in which people can be influential, and how we have thought about leadership, and the different approaches that are recognised and promoted (including in health), have evolved over the years.

The Evolution of Leadership Theories and Approaches

Interest in 'leaders' and 'leadership' has a long history, and how we think about leaders has changed significantly over the years (Fennell, 2021, Lord et al., 2017, Northouse, 2022, Stanley, 2022).

Stop and Think: Emotional Intelligence in Two Conversations

Take some time to consider the following two versions of a conversation and consider the role emotional intelligence has played in the outcome. The names below are fictitious but reflect conversations that you may have seen played out in actual practice.

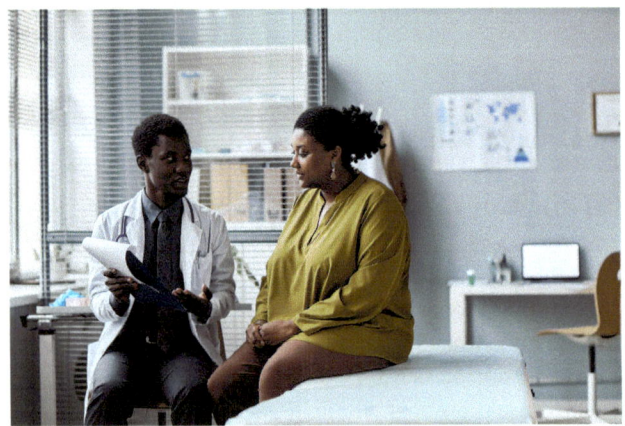

Source: Seventyfour/Adobe Stock Photos.

Conversation 1

Doctor Jones: Hi, how are you today? I know this has been a difficult time for you and imagine you have been feeling quite anxious.

Samira: I'm OK, thank you, but this is all I've been able to think about and I'm so worried that this will be bad news or worse than I had initially thought.

Doctor Jones: I can understand that Samira, and completely understand why you would be so worried. It's normal to feel that way. Perhaps if I talk you through the process that may help you?

Samira: I would really appreciate that. Thank you. I think it is not knowing that makes it so difficult.

Conversation 2

Doctor Jones: Good morning, Samira, how can I help?

Samira: I'm just so worried about this situation, it's all I can think about, and I'm so worried it's going to be worse than I thought.

Doctor Jones: Samira, as I have told you, I am still awaiting the result, so I am unable to provide any further information to you at this time and wouldn't want to jump to any conclusions.

Samira: Ok. I understand. It's just that the waiting is so difficult. It is really getting to me.

Doctor Jones: Look, Samira, I have lots of patients in a similar situation, and as I say to them, I can't change the speed by which these results are produced, so we'll just have to wait. I will contact you as soon as they are back and I have time.

Your reflections

Having read the two different conversations, we would like you to reflect on the following points.

- What was the difference between the two conversations? Did you recognise any examples of validation, emotional regulation or empathy in either example? Were there any elements that you were uncomfortable with? If so, why?

- How do you think each conversation might have affected Samira? Which conversation would you have more liked to have been on the receiving end of? Why?

A summary of the significant changes in how leaders and leadership are seen is provided in Table 18.2.

Lord et al. (2017) have highlighted three waves of leadership theory, which provides a useful overview of the evolution of ideas about leaders, who they are and what they do to influence and inspire others. Many social factors have influenced how we think about leaders and leadership, such as globalisation, new technologies, as well as the diversification of the workplace, which have shaped what leaders are expected or need to be able to do (i.e. who they are expected to influence and how), as well as who exactly can and should be a leader (Lord et al., 2017, Stanley, 2022).

Traits Approaches to Leadership

Traits and characteristic-based approaches focus on people's characteristics. They suggest that leaders have special, perhaps even superior 'traits' or 'qualities' that set them apart from followers and give them the ability to lead others (Fennell, 2021, Lord et al., 2017, Northouse, 2022, Stanley, 2022). These traits and characteristics can be incredibly diverse, for example, self-confidence, intelligence, integrity, determination and abundant reserves of energy (Stanley, 2022). Whilst

overtime traits-based approaches have generated less interest, they still at times form the basis of hiring and development practices (Lord et al., 2017).

Leadership Behaviours and Styles

Rather than looking at the specific traits of leaders, and claiming only those people with these can lead, behavioural models focus instead on the behaviours and actions that leaders use when they are influencing others (Fennell, 2021, Lord et al., 2017, Northouse, 2022, Stanley, 2022). In short, rather than considering the leader's traits, behavioural models focus on what leaders *do*. There are various leadership styles that range from high to low direction. These are summarised in Figure 18.3.

Situational Leadership

Seminal work has highlighted that managers (or leaders) tend to have preferential ways of working and leading, which may make them well-equipped to lead in certain situations (such as when working with a highly competent and

TABLE 18.2   Evolution of leadership theories.

Theory	Period	Summary
Great man theory	**Mid-1800s**	Individuals (usually men) are born leaders. They have certain characteristics that make them well-suited to lead. Leaders are born not made – i.e. 'he was a born leader'. Those without this 'birthright', must be led.
		This theory lacks evidence and has been replaced with theories that highlight anyone can lead.
Traits approach	**1930s**	Not hugely dissimilar to the great man theory. This suggested that leaders had certain 'traits' or 'characteristics', such as physical, social or personal characteristics that make them well-suited to lead. However, some traits can be developed (unlike great man theory).
		There is no definitive list of traits that make people good leaders. Some traits are often discussed as supporting leadership, such as extroversion and openness to experience. The list of traits a good leader was expected to have was significant and many highly effective leaders do not possess all identified traits.
Skills approach	**1940s**	Suggests that leadership skills can be learned – i.e. anyone can become a leader – setting it apart from traits and great man theories.
		It was however unclear how variations in skills led to different leadership performances.
Styles approach	**1940s**	These move beyond leader traits and skills, to consider how leaders behave (what they do, how they act and how people respond). Some examples are provided in Figure 18.3, though many different leadership styles have been proposed.
		Leaders can be task orientated or people (i.e. relational) orientated.
		Leaders may tend to lean more to one style, but no one style is appropriate in all contexts.
Situational leadership theory	**1960s**	Whilst leaders might have preferred ways of leading, the situational leadership theory, sometimes referred to as contingency theory, suggests that effective leaders can flex their approach to different situations (who is involved, what is involved, the organisational context, etc.). Good leadership requires flexibility – a one-size-fits-all approach is not appropriate. This theory highlights why some leaders do better in some situations than others, and why different team members may be better equipped to lead at different times.

Source: Adapted from Fennell (2021) and James and Bennett (2022).

Autocratic (high direction)		Democratic (low direction)	
Positive	Negative	Positive	Negative
Clarity regarding the decision maker	Staff are not able to contribute	Promotes team engagement	Lots of different opinions
Quick decisions can be made	Single point of knowledge / truth	People feel engaged and empowered	Finding a consensus can lead to frustration
Single point of contact and accountability	Stress and pressure held by one person	A range of perspectives can be considered	Can be time consuming
Clearly defined rules/procedures and processes	Can lead to low morale	Knowledge gaps can be avoided	Original goal can become lost or sidelined
Bureaucratic (high direction)		Laissez farie (low direction)	
Positive	Negative	Positive	Negative
Clearly defined hierarchy and individual roles	It is inflexible in its structure	People feel empowered	Only engagement is when there are problems. Reactive.
Works within a framework of policies and procedures	Limits freedom for creativity and innovation	Promotes creativity and innovation	Can be subject to communication challenges and miscommunication
Impersonal approach based on skills / expertise	Based on rules and regulations	Promotes a sense of autonomy	Lack of structure and clear guidance
Clear accountability	The rigidity of the approach can cause frustration	Reduced sense of "being managed"	Confusion re: accountability

FIGURE 18.3 Leadership high and low direction behaviours. **Source:** Adapted from Stanley (2022).

motivated team, all working in the same place), but less well equipped to lead in other situations (such as when working with a team who are inexperienced, and unsure of how to complete a task, and may not be co-located) (Fiedler, 1964, Hersey and Blanchard, 1969). In addition, certain leaders may be more likely to gel with certain followers and this is potentially influenced by all sorts of characteristics (such as age) (Lord et al., 2017). Whilst leaders might have preferred approaches to leadership, ranging from high through to low direction, it is unlikely that any one style will be appropriate for all situations, and this is particularly the case in healthcare, where environmental stressors and continuously evolving complexity require more dynamic and flexible approaches to be adopted, to meet the needs of different situations as they arise (Belrhiti et al., 2018). Situational leadership approaches essentially highlight the importance of leaders adapting their style in response to the context of those they are leading, and the context within which they are leading them (different situations, different needs of people in their teams, etc.) (Belrhiti et al., 2018, Hersey and Blanchard, 1969, Northouse, 2022, Vroom and Jago, 2007).

Transformational Leadership

The transformational leadership approach is now one of the most widely discussed and researched (Dinh et al., 2014, Lord et al., 2017, Northouse, 2022), including in the context of healthcare leadership (Fennell, 2021, Wu et al., 2024). Transformational leaders often have strong values and ideals that they hope to instil in others (Northouse, 2022). Transformational leadership gets its name through its role in changing (or transforming) people (both leaders and followers) (Northouse, 2022). This transformation can occur at micro (i.e. between individuals), meso (i.e. across an organisation or workgroup) or macro level (i.e. entire societies), and the transformations can be good and bad (often referred to as pseudo transformational leadership) (Bass, 1998, Fennell, 2021, Northouse, 2022).

Transformational leaders are often charismatic and visionary and can be highly effective in motivating individuals and teams towards doing more than expected (House and Howell, 1992, Northouse, 2022, Stanley, 2022). That this approach has the potential to motivate people to do more than expected, is perhaps why it has become so popular in healthcare contexts characterised by shortages, increased demands and the need to innovate and change (Wu et al., 2024). Motivation from transformational leadership is intrinsic (i.e. it comes from within), rather than extrinsic (such as being motivated by money or reward), setting transformational leadership apart from transactional leadership (I do this for you, you do this for me – a common influencing approach in much of society), and resulting in followers exceeding what is expected. Transformational leaders are said to focus on the needs of those they work with, recognising and valuing their contributions, building beliefs, morals, values, ethics and trust, and providing inspiration to increase individual and group moral decision-making and intrinsic motivation (Northouse, 2022, Zhu et al., 2011).

Criticisms of transformational leadership generally point towards its traits like heroic leadership features (especially in the context of charisma – suggesting it cannot be taught), that leaders might set people to change in harmful ways, as well as its lack of conceptual clarity (Fennell, 2021, Northouse, 2022, Stanley, 2022, van Knippenberg and Sitkin, 2013). The lack of conceptual clarity is largely because it has several components and activities, and whilst theoretical models exist about how these hang together, it is hard to capture and measure in a meaningful way. Scales do exist, such as the multifactor leadership questionnaire, though these have been criticised (Northouse, 2022). Some things are just hard to measure, though we all likely intuitively know a transformational when we see one, and can likely reflect on the powerful impact they have had on us and those around us. In the context of health, transformational leadership is highly studied, with around 41% of papers included in a recent review looking at it (Wu et al., 2024). Included papers suggested that transformational leadership within healthcare contexts may be important in creating positive safety cultures and high-quality care (Alloubani et al., 2019, Lappalainen et al., 2020, Seljemo et al., 2020), as well as promoting patient-centred care (Ree, 2020), and improving patient and staff satisfaction and staff retention (Labrague et al., 2020, Pishgooie et al., 2019, Wu et al., 2020, Xie et al., 2020). In addition, recent reviews have found that transformational leadership can increase organisational commitment in nursing staff and can improve retention (Conroy et al., 2023, Haoyan et al., 2023).

Leader-Member Exchange Theory

Leader-member exchange theory is a relationship-based approach to leadership, focusing on the relationships a leader has with their individual followers (Fennell, 2021, Lord et al., 2017, Northouse, 2022). It is largely set apart from other leadership theories, in that it essentially looks at the variance in relationships, particularly in the different leader–follower dyads, emphasising that each of these is unique and can sit on a high-quality, low-quality continuum (Lord et al., 2017, Northouse, 2022). Rather than leaders behaving in the same way with all their followers, leaders treat each of their followers differently, depending on their relationship quality with these (i.e. a unique leader–follower relationship), and how these might develop over time, for example, from strangers where

the groundwork is laid, to a relationship characterised by trust, mutual understanding and respect, fostering commitment and obligation (Lord et al., 2017, Northouse, 2022).

The characteristics of leaders and followers (or members) may have a role in how well relationships develop – for example, members who are extraverted and leaders who are agreeable, may well 'gel' better than those with less compatible characteristics (Lord et al., 2017, Northouse, 2022). This approach, which looks at social relationships, is not hugely dissimilar to some of the social network approaches discussed in chapter 15 and largely considers the relational quality and the outcomes associated with these (e.g. team effectiveness and job satisfaction). However, research looking at how these relationships evolve over time is sparse (Lord et al., 2017), unlike the trends increasingly seen in social network studies (explored in chapter 15). Leader-member exchange has been explored in healthcare contexts, for example, a recent student found that whilst leader-member exchanges clearly existed, these were influenced by the organisational culture and existing management practices (Hirvi et al., 2023).

Authentic Leadership

Increased interest in leaders being 'authentic' has been guided by societal concern about poor leadership practices in the public and private sectors (Lord et al., 2017, Northouse, 2022). Increasingly, publics want leaders who are transparent, who they can trust and whose motives and intentions are clear to them (Lord et al., 2017, Northouse, 2022). Whilst no uniform definition of authentic leadership exists, definitions generally point towards someone with good self-awareness (particularly in relation to their own values) and control (or self-regulation), with a strong moral compass, who is balanced in their analysis and decision-making, who is transparent, who has a clear purpose that they are passionate about and who can form trusted and empathetic relationships with others (Fennell, 2021, Lord et al., 2017, Northouse, 2022, Wu et al., 2024). Importantly, authentic leaders often have a desire to serve others and because of this have been shown to be particularly effective in leading teams (Lyubovnikova et al., 2017). You will likely be able to identify people you have worked with who have all these aspects and see how inspiring they can be. In the context of healthcare, a recent review highlighted significant recent interest in authentic leadership (Wu et al., 2024). In a healthcare context, authentic leadership likely increases the quality and safety of care provision, as well as creating care environments that are nice to work in, empowering and which people are less likely to want to leave (Wu et al., 2024).

Servant Leadership

One way to think about servant leadership is that it is an inverted approach to leadership. What we mean by this, is the relationship between leaders and followers is opposite to how this relationship has been traditionally seen. Essentially, servant leaders *serve* the needs of their teams and team members, rather than the other way around (Demeke et al., 2024, Fennell, 2021, Northouse, 2022, Stanley, 2022). They are essentially stewards, protecting those they serve, with power largely sitting with the team and its members (Fennell, 2021, Northouse, 2022, Stanley, 2022). The idea of servant leadership was first put forward by Robert Greenleaf (1904–1990) in several seminal texts (Greenleaf, 1977). Since then, interest in servant leadership, including in health has grown, as it has the potential to steer leadership efforts away from ones own interests to that of the team; their work, well-being and development (Demeke et al., 2024). In a healthcare context, servant leadership has been shown to increase individual, team and organisational performance (Demeke et al., 2024).

Distributive and Shared Leadership

Generally, distributive leadership is seen as a way of flattening hierarchy, with power and influence flowing downwards within an organisation (Currie and Lockett, 2011, Martin et al., 2015). This way of viewing leadership suggests that team members can lead each other towards goal accomplishment, with different members taking on leadership at the same or different times (Northouse, 2022, Stanley, 2022, Fennell, 2021). As we have shown, because leadership isn't tied to a specific person and the context of what needs to be led (especially in healthcare) is often fluid and changing, leadership can in fact be demonstrated by anyone within a team, with certain individuals being better placed to lead, depending on what *exactly* it is that is needing leadership. Essentially, shared or distributive leadership recognises that leadership can shift from one member of a team to another, depending on the task, and the needs of the team (Northouse, 2022, Stanley, 2022). Within healthcare contexts, interest has grown in relation to distributive/shared leadership, and its potential positive impacts, as well as some of the challenges it might present (Günzel-Jensen et al., 2018, Leach et al., 2021, Martin et al., 2015, Mitchell and Boyle, 2021).

Team Leadership

In the following chapter, we unpack teams and teamwork more fully. Leaders are generally seen as being important to teamwork and team effectiveness, as they are often the people who can set a vision, can define tasks and what is needing doing, and can monitor team relational behaviours, and where necessary take action to address these (Hill, 2022). As we explore in the following chapter, they are vitally important in terms of creating enabling structures, making resources available, buffering external challenges and setting the interpersonal climates that teams and team members operate within, which can have an impact on how able team members feel they can contribute or speak up if they are concerned (Edmondson and Bransby, 2023, Nembhard and Edmondson, 2006, Salas et al., 2018b).

Essentially, we can think of leaders as influencing the cognitive (what needs doing), motivational (wanting to do it) and affective (feeling good about doing it) and emergent states (how effective they are) of teams and team members (Hill, 2022). As we explore in the following chapter, teams (who increasingly work in complex multi-team systems) are now vital to delivering healthcare, and team leadership will continue to be important in adapting to the needs of the situation, and the needs of the team; through steering and influencing teams towards task and relational success.

Taking One Last SEIP

At the start of this chapter, we introduced you to the SEIPS model. Now in its third iteration (3.0), the model's iteration is largely in line with an increased focus on teams, and multi-team systems within healthcare, and the relevance of these to responding to people's increasingly complex needs, and the resultant complexity of care, in which people need to see multiple healthcare professionals, in multiple settings and across time (Carayon et al., 2020). The model emphasises the patient journey within healthcare's complex socio-technical systems, highlighting the importance of care being adaptive to changing needs over time, through learning and continuous improvement. Teams, teamwork and team effectiveness, as we will show in the next chapter, play a vitally important part in this continuous learning and improvement, as to do leaders, in the interpersonal climates that they set, and how they approach individuals and their teams. The most recent SEIPS model can be seen in Figure 18.4.

> ## Clinical Considerations
>
> - Healthcare professionals work within dynamic and complex systems. When work systems are poorly designed, human error can lead to mistakes, causing patient harm. An important consideration is designing work systems that are safe and effective.
> - Leadership is increasingly recognised as being important to the delivery of safe and effective care and several leadership approaches have been considered in the context of healthcare delivery, including transformational, authentic, servant and distributed leadership.

Conclusion

In this chapter, we introduced you to systems thinking, complexity, human factors and ergonomics. In reviewing the increasingly complex socio-technical environments in which healthcare is now typically delivered, the importance of

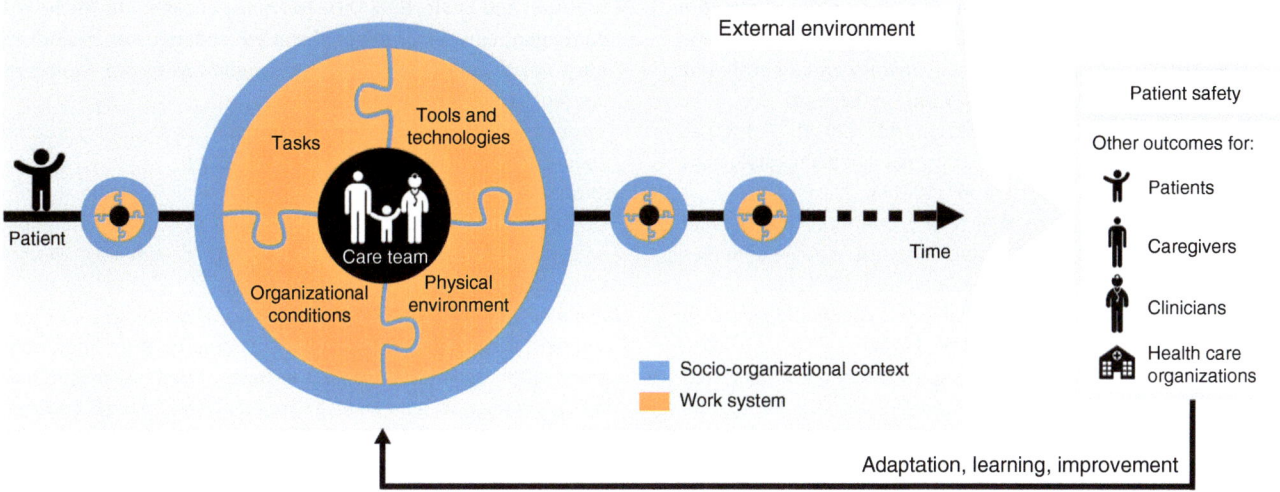

FIGURE 18.4 SEIPS 3.0 model: socio-technical systems approach highlighting a patient's journal and patient safety. **Source:** Carayon, P et al. (2020)/with permission of Elsevier.

effective leadership and management within healthcare has been emphasised. This chapter has introduced leadership as a social construct and social process. Some of the most important leadership theories have been introduced, alongside discussing their relevance to healthcare, including transformational, authentic, servant, distributed and team leadership. Finally, we returned to one useful model that can be used to consider the care environment, and how people interact with it, alongside the importance of healthcare systems being able to adapt to people's increasingly complex and changing healthcare needs. Teams and effective teamwork make this possible, which is the focus of our penultimate chapter.

References

Alloubani, A., Akhu-Zaheya, L., Abdelhafiz, I.M., and Almatari, M. (2019). Leadership styles' influence on the quality of nursing care. *International Journal of Health Care Quality Assurance* 32: 1022–1033.

Bass, B. (1998). The Ethics of Transformational Leadership. In: *Ethics: The Heart of Leadership* (ed. J. CIULLA). Praeger.

Belrhiti, Z., Nebot Giralt, A., and Marchal, B. (2018). Complex leadership in healthcare: a scoping review. *International Journal of Health Policy and Management* 7: 1073–1084.

Bennett, C.L. and James, A.H. (2022). Leadership and Management. In: *Clinical Leadership in Nursing and Healthcare*, Thirde (ed. D. Stanley, C.L. Bennett, and A.H. James). Wiley.

Carayon, P., Schoofs Hundt, A., Karsh, B.T. et al. (2006). Work system design for patient safety: the SEIPS model. *Quality & Safety in Health Care* 15 (Suppl 1): i50–i58.

Carayon, P., Wooldridge, A., Hoonakker, P. et al. (2020). SEIPS 3.0: human-centered design of the patient journey for patient safety. *Applied Ergonomics* 84: 103033.

Carayon, P., Xie, A., and Kianfar, S. (2014). Human factors and ergonomics as a patient safety practice. *BMJ Quality & Safety* 23: 196.

Conroy, N., Patton, D., Moore, Z. et al. (2023). The relationship between transformational leadership and staff nurse retention in hospital settings: a systematic review. *Journal of Nursing Management* 2023: 9577200.

Currie, G. and Lockett, A. (2011). Distributing leadership in health and social care: concerttive, conjoint or collective? *International Journal of Management Reviews* 13 (3): 286–300.

Demeke, G.W., Van Engen, M.L., and Markos, S. (2024). Servant leadership in the healthcare literature: a systematic review. *Journal of Healthcare Leadership* 1–14.

Dinh, J.E., Lord, R.G., Gardner, W.L. et al. (2014). Leadership theory and research in the new millennium: current theoretical trends and changing perspectives. *The Leadership Quarterly* 25: 36–62.

Dinh, J.V., Traylor, A.M., Kilcullen, M.P. et al. (2020). Cross-disciplinary care: a systematic review on teamwork processes in health care. *Small Group Research* 51: 125–166.

Donabedian, A. (1988). The quality of care: how can it be assessed? *JAMA* 260: 1743–1748.

Edmondson, A.C. and Bransby, D.P. (2023). Psychological safety comes of age: observed themes in an established literature. *Annual Review of Organizational Psychology and Organizational Behavior* 10: 55–78.

Fennell, K. (2021). Conceptualisations of leadership and relevance to health and human service workforce development: a scoping review. *Journal of Multidisciplinary Healthcare* 14: 3035–3051.

Fiedler, F. (1964). A Contingency Model of Leadership Effectiveness. In: *Advances in Experimental Social Psychology*. Academic Press.

Francis, R. 2013. Report of the mid staffordshire NHS foundation trust public inquiry. UK Government. Available online: https://assets.publishing.service.gov.uk/media/5a7ba0faed915d13110607c8/0947.pdf.

Goleman, D. (1998). What makes a leader? *Harvard Business Review* 76: 93–102.

Gopee, N. and Galloway, J. (2017). *Leadership and Management in Healthcare*. London: SAGE.

Greenleaf, R. (1977). *Servant Leadership: A Journey into the Nature of Legitimate Power and Greatness*. New York: Paulist Press.

Günzel-Jensen, F., Jain, A.K., and Kjeldsen, A.M. (2018). Distributed leadership in health care: the role of formal leadership styles and organizational efficacy. *Leadership* 14: 110–133.

Haoyan, X., Waters, D., Jinling, H. et al. (2023). Quantitative systematic review of the transformational leadership style as a driver of nurses' organisational commitment. *Nursing Open* 10: 4160–4171.

Hersey, P. and Blanchard, K.H. (1969). Life cycle theory of leadership. *Training and Development Journal* 23 (5): 26–34.

Hill, S. (2022). Team Leadership. In: *Leadership Theory and Practice* (ed. P. Northouse). Sage.

Hirvi, S., Laulainen, S., Junttila, K., and Lammintakanen, J. (2023). The dynamic nature of leader-member exchange relationships in health-care organizations. *Leadership in Health Services* 374–388.

Holden, R.J., Carayon, P., Gurses, A.P. et al. (2013). SEIPS 2.0: a human factors framework for studying and improving the work of healthcare professionals and patients. *Ergonomics* 56: 1669–1686.

Holmes, B.J., Best, A., Davies, H. et al. (2017). Mobilising knowledge in complex health systems: a call to action. *Evidence and Policy* 13: 539–560.

House, R.J. and Howell, J.M. (1992). Personality and charismatic leadership. *The Leadership Quarterly* 3: 81–108.

Institute of Medicine (IOM) (2000). *To Err is Human: Building a Safer Health System* (ed. L.T. Kohn, J.M. Corrigan, and M.S. Donaldson). Washington (DC): National Academies Press (US) Copyright 2000 by the National Academy of Sciences. All rights reserved.

James, A.H. and Bennett, C.L. (2022). Power, Politics, and Leadership. In: *Clinical Leadership in Nursing and Healthcare*, Thirde (ed. D. Stanley, C.L. Bennett, and A.H. James). Wiley.

Kapur, N., Parand, A., Soukup, T. et al. (2016). Aviation and healthcare: a comparative review with implications for patient safety. *JRSM Open* 7: 2054270415616548.

Kouzes, J.M. and Posner, B.Z. (1995). *The Leadership Challenge*. San Francisco: Jossey-Bass.

Labrague, L.J., Nwafor, C.E., and Tsaras, K. (2020). Influence of toxic and transformational leadership practices on nurses' job satisfaction, job stress, absenteeism and turnover intention: a cross-sectional study. *Journal of Nursing Management* 28: 1104–1113.

Lappalainen, M., Härkänen, M., and Kvist, T. (2020). The relationship between nurse manager's transformational leadership style and medication safety. *Scandinavian Journal of Caring Sciences* 34: 357–369.

Leach, L., Hastings, B., Schwarz, G. et al. (2021). Distributed leadership in healthcare: leadership dyads and the promise of improved hospital outcomes. *Leadership in Health Services* 34: 353–374.

Lord, R.G., Day, D.V., Zaccaro, S.J. et al. (2017). Leadership in applied psychology: three waves of theory and research. *Journal of Applied Psychology* 102: 434.

Lyubovnikova, J., Legood, A., Turner, N., and Mamakouka, A. (2017). How authentic leadership influences team performance: the mediating role of team reflexivity. *Journal of Business Ethics* 141: 59–70.

Martin, G., Beech, N., Macintosh, R., and Bushfield, S. (2015). Potential challenges facing distributed leadership in health care: evidence from the UK National Health Service. *Sociology of Health & Illness* 37: 14–29.

Mitchell, R. and Boyle, B. (2021). Too many cooks in the kitchen? The contingent curvilinear effect of shared leadership on multidisciplinary healthcare team innovation. *Human Resource Management Journal* 31: 358–374.

Monzani, L. and Van Dick, R. (2020). *Positive Leadership in Organizations*. Oxford Research Encyclopedia of Psychology.

Nembhard, I.M. and Edmondson, A.C. (2006). Making it safe: the effects of leader inclusiveness and professional status on psychological safety and improvement efforts in health care teams. *Journal of Organizational Behavior* 27: 941–966.

Northouse, P. (2022). *Leadership: Theory and Practice*. Sage.

Ockenden, D. 2022. Ockenden review: summary of findings, conclusions and essential actions. UK Government. Available online: https://www.gov.uk/government/publications/final-report-of-the-ockenden-review.

Pishgooie, A.H., Atashzadeh-Shoorideh, F., Falcó-Pegueroles, A., and Lotfi, Z. (2019). Correlation between nursing managers' leadership styles and nurses' job stress and anticipated turnover. *Journal of Nursing Management* 27: 527–534.

Plsek, P.E. and Greenhalgh, T. (2001). Complexity science: the challenge of complexity in health care. *BMJ* 323: 625–628.

Reason, J. (1990). *Human Error*. Cambridge: Cambridge University Press https://www.cambridge.org/highereducation/books/human-error/281486994DE4704203A514F7B7D826C0#overview.

Reason, J. (2000). Human error: models and management. *BMJ* 320 (768): 768–770.

Ree, E. (2020). What is the role of transformational leadership, work environment and patient safety culture for person-centred care? A cross-sectional study in Norwegian nursing homes and home care services. *Nursing Open* 7: 1988–1996.

Salas, E., Reyes, D.L., and Mcdaniel, S.H. (2018a). The science of teamwork: progress, reflections, and the road ahead. *The American Psychologist* 73: 593–600.

Salas, E., Zajac, S., and Marlow, S.L. (2018b). Transforming health care one team at a time: ten observations and the trail ahead. *Group & Organization Management* 43: 357–381.

Sanford, N., Lavelle, M., Markiewicz, O. et al. (2024). Decoding healthcare teamwork: a typology of hospital teams. *Journal of Interprofessional Care* 38: 602–611.

Seljemo, C., Viksveen, P., and Ree, E. (2020). The role of transformational leadership, job demands and job resources for patient safety culture in Norwegian nursing homes: a cross-sectional study. *BMC Health Services Research* 20: 799.

Shuffler, M.L. and Carter, D.R. (2018). Teamwork situated in multiteam systems: key lessons learned and future opportunities. *The American Psychologist* 73: 390–406.

Sinek, S. (2017). *Leaders Eat Last: Why Some Teams Pull Together and Other's Don't*. Penguin.

Spataru, A., Eiben, P., and Pluddemann, A. (2024). Performance of closed-loop systems for intravenous drug administration: a systematic review and meta-analysis of randomised controlled trials. *Journal of Clinical Monitoring and Computing* 38: 5–18.

Stanley, D., Bennett, C., and James, A.H. (2022). *Clinical Leadership in Nursing and Healthcare*, Thirde. Wiley.

Stanley, D. (2022). Leadership Theories and Styles. In: *Clinical Leadership in Nursing and Healthcare*, Thirde (ed. D. Stanley, C.L. Bennett, and A.H. James). Wiley.

Stewart, G.L., Courtright, S.H., and Manz, C.C. (2019). Self-leadership: a paradoxical core of organizational behavior. *Annual Review of Organizational Psychology and Organizational Behavior* 6: 47–67.

Van Knippenberg, D. and Sitkin, S.B. (2013). A critical assessment of charismatic—transformational leadership research: back to the drawing board? *The Academy of Management Annals* 7: 1–60.

Vroom, V.H. and Jago, A.G. (2007). The role of the situation in leadership. *American Psychologist* 62: 17.

Wiegmann, D.A., Wood, L.J., Cohen, T.N., and Shappell, S.A. (2022). Understanding the "swiss cheese model" and its application to patient safety. *Journal of Patient Safety* 18: 119–123.

Wu, X., Hayter, M., Lee, A.J. et al. (2020). Positive spiritual climate supports transformational leadership as means to reduce nursing burnout and intent to leave. *Journal of Nursing Management* 28: 804–813.

Wu, Y., Awang, S.R., Ahmad, T., and You, C. (2024). A systematic review of leadership styles in healthcare sector: insights and future directions. *Geriatric Nursing* 59: 48–59.

Xie, Y., Gu, D., Liang, C. et al. (2020). How transformational leadership and clan culture influence nursing staff's willingness to stay. *Journal of Nursing Management* 28: 1515–1524.

Zhu, W., Avolio, B.J., Riggio, R.E., and Sosik, J.J. (2011). The effect of authentic transformational leadership on follower and group ethics. *The Leadership Quarterly* 22: 801–817.

CHAPTER 19

Healthcare Teams, Team Effectiveness and Team Training

Chris Allen and Matt Flynn

School of Health Sciences, University of Southampton, Southampton, UK

Introduction

This chapter builds on the previous one which considered complexity and the importance of leadership and management to the delivery of safe and effective care. With care becoming increasingly complex, there is now a greater need for healthcare professionals to work in teams. In this chapter, we will review why teams are so important to healthcare delivery, as well as how teamwork in healthcare is seen and understood. We will introduce you to relevant models that can guide thinking about teams: what goes into them in terms of their inputs, what their teamwork processes are and what outcomes we might be interested in. We will consider the value of diversity in healthcare teams, as well as some of the challenges this can present. We will also examine psychological safety within the context of modern healthcare teams. Finally, this chapter will consider some evidence-based interventions that have been used to enhance teamwork and team effectiveness in healthcare settings.

LEARNING OUTCOMES

By the end of this chapter, you will be able to:

- Recognise the importance of effective teamwork in healthcare and be able to identify who forms part of a healthcare team.
- Consider the different types of healthcare teams and their memberships.
- Identify aspects contributing to team performance, such as team inputs and teamwork processes, using

models such as the Inputs-Processes-Outputs/ Inputs-Mediators- Outputs-Inputs (IPO/IMOI) model.
- Consider some of the ways teamwork processes can be enhanced, such as through team training, and how team performance can be assessed.

What Is a Team, and Why Do We Work in Them?

> **Key Terms and Definitions**
>
> **Team:** A group of people and social entity, who generally work together on shared goals and interdependent tasks.
>
> **Multi-team system:** Several teams, working together to achieve an overarching goal, often across different environments.
>
> **Interprofessional healthcare team:** A team composed of several different healthcare professionals or healthcare workers, for example, doctors, physios and nurses.

Teams are a social entity. In nearly every expertise-driven industry, effective teamwork has become a normal, even expected part of working life (Dinh et al., 2020, Salas et al., 2008, 2018a, Shuffler and Cronin, 2019). Work within

Social Sciences for Healthcare Professionals, First Edition. Edited by Chris Allen.
© 2026 John Wiley & Sons Ltd. Published 2026 by John Wiley & Sons Ltd.

every society and most industries is now far too complex to be carried out by a handful of co-acting individuals. Instead, it is common for people's work to be interdependent. By interdependent, we simply mean that people's work and their task accomplishments are tied to one another. Interdependence, as we will explore shortly, is a defining feature of teams (Salas et al., 2008, 2018a, Shuffler and Cronin, 2019). Players within a football team are interdependent. Their success is tied to the performance of one another. No one player (even a superstar) is likely to be able to achieve much on their own. The same can be said in most work contexts.

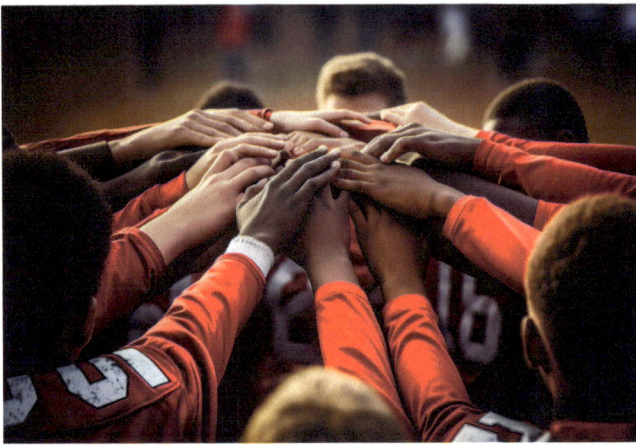

Source: Fabio/Adobe Stock Photos.

Interest in teams and teamwork is not new. Teams have been explored across industries, and the social sciences and the work of organisational studies, psychology, and sociology in particular, have provided rich insights into teams and teamwork (Mathieu et al., 2017, Salas et al., 2018a). In the context of healthcare, teams have become increasingly important due to increasing care complexity (Dinh et al., 2020, Sanford et al., 2024). Elsewhere in this book, we have highlighted the changes to populations that have resulted in people typically living longer, and with more complex, and longer-term healthcare needs (Omran, 2005). The increased recognition of the broader social determinants of health (covered in Chapter 8), amongst other things, has also widened the remit of healthcare (Marmot, 2010, Marmot et al., 2008, 2020).

This widened remit and complexity means that people's needs often cannot be met by generalists working in very small teams (in the example provided in the stop and think activity, just two people), by one professional, or by one profession working in isolation (Dinh et al., 2020, Sanford et al., 2024). Healthcare now commonly involves the coordinated involvement of multidisciplinary teams. Teams that are composed of multiple different professionals (such as nurses, physiotherapists, medics and occupational therapists), each with different skills and knowledge, that collectively, can meet people's increasingly diverse, complex and personalised care needs (Sanford et al., 2024). These multi-professional teams sit within a broader multi-team system (a system that involves multiple teams working together interdependently) that spans a full range of

inpatient and community care settings (such as district nursing teams, general practice teams and ward teams) (Salas et al., 2018a, Shuffler and Carter, 2018, Tu et al., 2024). This can lead to care that is fragmented – and to combat this, models of integrated care are being increasingly adopted to smooth transitions between services (Baxter et al., 2018, Davidson et al., 2021, Rocks et al., 2020).

Work with patients and their families is also becoming increasingly interdependent, with increased expectations being placed on individuals and their families to be more involved in their conditions management (see chapter 7), alongside increasing opportunities for the public to be more involved in the evaluation, design and delivery of the healthcare services they use (Brett et al., 2014, Ellis et al., 2017). So as with other complex work, healthcare teams now typically include a diverse mix of people, working interdependently across multiple care settings, in often challenging and unpredictable contexts (Dinh et al., 2020, Sanford et al., 2024).

All of these changes make effective teamwork necessary to deliver high-quality, safe and effective patient care. Put simply, more can be achieved by healthcare teams than solo practitioners, because healthcare teams typically draw on a broad range of people and professions, each with their different knowledge, skills and abilities (Rosen et al., 2018, Tu et al., 2024). However, when this interdependence is poorly coordinated, and where teams have inadequate teamwork processes (some of which we will explore later in this chapter), the result can be poor, fragmented, or even unsafe practice and care delivery, with ineffective teamwork and communication consistently being highlighted as a leading contributor to things going wrong and people being harmed (Manser, 2009, Rosen et al., 2018, Schot et al., 2020). Recognition of this has driven increased interest in how interprofessional teamwork and team effectiveness can be improved to benefit those accessing care, and those providing it (Rosen et al., 2018, Sanford et al., 2024, Schot et al., 2020).

Stop and Think: Why Do We Need to Work in Teams?

'My grandfather was a general practitioner in a small town in the USA in the mid Twentieth century. His medical team consisted of himself and a nurse (who was also my grandmother). He even served as his own pharmacist' (Thomas, 2011).

It is now uncommon for care to be provided by just two people. What changes have occurred, that have made the above example less likely?

Did you consider any of the following influencing factors?

- Changes in patient complexity
- Changes in patterns of health and disease
- Changes in levels of cognitive, physical, mental and sensory impairments in populations

- Advances in knowledge and understanding of health and disease, alongside its management
- Increased healthcare professional specialisation
- Increased focus on personalised, holistic care
- Increased understanding of the social determinants of health
- Increased use of technology, including digital technology
- Increased range of healthcare settings (such as acute and community), and range of care teams

People can work together, as part of a co-acting group, but may not be a 'real team'. 'Real teams' are a type of organisational unit that interdependently work towards shared goals, and who collectively reflect on performance and make necessary adjustments to improve on that performance (Lyubovnikova et al., 2015, Shuffler and Cronin, 2019). In the context of healthcare, teams that are 'real teams' are believed to be more likely to provide safe and effective care, and members of these teams are also more likely to be safer, and more satisfied in their roles (Lyubovnikova et al., 2015). Effective healthcare teams coordinate, adapt and can be flexible to changing demands (Dinh et al., 2020, Driskell et al., 2018, Rosen et al., 2018). They have shared mental models linked to the tasks that need to be completed, the team's overall objectives, and who members of the team are and what they are meant to be doing (essentially, putting all team members on the same page) (Dinh et al., 2020, Salas et al., 2005). They can reflect on performance and self-correct when mistakes or omissions are made, and they are cohesive (Dinh et al., 2020, Salas et al., 2005).

However, much of the teamwork literature has considered traditional teams with clear and obvious boundaries, and with relatively stable, and often exclusive memberships (i.e. team members are not also members of other teams). However, this is not the structure of most contemporary healthcare teams. They are fluid, their boundaries are not clear cut and their membership varies, with different people rotating in and out of the team, sometimes even on an hourly basis dependent on the specific knowledge and skills that are required (Kerrissey et al., 2023, Rosen et al., 2018, Sanford et al., 2024, Shuffler and Carter, 2018, Shuffler and Cronin, 2019). This can make healthcare teams challenging to study (Kerrissey et al., 2020, 2023, Sanford et al., 2024, Shuffler and Carter, 2018, Tu et al., 2024).

Despite this, recent work has highlighted that we now know a fair bit about healthcare teams, how they work, and how they can be best supported to deliver care that is safe, and that is high quality (Salas et al., 2018b). For example, we know that:

- Leadership matters. Whilst it can take many forms (some of which we discussed in the previous chapters), leadership steers, influences and motivates teams towards task accomplishment (Salas et al., 2018b).

- Effective teamwork can increase system resilience (e.g. in response to something unexpected happening) and can improve safety (Salas et al., 2018b).
- Psychological safety is important. Team members who feel psychologically safe are more likely to speak up if they see something that is concerning them, if they have an idea or if they believe they have solved a particular problem or issue (Salas et al., 2018b).
- Teamwork training, when well designed and delivered, can improve team effectiveness (Salas et al., 2018b).
- Bringing teams together through huddling and debriefing can improve team learning and future team performance (Salas et al., 2018b).

During this chapter, we will have the opportunity to unpick many of these points in more depth.

The focus of this chapter is on teams and teamwork within complex socio-technical systems (Carayon et al., 2020). We will explore how efforts to improve team effectiveness are highly relevant to improving the quality of care, and how other important parts of the system (e.g. those that we can use the previously introduced SEIPS model to identify) can influence care quality and safety (Carayon et al., 2020).

Whilst we suggest that effective teamwork is important, we also recognise that healthcare work is complex, and good teamwork alone will not result in all healthcare challenges being overcome. This is why it is important to look at teams within a social context.

But what exactly is a healthcare team and who is in it?

Healthcare Teams

When we think of 'teams' we often think of a social entity that has a clear and consistent boundary, who work together on common or shared goals (Salas et al., 2008, 2018a, Shuffler and Cronin, 2019). For example, a sports team will be made of a group of people, each with specific roles (or positions) and whilst everyone on the team may not be on the field during the game, they all play a part in the team's success. In healthcare teams, similar clear and consistent boundaries do not always exist, largely due to the levels of complexity and distributed interdependence, with care for one person sometimes involving the input of people across care settings (Kerrissey et al., 2020, 2023, Rosen et al., 2018, Sanford et al., 2024). Nearly every healthcare team is part of a multi-team system, and members of a healthcare team can belong to multiple other teams simultaneously (Kerrissey et al., 2023, Rosen et al., 2018, Sanford et al., 2024). On a day-to-day basis, healthcare teams are rarely stable and are rarely composed of the same individuals. Those living with multiple chronic conditions will likely see many different healthcare professionals throughout the year and these healthcare professionals will often have to talk to each other and work collaboratively. In addition, the average patient now may be required to see numerous different healthcare professionals, across many different healthcare settings and contexts (May et al., 2014, Rosen et al., 2018). This lack of stability and boundedness can make it hard to identify who is part of the 'team' and who isn't (Kerrissey et al., 2023, Salas et al., 2018b, Shuffler and Carter, 2018, Shuffler and Cronin, 2019).

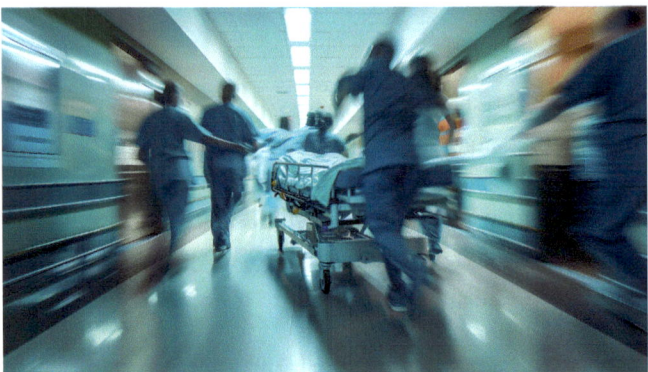

Source: safu designe/Adobe Stock Photos.

Stop and Think: What Is a 'Healthcare Team'?

What teams have you worked in?

Some teams you might have worked in include:

- A 'crash' or cardiac arrest team
- A ward team
- A rehabilitation team
- An integrated community team
- A specialist team
- A project team
- As just a few examples … you will likely have many more.

Which professionals were involved in this team and how were they involved?

How did these different professionals contribute to the availability of knowledge and skills within the team?

How dynamic was the team environment? Did different team members come and go in response to different service needs, or was team membership relatively stable and consistent?

How effective was the team in meeting the needs of those accessing care?

What made these teams effective?

What made these teams ineffective?

Increasingly the complexity and dynamism of care requires people to work with a much broader range of people and across multiple care settings, with team membership shifting in response to changing clinical contexts and challenges (Kerrissey et al., 2023, Rosen et al., 2018). Such shifts make it hard to pin down exactly who is in a healthcare team and

research has highlighted that even within the same care setting, different people within the same team can perceive their team's composition in very different ways, for example, in identifying different core team members, and different peripheral team members (Kerrissey et al., 2023). Prior research, much of which has studied more stable and consistent teams, suggests that stability and boundedness can help teams to establish an awareness of different members expertise, shared mental models, and ways of working together that are effective, as well as other important processes such as developing trust and developing cohesion (Salas et al., 2008).

It is recognised that it can be disruptive when team composition changes, and teams in healthcare can change quickly. The now seminal theory of group formation and its adaptions (Rickards and Moger, 2000, Tuckman, 1965), which you may well be familiar with (and is not without its critics), has for a long time provided a heuristic for thinking about how well formed a team is, and whether teamwork processes and ways of working together have yet been established. For many healthcare teams, the team is in a state of near-constant flux, and the extent to which this flux occurs, and the range and diversity of people that make up a team, is often constantly changing and varies from team to team. Therefore, according to Tuckman's seminal model, this means many contemporary healthcare teams operate in a continual state of 'forming' or 'storming', leading to challenges in teamwork processes that must be overcome.

In the context of hospital care teams, recent work has put forward a useful typology that can be used to identify five different types of hospital teams (Sanford et al., 2024), these are:

Structural teams: These are teams that have a relatively stable membership allowing trusting relationships to form that facilitate feedback, mutual performance monitoring, and team reflexivity (checking team performance and adjusting where necessary). An example of a structural team within a hospital setting is a ward-based team (e.g. an acute medicine for older people ward team), composed of multi-disciplinary team members, whose membership is relatively stable (albeit whose shift work means working with different members each day).

Hybrid teams: These are teams with less consistent membership that work between care settings and often include members who do not routinely work alongside each other and are not all co-located (i.e. they don't work in the same area). Hybrid teams can contain permanent members and these members are often relied upon by the team's transient team members for information and to help navigate complex processes.

Satellite teams: These are teams that often have a stable membership, but who are not co-located and will often work across multiple care settings. An example of a satellite team is a specialist team, which might have patients located all over the hospital in a variety of different wards. The nature of the specialist team influences its professional composition. For example, a tissue viability team might be uni-professional and compromised solely of nurses, whereas a surgical team may have greater professional diversity. Whilst these teams typically have a more stable core membership, working across a large geographical area can make communication challenging, which can impact on teamwork processes.

Responsive teams: These teams often do not have stable or consistent membership and are assembled quickly, generally in response to an urgent (often life-threatening) situation. An example of a responsive team is a cardiac arrest team, whose individual members might work in different clinical areas but be called upon to respond as a member of a cardiac arrest team anywhere within the hospital.

Coordinating teams: Finally coordinating teams, such as bed management teams. These may have some stable team members, but often draw on people from other teams (such as ward managers), to help solve organisational goals, such as ensuring patient flow and bed availability.

Except for structural teams, all other team types face significant challenges relating to teamwork processes. Even structural teams though can have fluctuating membership, both where the situation demands, as well as due to high turnover and workforce shortages, that may increase reliance on the use of non-permanent 'agency' or 'locum' team members. Therefore even in these teams, team members may not know one another particularly well, or even be familiar with the care setting (Griffiths et al., 2024, Zaranko et al., 2023).

The team types provided above fit within a multi-team system, in which even those working with structural teams may also be a member of another team, including sometimes teams in different care settings entirely (such as integrated care teams), and all hospital structural teams have interdependent relationships with other hospital care teams (Shuffler and Carter, 2018). One proposed way of thinking about such dynamic teams is 'teaming' or 'dynamic participation' which are terms used to describe the fluidity within which many contemporary teams' operate (Edmondson, 2012, Edmondson and Jean-Fracios, 2017, Kerrissey et al., 2023, Rosen et al., 2018). In the context of healthcare, adopting a 'role-based' approach can help us understand teams; what individuals within those teams should be doing, and how the team should be working together (Kerrissey et al., 2023, Valentine and Edmondson, 2015). For example, whilst each nurse will have different levels of experience, knowledge, skills and abilities, belonging to the 'profession' of nursing (explored in Chapter 6) means that a nurse should be able to fulfil the same roles within a team as other previously substituted in and out nurses, as they have had similar training and have similar value orientations. This extends to the other healthcare professions, and it is this role-based perception of teamwork in healthcare that has increased the focus on multi-professional/interprofessional team training – an approach that allows professionals to see the part of their profession within a team, as well as the part of other professionals, creating shared mental models about who does what, alongside standardised protocols, processes, closed loop communication and other strategies, such as ISBAR (Introduction, Situation, Background, Assessment,

Recommendation) (Burgess et al., 2020, Haig et al., 2006, Jiang et al., 2024, Müller et al., 2018, Rosen et al., 2018, Saragih et al., 2024).

Team Effectiveness: Inputs, Processes, Outcomes

The most common way to examine teams and what they entail is to break them down into their inputs (what we put into a team, such as who is in the team, how the team is structured and the team tasks), their processes (the teamwork processes – how the team thinks, what they do and how they feel – such as leadership, reflexivity and psychological safety, which we will shortly expand on) and their outputs (what the team can achieve in terms of its performance or how well the team develops) – this is commonly referred to as an 'IPO' model (Hackman, 1987, Mathieu et al., 2008, McGrath, 1964). These aspects are sometimes also broken down into inputs, mediators (which can include teamwork processes, and other emergent cognitive, affective and motivational states arising from team members interacting with one another) and outputs, with these outputs influencing what goes back into the team as an input, essentially an 'IMOI' model (Dinh et al., 2020, Ilgen et al., 2005). Both IPO and IMOI are examples of 'systems theories' and in this way are not dissimilar to the SEIPS model you were introduced to in the previous chapter, which is essentially also an IPO model (Aaberg et al., 2021, Carayon et al., 2020, 2006, Holden et al., 2013). IPO/IMOI models provide a useful heuristic, but they are not perfect and this is shown in more recent work, highlighting how different aspects of the model interact (Mathieu et al., 2018).

A clear distinction that is often made is that 'emergent states' make certain behaviours and ways of working more likely (such as trust), whereas the processes are what the team *actually* does (Dinh et al., 2020). Emergent states, often sit within processes, so for clarity, in the remainder of this chapter, we will refer to IPO as a useful heuristic and organising framework, through which we can consider teams, what we put into them and what supports their performance within organisations, including within healthcare (Dinh et al., 2020, Ilgen et al., 2005, McGrath, 1964). Some examples of inputs, processes and outputs are shown in Table 19.1 and you will have the opportunity to expand on some of these within the remainder of this chapter.

TABLE 19.1 Examples of inputs, processes and outputs relevant to health and care delivery.

Inputs	Processes	Outputs
Task	Communication	Care outcomes
Team composition	Reflexivity	Team outcomes
Team structure	Psychological safety	
	Conflict	
	Leadership	

Team Inputs

Team Member Characteristics

It is now widely recognised that a team of experts does not make an expert team, especially if people do not complement each other, and if teamwork processes (such as communication and collaboration) are poor (Salas, 2018). There are several things to consider when thinking about who should be in a team. We have already highlighted the importance of including a range of different professionals within your team, as this provides greater access to the knowledge and skills required to meet patients' increasingly complex needs (Rosen et al., 2018). In addition, personality traits might also help or hinder teams and can impact on team dynamics and team effectiveness (Bell et al., 2018). The impact of team member personality traits (we introduced some of these traits in Chapter 12), for example, conscientiousness, extraversion, openness to experience and agreeableness can have mixed impacts (Bell et al., 2018). Having conscientious team members makes it more likely that the team will complete tasks, but may result in team members taking over the tasks of underperformers (Bell et al., 2018). Extraverts are generally outgoing, and therefore often enjoy working in teams, but too many extroverted people within a team, might make it difficult for more introverted people to speak up and be heard (Bell et al., 2018). Unsurprisingly, agreeableness and emotional stability (which link to emotional intelligence discussed in the previous chapter) are also believed to contribute to positive team affective states and improved team cohesion (Bell et al., 2018). However, agreeableness may also limit task-related conflict, which can be important in helping teams come up with solutions to complex tasks as well as to innovation.

Diversity

Levels of cultural diversity in most western and developed nations are increasing and diverse teams create opportunities to bring people together who have a broad range of knowledge, skills and abilities, especially where they are also constitutionally diverse (e.g. in relation to team member age, gender, race, health, and level of impairment), knowledge and disciplinarily diverse (e.g. being composed of different professions) and culturally diverse (in terms of the range of people from different culturally and linguistically distinct groups). Teams with diversity in these aspects are arguably better equipped to meet most healthcare systems' current challenges. The team information processing theory in particular, highlights that diverse teams have more access to different knowledge, skills, abilities and viewpoints, and that this is generally advantageous (Bell et al., 2018). However, diverse teams may also experience increased challenges when drawing on such a wide range of views, knowledge, skills and experiences, and inclusive leadership can be important here in helping bridge conflicts and build team cohesion (Schmidt et al., 2023, Uman et al., 2023).

Creating inclusive environments through inclusive leadership practices that help people feel like they belong, whilst helping people to see the value in their own unique contributions, can help teams utilise the teams diversity, drawing on the teams unique insights and potential contributions, which are less available in more homogenous teams (Schmidt et al., 2023, Uman et al., 2023). Because of this, when diverse teams are integrated, and where people feel able to contribute, the teams' increased access to a wider range of knowledge, skills and perspectives can improve care (Schmidt et al., 2023, Uman et al., 2023). Research has also indicated that having diversity within a team, in terms of cultural and linguistic backgrounds can enhance cultural sensitivity, and help prevent misunderstandings, such as between professionals, or between professionals and those accessing care. In these situations, those with an understanding of different cultures are often able to act as 'bridge builders' (Schmidt et al., 2023, Uman et al., 2023).

Social Categorisation Perspective and 'Fault lines'

As we identified in Chapter 9, unconsciously, we tend to warm to those who are broadly like us (birds of a feather flock together), more than those who we see as being in some way 'different'. In the context of teams, differences can relate to many things. For example, multi-professional teams involve members with different professional orientations and focusses, as well as differential access to status, different reach and access to resources within organisations, as well as different demographic and personal characteristics (Carton and Cummings, 2012). As we explored above, this gives teams better access to a diverse range of knowledge, views and experiences, but it can also result in social categorisation and the emergence of 'fault lines' (Lau and Murnighan, 1998).

Fault lines are simply hypothetical dividing lines that split groups into subgroups based on members of the group having shared characteristics with one another (Lau and Murnighan, 1998). The concept of faultiness is closely linked to social identity theories (Lau and Murnighan, 1998). They can emerge where people group together based on shared characteristics, leading to the emergence of 'in groups' and 'out groups'. These differences can relate to many things, for example, a profession (such as nurses and doctors), work location (such as inpatient and community settings), as well as differences in individual demographic and personality traits. As just one example, a social category 'fault line' may result in the formation of subgroups, with one subgroup being composed of relatively young men (the ingroup), and one composed of older team members (the outgroup) (Lau and Murnighan, 1998). Obviously in very diverse teams, or in fully homogenous (very alike) teams, the emergence of ingroups and outgroups is far less likely (Lau and Murnighan, 1998). You may have seen this in your own teams. Do certain individuals with shared characteristics clump together and limit their interactions with other team members? If yes, they have likely formed a subgroup based on their homophily.

Ingroup and outgroup formations can create strong barriers to cooperation. Imagine you are on your break and you enter the staff room. In the staff room are several members of the team who share certain characteristics (e.g. profession, age, gender, etc.). They are *alike*, but very *unlike* you. In situations like these, you might find it hard to join in with their conversation. You are in the outgroup. To different degrees, we have all likely experienced being in both groups. Fault lines are generally believed to negatively impact on team effectiveness and can create us vs them mentalities, with different groups engaging in unproductive conflict, focusing on their own subgroups needs over the needs of the wider team, or not accepting the information or views of those outside their own subgroup at all (Bao et al., 2024). Sharing practices between different groups may be related to the power and status of different groups, and the level of interpersonal risk that sharing different views might bring (Bao et al., 2024). Teamwork processes such as communication, reflexivity and psychological safety, as we will explore, are important in promoting knowledge sharing. Where good knowledge-sharing practices exist and differences are valued, trust and cohesion can be built, allowing diverse knowledge and experience to be better utilised, and increasing team effectiveness.

Teamwork Processes

With such fluctuating team composition, establishing effective teamwork processes becomes even more essential in healthcare teams, with those teams engaging with effective processes being more likely to achieve higher levels of care quality and safety (LePine et al., 2008, Schmutz et al., 2019). Marks et al.'s (2001) seminal work on team actions highlights three main types of teamwork processes, these are:

Transition processes: What the team does *in-between* episodes of care or in-between tasks. This can include handovers, debriefs and closed-loop communication strategies that limit opportunities for important information to be missed (El-Shafy et al., 2018, Müller et al., 2018). Transition processes are important and are a known source of vulnerability, as they involve processes that when not effective can lead to missed information, errors and patient harm (Arbaje et al., 2014, Carayon et al., 2020, Wears et al., 2011).

Action processes: These are the team's actions *during* episodes of care. These relate to communication and coordination of team activities, and the ongoing monitoring of team performance, the team's collective actions, adaptability and 'back up' behaviours (Salas et al., 2005).

Interpersonal processes: These are essentially the actions that are taken to manage the *relationships* within the team (Dinh et al., 2020). We will unpack many of these interpersonal processes shortly, including the promotion of inclusive, psychologically safe working environments, and taking steps to meet a team's relational needs.

Communication

The quality of communication is often seen as being more important than its regularity (Marlow et al., 2018). High-performing teams generally have better communication processes than lower-performing teams (Dinh et al., 2020, LePine et al., 2008, Marlow et al., 2018, Salas et al., 2018b), and in the context of healthcare, poor communication can result in harm (Dinh et al., 2020, Rosen et al., 2018). An example of where harm can easily occur is when communication is poor, key information is missed at handovers, members of the team do not understand what has been said, or patients do not understand the instructions they have been given. Establishing effective communication in very large teams and multi-team systems can be particularly challenging (Shuffler and Carter, 2018, Shuffler and Cronin, 2019). As you can see in Figure 19.1, larger teams have more needed linkages between team members – this has been referred to as the 'law of n-Squared' (Krackhardt, 2003). Increasing the number of team members increases the number of needed linkages quite rapidly. For example, 4 team members need to maintain 6 links between them. Increasing the team to 8 increases the number of links to 28. Essentially, as the number of people in a team grows, the number of links needed grows at a faster pace, and this can quickly outrun a team's cognitive capacity to communicate with one another effectively (Krackhardt, 2003, Tu et al., 2024).

Clearly team size and configuration are important to how well a team can communicate. Various communication interventions exist, some of which are discussed later in this chapter.

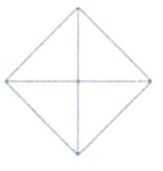
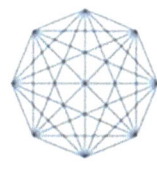
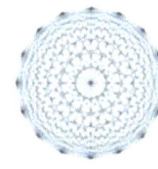
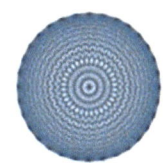

| 4 members | 8 members | 16 members | 32 members |
| 6 links | 28 links | 120 links | 496 links |

FIGURE 19.1 Law of *n*-squared. As the number of team members increases, the number of potential linkages between team members rises rapidly. **Source:** Tu et al., (2024) / With permission of John Wiley & Sons.

Psychological Safety and Conflict

Since first being discussed as a loose concept in the 1960s (notably in the work of Shein and Bennis, 1965), interest in psychological safety within organisations has grown substantially (Edmondson and Bransby, 2023), and studies consistently highlight the importance of psychological safety in work settings that are complex and dynamic, such as healthcare (Dietl et al., 2023, Edmondson et al., 2016, Nembhard and Edmondson, 2006, O'Donovan and McAuliffe, 2020a, 2020b).

But what does it mean to be psychologically safe at work?

Psychological safety is challenging to define, but we can likely all intuitively relate to what it means to be 'psychologically safe'. It is sometimes useful to think about this concept in relation to the spread of norms and behaviours within a team. When you work in a team, even if you only work in that team very briefly, you will have likely identified how that team works and what the norms are. This can include for example, what is and what is not tolerated, either by peers or by those in managerial or supervising positions, or other roles that might imply leadership. For example, to what extent is deviance or dissent tolerated? To what extent is feedback asked for and received? To what extent can you challenge upwards, laterally or downwards? To what extent are requests for help acceptable and how forthcoming is that help, when it is requested? Professor Amy Edmondson, a leading academic in this area, highlights these norms and values form the basis of the team's shared interpersonal climate (Edmondson and Bransby, 2023). This climate can lead to people either having a voice or being silenced and this can be the difference between someone identifying and highlighting to the team that the wrong leg has been marked prior to surgery, or being silent and exposing a patient to significant harm. When the team is facing a challenge they cannot overcome, this climate can also be the difference between someone with an idea that might help the team overcome it speaking up, or being silent. Clearly, for healthcare teams to be safe and effective, people need to be able to speak up and feedback loops are vital in improving work systems and processes (Carayon et al., 2020). Psychological safety relates to the extent to which individuals working within a team (generally in a work context), feel safe to express themselves, give suggestions or speak up. Essentially, how much they feel able to take interpersonal risks (Dietl et al., 2023, Nembhard and Edmondson, 2006, O'Donovan and McAuliffe, 2020a, 2020b).

Historical issues such as power and status imbalance between professional groups (more on this in Chapter 6) have meant that healthcare settings have not always been the most psychologically safe environments to work in. Particularly where hierarchies are very steep, lower-status team members may be more hesitant to speak up about their concerns (Edmondson and Bransby, 2023, Nembhard and Edmondson, 2006). However, when supportive interpersonal climates are created, team members are far more likely to open up and share mistakes or near misses in clinical environments, and it is this increased voice that creates opportunities for adverse incidents to be addressed through team learning, allowing safeguards to put in place to reduce risk of reoccurrence (Dietl et al., 2023, Nembhard and Edmondson, 2006, O'Donovan and McAuliffe, 2020a). Because working in a healthcare team involves a high degree of complex, interdependent work where mistakes can result in significant harm to patients and even death, there is now significant interest in how to create psychologically safe working environments that enhance safety and team effectiveness (Dietl et al., 2023, O'Donovan and McAuliffe, 2020a, 2020b).

As we have alluded to, it is also recognised that interpersonal environments that allow people to speak up, can lead to increased innovation and creativity, by facilitating task-related conflicts that can allow team members the opportunity to play with different ideas, and creative ways of solving complex problems without fear of being judged, or looking stupid. Particularly in relation to complex tasks, diverse teams (because of the wide range of opinions, expertise, professional judgements, etc. that are available) with good psychological safety, who can engage in constructive task-related conflict, generally have improved decision making and often outperform teams with no conflict (Edmondson, 2018, 2023, Edmondson and Besieux, 2021). However, both diversity and psychological safety are important here. For example, a very homogenous team (i.e. a team whose members are very alike) with good psychological safety, may result in an echo chamber – people can speak up, but because people are so similar, their contributions will likely also be pretty similar.

Incivility

In contrast to the positive working environments that psychological safety can create, incivility between colleagues and between those accessing care, and those delivering it, can result in disharmony, reduced safety and reduced care quality (Freedman et al., 2024). Workplace incivility is generally defined as a low-intensity deviant behaviour that breaks the civil norms of a workplace environment and may or may not be intended to cause harm (Freedman et al., 2024). Incivility can include behaviours that are directed at one another that are uncivil, rude or discourteous, and this is usually underpinned by a lack of respect for one another, but unlike bullying, may not have a clear target, or even be intended to cause harm (Freedman et al., 2024). There are many examples of incivility and you may have seen or been exposed to some of these – in fact, a recent review suggests around 25% of healthcare professionals have experienced uncivil behaviour from a range of people (though most commonly medics and supervisors – further highlighting challenges of hierarchy in healthcare) (Freedman et al., 2024). Other reviews have suggested an even higher incidence (Shoorideh et al., 2021). Generally, these behaviours break social norms for what behaviours are seen as acceptable. They can include gossiping, yelling or swearing at others, interrupting and ignoring. Essentially behaviours that are disharmonious, break social norms for how people should behave in a work context, and that are not nice to be on the receiving end of. Incivility can have a significant impact on teams, including impacting on patients, safety, worker well-being and overall organisational culture (Freedman et al., 2024).

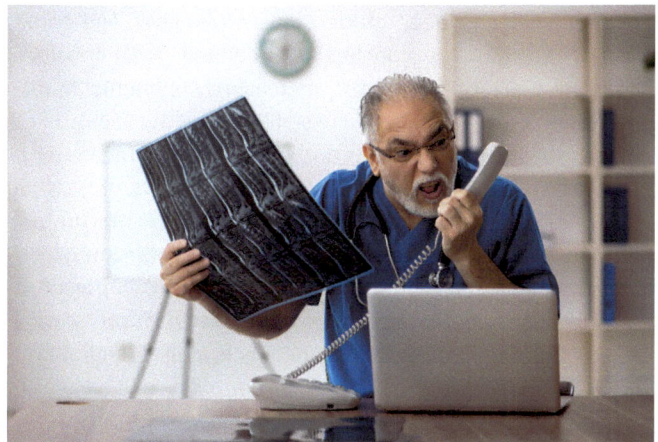

Source: Elnur / Adobe Stock Photos.

Team members being compassionate with one another (something that a leader's own behaviour often has a role in shaping) is not just a 'nice to have' but is intrinsically tied to care quality and patient safety (Freedman et al., 2024, Wang et al., 2024). In the previous chapter, we introduced you to the concept of emotional intelligence, and the self-regulation component of this can influence how civil members within a team are likely to be to one another, particularly during difficult situations.

Group Think

Human decision-making is complex. There is a considerable body of evidence that considers *individual* decision-making processes (Kahneman, 2012, Tversky and Kahneman, 1974), alongside research examining *group* decision-making processes (DiPierro et al., 2022). As we have highlighted above, creating the right environment and flattening hierarchies can encourage teams to share information and draw on each other's knowledge to arrive at sensible decisions. But as with individual decision-making processes, group decision-making processes can be flawed and can be subject to unintentional implicit (and sometimes even deliberate or explicit) bias (explored in Chapter 9).

Groupthink is one theory that seeks to explain the systematic bias in decision-making that can emerge from groups (or work teams) (DiPierro et al., 2022). As a theory, groupwork arose in the 1970s, in the seminal work of psychologist Irving Janis (1918–1990), to understand how a group (or teams) decision-making can be influenced (Janis, 1972). Groupthink is more likely to happen in groups that are highly cohesive and can lead to poor decision-making (DiPierro et al., 2022). Returning to the example of someone in the team not challenging the wrong leg being marked prior to surgery. Failure to voice a concern such as this, due to the assumption that the team must be right, and you must be wrong, is an example of groupthink. The desire to maintain group harmony, or harmony with individuals, overrides the desire to speak up (Pype et al., 2018). There are a range of

factors that can contribute to groupthink in healthcare teams. These include team members being homogenous (which is common in healthcare teams due to professional orientations and people often having similar backgrounds), hierarchy (which is also common in healthcare teams and can relate to the different statuses and power held by different professions), inflexibility and the sometimes highly stressful decision-making environments, where decisions must be made quickly and people have to 'think on their feet' (DiPierro et al., 2022). In addition, whilst it might be beneficial to seek the views of the whole interprofessional team to guide decision-making processes, in many contexts, professionals still make decisions in isolation (DeKeyser Ganz et al., 2016) and groupthink limits opportunities for these decisions to be constructively challenged.

Reflexivity

As healthcare professionals, you will likely be very familiar with individual reflective practice, which is a common requirement across the professions, and often emphasised as an expectancy in professional standards and codes (HCPC, 2023, NMC, 2019). However, team reflexivity in healthcare is arguably less practiced, and less understood. Various approaches have been considered to enhance team-level reflexivity including simulation-based education and providing team members peer review opportunities, with debriefing sessions typically focusing on technical and nontechnical skills and improvement (McHugh et al., 2020). In addition, teams can make use of video reflective ethnography, which involves recording aspects of practice and having the opportunity to review these, consider what works well and what doesn't work so well, and decide if the team needs to do anything differently moving forward (McHugh et al., 2020). Reviews have suggested such approaches can promote social learning and lead to service improvement (McHugh et al., 2020).

Understanding Team Performance (Outputs)

As we discussed in Chapter 5, understanding what aspects of a healthcare system's performance are important can be challenging. There is no catch-all outcome measure for healthcare team effectiveness (Dinh et al., 2020, Schmutz et al., 2019). In terms of team outputs, the IPO model generally prompts us to consider team performance, as well as the team health (i.e. how likely it is that the team will continue to work together collaboratively). In terms of team performance, different teams will aspire to different outcomes as measures of their success (Dinh et al., 2020, Schmutz et al., 2019). For example, in examining how well a surgical team performs, measures such as mortality or the rates of surgical complications will be important. However, these may be less useful in other care settings where death is less common, and where people do not have surgery and therefore do not typically experience these types of

TABLE 19.2	Outputs that are often used to assess performance, specifically related to health.
Category	**Examples**
Patient safety	For example, medication and diagnostic safety, safety related to ongoing follow up and monitoring of treatment, reduction of iatrogenic harms such as hospital acquired infections, pressure sores etc.
Patient outcomes	For example, physical and mental health outcomes and general wellbeing, care efficiency and effectiveness, levels of treatment related burden and stress, experience and satisfaction
Caregiver outcomes	For example, physical and mental health outcomes and general wellbeing, care giver stress and burden.
Healthcare professional outcomes	For example, occupational health and safety, job satisfaction, fatigue, burnout etc.
Organizational outcomes	For example, organizational performance against targets and objectives, turnover, staff sickness and absence etc.

Source: Adapted from: Carayon et al. (2020).

complications. Whilst how success is defined can look different in different contexts, what people are often most concerned about are patient health-related outcomes and adverse events. Work relating to the SEIPS 3.0 model (Carayon et al., 2020) that we introduced you to in the previous chapter, highlights the following categories and outcomes as being increasingly relevant in assessing health system performance (Table 19.2).

Teamwork Training and Teamwork Interventions

Even with the right combination of people in a team, teams can need support to function effectively. Teamwork training and team development interventions necessarily focus on teamwork processes (i.e. the P within the IPO model). There is a growing body of evidence supporting team training, and team development interventions can improve team effectiveness, and ultimately care outcomes (Hughes et al., 2016, Salas et al., 2018b). When considering the value of team training to improve team effectiveness, an obvious starting point is to consider what team behaviours and processes the training should seek to address, and how these might help healthcare teams to overcome whatever teamwork challenges they are facing. Well-designed team training interventions have been shown to increase team effectiveness in a range of contexts, and may even reduce mortality (Hughes et al., 2016, Salas et al., 2018b, Weaver et al., 2014). TeamSTEPPS™, which is arguably one of the most well-known

evidence-based team training interventions in healthcare (others do exist), has been shown to reduce error and enhance attitudes towards teamwork and teamwork processes including communication (Karlsen et al., 2022, Parker et al., 2019). TeamsSTEPPS™ has been around for a while now, and some have argued new approaches are needed that consider healthcare delivery within the increasingly dynamic multi-team systems that we have discussed (Ingels et al., 2023).

Team-based interventions and training in healthcare tend to emphasise the needs for different professions to be able to communicate and work together effectively in interprofessional teams. They often aim to guide understanding of different professional roles and responsibilities, and can lead to improved care outcomes and staff satisfaction (Franz et al., 2020, Saragih et al., 2024, Van Diggele et al., 2020).

'Huddle Up' – Team Huddles

By looking at transition and action processes, several concrete interventions have been identified that reduces the risk of important information being missed, including when care moves between different providers (such as at shift change). Team huddles are common in high-risk industries, such as aviation, nuclear power and increasingly healthcare (Rowan et al., 2022). Huddles are essentially a structured brief communication between team members that lasts around 5–15 minutes and can happen multiple times a day (Franklin et al., 2020, Rowan et al., 2022). Research has suggested that team huddles in healthcare can help flatten hierarchy, increase communication between team members, and lead to greater shared responsibility across the team, increasing care quality and safety (Franklin et al., 2020, Rowan et al., 2022). Essentially, these activities provide a 'touch point' and allocate time for team reflexivity to occur. However, exactly what huddling entails can differ and can mean different things to different people. It can also be referred to by several other similar terms, such as 'meetings', 'rounds', 'briefings' and 'reviews' and recent work has reviewed the literature and presented a proposed taxonomy (Franklin et al., 2020), which may in time help create more standardisation in team huddling processes to aid in their evaluation.

Teamwork and Innovation

Innovation relies on teamwork. This not only because some of the best ideas lie at the intersection of diverse experiences and perspectives (Syed, 2021) but also because teams are often needed for the implementation of new innovations (McGuier et al., 2024). In the following chapter, we introduce technology and innovation, highlighting its increasing importance in meeting the many and varied challenges most healthcare systems around the world are currently facing.

In the context of implementation, new innovations require individuals to work together to adapt to any changing demand or expectancy that a new technology or innovation may create (McGuier et al., 2024). Essentially, alongside the other factors that are discussed in the following chapter in more depth, whether a new technology can be successfully embedded within a clinical setting, is likely to relate to a range of teamwork processes, and a recent review has demonstrated that highly adaptive teams tend to have more success implementing new innovations than teams with negative affect (emotions), and poor teamwork processes (McGuier et al., 2024).

Importantly, the study of new innovations, such as electronic health records and virtual wards (covered in more depth in the following chapter), have the potential to contribute to our understanding of multi-team systems, as well as having the potential to improve team effectiveness by increasing needed access to information across teams, particularly in terms of the care that can be delivered in increasingly complex multi-team systems (Shuffler and Carter, 2018, Tu et al., 2024).

Clinical Considerations

- Healthcare teams are typically large and diverse, as well as very fluid, with frequently changing compositions. This can make some teamwork processes challenging.
- The adoption of standardised communication approaches, such as ISBAR, can help teams communicate effectively, especially where team members may be less familiar with one another.

- Creating psychologically safe clinical environments, enhances patient safety, by supporting people to speak up when they see something that might be a risk. Conversely, incivility can contribute to poor working environments, and poor safety cultures.
- Teamwork training can be effective in improving teamwork and teamwork processes.

Conclusion

In this chapter, we have considered teams and teamwork. We have highlighted the importance of healthcare teams in responding to the challenges most healthcare systems are currently facing. We have reviewed the teamwork literature, and in doing so, have highlighted that healthcare teams are generally very different to the bounded teams that have been examined in much of the teamwork literature. A few models for considering the different components of teams and team effectiveness have been discussed, alongside some relevant interventions that can be used to improve team performance. Finally, this chapter considered the role of teams to innovation and implementation, the subject of this book's final chapter.

References

Aaberg, O. R., Hall-Lord, M. L., Husebø, S. I. E. & Ballangrud, R. 2021. A human factors intervention in a hospital – evaluating the outcome of a TeamSTEPPS program in a surgical ward. *BMC Health Services Research*, 21, 114.

Arbaje, A. I., Kansagara, D. L., Salanitro, A. H., Englander, H. L., Kripalani, S., Jencks, S. F. & Lindquist, L. A. 2014. Regardless of age: Incorporating principles from geriatric medicine to improve care transitions for patients with complex needs. *Journal of General Internal Medicine*, 29, 932–939.

Bao, X., Dai, Y., Wu, Q., Nie, W. & Tao, H. 2024. Primary health care team faultlines and team performance: the mediating role of knowledge sharing. *Frontiers in Psychology*, 15.

Baxter, S., Johnson, M., Chambers, D., Sutton, A., Goyder, E. & Booth, A. 2018. The effects of integrated care: a systematic review of UK and international evidence. *BMC Health Services Research*, 18, 350.

Bell, S. T., Brown, S. G., Colaneri, A. & Outland, N. 2018. Team composition and the ABCs of teamwork. *American Psychologist*, 73, 349.

Brett, J., Staniszewska, S., Mockford, C., Herron-Marx, S., Hughes, J., Tysall, C. & Suleman, R. 2014. Mapping the impact of patient and public involvement on health and social care research: a systematic review. *Health Expectations*, 17, 637–650.

Burgess, A., Van Diggele, C., Roberts, C. & Mellis, C. 2020. Teaching clinical handover with ISBAR. *BMC Medical Education*, 20, 459.

Carayon, P., Schoofs Hundt, A., Karsh, B. T., Gurses, A. P., Alvarado, C. J., Smith, M. & Flatley Brennan, P. 2006. Work system design for patient safety: the SEIPS model. *Quality & Safety in Health Care*, 15(Suppl 1), i50–i58.

Carayon, P., Wooldridge, A., Hoonakker, P., Hundt, A. S. & Kelly, M. M. 2020. SEIPS 3.0: human-centered design of the patient journey for patient safety. *Applied Ergonomics*, 84, 103033.

Carton, A. M. & Cummings, J. N. 2012. A theory of subgroups in work teams. *Academy of Management Review*, 37, 441–470.

Davidson, L., Scott, J. & Forster, N. 2021. Patient experiences of integrated care within the United Kingdom: a systematic review. *International Journal of Care Coordination*, 24, 39–56.

Dekeyser Ganz, F., Engelberg, R., Torres, N. & Curtis, J. R. 2016. Development of a model of interprofessional shared clinical decision making in the ICU: a mixed-methods study. *Critical Care Medicine*, 44, 680–689.

Dietl, J. E., Derksen, C., Keller, F. M. & Lippke, S. 2023. Interdisciplinary and interprofessional communication intervention: how psychological safety fosters communication and increases patient safety. *Frontiers in Psychology*, 14, 1164288.

Dinh, J. V., Traylor, A. M., Kilcullen, M. P., Perez, J. A., Schweissing, E. J., Venkatesh, A. & Salas, E. 2020. Cross-disciplinary care: a systematic review on teamwork processes in health care. *Small Group Research*, 51, 125–166.

Dipierro, K., Lee, H., Pain, K. J., Durning, S. J. & Choi, J. J. 2022. Groupthink among health professional teams in patient care: a scoping review. *Medical Teacher*, 44, 309–318.

Driskell, J. E., Salas, E. & Driskell, T. 2018. Foundations of teamwork and collaboration. *The American Psychologist*, 73, 334–348.

Edmondson, A. 2012. *Teaming: How Organizations Learn, Innovate, and Compete in the Knowledge Economy*, Wiley.

Edmondson, A. 2018. *The fearless organization: Creating Psychological Safety in the Workplace for Learning, Innovation, and Growth*, Wiley.

Edmondson, A. 2023. *Right kind of wrong: Why learning to fail can teach us to thrive*, Cornerstone Press.

Edmondson, A. C. & Besieux, T. 2021. Reflections: voice and silence in workplace conversations. *Journal of Change Management*, 21, 269–286.

Edmondson, A. C. & Bransby, D. P. 2023. Psychological safety comes of age: observed themes in an established literature. *Annual Review of Organizational Psychology and Organizational Behavior*, 10, 55–78.

Edmondson, A. C., Higgins, M., Singer, S. & Weiner, J. 2016. Understanding psychological safety in health care and education organizations: a comparative perspective. *Research in Human Development*, 13, 65–83.

Edmondson, C. & Jean-Fracios, H. 2017. *Extreme Teaming: Lessons in Complex, Cross-Sector Leadership*, Emerald Group Publishing.

El-Shafy, I. A., Delgado, J., Akerman, M., Bullaro, F., Christopherson, N. A. M. & Prince, J. M. 2018. Closed-loop communication improves task completion in pediatric trauma resuscitation. *Journal of Surgical Education*, 75, 58–64.

Ellis, J., Boger, E., Latter, S., Kennedy, A., Jones, F., Foster, C. & Demain, S. 2017. Conceptualisation of the 'good' self-manager: a qualitative investigation of stakeholder views on the self-management of long-term health conditions. *Social Science & Medicine*, 176, 25–33.

Franklin, B. J., Gandhi, T. K., Bates, D. W., Huancahuari, N., Morris, C. A., Pearson, M., Bass, M. B. & Goralnick, E. 2020. Impact of multidisciplinary team huddles on patient safety: a systematic review and proposed taxonomy. *BMJ Quality & Safety*, 29, 1.

Franz, S., Muser, J., Thielhorn, U., Wallesch, C. W. & Behrens, J. 2020. Inter-professional communication and interaction in the neurological rehabilitation team: a literature review. *Disability and Rehabilitation*, 42, 1607–1615.

Freedman, B., Li, W. W., Liang, Z., Hartin, P. & Biedermann, N. 2024. The prevalence of incivility in hospitals and the effects of incivility on patient safety culture and outcomes: a systematic review and meta-analysis. *Journal of Advanced Nursing*.

Griffiths, P., Saville, C., Ball, J., Culliford, D., Jones, J., Lambert, F., Meredith, P., Rubbo, B., Turner, L., Dall'ora, C. & Workforce Health Outcomes Study Group 2024. Nursing team composition and mortality following acute hospital admission. *JAMA Network Open*, 7, e2428769–e2428769.

Hackman, J. R. 1987. The design of work teams. *In:* Lorsch, J. W. (ed.) *Handbook of Organizational Behavior*, Prentice-Hall, 315–342.

Haig, K. M., Sutton, S. & Whittington, J. 2006. SBAR: a shared mental model for improving communication between clinicians. *The Joint Commission Journal on Quality and Patient Safety*, 32, 167–175.

HCPC. 2023. Physiotherapists: The standards of proficiency for physiotherapists. [Online]. Health & Care Professions Council. Available: https://www.hcpc-uk.org/standards/standards-of-proficiency/physiotherapists/ [Accessed].

Holden, R. J., Carayon, P., Gurses, A. P., Hoonakker, P., Hundt, A. S., Ozok, A. A. & Rivera-Rodriguez, A. J. 2013. SEIPS 2.0: a human factors framework for studying and improving the work of healthcare professionals and patients. *Ergonomics*, 56, 1669–1686.

Hughes, A. M., Gregory, M. E., Joseph, D. L., Sonesh, S. C., Marlow, S. L., Lacerenza, C. N., Benishek, L. E., King, H. B. & Salas, E. 2016. Saving lives: a meta-analysis of team training in healthcare. *The Journal of Applied Psychology*, 101, 1266–1304.

Ilgen, D. R., Hollenbeck, J. R., Johnson, M. & Jundt, D. 2005. Teams in organizations: from input-process-output models to IMOI models. *Annual Review of Psychology*, 56, 517–543.

Ingels, D. J., Zajac, S. A., Kilcullen, M. P., Bisbey, T. M. & Salas, E. 2023. Interprofessional teamwork in healthcare: observations and the road ahead. *Journal of Interprofessional Care*, 37, 338–345.

Janis, I. L. 1972. *Victims of groupthink: A Psychological Study of Foreign-Policy Decisions and Fiascoes*, Houghton Mifflin.

Jiang, Y., Cai, Y., Zhang, X. & Wang, C. 2024. Interprofessional education interventions for healthcare professionals to improve patient safety: a scoping review. *Medical Education Online*, 29, 2391631.

Kahneman, D. 2012. *Thinking, Fast and Slow*, Penguin.

Karlsen, T., Hall-LORD, M. L., Wangensteen, S. & Ballangrud, R. 2022. Bachelor of nursing students' attitudes toward teamwork in healthcare: the impact of implementing a teamSTEPPS® team training program – a longitudinal, quasi-experimental study. *Nurse Education Today*, 108, 105180.

Kerrissey, M., Novikov, Z., Tietschert, M., Phillips, R. & Singer, S. J. 2023. The ambiguity of "we": perceptions of teaming in dynamic environments and their implications. *Social Science & Medicine*, 320, 115678.

Kerrissey, M. J., Satterstrom, P. & Edmondson, A. C. 2020. Into the fray: adaptive approaches to studying novel teamwork forms. *Organizational Psychology Review*, 10, 62–86.

Krackhardt, D. 2003. *Constraints on the Interactive Organization as an Ideal Type. Networks in the Knowledge Economy*, Oxford Academic: New York.

Lau, D. C. & Murnighan, J. K. 1998. Demographic diversity and faultlines: the compositional dynamics of organizational groups. *Academy of Management Review*, 23, 325–340.

Lepine, J. A., Piccolo, R. F., Jackson, C. L., Mathieu, J. E. & Saul, J. R. 2008. A meta-analysis of teamwork processes: tests of a multidimensional model and relationships with team effectiveness criteria. *Personnel Psychology*, 61, 273–307.

Lyubovnikova, J., West, M. A., Dawson, J. F. & Carter, M. R. 2015. 24-Karat or fool's gold? Consequences of real team and co-acting group membership in healthcare organizations. *European Journal of Work and Organizational Psychology*, 24, 929–950.

Manser, T. 2009. Teamwork and patient safety in dynamic domains of healthcare: a review of the literature. *Acta Anaesthesiologica Scandinavica*, 53, 143–151.

Marks, M. A., Mathieu, J. E. & Zaccaro, S. J. 2001. A temporally based framework and taxonomy of team processes. *The Academy of Management Review*, 26, 356–376.

Marlow, S. L., Lacerenza, C. N., Paoletti, J., Burke, C. S. & Salas, E. 2018. Does team communication represent a one-size-fits-all approach?: A meta-analysis of team communication and performance. *Organizational Behavior and Human Decision Processes*, 144, 145–170.

Marmot, M., Allen, J., Boyce, T., Goldblatt, P. & Morrison, J. 2020. Health Equity in England: The Marmot Review 10 Years On [Online]. The Health Foundation Available: https://www.health.org.uk/publications/reports/the-marmot-review-10-years-on [Accessed].

Marmot, M., Friel, S., Bell, R., Houweling, T. A. J. & Taylor, S. 2008. Closing the gap in a generation: health equity through action on the social determinants of health. *The Lancet*, 372, 1661–1669.

Marmot, M. G. 2010. Fair society, healthy lives: the Marmot Review: strategic review of health inequalities in England post- 2010.

Mathieu, J., Maynard, M. T., Rapp, T. & Gilson, L. 2008. Team effectiveness 1997-2007: a review of recent advancements and a glimpse into the future. *Journal of Management*, 34, 410–476.

Mathieu, J. E., Hollenbeck, J. R., Van Knippenberg, D. & Ilgen, D. R. 2017. A century of work teams in the Journal of Applied Psychology. *Journal of Applied Psychology*, 102, 452–467.

Mathieu, J. E., Wolfson, M. A. & Park, S. 2018. The evolution of work team research since Hawthorne. *The American Psychologist*, 73, 308–321.

May, C. R., Eton, D. T., Boehmer, K., Gallacher, K., Hunt, K., Macdonald, S., Mair, F. S., May, C. M., Montori, V. M., Richardson, A., Rogers, A. E. & Shippee, N. 2014. Rethinking the patient: using burden of treatment theory to understand the changing dynamics of illness. *BMC Health Services Research*, 14, 281.

McGrath, J. 1964. *Social Psychology: A Brief Introduction*, New York: Holt, Rinehart, and Winstone.

McGuier, E. A., Kolko, D. J., Aarons, G. A., Schachter, A., Klem, M. L., Diabes, M. A., Weingart, L. R., Salas, E. & Wolk, C. B. 2024. Teamwork and implementation of innovations in healthcare and human service settings: a systematic review. *Implementation Science*, 19, 49.

McHugh, S. K., Lawton, R., Hara, J. K. & Sheard, L. 2020. Does team reflexivity impact teamwork and communication in interprofessional hospital-based healthcare teams? A systematic review and narrative synthesis. *BMJ Quality Safety*, 29, 672.

Müller, M., Jürgens, J., Redaèlli, M., Klingberg, K., Hautz, W. E. & Stock, S. 2018. Impact of the communication and patient hand-off tool SBAR on patient safety: a systematic review. *BMJ Open*, 8, e022202.

Nembhard, I. M. & Edmondson, A. C. 2006. Making it safe: the effects of leader inclusiveness and professional status on psychological safety and improvement efforts in health care teams. *Journal of Organizational Behavior*, 27, 941–966.

NMC. 2019. The Code: Professional standards of practice and behaviour for nurses, midwives and nursing associates [Online]. Available: https://www.nmc.org.uk/standards/code/ [Accessed].

O'Donovan, R. & McAuliffe, E. 2020a. A systematic review exploring the content and outcomes of interventions to improve psychological safety, speaking up and voice behaviour. *BMC Health Services Research*, 20, 1–11.

O'Donovan, R. & McAuliffe, E. 2020b. A systematic review of factors that enable psychological safety in healthcare teams. *International Journal for Quality in Health Care*, 32, 240–250.

Omran, A. R. 2005. The epidemiologic transition: a theory of the epidemiology of population change. 1971. *The Milbank Quarterly*, 83, 731–757.

Parker, A. L., Forsythe, L. L. & Kohlmorgen, I. K. 2019. TeamSTEPPS(®) : an evidence-based approach to reduce clinical errors threatening safety in outpatient settings: an integrative review. *Journal of Healthcare Risk Management*, 38, 19–31.

Pype, P., Mertens, F., Helewaut, F. & Krystallidou, D. 2018. Healthcare teams as complex adaptive systems: understanding team behaviour through team members' perception of interpersonal interaction. *BMC Health Services Research*, 18, 570.

Rickards, T. & Moger, S. 2000. Creative leadership processes in project team development: an alternative to Tuckman's stage model. *British Journal of Management*, 11, 273–283.

Rocks, S., Berntson, D., Gil-Salmerón, A., Kadu, M., Ehrenberg, N., Stein, V. & Tsiachristas, A. 2020. Cost and effects of integrated care: a systematic literature review and meta-analysis. *The European Journal of Health Economics*, 21, 1211–1221.

Rosen, M. A., Diazgranados, D., Dietz, A. S., Benishek, L. E., Thompson, D., Pronovost, P. J. & Weaver, S. J. 2018. Teamwork in healthcare: key discoveries enabling safer, high-quality care. *The American Psychologist*, 73, 433–450.

Rowan, B. L., Anjara, S., de Brún, A., Macdonald, S., Kearns, E. C., Marnane, M. & Mcauliffe, E. 2022. The impact of huddles on a multidisciplinary healthcare teams' work engagement, teamwork and job satisfaction: a systematic review. *Journal of Evaluation in Clinical Practice*, 28, 382–393.

Salas, E. 2018. *The Science of Teamwork: Progress, Reflections, and the Road Ahead*, American Psychologist.

Salas, E., Cooke, N. J. & Rosen, M. A. 2008. On teams, teamwork, and team performance: discoveries and developments. *Human Factors*, 50, 540–547.

Salas, E., Reyes, D. L. & Mcdaniel, S. H. 2018a. The science of teamwork: progress, reflections, and the road ahead. *The American Psychologist*, 73, 593–600.

Salas, E., Sims, D. E. & Burke, C. S. 2005. Is there a "big five" in teamwork? *Small Group Research*, 36, 555–599.

Salas, E., Zajac, S. & Marlow, S. L. 2018b. Transforming health care one team at a time: ten observations and the trail ahead. *Group & Organization Management*, 43, 357–381.

Sanford, N., Lavelle, M., Markiewicz, O., Reedy, G., Rafferty, D. A. M., Darzi, L. A. & Anderson, J. E. 2024. Decoding healthcare teamwork: a typology of hospital teams. *Journal of Interprofessional Care*, 38, 602–611.

Saragih, I. D., Hsiao, C.-T., Fann, W.-C., Hsu, C.-M., Saragih, I. S. & Lee, B.-O. 2024. Impacts of interprofessional education on collaborative practice of healthcare professionals: A systematic review and meta-analysis. *Nurse Education Today*, 136, 106136.

Schein, E. & Bennis, W. G. 1965. *Personal and Organizational Change Through Group Methods: The Laboratory Approach*, Wiley.

Schmidt, M., Steigenberger, N., Berndtzon, M. & Uman, T. 2023. Cultural diversity in health care teams: a systematic integrative review and research agenda. *Health Care Management Review*, 48, 311–322.

Schmutz, J. B., Meier, L. L. & Manser, T. 2019. How effective is teamwork really? The relationship between teamwork and performance in healthcare teams: a systematic review and meta-analysis. *BMJ Open*, 9, e028280.

Schot, E., Tummers, L. & Noordegraaf, M. 2020. Working on working together. a systematic review on how healthcare professionals contribute to interprofessional collaboration. *Journal of Interprofessional Care*, 34, 332–342.

Shoorideh, F. A., Moosavi, S. & Balouchi, A. 2021. Incivility toward nurses: a systematic review and meta-analysis. *Journal of Medical Ethics and History of Medicine*, 14, 15.

Shuffler, M. L. & Carter, D. R. 2018. Teamwork situated in multiteam systems: key lessons learned and future opportunities. *The American Psychologist*, 73, 390–406.

Shuffler, M. L. & Cronin, M. A. 2019. The challenges of working with "real" teams: challenges, needs, and opportunities. *Organizational Psychology Review*, 9, 211–218.

Syed, M. 2021. *Rebel ideas: The Power of Thinking Differently*, John Murray.

Thomas, E. J. 2011. Improving teamwork in healthcare: current approaches and the path forward. *BMJ Quality Safety*, 20, 647.

Tu, S. P., Garcia, B., Zhu, X., Sewell, D., Mishra, V., Matin, K. & Dow, A. 2024. Patient care in complex Sociotechnological ecosystems and learning health systems. *Learning Health Systems*, 8, e10427.

Tuckman, B. W. 1965. Developmental sequence in small groups. *Psychological Bulletin*, 63, 384.

Tversky, A. & Kahneman, D. 1974. Judgment under uncertainty: heuristics and biases: biases in judgments reveal some heuristics of thinking under uncertainty. *Science*, 185, 1124–1131.

Uman, T., Edfors, E., Padoan, S. & Edberg, A.-K. 2023. Contribution of an inclusive climate to the work of culturally diverse healthcare teams: a qualitative descriptive design. *Nordic Journal of Nursing Research*, 43, 20571585211070381.

Valentine, M. A. & Edmondson, A. C. 2015. Team scaffolds: how mesolevel structures enable role-based coordination in temporary groups. *Organization Science*, 26, 405–422.

Van Diggele, C., Roberts, C., Burgess, A. & Mellis, C. 2020. Interprofessional education: tips for design and implementation. *BMC Medical Education*, 20, 455.

Wang, K. L., de Montemas, W., Dey, S., Johnson, A., Nguyen, H., Tuqiri, K., Crawford, B. & Murray, S. 2024. Not just a 'nice to have': team compassionate care behaviours and patient safety. *Australian Journal of Management*, 0, 03128962241270743.

Wears, R. L., Perry, S. J. & Patterson, E. S. 2011. Handoffs and transitions of care. *In:* Carayon, P. (ed.) *Handbook of Human Factors and Ergonomics in Health Care and Patient Safety*, 2nd Edition, Mahwah: Lawrence Erlbaum Associates, 163–171.

Weaver, S. J., Dy, S. M. & Rosen, M. A. 2014. Team-training in healthcare: a narrative synthesis of the literature. *BMJ Quality and Safety*, 23, 359–372.

Zaranko, B., Sanford, N. J., Kelly, E., Rafferty, A. M., Bird, J., Mercuri, L., Sigsworth, J., Wells, M. & Propper, C. 2023. Nurse staffing and inpatient mortality in the English national health service: a retrospective longitudinal study. *BMJ Quality & Safety*, 32, 254.

CHAPTER 20

Digital and Technological Innovation in Complex Healthcare Systems

Chris Allen[1], Eloise Monger[1], and Cheryl Metcalf[2]

[1] *School of Health Sciences, University of Southampton, Southampton, UK*
[2] *School of Healthcare Enterprise and Innovation, University of Southampton, Southampton, UK*

Introduction

In this chapter, you will be introduced to technology; what it is, the ways in which it is implemented, and what considerations there are for the delivery of safe, effective and equitable care. Technologies of various kinds are increasingly being seen as important in overcoming some of society's greatest challenges, including in health. Many technologies have the potential to improve care. But they can also have a potentially disruptive impact and result in unintended consequences, as well as exacerbating inequalities. It is therefore vital that the development of technologies consider the intended users and the broader social contexts in which the technology will be used. Building on earlier chapters, we highlight the impacts of innovations on those delivering and receiving healthcare; considering how new technologies can change how we make decisions, how we think about health, who is involved in a conditions' management and what involvement they have. Technologies are increasingly reshaping care pathways and processes, and the experiences of those delivering and receiving healthcare.

LEARNING OUTCOMES

By the end of this chapter, you will be able to:

- Explain the importance of technology and digital technology in overcoming some of the current healthcare challenges that healthcare systems around the world are experiencing.

- Recognise the potentially disruptive impact of new technologies on care and how these can be reduced.

- Understand the importance of technologies being designed and implemented with users (patients and staff), and an understanding of the clinical context it will be introduced to.

- Identify some of the most important ways that new digital technologies are changing how care is being thought about and delivered.

- Recognise the potential impact of new technologies on exacerbating existing inequalities and disadvantages.

Social Sciences for Healthcare Professionals, First Edition. Edited by Chris Allen.
© 2026 John Wiley & Sons Ltd. Published 2026 by John Wiley & Sons Ltd.

The Social Sciences, Technology, Innovation and Digital Health

> ### Key Terms and Definitions
>
> **Innovation:** Generally refers to a new idea, method or device.
>
> **Health technology:** The health products of human knowledge and skills, for example, devices, medicines and procedures.
>
> **Digital health technology:** Essentially any technology that uses digital tools to respond to a health need.
>
> **Telehealth:** Providing healthcare remotely through various technologies such as videoconferencing software and hardware.
>
> **Artificial intelligence (AI):** Computational techniques that make use of data and imitate human intellect.
>
> **Machine learning (ML):** Algorithms that build models based on data to either predict or make decisions.
>
> **Digital literacy:** Whether someone can use digital tools to solve problems, communicate and potentially even create.

The discipline of Science and Technology Studies (STS) is relatively new (Knopes, 2019). It is a truly inter-and multidisciplinary field, drawing on the work of social scientists, historians and philosophers (Knopes, 2019). The now seminal work of Latour and Woolgar (1979) and more recently Law (2002) highlighted the inseparability of science, technology and society. Put simply, technologies are products of our societies (i.e. they are normally created in response to something society either needs or demands), and once created they are then used within that society (Knopes, 2019).

Increasingly, technologies (including digital health technologies) are being explored at the intersection of Science, Technology, Health and the Social Sciences (Henwood and Marent, 2019). Whilst STS is a specific discipline within the social sciences, other social sciences have made important contributions in helping us understand more about technologies' impacts on individuals and on society more generally. Psychology, for example, often considers how technologies can influence an individual's behaviour (we cover this more in Chapter 13 in the context of behaviour change interventions) and Sociology (including its subdiscipline Medical Sociology) has helped us understand the social context of technologies, helping us understand intended use and likely success, alongside the social structures that may help or hinder a technologies adoption and diffusion, as well as the impact they may have on inequalities.

Whilst much can be gained from new technologies, they can also be ineffective and sometimes even unsafe, leading to unintended and unpredictable consequences to individuals and wider society. Recent history is full of examples of attempts to innovate that have ended up failing, such as the National Health Service (NHS) National Programme for IT (NPfIT) and other failed digital transformations (Greenhalgh et al., 2011, Wachter, 2016). As we explore throughout this chapter, approaching technology through the lens of the social sciences and understanding its impact, helps ensure that technologies are useful, equitable, responsibly designed, regulated and solution-focused; making technology far more likely to be beneficial to people and societies.

The Case for Innovation in Health

As we highlighted in Chapters 5–7, healthcare systems around the world are facing increased strain in the face of demographic and epidemiological transitions, as more people are living longer, with more complex health and social care needs. Technological advancements have had a significant role in these transitions, by improving population health and creating new ways through which diseases can be prevented, identified and treated. The relatively rapid improvements of medical science in the 20th century has increased average human longevity, resulting in an increased prevalence of chronic illness (associated with increasing age and modern lifestyles) and increased care complexity (see Chapters 18 and 19). Alongside a rise in those needing care, there are sustained global healthcare professional shortages (see Chapter 6) and reduced resources. In this context, healthcare systems, and you as healthcare professionals working within them, will increasingly need to do more, with less. This will inevitably necessitate the use of new technologies, alongside adopting fundamentally new ways of working and thinking about care. Technology has been increasingly seen as a 'magic pill' or panacea for addressing the key healthcare challenges societies will face. But as we will explore, they need to be developed responsibly, with users in mind and with an appreciation of the complex social contexts they will be deployed in.

To do this, we first need to consider what a health technology is.

What Is a Health Technology?

In 2007, the World Health Organization (WHO) defined Health Technology as:

'The application of organized knowledge and skills in the form of devices, medicines, vaccines, procedures, and systems developed to solve a health problem and improve quality of life' (WHO, 2007).

As a term, it is used interchangeably with healthcare technology. Taken broadly, health technologies influence care and the way it is delivered in several ways, and we will have the opportunity to explore some of these in this chapter.

Stop and Think: Healthcare Technologies in Practice

We would like you to take a moment to think about the health technologies that you are familiar with and that you have used, either as a healthcare professional or as someone receiving care.

- Why did you use it?
- Who referred you to it?
- What did it do?
- Were you happy with the outcome?
- Could a different technology have been used and would using a different technology have resulted in a different outcome?

What Is a Digital Health Technology?

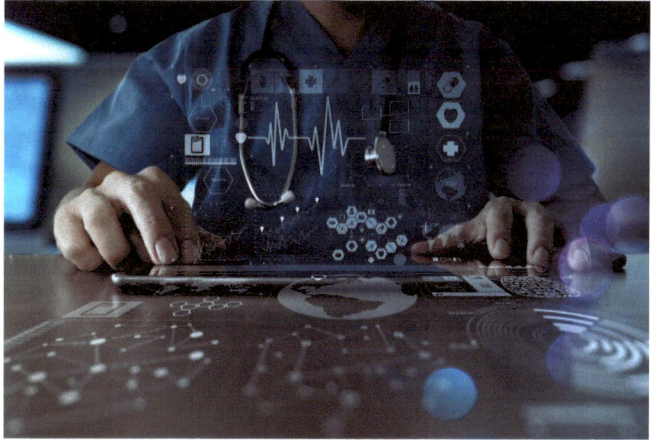

Source: everythingpossible/Adobe Stock Photos.

In 2021, the WHO emphasised digital healthcare as a strategic priority for achieving the United Nations Sustainable Development Goals (covered more in Chapter 5) (WHO, 2021). Digital health technologies can take the form of a broad range of technologies that make use of digital tools which can include those that facilitate data capture and storage such as electronic health records. These are increasing the ease of access, and levels of information available to healthcare professionals, as well as increasingly to those wanting to access more information about their own health and care (Dowding et al., 2024). They can also include those technologies that increase the personalisation of care and that allow people to be more involved in the management of their own health daily (such as self-management applications and online peer support) and on a more even footing with healthcare professionals (Allen et al., 2020, Topol, 2016). In addition, they can include those technologies that allow healthcare to be delivered at a distance, such as the software and hardware that underpins virtual consultations and remote monitoring (Gilbert et al., 2018, 2019, Wells, 2024, Wherton et al., 2021). Finally, they can include those technologies that have the potential to accelerate the use of data and evidence into clinical practice, as well as support healthcare decision-making and diagnosis, through the use of emerging computer science technologies such as AI and ML (O'Connor, 2024, O'Connor et al., 2023, Topol, 2019, WHO, 2021).

In summary, you will have likely seen and made use of a range of innovations and digital tools, either as a user of healthcare services or as a healthcare professional. You may have had some positive experiences with these. After all, most are fundamentally intended to improve care, by making care more effective, efficient, convenient, personalised and safe (Topol, 2019, WHO, 2021). However, you may have also encountered new technologies that don't work, don't address a clear need, negatively disrupt care processes and pathways, or lead to situations that are unsafe. In these situations, you might feel like you are stuck with technology when what you want is a technology that works. By considering the potential benefits of new technologies, alongside their associated evidence bases, societies need to identify which technologies are likely to be beneficial now, which technologies are desirable for future application, and equally, which technologies may be harmful and unwanted.

When new technologies and ways of working are being considered, it is important to understand the technology, its likely impact on those delivering and receiving care, as well as its likely impact on the wider healthcare system and society more generally.

There are some important questions to consider here, including:

- How does the technology work? Is it easy to use, reliable and safe? Are there appropriate safeguards in place?
- Will the technology change existing care pathways and processes that have often become embedded over many years, and which people value and are accustomed to? What will the impact of these changes be?
- What knowledge and skills are required to use the technology safely and effectively? Are they present within the existing workforce or will further training and support be required?
- Will the technology create new roles?
- Will the technology deskill the current workforce and make existing roles irrelevant?
- Will the target population be able to access and use the technology equitably? Or will some be disadvantaged and further marginalised by the technology?
- Will the technology create dependence? Is there a risk to service delivery if the technology breaks?
- Can the technology be sustained over time? Is there adequate and stable funding available to ensure its continued use?

Understanding What Makes Us Unwell

Health technologies used to support diagnosis influence the way healthcare professionals and society come to understand health and disease in several ways (see Chapter 3). In turn, this can influence how care is accessed and delivered (Hofmann and Svenaeus, 2018). As technology has improved, we are now better able to detect abnormalities that may predict future disease. Many years ago, the scalpel, which can be defined as a technology, enabled the first systematic dissections of human bodies which paved the way for an improved understanding of human anatomy and physiology. More recent technology, for example, medical imaging technologies such as computed tomography (CT), magnetic resonance imaging (MRI), positron emission tomography (PET) and ultrasound scans tell us even more about our body's inner workings and therefore have changed how healthcare is delivered and experienced. Such imaging can be powerful, for example, the use of ultrasound scans has changed how maternity care is delivered, how it is experienced, and how people first connect with their unborn children (Lumley, 1990, Øyen and Aune, 2016). These technologies can also change who gets care. Routine screening (now a mainstay public health secondary prevention intervention) may detect a sign or marker of disease in someone who is otherwise presenting as well, changing the way they are seen and see themselves from being healthy to being sick and in need of treatment. Improved detection of abnormalities, whilst having the potential to improve health, may also result in issues that may be relatively benign, becoming subject to aggressive and potentially life-changing interventions (see overdiagnosis in Chapter 3).

New technologies also influence how people see and monitor their own health. Commercial products, such as health monitoring apps on smartphones and consumer genetic testing, can provide opportunities for people to monitor their estimated likelihood of developing a disease (Laranjo et al., 2021, Nolan and Ormondroyd, 2023). This access to personal health-related data (often in real time) enables and empowers individuals to take responsibility and potentially corrective action. For example, an individual may change health behaviours if results suggest that they might be at a high risk of disease (Majumder et al., 2021, Panacer, 2023). This may be hugely beneficial if it leads to improved longer-term outcomes, but it could also potentially lead to an increase in health anxiety and consequential increased demands on health systems from people not requiring care.

A Helping Hand: Decision Support, Artificial Intelligence (AI) and Machine Learning (ML)

Two main categories of AI tools are likely to have an increasing impact on healthcare delivery, these are:

Generative AI: 'Generates' text from a brief or instruction and may increasingly be used to free up the time taken on administrative tasks, such as writing clinical notes, letters and reports. Generative AI can do this in seconds, rather than the many hours of human effort that have traditionally been required for such activities, freeing up time for tasks that more specifically require human input (O'Connor, 2024, O'Connor et al., 2023, Topol, 2019, Woodnutt et al., 2024).

Predictive AI: Predictive analytics have been used in healthcare for some time, as a way of assessing likely outcomes and risks (O'Connor, 2024). Advancements in ML have allowed for predictive modelling that may influence care in several ways, such as genetic profiling, reducing the risk of human error (e.g. through automatic image interpretation highlighting where there may be suspected abnormalities), as well as predicting how individual patients are likely to respond to certain treatments (O'Connor, 2024, Topol, 2019). AI and ML alongside an improved understanding of genetics are likely to open the door to truly personalised, precision medicine and care (Dias and Torkamani, 2019, Johnson et al., 2021). Instead of one pill and dose being offered to everyone in at-risk populations, new technologies may allow people to be offered *the precise* treatment that someone with their specific constitutional factors is most likely to positively respond to (Johnson et al., 2021).

AI has some significant limitations. It makes a 'best guess', based on algorithms and the use of training datasets, and these may introduce bias resulting in inequitable decision-making. This is especially true for those who are less represented in the datasets that it uses, such as marginalised groups (explored later in this chapter) (Whitehead et al., 2024). In addition, AI is currently incapable of making the complex judgements that humans can. Whilst AI and ML might be a helpful hand in highlighting abnormal skin changes, blood results, or imaging, and in producing decision support tools (O'Connor, 2024, Topol, 2019), a trained human is still generally needed to interpret and act on these findings in context.

Health and Self-Management Tools

Research has demonstrated that digital health apps can be acceptable to those using them (North et al., 2020). There is some evidence that self-management apps may be effective in reducing hospital admissions, by helping people manage their condition and any acute exacerbation from home, often with limited or no professional involvement (Alwashmi et al., 2016, Yang et al., 2018).

As the number of health apps available continues to grow, international and national regulators are struggling to keep pace with their proliferation, and apps can vary considerably in quality and efficacy (Chib and Lin, 2018). There are, as with other fast-moving areas of innovation, challenges to creating a robust evidence base (Gordon et al., 2020). App development and deployment is quick, and evidence generation is typically slow, largely due to the necessary rigors and safeguards of research, particularly clinical research (Gordon et al., 2020). A lack of evidence does not necessarily mean that a digital health app is not useful or safe, especially to those who find that they benefit from them; it just means use should be approached with caveats and cautions, particularly in the context of healthcare professional prescription or recommendation (Akbar et al., 2020).

Various technologies, including lay access to electronic health records and the increase in individuals' use of health apps, mean people will have more opportunities to self-manage their health and this necessitates healthcare professionals adopting and developing their clinical practices to support this shift in responsibility (Topol, 2016, 2019). This will require working with patients and potentially using patients' own personally generated and held data[1] to offer personalised support in clinical consultations (Strudwick, 2024, Topol, 2016). It has been suggested for some time that new technologies have the potential to change patient/provider relationships through increased lay access to information, and where those accessing care may have more access to data about their own health than their healthcare professionals. This may reduce medical hegemony and increase patient autonomy over the management of their conditions (Hardey, 1999). However, the increased opportunities people have to self-manage their health will generally require digital and health literacy, which has the potential to place those with lower literacies at a disadvantage (Arias López et al., 2023).

Remote Access, Video Consultations and Virtual Wards

New technologies can provide opportunities to deliver healthcare at a distance. This has potential benefits to healthcare providers and those accessing care; for example, by increasing efficiency, minimising the environmental impact of travel, and potentially even decreasing the need for some physical estates and facilities.

Whilst the technology has been available for some time and has been examined in a range of different clinical contexts (Gilbert et al., 2018, 2019, Wells, 2024, Wherton et al., 2021), the COVID-19 pandemic provided something of an opportunity (in crisis) for the rapid deployment of remote consultation, including video consultation in the United Kingdom (Wherton et al., 2021), and other countries (Møller et al., 2024, Peeters et al., 2024). In the context of the pandemic, the primary motivation for such rapid deployment was to allow healthcare access to continue where physical access wasn't required, or where it might put people at risk of contracting COVID-19 (Jiménez-Rodríguez et al., 2020).

Remote access to care is likely to become increasingly common. In the NHS in England, for example, 'virtual wards' have been rolled out in several care settings (Wells, 2024). Evidence suggests that virtual wards and hospital-at-home services have the potential to improve outcomes by extending acute care provision into people's homes, reducing the iatrogenic risks associated with acute hospital care (such as hospital acquired infections), improving people's experiences of care and reducing the burden of treatment (Chauhan and McAlister, 2022, Lin et al., 2024).

> ### Stop and Think: Technologies and Current Use in Practice
>
> Recent reviews, such as the Topol (2019) review, have highlighted that some technologies will have a significant impact on healthcare professional roles and how care is delivered.
>
> Health technology is moving forward at pace. The tools that you will be using in your practice and how you are using them (e.g. on who) will continue to evolve over time. With some of the examples of different technologies above, can you identify specific examples of their use in your current practice?
>
> You might want to consider the following in your reflections:
>
> - How was the technology used?
> - Who was the technology used by? Was it intended to be used in a specific condition or by a specific group?
> - Did the technology meet the needs of those using it?
> - Did the technology lead to improved care?
> - Were there any aspects of the technology that were unhelpful, or made things more difficult for you, or for those accessing care?
>
> | Technology | Examples you have seen |
> |---|---|
> | Telemedicine | |
> | Smartphone applications | |
> | Sensors and wearables for diagnostics and remote monitoring | |
> | Virtual and augmented reality | |
> | Automated image interpretation using artificial intelligence (AI) | |
> | Predictive analytics using AI | |

---

[1]Increasingly, patients will have data about their health that healthcare professionals do not. For example, the data held by self-trackers, and data collected by medical devices, such as glucometers in self-managing diabetes.

Preparing Healthcare Professionals for the Digital Future

The Topol (2019) Review made recommendations on how to support the healthcare workforce to make use of digital innovations to improve healthcare delivery, particularly in relation to safety and efficiency (Topol, 2019). Alongside the NHS Long Term plan (NHS, 2019) and Long Term Workforce plan (NHS, 2023), there is a recognition in the United Kingdom that digital technologies will become an increasingly central feature of how care is thought about and delivered, alongside a recognition that some healthcare systems, such as the NHS, have been slow to adapt and make use of new technologies (Darzi, 2024). The COVID-19 pandemic demonstrated that healthcare professionals do have the ability, often very quickly, to adopt new ways of working. However, the arrival of new technologies, in particular the embedding of new digital technologies into clinical practice, raises important questions about how they should be evaluated, implemented and used safely to augment and improve the care that is provided by healthcare professionals.

In Chapter 6, we highlighted the challenges in defining what is and what is not a 'healthcare professional'. In the context of technology adoption and improvement, everyone working in healthcare should be encouraged to be agents of change, especially where changes can make a meaningful impact on the quality of care. Whilst recognising all those working in healthcare are important in supporting adoption, Professional Statutory and Regulatory Bodies such as in the United Kingdom: the Nursing and Midwifery Council (NMC, 2019), General Medical Council (GMC, 2017) and the Health and Care Professions Council (HCPC, 2023), are stipulating the importance of their registered healthcare professionals being able to demonstrate the numeracy, literacy, digital and technological skills that are needed to meet people's increasingly complex needs in a safe, secure and effective way.

Healthcare professionals having the knowledge and skills to use the full range of technologies that support care, is clearly important. Often overlooked is the interaction of healthcare professionals with these technologies, how the technologies are designed and how they impact on clinical workflows. In the previous chapters, we introduced you to the Systems Engineering Initiative for Patient Safety (SEIPS) model, highlighting that you work in a complex system and the quality of care that you are able to provide is shaped by many things. This includes the various tools and technologies that you use, which can either help or hinder you depending on how well they are designed around your needs, the needs of those accessing care and the healthcare system more generally (Carayon et al., 2006).

Technologies, when designed well, can free up your time, giving you more time to spend with those accessing care

(Bingham et al., 2021). They can also increase safety, for example, closed-loop medication administration systems[2] that mitigate risks caused by human error (Shah et al., 2016). However, they can also pull you away from patients (e.g. by forcing you to look at a computer) (Forde-Johnston et al., 2023), and this can be especially the case whilst you are building up confidence using something new. Increasing confidence and competence to use something new requires knowledge and trust in the technology itself, alongside baseline digital, social and communication skills[3] (Konttila et al., 2019). Competence and confidence to use a technology are generally influenced by several things, such as positive or negative experiences of using technology in the past (Konttila et al., 2019).

Where healthcare professionals lack the required competence to use new technologies, especially where the technology is also poorly designed and challenging to use, patient harm is more likely (Salahuddin and Ismail, 2015). The interaction of healthcare professionals, with technologies within a complex system, makes it necessary for healthcare professionals to be included in the development of the new technologies that they will be required to use, as this allows the technology to fit within clinical workflows (Kruse et al., 2016). However, technology is often something that is 'done to', rather than 'done with' healthcare professionals. Where healthcare professionals have been excluded from their development, innovations can hinder or increase work which in turn increases the likeliness that the technology won't be used, or 'workarounds' will be adopted (Fraczkowski et al., 2020, Wisner et al., 2019).

Stop and Think: Technology, Help or Hindrance?

Thinking about your own clinical practice, can you identify the use of technology which has:

1. Decreased the time taken to perform a basic, or complex administrative task. In what ways did it improve efficiency?

2. Increased the time taken to perform a basic, or complex administrative task. In what ways did the technology increase the amount of time taken?

3. Released time for you to provide more direct patient care. How did the technology facilitate this and what was the impact?

4. Taken time away from direct patient care. How did the technology cause this and what was the impact?

5. Made a task more efficient. In what way did the technology make a task more efficient?

---

[2]You may well have seen or used these. This is essentially where barcodes for patients and their drugs are scanned, to ensure the right patient, receives the right drug, at the right time.

[3]Because interacting with someone over a video consultation, for example, is very different to interacting with someone in person.

6. Made a task less efficient. In what way did the technology make a task less efficient?

7. Increased patient safety. How did the technology contribute to this?

8. Made care more unsafe. In what way did the technology contribute to care that was more unsafe?

9. Improved a key patient outcome: such as reducing the number and severity of complications or reducing someone's length of stay.

10. Made no difference to key patient outcomes. Why do you think this was the case?

11. Led to worse patient outcomes. Why do you think this was the case?

Healthcare professionals should not just be intended users of new innovations. Alongside patients and service users, they can contribute significant clinical knowledge about what technologies are needed and can themselves be the innovators. Creating psychologically safe environments (covered in the previous chapter) allows healthcare professionals to be increasingly entrepreneurial and make suggestions for innovations that might improve care and health outcomes (Hatton and Stanmore, 2024). In the next section, we consider the importance of needs-led, responsible innovation which healthcare professionals should have increasing opportunities to be involved with, either as the creators of such innovations or as significant contributors, alongside other stakeholders, to their design and deployment.

What Does Success Look Like? Needs Led and Responsible Innovation

New technologies can emerge at pace from a rapidly expanding, and often financially lucrative MedTech sector. Government Institutions do not have the resources to do this innovation alone and these industries are becoming an increasingly important partner in addressing the healthcare challenges that we face. Many companies have solid commitments to corporate social responsibility, a concept that you were introduced to in Chapter 12. However, a desire to push the boundaries of technology (creating new stuff) and the need for private companies to be profitable, can lead to new technologies being pushed out into healthcare systems that are not needed, not useful, not valued, and not socially responsible. In this section, we outline the importance of engaging with a range of stakeholders and users, including those from marginalised groups, to ensure innovations are developed responsibly to fit the needs, demands and constraints of those who will be using them

(including lay people and healthcare professionals), wider stakeholders, healthcare systems, society and importantly our planet (Lehoux et al., 2022, Pacifico Silva et al., 2018).

Doing this well involves fully understanding the issue that the technology seeks to address from all perspectives, for example:

- How does it affect those accessing and receiving care?

- How do healthcare professionals manage patient care and what problems does the innovation seek to address for them?

- Will the new technology replace an existing activity or whole set of activities, and if it will, what are the likely consequences and who will be affected?

- Will there be any impacts to other parts of the healthcare system and what needs to change elsewhere in the system (including at the macro level of policy and regulation) to ensure new solutions are compliant with the relevant legislation?

- Will the new technology replace or simply augment healthcare workers?

- Will people need new skills or will they be deskilled by the technology?

- And then there is the question of who pays for it, and how is it funded.

Whatever the innovation, it is important that it adds value, that it does not further exacerbate the issues it seeks to address, and that any unintended consequences can be safely managed (Lehoux et al., 2022, Pacifico Silva et al., 2018). Stilgoe et al.'s (2013) seminal Responsible Research Innovation (RRI) framework highlights four important considerations that should increasingly guide responsible innovation; these are:

Anticipation: Emerging technologies often pop up in markets that have no appropriate regulatory frameworks or rules that govern them. For example, the availability of generative AIs such as Chat-GPT saw various institutions scramble to create rules and regulations to contain their use. Where regulatory frameworks fail to create adequate safeguards and governance, patient harm can follow (Carreyrou, 2023). It is therefore necessary to horizon scan, consider which technologies might become important in the future and ensure rules and regulations are responsive to them when they emerge.

Reflexivity: This involves innovators considering their own activities and behaviours, being mindful that there may be limits to what they know, and being mindful that how they see an innovation (in terms of its value, importance, etc.), may not be how others see it. It is important for innovators to be able to challenge their own bias and preconceptions. After all, it's natural to be excited about something we have created or a problem that we believe we have solved (especially when significant time and resource have already been invested), and it is important to be able to reflect on this, in the context of what it might be able to do for others and for society. Codes of conduct and commitments to corporate social responsibility can help steer such reflection.

Inclusion: This emphasises the importance of seeking a wide range of views, from a diverse range of people. For example, requiring the inclusion of lay members on advisory committees and overt efforts to involve those whose voices are seldom heard, such as those from marginalised groups. In combination with reflexivity, engagement with a broad range of views helps innovators challenge their assumptions and can lead to increased creativity. There are several existing ways to engage those from diverse backgrounds through increasing patient and public involvement and engagement (PPIE) opportunities, such as through youth panels and disability forums (Metcalf et al., 2024).

Responsiveness: This emphasises the importance of being able to change course based on new knowledge or norms, or on feedback, for example, if an intended user or stakeholder says something won't work. It also highlights the importance of being responsive to new challenges when they emerge.

Many aspects of this framework overlap, for example, increased anticipation can lead to increased inclusion, where a diverse range of views are sought as to how an emergent technology should be governed. Inclusion, when done well, can also promote reflexivity (as it broadens access to different viewpoints), which might, in turn, lead to increasing responsiveness. Importantly, underpinning all these dimensions, engaging intended users alongside stakeholders is emphasised.

Intended User and Stakeholder Engagement

In your practice, but also in your daily lives, you will have seen technologies that work well and respond to a clear need. It is likely that these are technologies that you value and therefore continue to use, even without being told you have to. In contrast, you will have also seen technologies that are clunky, do not really work or do not really address any significant issues that you are experiencing. It is less likely that you value this type of technology and you have probably stopped using it altogether, or if you were forced to use it, you have likely developed some workarounds or shortcuts to minimise its impact on you.

Innovations are far more likely to be successfully embedded when people see value in them (Sinek, 2009). For any technology to be useful (and therefore valued), it needs to be developed with its intended users (this can include service users and healthcare professionals), with input from other stakeholders and with a full appreciation and understanding of the social context in which the technology will be deployed (Dickinson et al., 2019).

For an innovation, understanding the social context involves consideration of the likely barriers and facilitators of the innovations design and development, including whether the technology will be integrated into an existing complex system or change the system entirely (Pereno and Eriksson, 2020, Yazdi and Acharya, 2013). Stakeholder engagement is an important and often overlooked step in needs-led innovation (Pacifico Silva et al., 2018). One of the authors' previous work (Metcalf et al., 2024), involved developing an engagement methodology to help guide this and highlighted the following important steps:

1. Understanding who the stakeholders are – this involves stakeholder mapping.
2. Understanding the perspectives and influences of stakeholders, such as through using the Mendelow matrix[4] (Mendelow, 1991).
3. Having conversations with relevant stakeholders.
4. Understanding and presenting commonality by creating a Barriers and Opportunities Map.

By considering social context and by engaging with those likely to be using the technology (healthcare professionals and those accessing care), as well as other key stakeholders, it is far more likely that a technology will address people's needs and will be more likely to be valued, and subsequently used. After all, needs-led innovations are far more likely to be successfully implemented in practice and improve healthcare delivery than technology-led innovations where something new is created, simply because it can be (Dickinson et al., 2019).

In Chapter 12, we introduced you to Everett Roger's (1931–2004) Diffusion of Innovations Theory (Rogers, 2003, Rogers et al., 2014), which is a seminal theory in the social sciences, highlighting that when a new idea or innovation is first introduced, it can take time before it gains momentum and takes off, diffusing beyond those keen early adopters to others within a social system. Diffusion of an innovation across a social system depends on many things. Whilst there will always be early adopters and conversely laggards, who adopt the technology later, the rate at which an innovation diffuses (if it diffuses at all) is influenced by several things, including its:

Relative advantage: Is it better than what already exists? Engagement with intend users and all relevant stakeholders can help innovators better understand what is already available and if their proposed solution is any better.

Compatibility: How compatible is the innovation with the social systems' values and processes? Engagement, with intended users and all relevant stakeholders, can help innovators determine how well their proposed solution will fit within the existing social system.

Complexity: How straightforward is the innovation to use – no one likes something that is unnecessarily complicated and hard to use.

---

[4]The Mendelow matrix is quadrant figure, with a stakeholder's power (low to high) mapped against their interest (also low to high). Once mapped, this tool can be used to prioritise and plan when, how and from what perspective to engage with different stakeholders.

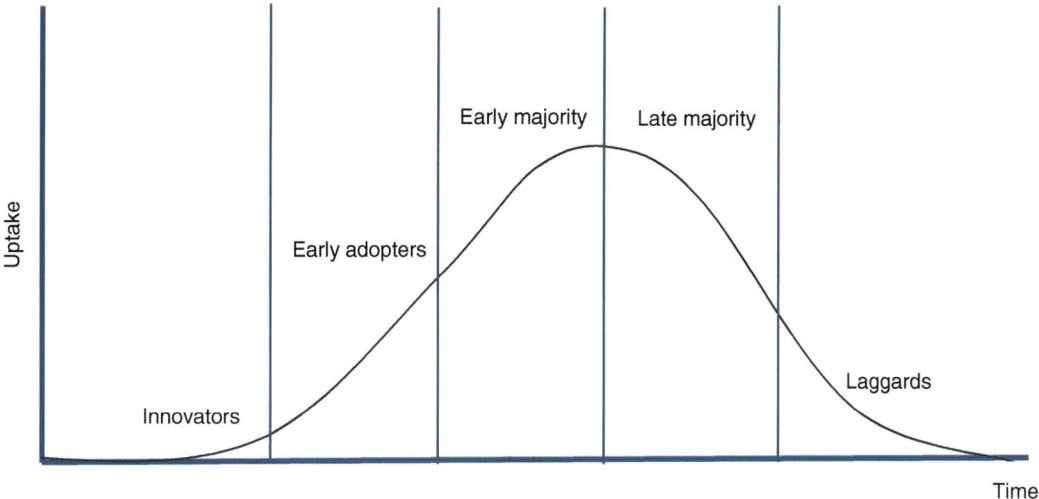

FIGURE 20.1   Diffusion of innovation curve. **Source:** Adapted from: Rogers (2003).

Trialability: Can intended users and stakeholders test, inter-act, or 'play' with the innovation before they make deci-sions about it. Allowing intended users and stakeholders to do this can also elicit valuable feedback.

Observability: Can outcomes be observed? Does using the technology result in tangible, visible benefits?

Ultimately, it is important to understand the target popu-lation, as well as the full range of factors (i.e. the social context), that are likely to influence the adoption and diffusion (or spread) of an innovation within a social system. Engaging with those who will be using the technology and ensuring they have the opportunity to contribute to its design, may encourage them to become early adopters (as shown in the now seminal diffusion of the innovation curve in Figure 20.1) and promote the spread and scalability of the innovation in your clinical set-ting (Rogers and Shoemaker, 1971).

There is now a range of systematic approaches and formal methods such as design thinking, user-led design, co-development and PPIE that can help to ensure intended end users and wider key stakeholders are directly involved in the development and deployment of new health technologies.

Adoption: Moving Beyond Creation

What we have just considered increases the likeliness that what is created is valued, needed and wanted, and that it fits the needs of healthcare (professionals and patients) in a socially responsible way. All of this improves the chances of an innova-tion being adopted and sustained in clinical practice.

The Non-adoption, Abandonment, Scale-up, Spread and Sustainability (NASSS) framework proposed by Greenhalgh et al. (2017) (See Figure 20.2) is useful in guiding our thinking and con-versations around the adoption of new technologies into clinical practice. Greenhalgh and colleague's work involved systemati-cally reviewing a range of empirical case studies that considered the adoption of new technologies and identifying what factors impacted on their mainstreaming and continued use.

The NASSS framework can be used alongside the considera-tions for responsible innovations that we have outlined earlier. Using the NASSS framework, you are encouraged to consider:

The condition: The first consideration the framework consid-ers is the condition that the technology will address. In their work, the authors found that it was common for clinicians to not use technologies where concerns existed around the complexity of patient needs, such as their high levels of morbidity, their overall cognition (especially where this is impaired) and broader concerns around their socio-economic position and general health literacy (Greenhalgh et al., 2017).

The technology: The next consideration is the technology itself, including its features (both material and technical), its interoperability (which is discussed later), its ongoing sustainability (in terms of sources of funding and relation-ships with suppliers) and how these translate into ease of use. Technologies that are challenging to use, change pro-fessional roles, have poor aesthetics, are unreliable or diffi-cult to interpret (especially when the stakes are high), are less likely to be adopted and become mainstreamed (ibid).

Value proposition: This links to what we have discussed already and considers whether the technology is value-led and solutions-focused and whether it adequately addresses the challenges people are concerned about (ibid).

Adopter system: This considers the readiness and the atti-tudes of those who are going to be using the technology: such as patients, their caregivers, and staff. Staff may be concerned about the impact of the technology on their patients, or about the impact of the technology on their role, or even their job security. Healthcare professionals, as well as patients, may not trust new technologies (Adjekum et al., 2018), may lack the necessary skills to use them and

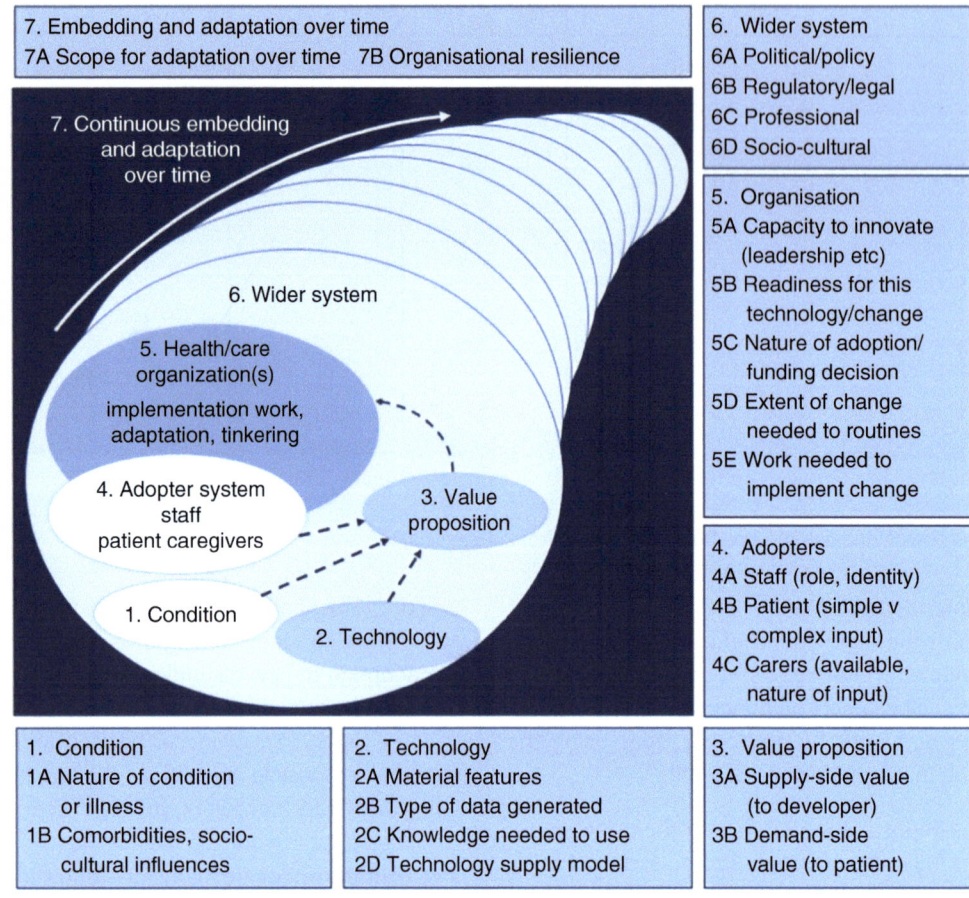

FIGURE 20.2   The NASSS framework – a useful framework for considering the various system influences that relate to how likely a technology is likely to be adopted into clinical practice. **Source:** Greenhalgh et al. (2017)/JMIR Publications/CC BY 4.0.

have limited resources and social support to help them adjust to changes in life routines that new technologies invariably present (Reidy et al., 2020).

Organisation: The long-term sustainability of any new technology requires a financial commitment from healthcare providers. Understanding the full economic impact of any new deployment can be challenging, as costs need to be considered beyond those involved in simply buying the technology. Cost and savings are not always easy to predict, as it is not always clear what uptake will be like, and how much can be saved/or lost through improved or worsening efficiency elsewhere in the system.

The wider context: These are often the macro-level features of society that make such innovations relevant (or irrelevant), such as the broader policy, regulatory body approval and funding arrangements of the technologies, and acceptance of those who will be working with them (such as professional regulatory bodies).

And finally; the interaction between these domains, and the technologies ongoing adoption overtime (Greenhalgh et al., 2017) (Figure 20.2).

Healthcare Systems Readiness for Innovations

Where technologies have the potential to address significant societal issues and improve care for individuals and populations, a lack of health system readiness or clear implementation strategy can significantly impact the likelihood of any new technology being safely and effectively adopted into mainstream clinical practice (Greenhalgh et al., 2017).

Some further important considerations include:

- Contingency planning (what must be done to continue to deliver safe and effective care, if the technology fails).
- Interoperability (how well different technologies work together).
- Security and information governance.

Contingency Planning

New technologies are generally rolled out as either a 'big bang' (i.e. all at once) or incrementally (which can be safer but can result in more than one process existing within the same health system) (Maguire et al., 2018). Once fully embedded within a system, the change often becomes irreversible quickly. For example, you will likely now be very used to electronic prescribing systems, but not that long ago, prescriptions were largely paper based. With electronic prescribing systems now such a mainstay in clinical practice in so many settings, it would require a significant and coordinated effort to go back to exclusively paper-based prescribing in most clinical settings. Healthcare services, other processes, staff and patients themselves in many settings have become so accustomed to and dependent upon electronic prescribing, that if the technology were to now fail, it would be highly disruptive. Acceptable contingencies need to be considered and adopted to ensure continued safe and effective care in the event of technological failure.

Interoperability

Think about your current or recent clinical role. Do those accessing the service have to repeatedly tell you and other healthcare professionals the same information as they move between services, or even between different aspects of the same service? In most healthcare systems, the answer is probably yes. This is often because the various information systems that healthcare delivery is reliant on are unable to interface with one another. This is often referred to as 'interoperability' (Mistry et al., 2022). The rapid emergence of tools that capture and store health data, sometimes with limited consideration as to how they will work with existing technologies, work systems and processes, has meant that often data exists in multiple settings and contexts, in different formats, states of completeness and with differing levels of access between providers and patients. For example, multiple systems for electronic prescribing, patient monitoring, clinical imaging and laboratory result reporting exist (sometimes even within the same healthcare system) but they often don't link together or share data, and this can result in care feeling disjointed, as well as being ineffective and potentially unsafe (Janakiraman et al., 2023, Li et al., 2022).

Security

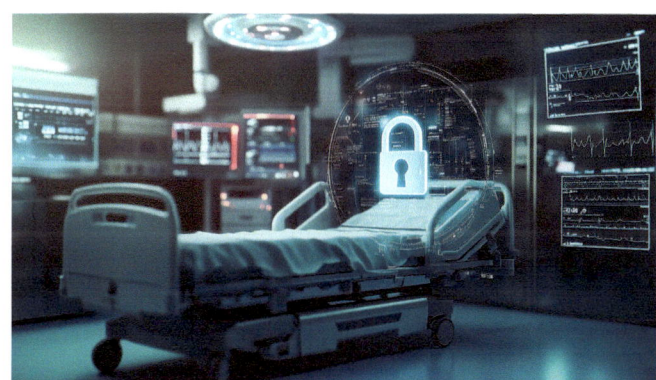

Source: andyaziz6/Adobe Stock Photos.

New technologies continue to test security and information governance processes. With the increasing number of systems being supported by digital tools, the Internet of Things (IoT) and even more relevant the Internet of Medical Things (IoMT) (De Michele and Furini, 2019), alongside the increased need to share information between different systems (sometimes with different data owners), the vulnerability to and incidence of unauthorised access, tampering and various other forms of 'cyber-attack' have increased (Alajlan et al., 2023, Dickson, 2024, Tarikere et al., 2021). The nature of these threats and the risks that they create for healthcare systems is continuing to evolve. Recent challenges have included the publishing of confidential patient data on the internet and the prolonged and widespread disruption caused by cyberattacks. For the potential benefits of new digital technologies to be realised, without unintended harms emerging through such threats, governments, healthcare systems and the creators of digital innovations will increasingly need to work together to manage risk and mitigate harm.

Poor information governance has been identified in several digital health applications, including those with specific endorsements from healthcare providers. For example, research into the applications that were promoted within the since-retired NHS Apps Library found that promoted applications poorly protected user's identities and personal information (Huckvale et al., 2015).

> **Stop and Think: NASSS Framework**
>
> Using the outline of the NASSS framework provided, consider an innovation in your current practice setting.
>
> To what extent were the following considerations made, prior to the technology being adopted?
>
> What impact did these have, and how have they resulted in the technology continuing to be used, or being abandoned?
>
> - The condition
> - The technology
> - The value proposition
> - The adopter system
> - The organisation
> - The wider context

Technologies, Inequality and Their Impact on Health

Various digital technologies, such as contract tracing apps, and video consultations, as well as technologies used by people to carry out everyday tasks such as working from home, shopping and connecting digitally with socially distanced friends and family, helped to stem the spread of the COVID-19 virus and protect those most vulnerable. The swiftness within which such technologies became so widespread in their use and have since continued to be used, serves to underline the increasing relevance of digital technologies to many aspects of our everyday lives. For many, the increasing ubiquity of digital technologies in everyday life expands people's opportunities, by reducing barriers to knowledge (including that related to health) (Litchman et al., 2019, Kingod et al., 2017), as well as helping people to extend and maintain their social networks through, for example, social media applications (Allen et al., 2020). However, alongside the new opportunities digital technologies may create, there are new types of inequality. In terms of the internet, these inequalities principally reveal themselves in two ways:

- Either people lack access to the technology altogether,
- Or, they have access but do not have the necessary knowledge or skills to use the technology in ways that are meaningful or beneficial to them.

Assumptions that all have access can often underpin digital health interventions, consequently, their deployment can exacerbate inequalities, where people do not have access or do not have the skills to access and use them in meaningful or beneficial ways. The rising importance of the internet, and its impact on inequality, has led to academics calling for revisions to the Rainbow Model (first introduced in chapter 8) (Jahnel et al., 2022, Morley et al., 2020, Rice and Sara, 2019). One argument is that rather than recreating the model with an extra layer, we recognise that some degree of digital transformation

has permeated into most aspects of our daily lives, and therefore, its influence should be considered within the layers of the existing model (Jahnel et al., 2022). This is shown in the digital rainbow in Figure 20.3.

One example of this, which has relevance to how much patients can reasonably be expected to take on greater responsibility for the management of their conditions (as we discussed earlier), is access to personal health data (Jahnel et al., 2022). Whilst in the United Kingdom (alongside many other countries) people have had a right to access data about their health for some time, accessing this has not been straightforward. Providing the public with easy access to their own health information (such as through electronic health records) has been an ambition of many countries for some time and has been noted as a significant achievement for some countries in promoting patient empowerment (Britnell, 2015). At the macro level, a country's general socioeconomic and cultural conditions (the outer ring on the Dahlgren and Whitehead model) ultimately determines how much effort is put into achieving such ambitions, and how much is invested in supporting access to new technologies that may benefit individuals and populations (Dahlgren and Whitehead, 2021, Whitehead and Dahlgren, 1991).

In addition, digital technology also shapes our living and working conditions. The internet is increasingly used to access good (and bad) quality health information and healthcare (both physically e.g. booking appointments and online) (Arias López et al., 2023), as well as access to and attainment from other institutions that relate to our health, such as education and employment (both of which are important determinants of health as explored in Chapter 8, and both are important in terms of

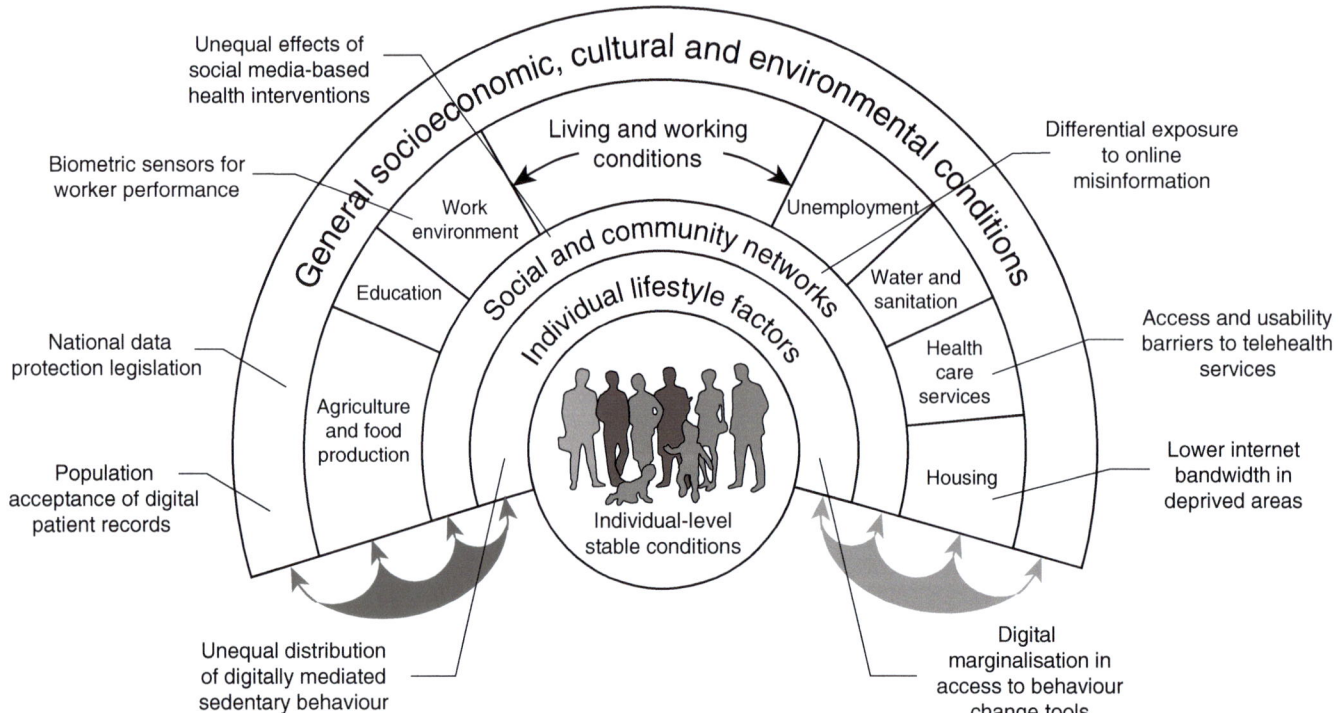

FIGURE 20.3 Adapted Dahlgren and Whitehead model, highlighting the relevance of digital domains of everyday life to social determinants of health and inequalities. **Source:** Jahnel et al (2022) / with permission of SAGE Publications.

supporting digital literacy and health literacy more generally). Thus where marginalised groups face poorer access, existing inequalities may be further exacerbated by such technologies (Arias López et al., 2023). As a further example, the use of video consultations can both increase access, particularly for those in remote areas, or those who are unable to take time off work or from caring responsibilities (Wherton et al., 2021), but may significantly disadvantage others (such as those without a compatible device, those without adequate internet connection, those without the necessary knowledge and skills, or those who are unable to access a private space to have sensitive discussions in), especially if physical face to face options are not retained, such as when processes become 'digital by default'. Those disadvantaged and socially excluded in other ways are likely to experience greater challenges accessing and using digital technologies in a beneficial way (Ragnedda et al., 2022); and multiple forms of disadvantage often intersect (see Chapter 8) (Husain et al., 2022).

Healthcare devices can also result in some groups being disadvantaged. For example, a recent independent review of medical devices, commissioned by the UK Government, found inequities in the accuracy of blood oxygen saturation measurements using pulse oximetry in those with darker skin tones (Whitehead et al., 2024). The review also highlighted the impacts of a lack of diversity in the data AI is trained on, with much of the data coming from white men which results in an inherent bias in AI's recommendations. This means that use may negatively impact the care and safety of those with different personal characteristics (Whitehead et al., 2024). There are also significant differences in the health technologies that people can access. As we highlighted in Chapter 5, in most sectors, consumers drive sales and therefore have some degree of autonomy in the choices that they make about what technologies they access. In contrast, access to healthcare innovations varies considerably between different healthcare systems, as care is financed, organised and regulated in different ways. Where you live, whether you have access to free healthcare like the NHS or other forms of universal health coverage, voluntary or compulsory health insurance, and your socio-economic status, often determine what healthcare services you can access, and through these, what technologies you can make use of. Differences exist, even within the same healthcare system, for example, in the United Kingdom there are postcode-related differences in access to in vitro fertilisation (IVF) and devices that help people with diabetes track their blood sugar levels (Hamper and Perrotta, 2023, Iacobucci, 2018).

Clinical Considerations

- New technologies, when designed well and with their intended users, can make care safer and more efficient.

- However, new technologies can also be very disruptive and may make delivering safe and effective care challenging, especially where users or existing care processes have not been considered.

- Digital literacy is being recognised as increasingly important in terms of people being able to make use of digital tools to be able to support their own health and well-being.

- New technologies can exacerbate existing inequalities, with those most likely to be disadvantaged by them being more likely to be from already socially excluded groups.

Conclusion

In this chapter, we have outlined the case for the need for innovation to address global healthcare challenges. Many of the new technologies that we discussed have the potential to improve care. But if the groundwork is not done first, they can also be disruptive, potentially placing people at risk. We have highlighted several technologies, including digital technologies, that are increasingly impacting on health and care, and changing the roles of, and relationships between healthcare professionals and healthcare users. The place of needs-led, responsible innovation has been explored, and the potential impacts of new technologies have on worsening inequalities have been considered. Many of these technologies are best seen as enablers, having the potential to increase the quality and effectiveness of care, freeing up time for people to be able to provide excellent care. In the context of such rapid technological advances, human knowledge and compassion continue to be vitally important in the delivery of care.

References

Adjekum, A., Blasimme, A. & Vayena, E. 2018. Elements of trust in digital health systems: scoping review. *Journal of Medical Internet Research*, 20, e11254.

Akbar, S., Coiera, E. & Magrabi, F. 2020. Safety concerns with consumer-facing mobile health applications and their consequences: a scoping review. *Journal of the American Medical Informatics Association*, 27, 330–340.

Alajlan, R., Alhumam, N. & Frikha, M. 2023. Cybersecurity for blockchain-based IoT systems: a review. *Applied Sciences*, 13, 7432.

Allen, C., Vassilev, I., Kennedy, A. & Rogers, A. 2020. The work and relatedness of ties mediated online in supporting long-term condition self-management. *Sociology of Health & Illness*, 42, 579–595.

Alwashmi, M., Hawboldt, J., Davis, E., Marra, C., Gamble, J. M. & Abu Ashour, W. 2016. The effect of smartphone interventions on patients with chronic obstructive pulmonary disease exacerbations: a systematic review and meta-analysis. *JMIR mHealth and uHealth*, 4, e105.

Arias López, M. D. P., Ong, B. A., Borrat Frigola, X., Fernández, A. L., Hicklent, R. S., Obeles, A. J., Rocimo, A. M. & Celi, L. A. 2023. Digital literacy as a new determinant of health: a scoping review. *PLOS Digital Health*, 2, e0000279.

Bingham, G., Tong, E., Poole, S., Ross, P. & Dooley, M. 2021. A longitudinal time and motion study quantifying how implementation of an electronic medical record influences hospital nurses' care delivery. *International Journal of Medical Informatics*, 153, 104537.

Britnell, M. 2015. *In Search of the Perfect Health System*, Palgrave Macmillan.

Carayon, P., Schoofs Hundt, A., Karsh, B. T., Gurses, A. P., Alvarado, C. J., Smith, M. & Flatley Brennan, P. 2006. Work system design for patient safety: the SEIPS model. *Quality & Safety in Health Care*, 15(1), i50–i58.

Carreyrou, J. 2023. *Bad Blood: Secrets and Lies in a Silicon Valley Startup*, Picador.

Chauhan, U. & Mcalister, F. A. 2022. Comparison of mortality and hospital readmissions among patients receiving virtual ward transitional care vs usual postdischarge care: a systematic review and meta-analysis. *JAMA Network Open*, 5, e2219113.

Chib, A. & Lin, S. H. 2018. Theoretical advancements in mHealth: a systematic review of mobile apps. *Journal of Health Communication*, 23, 909–955.

Dahlgren, G. & Whitehead, M. 2021. The dahlgren-whitehead model of health determinants: 30 years on and still chasing rainbows. *Public Health*, 199, 20–24.

Darzi, A. 2024. *Independent Investigation of the National Health Service in England*, UK Government.

De Michele, R. & Furini, M. 2019. Iot healthcare: benefits, issues and challenges. *Proceedings of the 5th EAI International Conference on Smart Objects and Technologies for Social Good*, 160–164.

Dias, R. & Torkamani, A. 2019. Artificial intelligence in clinical and genomic diagnostics. *Genome Medicine*, 11, 70.

Dickinson, A., Donovan-Hall, M., Kheng, S., Wiegand, S., Wills, G., Ostler, C., Srors, S., Tech, A., Granat, M. & Kenney, L. 2019. Technologies to enhance quality and access to prosthetics and orthotics: the importance of a multidisciplinary, user-centred approach. *World Health Organization*, 54–70.

Dickson, J. 2024. Information Governance and Cyber Security. *In:* Phillips, N., Stacey, G. & Dowding, D. (eds.) *Harnessing Digital Technology and Data for Nursing Practice*, Elsevier.

Dowding, D., Grogan, L. & Newcombe, S. 2024. Information governance and security. *In:* Phillips, N., Stacey, G. & Dowding, D. (eds.) *Harnessing Digital Technology and Data for Nursing Practice*, Elsevier.

Forde-Johnston, C., Butcher, D. & Aveyard, H. 2023. An integrative review exploring the impact of Electronic Health Records (EHR) on the quality of nurse-patient interactions and communication. *Journal of Advanced Nursing*, 79, 48–67.

Fraczkowski, D., Matson, J. & Lopez, K. D. 2020. Nurse workarounds in the electronic health record: an integrative review. *Journal of the American Medical Informatics Association*, 27, 1149–1165.

Gilbert, A. W., Jaggi, A. & May, C. R. 2018. What is the patient acceptability of real time 1:1 videoconferencing in an orthopaedics setting? A systematic review. *Physiotherapy*, 104, 178–186.

Gilbert, A. W., Jaggi, A. & May, C. R. 2019. What is the acceptability of real time 1:1 videoconferencing between clinicians and patients for a follow-up consultation for multi-directional shoulder instability? *Shoulder & Elbow*, 11, 53–59.

GMC. 2017. *Generic professional capabilities framework* [Online]. General Medical Council. Available online at: https://www.gmc-uk.org/-/media/documents/generic-professional-capabilities-framework--2109_pdf-70417127.pdf [Accessed].

Gordon, W. J., Landman, A., Zhang, H. & Bates, D. W. 2020. Beyond validation: getting health apps into clinical practice. *NPJ Digital Medicine*, 3, 14.

Greenhalgh, T., Russell, J., Ashcroft, R. E. & Parsons, W. 2011. Why national eHealth programs need dead philosophers: Wittgensteinian reflections on policymakers' reluctance to learn from history. *The Milbank Quarterly*, 89, 533–563.

Greenhalgh, T., Wherton, J., Papoutsi, C., Lynch, J., Hughes, G., A'court, C., Hinder, S., Fahy, N., Procter, R. & Shaw, S. 2017. Beyond adoption: a new framework for theorizing and evaluating nonadoption, abandonment, and challenges to the scale-up, spread, and sustainability of health and care technologies. *Journal of Medical Internet Research*, 19, e367.

Hamper, J. & Perrotta, M. 2023. Blurring the divide: navigating the public/private landscape of fertility treatment in the UK. *Health & Place*, 80, 102992.

Hardey, M. 1999. Doctor in the house: the Internet as a source of lay health knowledge and the challenge to expertise. *Sociology of Health & Illness*, 21, 820–835.

Hatton, S. & Stanmore, E. 2024. Entrepreneurship in Nursing. *In:* Phillips, N., Stacey, G. & Dowding, D. (eds.) *Harnessing Digital Technology and Data for Nursing Practice*, Elsevier.

HCPC. 2023. *Physiotherapists: the standards of proficiency for physiotherapists* [Online]. Health & Care Professions Council. Available online at: https://www.hcpc-uk.org/standards/standards-of-proficiency/physiotherapists/ [Accessed].

Henwood, F. & Marent, B. 2019. Understanding digital health: productive tensions at the intersection of sociology of health and science and technology studies. *Sociology of Health & Illness*, 41, 1–15.

Hofmann, B. & Svenaeus, F. 2018. How medical technologies shape the experience of illness. *Life Sciences, Society and Policy*, 14, 3.

Huckvale, K., Prieto, J. T., Tilney, M., Benghozi, P.-J. & Car, J. 2015. Unaddressed privacy risks in accredited health and wellness apps: a cross-sectional systematic assessment. *BMC Medicine*, 13, 214.

Husain, L., Greenhalgh, T., Hughes, G., Finlay, T. & Wherton, J. 2022. Desperately seeking intersectionality in digital health disparity research: narrative review to inform a richer theorization of multiple disadvantage. *Journal of Medical Internet Research*, 24, e42358.

Iacobucci, G. 2018. NHS England tells CCGs to end postcode lottery over diabetes glucose devices. *BMJ*, 363, k4812.

Jahnel, T., Dassow, H. H., Gerhardus, A. & Schüz, B. 2022. The digital rainbow: digital determinants of health inequities. *Digit Health*, 8, 20552076221129093.

Janakiraman, R., Park, E., Demirezen, E. M. & Kumar, S. 2023. The effects of health information exchange access on healthcare quality and efficiency: an empirical investigation. *Management Science*, 69, 791–811.

Jiménez-Rodríguez, D., Santillán García, A., Montoro Robles, J., Rodríguez Salvador, M. D. M., Muñoz Ronda, F. J. & Arrogante, O. 2020. Increase in video consultations during the COVID-19 pandemic: healthcare professionals' perceptions about their implementation and adequate management. *International Journal of Environmental Research and Public Health*, 17, 5112.

Johnson, K. B., Wei, W. Q., Weeraratne, D., Frisse, M. E., Misulis, K., Rhee, K., Zhao, J. & Snowdon, J. L. 2021. Precision medicine, AI, and the future of personalized health care. *Clinical and Translational Science*, 14, 86–93.

Kingod, N., Cleal, B., Wahlberg, A. & Husted, G. R. 2017. Online peer-to-peer communities in the daily lives of people with chronic illness: a qualitative systematic review. *Qualitative Health Research*, 27, 89–99.

Knopes, J. 2019. Science, technology, and human health: the value of STS in medical and health humanities pedagogy. *The Journal of Medical Humanities*, 40, 461–471.

Konttila, J., Siira, H., Kyngäs, H., Lahtinen, M., Elo, S., Kääriäinen, M., Kaakinen, P., Oikarinen, A., Yamakawa, M., Fukui, S., Utsumi, M., Higami, Y., Higuchi, A. & Mikkonen, K. 2019. Healthcare professionals' competence in digitalisation: a systematic review. *Journal of Clinical Nursing*, 28, 745–761.

Kruse, C. S., Kristof, C., Jones, B., Mitchell, E. & Martinez, A. 2016. Barriers to electronic health record adoption: a systematic literature review. *Journal of Medical Systems*, 40, 252.

Laranjo, L., Ding, D., Heleno, B., Kocaballi, B., Quiroz, J. C., Tong, H. L., Chahwan, B., Neves, A. L., Gabarron, E., Dao, K. P., Rodrigues, D., Neves, G. C., Antunes, M. L., Coiera, E. & Bates, D. W. 2021. Do smartphone applications and activity trackers increase physical activity in adults? Systematic review, meta-analysis and metaregression. *British Journal of Sports Medicine*, 55, 422.

Latour, B. & Woolgar, S. 1979. *Laboratory Life: The Construction of Scientific Facts*, Princton University Press.

Law, J. 2002. *Aircraft Stories: Decentering the Object in Technoscience*, Duke University Press.

Lehoux, P., Rivard, L. & Silva, H. P. 2022. *Responsible Innovation in Health: Concepts and Tools for Sustainable Impact*, Springer Nature.

Li, E., Clarke, J., Ashrafian, H., Darzi, A. & Neves, A. L. 2022. The impact of electronic health record interoperability on safety and quality of care in high-income countries: systematic review. *Journal of Medical Internet Research*, 24, e38144.

Lin, L., Cheng, M., Guo, Y., Cao, X., Tang, W., Xu, X., Cheng, W. & Xu, Z. 2024. Early discharge hospital at home as alternative to routine hospital care for older people: a systematic review and meta-analysis. *BMC Medicine*, 22, 250.

Litchman, M. L., Walker, H. R., Ng, A. H., Wawrzynski, S. E., Oser, S. M., Greenwood, D. A., Gee, P. M., Lackey, M. & Oser, T. K. 2019. State of the science: a scoping review and gap analysis of diabetes online communities. *Journal of Diabetes Science and Technology*, 13, 466–492.

Lumley, J. 1990. Through a glass darkly: ultrasound and prenatal bonding. *Birth*, 17, 214–217.

Maguire, D., Honeyman, M., Omojomolo, D. & Evans, H. 2018. Digital Change in Health and Social Care. The King's Fund. Available online at: https://www.kingsfund.org.uk/insight-and-analysis/reports/digital-change-health-social-care.

Majumder, M. A., Guerrini, C. J. & Mcguire, A. L. 2021. Direct-to-consumer genetic testing: value and risk. *Annual Review of Medicine*, 72, 151–166.

Metcalf, C. D., Ostler, C., Thor, P., Kheng, S., Srors, S., Sann, R., Worsley, P., Gates, L., Donnovan-Hall, M., Harte, C. & Dickinson, A. 2024. Engaging multisector stakeholders to identify priorities for global health innovation, change and research: an engagement methodology and application to prosthetics service delivery in Cambodia. *Disability and Rehabilitation*, 46, 685–696.

Mistry, P., Maguire, D., Chikwira, L. & Lindsay, T. 2022. Interoperability is more than technology. The King's Fund. Available online at: https://www.kingsfund.org.uk/insight-and-analysis/reports/digital-interoperability-technology.

Møller, O. M., Vange, S. S., Borsch, A. S., Dam, T. N., Jensen, A. M. & Jervelund, S. S. 2024. Medical specialists' use and opinion of video consultation in Denmark: a survey study. *BMC Health Services Research*, 24, 516.

Morley, J., Cowls, J., Taddeo, M. & Floridi, L. 2020. Public health in the information age: recognizing the infosphere as a social determinant of health. *Journal of Medical Internet Research*, 22, e19311.

NHS. 2019. *The NHS long term plan* [Online]. NHS. Available online at: https://www.longtermplan.nhs.uk/publication/nhs-long-term-plan/ [Accessed].

NHS. 2023. *NHS long term workforce plan* [Online]. Available online at: https://www.england.nhs.uk/publication/nhs-long-term-workforce-plan/ [Accessed].

NMC. 2019. *Standards of proficiency for registered nurses* [Online]. Nursing & Midwifery Council. Available online at: https://www.nmc.org.uk/standards/standards-for-nurses/standards-of-proficiency-for-registered-nurses/ [Accessed].

Nolan, J. J. & Ormondroyd, E. 2023. Direct-to-consumer genetic tests providing health risk information: a systematic review of consequences for consumers and health services. *Clinical Genetics*, 104, 3–21.

North, M., Bourne, S., Green, B., Chauhan, A. J., Brown, T., Winter, J., Jones, T., Neville, D., Blythin, A., Watson, A., Johnson, M., Culliford, D., Elkes, J., Cornelius, V. & Wilkinson, T. M. A. 2020. A randomised controlled feasibility trial of E-health application supported care vs usual care after exacerbation of COPD: the RESCUE trial. *NPJ Digital Medicine*, 3, 145.

O'connor, S., Yan, Y., Thilo, F. J. S., Felzmann, H., Dowding, D. & Lee, J. J. 2023. Artificial intelligence in nursing and midwifery: a systematic review. *Journal of Clinical Nursing*, 32, 2951–2968.

o'connor, S. 2024. Artificial Intelligence in Nursing. *In:* Phillips, N., Stacey, G. & Dowding, D. (eds.) *Harnessing Digital Technology and Data for Nursing Practice*, Elsevier.

Øyen, L. & Aune, I. 2016. Viewing the unborn child – pregnant women's expectations, attitudes and experiences regarding fetal ultrasound examination. *Sexual & Reproductive Healthcare*, 7, 8–13.

Pacifico Silva, H., Lehoux, P., Miller, F. A. & Denis, J.-L. 2018. Introducing responsible innovation in health: a policy-oriented framework. *Health Research Policy and Systems*, 16, 90.

Panacer, K. S. 2023. Ethical issues associated with direct-to-consumer genetic testing. *Cureus*, 15, e39918.

Peeters, K. M. M., Reichel, L. A. M., Muris, D. M. J. & Cals, J. W. L. 2024. Family physician–to–hospital specialist electronic consultation and access to hospital care: a systematic review. *JAMA Network Open*, 7, e2351623–e2351623.

Pereno, A. & Eriksson, D. 2020. A multi-stakeholder perspective on sustainable healthcare: from 2030 onwards. *Futures*, 122, 102605.

Ragnedda, C., Ruiu, M. L. & Addeo, F. 2022. The self-reinforcing effect of digital and social exclusion: the inequality loop. *Telematics and Informatics*, 72, 101852.

Reidy, C., Foster, C. & Rogers, A. 2020. A novel exploration of the support needs of people initiating insulin pump therapy using a social network approach: a longitudinal mixed-methods study. *Diabetic Medicine*, 37, 298–310.

Rice, L. & Sara, R. 2019. Updating the determinants of health model in the information age. *Health Promotion International*, 34, 1241–1249.

Rogers, E. 2003. *Diffusion of Innovations*, New York: Free Press.

Rogers, E. & Shoemaker, F. 1971. *Communication of Innovation*, New York: The Free Press.

Rogers, E. M., Singhal, A. & Quinlan, M. M. 2014. Diffusion of Innovations. *In:* Stacks, D. W. & Salwen, M. B. (eds.) *An Integrated Approach to Communication Theory and Research*, Routledge.

Salahuddin, L. & Ismail, Z. 2015. Classification of antecedents towards safety use of health information technology: a systematic review. *International Journal of Medical Informatics*, 84, 877–891.

Shah, K., Lo, C., Babich, M., Tsao, N. W. & Bansback, N. J. 2016. Bar code medication administration technology: a systematic review of impact on patient safety when used with computerized prescriber order entry and automated dispensing devices. *The Canadian Journal of Hospital Pharmacy*, 69, 394–402.

Sinek, S. 2009. *Start with Why: How Great Leaders Inspire Everyone to Take Action*, Portfolio.

Stilgoe, J., Owen, R. & Macnaghten, P. 2013. Developing a framework for responsible innovation. *Research Policy*, 42, 1568–1580.

Strudwick, G. 2024. People Taking Control of Their Own Health Information. *In:* Phillips, N., Stacey, G. & Dowding, D. (eds.) *Harnessing Digital Technology and Data for Nursing Practice*, Elsevier.

Tarikere, S., Donner, I. & Woods, D. 2021. Diagnosing a healthcare cybersecurity crisis: the impact of IoMT advancements and 5G. *Business Horizons*, 64, 799–807.

Topol, E. 2016. *The Patient Will See You Now: The Future of Medicine Is in Your Hands*, Basic Books.

Topol, E. 2019. *Preparing the healthcare workforce to deliver the digital future* [Online]. NHS Health Education England. Available online at: https://topol.hee.nhs.uk/ [Accessed].

Wachter, R. 2016. Making IT Work: Harnessing the Power of Health Information Technology to Improve Patient Care. Report of the National Advisory Group on Health Information Technology to Improve Care in England.

Wells, E. 2024. Remote Care and Virtual Wards: Transforming Nursing Practice. *In:* Phillips, N., Stacey, G. & Dowding, D. (eds.) *Harnessing Digital Technology and Data for Nursing Practice*, Elsevier.

Wherton, J., Greenhalgh, T. & Shaw, S. E. 2021. Expanding video consultation services at pace and scale in Scotland during the COVID-19 pandemic: national mixed methods case study. *Journal of Medical Internet Research*, 23, e31374.

Whitehead, M., Ali, R., Carrol, E., Holmes, C. & Kee, F. 2024. *Equity in Medical Devices: Independent Review*, UK Government.

Whitehead, M. & Dahlgren, G. 1991. What can be done about inequalities in health? *The Lancet*, 338, 1059–1063.

WHO 2007. *Health Technologies. Sixtieth World Health Assembly*, World Health Organization.

WHO 2021. *Global Strategy on Digital Health 2020–2025*, World Health Organization.

Wisner, K., Lyndon, A. & Chesla, C. A. 2019. The electronic health record's impact on nurses' cognitive work: an integrative review. *International Journal of Nursing Studies*, 94, 74–84.

Woodnutt, S., Allen, C., Snowden, J., Flynn, M., Hall, S., Libberton, P. & Purvis, F. 2024. Could artificial intelligence write mental health nursing care plans? *Journal of Psychiatric and Mental Health Nursing*, 31, 79–86.

Yang, F., Wang, Y., Yang, C., Hu, H. & Xiong, Z. 2018. Mobile health applications in self-management of patients with chronic obstructive pulmonary disease: a systematic review and meta-analysis of their efficacy. *BMC Pulmonary Medicine*, 18, 147.

Yazdi, Y. & Acharya, S. 2013. A new model for graduate education and innovation in medical technology. *Annals of Biomedical Engineering*, 41, 1822–1833.

Index

Social Sciences for Healthcare Professionals, First Edition. Edited by Chris Allen.
© 2026 John Wiley & Sons Ltd. Published 2026 by John Wiley & Sons Ltd.